Physiotherapy in Mental Health and Psychiatry

For Elsevier

Senior Content Strategist: Rita Demetriou-Swanwick
Content Development Specialist: Jo Collett
Project Manager: Julie Taylor
Designer/Design Direction: Margaret Reid
Illustration Manager: Karen Giacomucci

Physiotherapy in Mental Health and Psychiatry

A SCIENTIFIC AND CLINICAL BASED APPROACH

Edited by

PROF. DR. MICHEL PROBST, PT, PhD
University of Leuven, KU Leuven, Leuven, Belgium

PROF. LIV HELVIK SKJAERVEN, MSc, PT
Western Norway University of Applied Sciences, Bergen, Norway

ELSEVIER   Edinburgh   London   New York   Oxford   Philadelphia   St Louis   Sydney   Toronto

ELSEVIER

ISBN 978-0-7020-7268-0

Notices
Knowledge and best practice in this field are constantly changing. As new research and experience broaden our understanding, changes in research methods, professional practices, or medical treatment may become necessary.

Practitioners and researchers must always rely on their own experience and knowledge in evaluating and using any information, methods, compounds, or experiments described herein. In using such information or methods they should be mindful of their own safety and the safety of others, including parties for whom they have a professional responsibility.

With respect to any drug or pharmaceutical products identified, readers are advised to check the most current information provided (i) on procedures featured or (ii) by the manufacturer of each product to be administered, to verify the recommended dose or formula, the method and duration of administration, and contraindications. It is the responsibility of practitioners, relying on their own experience and knowledge of their patients, to make diagnoses, to determine dosages and the best treatment for each individual patient, and to take all appropriate safety precautions.

To the fullest extent of the law, neither the Publisher nor the authors, contributors, or editors, assume any liability for any injury and/or damage to persons or property as a matter of products liability, negligence or otherwise, or from any use or operation of any methods, products, instructions, or ideas contained in the material herein.

your source for books,
journals and multimedia
in the health sciences
www.elsevierhealth.com

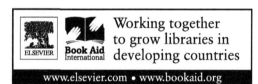

Working together
to grow libraries in
developing countries

www.elsevier.com • www.bookaid.org

The
publisher's
policy is to use
paper manufactured
from sustainable forests

CONTENTS

CONTRIBUTORS LIST

BEELEKE BREDERO, MSc, PT
Department of Rehabilitation Sciences, University of
Leuven, KU Leuven, Leuven, Belgium

EMANUEL BRUNNER, MSc, PT
Department of Rehabilitation Sciences, University of
Leuven, KU Leuven, Leuven, Belgium
Kantonsspital Winterthur, Institute of Physiotherapy,
Winterthur, Switzerland

JOERI CALSIUS, PhD
Clinical Psychologist, Psychotherapist and PT
University of Hasselt, Belgium
Therapy Center Daimon, Belgium

DANIEL CATALÁN-MATAMOROS, PhD, MBA, PT
Member of the Research Group CTS 451 Health
Sciences, Department of Nursing Science,
Physiotherapy and Medicine, University of
Almeria, Spain
Associate Professor, University Carlos III of Madrid,
Spain
President of the Spanish Association of
Physiotherapists in Mental Health

MARIT DANIELSEN
Department of Neuroscience, Faculty of Medicine,
Norwegian University of Science and Technology,
Trondheim, Norway

JOANNE CONNAUGHTON, DPhysioRes,
BAppSc(Physio)
School of Physiotherapy, The University of Notre
Dame Australia, Fremantle, Australia

WIM DANKAERTS, PhD, PT
Department of Rehabilitation Sciences, University of
Leuven, KU Leuven, Leuven, Belgium

URSULA DANNER, PhD, PT
Department Health Sciences, FH Campus Wien,
University of Applied Sciences, Vienna, Austria
Department of Psychiatry and Psychotherapeutic
Medicine, Medical University of Graz, Austria
Department Health Studies/Physiotherapy, FH
Joanneum, University of Applied Sciences, Graz,
Austria

ANNET DE JONG, MSc, PT
Department of Psychosomatic Physiotherapy,
University of Applied Sciences, Hogeschool
Utrecht, Utrecht, The Netherlands

JOLIEN DIEDENS, MSc, PT
University Psychiatric Centre KU Leuven, Leuven,
Belgium
Department of Rehabilitation Sciences, University of
Leuven, KU Leuven, Leuven, Belgium

TOVE DRAGESUND, PhD, PT
Department of Global Public Health and Primary
Care, University of Bergen, Bergen, Norway

KIRSTEN EKERHOLT, MSc, PT
Faculty of Health Sciences, Oslo and Akershus
University College of Applied Sciences, , Oslo,
Norway

WILLEMIEN FOKKE, MSc, PT
Psychosomatic Physiotherapy, University of Applied
  Sciences Utrecht, Utrecht, The Netherlands

LAUREN FORDHAM, MSc, PT
Derbyshire Healthcare NHS Foundation Trust,
  Derbyshire, United Kingdom

APRIL GAMBLE, DPT
The Centre for Victims of Torture, Minneapolis, MN,
  USA

GUNVOR GARD, PhD, PT
Professor, Faculty of Medicine, Lund University,
  Lund, Sweden

ANTONIA GÓMEZ-CONESA, PhD, PT, Psych
Professor, Department of Physiotherapy, Faculty of
  Medicine, University of Murcia, Spain

ANNE GRETLAND, MSc, PT
Department of Health and Care Sciences, UiT The
  Arctic University of Norway, Tromsø, Norway

LAURA PIZER GUERON, MPH, DPT
The Centre for Victims of Torture, Minneapolis, MN,
  USA

AMANDA LUNDVIK GYLLENSTEN, PhD, PT
Associate Professor, Department of Physical Therapy,
  Lund University, Lund, Sweden

A. HAGEN, MSc, PT
University of Applied Sciences Utrecht, Utrecht, The
  Netherlands; Physiotherapy Van Breestraat,
  Amsterdam, The Netherlands

LENA HEDLUND, PhD, PT
Department of Physical Therapy, Lund University,
  Lund, Sweden

EVELINE C. KEMPENAAR, MSc, PT
Praktijk voor Psychosomatische Fysiotherapie,
  Hillegom, The Netherlands

JEPKEMOI JOANNE KIBET, MSc, PT
The Centre for Victims of Torture, Minneapolis, MN,
  USA

JAN KNAPEN, PhD, PT
Local Multidisciplinary Network in Primary Health
  Care, Sint-Truiden, Belgium; AZERTIE, Zonhoven,
  Belgium

ALICE KVÅLE, PhD, PT
Department of Physiotherapy, Western Norway
  University of Applied Sciences, Bergen, Norway

YANNICK MARCHAL, MSc
Local Multidisciplinary Network in Primary Health
  Care, Sint-Truiden, Belgium
Department of Family Medicine, Vrije Universiteit
  Brussel, Brussels, Belgium

DANIELLE M. MATTO, MA, PT
Kracht Door Balans, Amersfoort, Netherlands

MONICA MATTSSON, PhD, PT
Department of Psychiatry, University of Umeå,
  Umeå, Sweden

YVES MORIËN, MSc
AZERTIE, Zonhoven, Belgium

LENE NYBOE, PhD, PT
Aarhus University Hospital, Aarhus, Denmark

AUD MARIE ØIEN, PhD, PT
Faculty of Social Sciences, Western Norway
  University of Applied Sciences, Sogndal, Norway

CLAIRE O'REILLY, PT
The Centre for Victims of Torture, Minneapolis, MN,
  USA

ANNE REITAN PARKER, PT
Department of Physiotherapy, Royal Edinburgh
  Hospital, Edinburgh, Scotland, United Kingdom

MICHEL PROBST, PhD, PT, Prof
Department of Rehabilitation Sciences, University of Leuven, KU Leuven, Leuven, Belgium
University Psychiatry Center, KU Leuven, Leuven, Belgium

GRACIELA ROVNER, PhD, PT
ACT Institutet Sweden, Gothenburg, Sweden
Center for Psychiatry Research, Karolinska Institutet, Stockholm, Sweden

MARYANN DE RUITER, MSc, PT
The Centre for Victims of Torture, Minneapolis, MN, USA

MATTHIJS RÜMKE, MSc, PT
Social Factory, Rotterdam, The Netherlands

MERJA SALLINEN, PhD, PT
Satakunta University of Applied Sciences, Pori, Finland

JOHAN SIMONS, PhD, PT
Department of Rehabilitation Sciences, University of Leuven, KU Leuven, Leuven, Belgium

MATTHEW D. SKINTA, PhD, ABPP
Sexual & Gender Identity Clinic, Gronowski Center, Palo Alto University, Palo Alto, CA, USA

LIV HELVIK SKJAERVEN, MSc, PT
Department of Occupational Therapy, Physiotherapy and Radiography, Faculty of Health and Social Sciences, Western Norway University of Applied Sciences, Bergen, Norway

LINDA SLOOTWEG, MSc, PT
Psychosomatic Physiotherapy, University of Applied Sciences, Utrecht, The Netherlands

ANDREW SOUNDY, PhD, PT
School of Sport, Exercise and Rehabilitation Sciences, University of Birmingham, Birmingham, United Kingdom

LIV INGER STRAND, PhD, PT
Department of Global Public Health and Primary Care, Physiotherapy Research Group, University of Bergen, Bergen, Norway

MARIA STRÖMBÄCK, PhD, PT
Community Medicine and Rehabilitation, Physiotherapy, Umeå University, Umeå, Sweden; Clinical Science, Psychiatry, Umeå University, Umeå, Sweden

BRENDON STUBBS, PhD, PT
Health Services & Population Research and Psychosis Studies, King's College London, London, United Kingdom

MARY-ANNE SUNDAL, MSc, PT
Department of Occupational Therapy, Physiotherapy and Radiography, Faculty of Health and Social Sciences, Bergen University College, Bergen, Norway

EVELIEN SWIERS, MSc, PT
Department of Pychosomatic Physiotherapy, Hogeschool Utrecht, Utrecht, The Netherlands

ELINE THORNQUIST, PhD, PT
Department of Occupational Therapy, Physiotherapy and Radiography, Faculty of Health and Social Sciences, Western Norway University of Applied Sciences, Bergen, Norway
Department of Health and Care Sciences, University of Tromsø, Tromsø, Norway

MIEKE VAN WIJK-ENGBERS, MSc, PT
University of Applied Sciences, Institute of Movement Studies Master Physiotherapy, Utrecht, The Netherlands

TINE VAN DAMME, PhD, PT
Department of Rehabilitation Sciences, University of Leuven, KU Leuven, Leuven, Belgium

DAVY VANCAMPFORT, PhD, PT
Department of Rehabilitation Sciences, University of Leuven, KU Leuven, Leuven, Belgium
University Psychiatric Centre, KU Leuven, Leuven-Kortenberg, Belgium

MARIA WIKLUND, PhD, PT
Community Medicine and Rehabilitation, Physiotherapy, Umeå University, Umeå, Sweden

Section 1

INTRODUCTION

1

INTRODUCTION TO PHYSIOTHERAPY IN MENTAL HEALTH AND PSYCHIATRY

MICHEL PROBST ■ LIV HELVIK SKJAERVEN

SUMMARY

Physiotherapy in mental health care and psychiatry offers a rich variety of observation and evaluation tools as well as a range of interventions related to a patient's physical and mental health problems, based on a 50-year-long history. Physiotherapy in mental health care addresses human movement, function, physical activity and exercise in individual and group therapeutic settings and bridges the physical and mental health needs of humans. This chapter offers some general reflections on mental health, the evolution of physiotherapy in mental health care and the scope of interventions, stigma and physiotherapy research. Physiotherapy in mental health care and psychiatry can offer added and beneficial value in the treatment of people with mental health problems.

KEY POINTS

■ What can physiotherapy in mental health provide to individuals with mental health problems?

■ General knowledge and challenges associated with application of physiotherapy to mental health.

■ The role of a physiotherapist in mental health is a healthcare provider, healthcare manager, professional developer and scientific researcher.

LEARNING OBJECTIVES

■ To be aware of the fundamentals of physiotherapy in mental health care and psychiatry, responding to the need in society.

■ To reflect on general topics related to physiotherapy in mental health care and psychiatry.

■ To develop a professional identity of physiotherapy in mental health care and psychiatry.

INTRODUCTION

The implementation of physiotherapy in mental health care and psychiatry has a long and strong tradition of more than 50 years in education and clinical practice, and in several countries it receives government support. Unfortunately, this is not the case in all countries. In some countries, mental healthcare settings even ignore the potential value of physiotherapy. The use of physiotherapy in mental health care and psychiatry is not common and is often overlooked.

Physiotherapists who specialize in mental health psychiatry are regularly confronted with a type of dualism. On the one hand, physiotherapists are respected because they are healthcare providers who have close contact with patients. They support patients within the physiotherapy framework in dealing with their emotions and past experiences rather than addressing only their medical conditions. On the other hand, a physiotherapist working in mental health care may also experience considerable scepticism due to ignorance and a lack of knowledge of what the profession can provide.

Therefore, the aim of this book is twofold. First, the book presents different existing perspectives on and information about physiotherapeutic interventions in mental health care and psychiatry. Second, it highlights the best clinical practice of physiotherapy in mental health care today. As a consequence, this book also aims to inform and convince colleagues about the opportunities associated with this quickly developing specialty in physiotherapy.

This book illustrates new developments in physiotherapy methods and applications in the fields of mental health and psychiatry, including innovative and effective strategies to address today's complex health challenges, such as long-lasting musculoskeletal disorders, chronic pain, psychosomatic disorders and mental health problems. This book also focuses on the effect of exercise, body and movement awareness and psychomotor physiotherapy interventions to improve mental health and increase well-being. The book reveals current scientific research on the effect of physiotherapy on mental health disorders, such as depression, anxiety, schizophrenia, eating disorders, bipolar disorders and dementia, over the course of a person's life. Moreover, newly introduced topics have been included, such as the integration of psychological interventions in physiotherapy and the role of physiotherapy in individuals suffering from the effects of torture or violence, with special attention to the refugee crises. These topics demonstrate how mental health physiotherapy meets the needs of the currently changing society.

Physiotherapists have specific and unique expertise in both a person's 'body' and a person's 'body in movement', two important issues that are integral in psychopathology. It is an intriguing finding that this expertise is not always a sufficient reason to award both aspects a full place in mental health care.

Physiotherapists specialized in mental health care and psychiatry receive specific physical and mental health training to become qualified to bridge the gap between the physical and mental health needs of patients. Based on clinical practice and the current scientific evidence, a rationale and clinical guidance for incorporating physiotherapy into health promotion, prevention, treatment and rehabilitation for patients with mental health problems are presented.

It is important for the purpose of communication with practitioners of other medical and paramedical professions to understand what physiotherapists in mental health care can offer. Physiotherapists in mental health care aim to bring the content and value of professional interventions as well as the different indications for their use into the spotlight. Over the last five

decades, physiotherapy in mental health care has evolved based on evidence to include a wide range of treatment modalities for both individual and group physiotherapy. In addition to applying a physiotherapy approach for health benefits, the presence of the therapeutic relationship and the focus on the therapeutic process are crucial in physiotherapy for mental health applications.

This introduction offers some general reflections on mental health and psychiatry (e.g., mental health and mental health problems/disorders, stigma, physical activity and mental health) and specific topics related to physiotherapy in mental health care and psychiatry (e.g., definition, scope of interventions, research). This introduction does not aim to offer answers to the various issues; rather, the aim is to stimulate reflection and open a discussion regarding a specialty within the physiotherapy field.

NO HEALTH WITHOUT MENTAL HEALTH

According to the World Health Organization (WHO) health is defined as 'a state of complete physical, mental and social well-being and not merely the absence of disease or infirmity' (Preamble to the Constitution of the World Health Organization as adopted by the International Health Conference, New York, 19–22 June, 1946; signed on 22 July 1946 by the representatives of 61 States [Official Records of the World Health Organization, no. 2, p. 100] and entered into force on 7 April 1948).

Mental health is defined as a condition that permits a state of optimal physical, mental and social well-being and is not merely the absence of disease. Mental health is related to the promotion of well-being, the prevention of mental disorders and the treatment and rehabilitation of people affected by mental disorders (WHO, 2010) (Box 1).

After a long period of unimportance, mental health is now a high priority for most policymakers worldwide. This emphasis on mental health has resulted in an increasing amount of scientific and non-scientific literature focused on physical activity, exercises, movement-related activities, body and movement awareness and well-being for individuals with mental health problems.

The International Organization of Physiotherapy in Mental Health (IOPTMH) implemented the recommendations of WHO in 2005 as part of its mission as a guideline for the future.

If physiotherapists want to be part of a successful mental health service, it is a precondition *sine qua non* to further develop high-quality and innovative clinical practices, education and research in agreement with these recommendations.

These recommendations are translated into the field of physiotherapy for clinical practice, education and research:

1. to improve physiotherapy mental health care;
2. to organize specific physiotherapy care for people of different ages, including children, adolescents and the elderly, and for high-risk groups;
3. to ensure access to primary physiotherapy care for people with mental health problems;
4. to provide treatment in community-based physiotherapy services for individuals with severe mental health problems;
5. to disseminate quality information/knowledge and skills regarding mental health in physiotherapy education;
6. to promote mental health because mental health and well-being are fundamental to the quality of life of all citizens;
7. to be sufficiently informed to combat stigmatization of and discrimination against individuals with mental health problems;
8. to provide adequate specialized education and competent professionals in physiotherapy;
9. to participate and engage in a multidisciplinary approach;
10. to engage in evaluating the effectiveness of physiotherapy care and promoting new evidence-based guidelines.

Good mental health is more than the absence of diagnosable mental health problems. A person's mental health affects different aspects of life. For example, in terms of relationships, mental health involves having a good relationship with family and having supportive friends with the ability to reflect upon and share feelings. Regarding leisure time, mental health involves having hobbies, exercising on a regular basis and having regular vacation time. Furthermore, it is important to follow a healthy lifestyle that includes healthy eating habits, not smoking or drinking, not taking drugs and being able to achieve some goals in life.

In the literature, a distinction is made between mental health problems and mental illness. A mental health problem interferes with emotional and/or social abilities. It is a negative mental experience that is part of everyday life. It can happen to anyone at any time and covers a broad range of mild problems that are less severe than those associated with a mental illness. Individuals with a mental illness have a growing imbalance in the abilities mentioned previously. Mental illness or disorder is defined as a syndrome characterized by a clinically significant disturbance in an individual's cognition, emotion regulation or behaviour. The condition reflects dysfunction of the psychological, biological or developmental processes underlying mental functioning (American Psychiatric Association, 2013). In clinical practice, disorders occur in a variety of forms and symptoms can overlap. Distinctions are made between mild, moderate and severe mental illness.

Mental ill-health accounts for approximately 20% of illnesses, and mental health problems account for almost 25% of general practice consultations. When mental illness or a mental health problem leads to work absenteeism or the inability to find employment, it has a great impact on social services. Different cultures worldwide have different approaches to mental health and mental illness.

It is important for colleagues to have a basic understanding of the most common mental disorders and illnesses and the mechanism by which they may influence the approach and clinical judgement of a physiotherapist.

MENTAL HEALTH AND STIGMA

Stigma is a mark of disgrace associated with a particular circumstance, quality or person (Stevenson, 2015). Another term for stigma is *prejudice* based on negative stereotyping (Corrigan, 2004). Stigma is primarily observed in mental health. The pain of mental illness is significant, but the added layer of stigma affects personal well-being, economic productivity and public health, fuelling a vicious cycle of lowered expectations, deep shame and hopelessness (Hinshaw, 2007).

People suffering from mental disorders struggle with the disease itself, as well as with the associated prejudice and discrimination. These two issues are important for physiotherapists working with people with mental disorders, as they can affect the treatment and quality of care. To decrease stigma in mental health, it is important to inform people more about mental health, mental health problems and the consequences for the person in daily life, given that stigmatization is partly due to a lack of understanding and insight. Physiotherapists generally also have the important role of informing people in a correct manner. To decrease stigmatization, several steps can be taken:

1. help identify and eliminate misconceptions about mental illness;
2. contribute to the prevention of mental health problems;
3. inform individuals adequately about mental health and refer them when necessary to specialized professionals in mental health and psychiatry;
4. offer physiotherapy interventions to individuals with unstable mental health.

Although there is an increasing body of evidence directed towards the implementation of physiotherapy in mental health and psychiatry, considerable stigmatization and taboos remain in this area. Studies in Belgium (Probst & Peuskens, 2010), Turkey (Yucel & Acar, 2016), Switzerland (Schwank & Brunner, 2016) and Australia (Connaughton & Gibson, 2016; Stewart et al., 2016) investigated attitudes and beliefs regarding mental illness in physiotherapy students. Some of the key findings were the following:

- Physiotherapy students have a moderately positive attitude towards psychiatry.
- Female students have a more positive attitude than male students.
- Students without prior experience with mental illness have a more positive belief or attitude.
- The attitudes towards psychiatry improved after courses in this domain.

The studies underlined the necessity of implementing courses, lectures, testimony, skill training and clinical practices related to mental health and psychiatry in the global curricula of physiotherapy education. This implementation will improve professional attitudes and beliefs directed towards mental illnesses and prevent stigmatization in clinical practice. Even if physiotherapy students will never work with psychiatric patients, such courses will broaden their minds and strengthen their interventions.

'NO MENTAL HEALTH WITHOUT PHYSICAL ACTIVITY' AND 'EXERCISE IS MEDICINE'

Currently, the importance of physical activities for people with mental illness is receiving considerable attention in the scientific and nonscientific literature. The relationship between mental health and physical activity is supported by a growing number of articles concerning the importance of physical activity in mental health and psychiatric rehabilitation (Vancampfort et al., 2012a,b). These research findings have very slowly become integrated into clinical practice. Physical activity is not considered a worthwhile strategy by many mental health professionals. The discrepancy between theory and practice is intriguing, because: (1) approximately a quarter of the population is faced with mental dysfunction of some type and (2) physical activities and body health are 'hot topics' in our society.

Physical activity enhances the effectiveness of psychological therapies. There is evidence that exercise has a positive effect on individuals with mental health problems. Exercise is an important component in improving quality of life and symptom management for people with a wide range of mental health problems. Physical activity has an added benefit, because people with mental health problems are also at increased risk of a range of physical health problems, including cardiovascular diseases, endocrine disorder and obesity (Vancampfort et al., 2012a,b). Today, more psychiatrists are slowly becoming convinced that medication, psychotherapy and physical activity are the basic standards for therapy in mental illness.

An international comparison is somewhat difficult given that the domain of physical activity in mental health is claimed by several healthcare providers with different names and educational backgrounds in different countries.

Australian healthcare providers developed an international concept called Healthy Active Lives (HeAL) a few years ago to address the problems of physical inactivity and mental illnesses. The HeAL statement reflects the international consensus on a set of key principles, processes and standards. It aims to combat the stigma, discrimination and prejudice that prevents young people experiencing psychosis from leading healthy, active lives and to confront the perception that poor physical health is inevitable (http://www.iphys.org.au). It also aims to reverse the trend of people with severe mental illness dying early as a result of their lifestyle (e.g., physical inactivity, unhealthy eating habits). Essentially, the developers of the HeAL programme want people with severe mental illness to enjoy the same health as their young peers and not to experience a double disability of mental illness and obesity. This book includes several chapters that demonstrate the importance of physical activity in mental health and the role of the physiotherapist.

PHYSIOTHERAPY AND MENTAL HEALTH

The literature on this topic is sparse and mostly limited to a country-specific approach, potentially explaining why a physiotherapy approach to mental health unfortunately often receives little respect in institutions and healthcare systems in some countries. Hare (1986) was the first author to write a book in English about 'physiotherapy in psychiatry'. However, more than two decades earlier, Ueberschlag (1960) had written an essay in French about physiotherapy in psychiatry. Later, Everett et al. (2003), with occupational therapists from the UK, published a new book. Books were also published outlining Belgian, German and Scandinavian perspectives (Bunkan & Thornquist, 1985; Roxendal, 1985; Probst & Bosscher, 2001; Skjaerven, 2003; Hütter-Becker & Dölken, 2004; Biguet et al., 2012; Ianssen, 2012). However, most of these books were not written in English and focus on selected aspects of physiotherapy in mental health care.

This professional literature is important with regard to the development of the field of physiotherapy in mental health care. However, it is now time to consolidate the knowledge obtained from various views and resources. This book should be considered as a next step in the evolution of physiotherapy in mental health care and psychiatry that stretches beyond national borders (Fig. 1). The aim of the book is to develop a global perspective on the role of physiotherapy in mental health care. This summary of the broad scope of interventions will also strengthen our credibility, not only with patients and in the medical field, but even at government level. This book also intends to strengthen the identity of physiotherapists working in mental health care.

This book is based on the European idea of collaboration and exchange of knowledge. The proposed principles are, of course, not limited to Europe; they need to be transferred and adapted to different cultures. This book is a result of the collaboration of physiotherapists working in the field of mental health in different countries. It aims to foster, for the first time, a clear and detailed description of the diversity of the specialty of physiotherapy in mental health care in 2017. Diversity broadens our minds and offers appropriate guidance.

The content of this book is organized into sections. After the introduction, in the first section, physiological and psychological models implemented in physiotherapy and mental health are described and discussed. Second, an overview is presented of different methodologies that are frequently used within the field of physiotherapy in mental health and psychiatry. The book continues with a presentation of a variety of internal and external observation and evaluation tools for the physiotherapy profession. Subsequently, this book also includes a focus on the clinical role and potential indications for physiotherapy in the treatment of several disorders. Attention is paid to specific mental health problems according to age. In general, the perception of physiotherapy in mental health care and psychiatry mostly relates to treating individuals with mental illnesses suffering from physical disabilities. This view does not correspond to the complete scope of physiotherapy in mental health. Physiotherapists offer an additional contribution, given that they have knowledge of human movement. This book reflects a rich variety of approaches within physiotherapy in mental health care and psychiatry worldwide.

Together with occupational therapists, physiotherapists, as partners in a multidisciplinary team, can

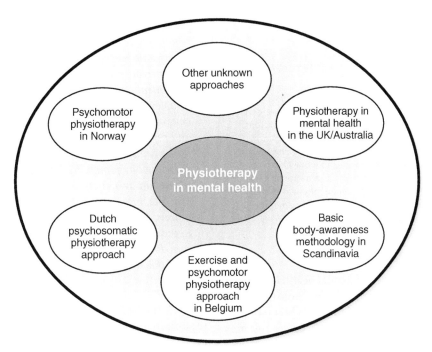

FIGURE 1 ■ Physiotherapy in mental health: a state-of-the-art approach.

improve the quality of life of a person with mental health problems. In some countries, occupational therapy colleagues are more involved in and integrated into mental health care and psychiatry services depending on their tradition. In other countries, the situation differs according to national policy. There has been a growing tendency, however, for the physiotherapist to be regarded as a necessary member of mental health care.

HISTORY OF THE INTERNATIONAL ORGANIZATION OF PHYSICAL THERAPY IN MENTAL HEALTH

The idea of developing an identity for physiotherapists working in mental health internationally and professionally emerged in 2004 in Belgium during meetings with Scandinavian colleagues (Probst, 2012). The idea became more concrete and led to the organization of the first international research conference on physiotherapy in psychiatry and mental health, at Leuven University (KU Leuven, Belgium, 2006). The proposal to organize further conferences and to develop

a professional organization gained genuine support, leading to conferences taking place every 2 years in Bergen (University College Bergen, Norway, 2008), Lund (Lund University, Sweden, 2010), Edinburgh (Edinburgh Royal Psychiatric Hospital, UK, 2012), Utrecht (University of Applied Sciences Utrecht, The Netherlands, 2014) and Madrid (University of Carlos III of Madrid, Spain, 2016). For the abstracts of all these conferences, refer to http://www.icppmh.org.

Between 2006 and 2011, the provisional executive committee developed into a professional organization. After 7 years of development, and with support from the Norwegian subsection of psychiatric and psychosomatic physiotherapy, the World Confederation for Physical Therapy (WCPT) recognized the International Organization of Physical Therapists in Mental Health (IOPTMH) as an official subgroup. In Amsterdam in 2011, a new international organization, the IOPTMH, was born. The IOPTMH is an international nongovernmental organization with specific interest in the area of mental health that is recognized as a subgroup of the WCPT (Box 2). Countries with physiotherapists interested in promoting the use of physiotherapy to improve the mental health of people worldwide can apply for membership (Probst, 2012).

The overriding objectives of the IOPTMH (see the IOPTMH constitution at http://www.iccpmh.org) are to foster collaboration between physiotherapists practising in mental health worldwide, to encourage improved standards and clinical consistency of physiotherapy in mental health care and to advance practice, education and research by communicating and exchanging information. One of the objectives of the IOPTMH is to organize an International Conference of Physiotherapy in Psychiatry and Mental Health (ICPPMH) every 2 years.

PHYSIOTHERAPY IN MENTAL HEALTH: DEFINITION

The IOPTMH developed a definition that describes in general the field of physiotherapy in mental health, with the aim of being recognizable to colleagues worldwide:

> *Physiotherapy in mental health is a specialty within physiotherapy. It is implemented in different health and mental health settings, psychiatry and psychosomatic medicine. It is person-centred and provided for children, adolescents, adults and older people with mild, moderate and severe, acute and chronic mental health problems, in primary and community care, inpatients and outpatients. Physiotherapists in mental health provide health promotion, preventive health care, treatment and rehabilitation for individuals, groups and in group therapeutic settings. Physiotherapists in mental health create a therapeutic relationship to provide assessment and services specifically related to the complexity of mental health within a supportive environment applying a model including biological and psychosocial aspects. Physiotherapy in mental health aims to optimize wellbeing and empower the individual by promoting functional movement, movement awareness, physical activity and exercises, bringing together physical and mental aspects. Physiotherapists in mental health contribute to the multidisciplinary team and interprofessional care. Physiotherapy in mental health is based on the available scientific and best clinical evidence.*
>
> **Probst et al. (2015)**

In 2005, the WHO published their recommendations regarding mental health. The IOPTMH further developed this recommendation for the specialty of physiotherapy (see also Box 1):

1. to improve physiotherapy mental health care, health promotion and preventive health care;
2. to organize specific physiotherapy care for people of all ages, including children, adolescents and the elderly, and for high-risk groups, such as individuals with eating disorders and psychotic disorders;
3. to ensure access to primary physiotherapy care for people with mental health problems;
4. to provide treatment in community-based physiotherapy services for individuals with severe mental health problems (Box 3).

Physiotherapists in mental health also use the International Classification of Functioning, Disability and Health (ICF) (WHO, 2001). This classification uses a biopsychosocial model and differs from other diagnostic systems that are mostly based on a biomedical model. Vroman & Arthanat (2010) demonstrated the applicability of the ICF as a conceptual framework and a classification system. The use of the ICF enables practitioners to evaluate and interpret chronic mental health disorders within different populations and at varying levels of disabilities and function (Ewert et al., 2004). The ICF provides a broad, transdisciplinary

BOX 3

BOX 3

THE QUALITY OF PHYSIOTHERAPY
INTERVENTIONS IN MENTAL
HEALTH

Physiotherapy is recognized within medicine; physiotherapists obtain in-depth knowledge and training regarding the human body as well as human movement and function, physical activity and physical training; and physiotherapists in mental health are trained in acquiring therapeutic competency. This starting point is the basis of our quality warranty.

Physiotherapy interventions in mental health should fulfil at least four minimal criteria:

1. The nature of the interventions should be clearly described.
2. The claimed benefits of the services must be explicitly stated.
3. These claimed benefits must be scientifically validated.
4. Individual risks that may outweigh benefits must be disclosed.

framework for planning treatment, defining goals, assessing progress and outcomes and allocating resources for people with mental disorders (Reed et al., 2009).

THE PROFESSIONAL STATUS OF PHYSIOTHERAPY IN MENTAL HEALTH CARE

The professional status of physiotherapy is accepted worldwide as a conventional approach, which suggests that the approach is consistent with internationally accepted standard models or traditions that are primarily grounded on an evidence-based approach.

The professional borders are very clear and are defined by deontological rules. Depending on various traditions, physiotherapists in mental health care include complementary or alternative approaches in their physiotherapy interventions (Box 4). In many cultures, mental health is closely associated with religion and spirituality. In other cultures, some

BOX 4

CONVENTIONAL THERAPY VERSUS COMPLEMENTARY THERAPY VERSUS
ALTERNATIVE THERAPY

Conventional therapy can be described as therapy practised by medical doctors and their allied health professionals, such as physiotherapists. Complementary therapy (CT) lies outside the domain of the conventional approach but is used together with conventional therapies. It is a broad domain of healing resources that encompasses all health systems and promotes health and well-being. CTs refer to therapies that can be used to supplement biomedical treatment to support prevention and treatment. These therapies are considered as additional to other conventional approaches (Eisenberg et al., 2001; Barnes et al., 2004; Saad & Medeiros, 2012).

It is difficult to define CTs because the field is very broad and constantly changing. Furthermore, the list of what is considered to be CT changes continually, and therapies for which safety and effectiveness are demonstrated may become part of conventional medicine. The number of patients asking their general practitioners about CTs is continuously increasing. These therapies are complementary because they enhance the effects of conventional medicine, and fulfil demands that cannot be achieved by a standard approach (this is the definition of complementary medicine adopted by the Cochrane Collaboration).

CTs aim to achieve a broader cure (physical, mental, emotional, social and spiritual) (Deutsch & Anderson, 2007). The classical conventional approach can be combined with CTs, and some high-quality evidence supports their safety and effectiveness. The combination of a CT and a conventional approach is called *integrative medicine*. More studies are required to broaden the therapeutic options, strengthen public preferences and clarify the language and outcomes associated with CT.

Alternative therapies are defined as unconventional, unorthodox and unproven therapies that are used instead of conventional medicine, mostly as a stand-alone approach. These are approaches that have not been developed by the use of generally accepted methods or by validating their effectiveness (Angell & Kassirer, 1998; Beyerstein, 2001). CT differs from alternative therapy because alternative therapy/medicine is used instead of conventional medicine. Some treatments have not been investigated or approved by regulatory agencies (Eisenberg et al., 2001).

The borders between conventional and complementary approaches and between complementary and alternative approaches are very small in mental health (Richardson, 2004).

physiotherapists believe that integrating such complementary or alternative therapies would diminish the professional status of physiotherapy in mental health. Similar to other care providers, physiotherapists in mental health care must be cautious about including alternative and complementary approaches in their physiotherapy interventions. The Patient Intervention Comparison Outcomes (PICO) criteria can be helpful in analysing whether an alternative approach is scientifically well founded (Deutsch & Anderson, 2007). These criteria include the following questions: Who are the relevant patients (P)? What is the intervention strategy (I)? Is there a control strategy (C)? What are the patients' relevant consequences (O)? Physiotherapists in mental health must guarantee the credibility of physiotherapy interventions.

Occasionally exercises derived from other fields, such as yoga, tai chi, qi-gong, Pilates and mindfulness are used. However, physiotherapists are not yoga trainers and mindfulness experts unless they undergo specific training. It is acceptable to include these exercises to improve mental health and physical fitness. The question is when these exercises become of benefit to the patient and when these exercises become useful in the profession of physiotherapy in mental health care.

In mental health and psychiatry, physiotherapy primarily involves a multidisciplinary or interdisciplinary team. Multidisciplinary or pluridisciplinary means that the various interventions are provided in isolation and that one or more disciplines work collaboratively but do not have mutual contact with each other. This approach recognizes the importance of different disciplines and involves professionals operating within the boundaries of their profession towards discipline-specific goals while recognizing the important contributions from other disciplines (European Region of the World Confederation for Physical Therapy, 2003). Interdisciplinary refers to mutual contact between different care providers. Transdisciplinary is a relatively new term in health care that indicates that various caregivers participate in each other's domains.

RESEARCH IN PHYSIOTHERAPY AND MENTAL HEALTH CARE

Physiotherapy in mental health care and psychiatry is a relatively new, small, but quickly developing specialty that is based on a combination of clinical and scientific evidence. Despite the complexity of research in mental health, evidence-based practice has become a central aspect of physiotherapy today (Herbert et al., 2011). An increasing number of articles within and outside international physiotherapy journals provide the foundation for this field. Currently, increasing evidence suggests that physiotherapy, with its specific approach and therapeutic interventions, can make significant contributions to well-being and mental health. To bridge the gap between clinicians and researchers, scientific findings must be translated into a more clinical-based language (see Table 1).

To develop high-quality care, research is needed that provides evidence for a prominent role of physiotherapy in mental health care, with themes including the efficient positive contribution of physiotherapy to the treatment process, the potential changes in quality of life in the long term, the contribution to well-being and mental health, patient satisfaction with the treatment, the cost–benefit analysis of the interventions in a time of economic crisis, the evaluation of the side effects and the development of specific clinical physiotherapy measurements. To preserve or acquire a professional platform in the long term, to present a distinct profile of physiotherapy in mental health to policymakers and to distinguish the specialty

TABLE 1		
Scientifically and Clinically Derived Knowledge		
Source of Knowledge	**Strengths**	**Limitations**
Scientifically Derived		
A set of interrelated facts presenting a systematic view of a phenomenon to describe, explain and predict its future occurrence	Highly reliable Systematic and controlled Objective and unbiased	Reductionist, conservative and often slow to evolve Lack of focus on external validity (practicability)
Professional Practice		
Knowledge gained through experience	Holistic Innovative Immediate	Less reliable Lack of explanations Increased susceptibility to bias

from 'alternative' healthcare providers, mental health physiotherapists must prove that what they do is well founded and provides significant additional value to the person who requests aid. Therefore research in this field is important and even vital. In this book, different authors underpin their clinical practice by describing quantitative and qualitative research.

THE FUTURE

Physiotherapy in mental health care contributes to the improvement of well-being and autonomy in people with physical needs associated with mental health, people with psychological disorders and people with learning disabilities by using physical approaches to influence their mental health.

To further develop and build a high-standard quality framework for physiotherapy in mental health care, the following points of interest will be elaborated in the short and long term: (1) stimulating physiotherapy education to include mental health courses in the curriculum, (2) improving clinical physiotherapy practice in mental health care, (3) encouraging physiotherapy in preventive (mental) health care and (mental) health promotion and (4) stimulating a research attitude and collaborating with other specialties within and outside physiotherapy.

Physiotherapists working in mental health care are in a unique position to provide an extensive range of therapeutic approaches aimed at relieving symptoms, boosting confidence and improving the quality of daily life. This is why and how mental health is an exciting and constantly evolving field for physiotherapists.

Together with the growing number of articles published in and outside physiotherapy journals, this book can be considered as the first international reference book of physiotherapy in mental health care. It provides an overview of the existing physiotherapy approaches in mental health care and psychiatry. The editors and the authors of the different chapters wish you pleasurable reading.

REFERENCES

American Psychiatric Association, 2013. Diagnostic and Statistical Manual of Mental Disorders (DSM-V), fifth ed. APA Press, Washington DC.

Angell, M., Kassirer, J., 1998. Alternative medicine—the risks of untested and unregulated remedies. NEJM 339, 839–841.

Barnes, P., Powell-Grineer, E., McFann, K., Nahim, R.L., 2004. Complementary and alternative medicine use among adults: USA 2002. Advance data from vital and health statistics 343. National Center for Health Statistics, Hyattsville, MD.

Beyerstein, B.L., 2001. Alternative medicine and common errors of reasoning. Acad. Med. 76, 230–237.

Biguet, G., Keskinen-Rosenqvist, R., Levy Berg, A., 2012. Att Förstå Kroppens Budskap—Sjukgymnastiska Perspektivand [To Understand the Message of the Body—Physiotherapy Perspectives]. Karolinska Institutet, Stockholm.

Bunkan, B., Thornquist, E., 1985. Hva er Psykomotorisk Fysioterapi? [What is Psychomotor Physiotherapy?]. Universitetsforlaget, Oslo.

Connaughton, J., Gibson, W., 2016. Physiotherapy students' attitudes toward psychiatry and mental health: a cross-sectional study. Can. J. Physiother. 68, 172–178.

Corrigan, P., 2004. How stigma interferes with mental health care. Am. Psychol. 59, 614–625.

Deutsch, J.E., Anderson, E.Z., 2007. Complementary Therapies for Physical Therapy: A Clinical Decision-Making Approach. Saunders, Philadelphia.

Eisenberg, G.M., Kessler, R.C., Van Rompay, M.I., et al., 2001. Perceptions about complementary therapies relative to conventional therapies among adults who use both: results from a national survey. Ann. Intern. Med. 135, 344–351.

European Region of the World Confederation for Physical Therapy, 2003. European physiotherapy benchmark statement. ER-WCPT, Brussels, Belgium. Retrieved from: http://www.physio-europe.org/index.php?action=80.

Everett, T., Donaghy, M., Fever, S., 2003. Interventions for Mental Health: An Evidence Based Approach for Physiotherapists and Occupational Therapists. Butterworth Heinemann, Edinburgh.

Ewert, T., Fuessl, M., Cieza, A., et al., 2004. Identification of the most common patient problems in patients with chronic conditions using the ICF checklist. J. Rehabil. Med. 36, 22–29.

Hare, M., 1986. Physiotherapy in Psychiatry. Heineman, London.

Herbert, R., Jamtvedt, G., Hagen, K.B., Mead, J., 2011. Practical Evidence-Based Physiotherapy. E-book, second ed. Elsevier, London.

Hinshaw, S.P., 2007. The Mark of Shame: Stigma of Mental Illness and an Agenda for Change. Oxford University Press, New York.

Hütter-Becker, A., Dölken, M., 2004. Physiotherapie in der Psychiatrie. Thieme Verlag, Stuttgart.

Ianssen, B., 2012. Norwegian Psychomotor Physiotherapy. Movements of Life. Fagtrykk, Trondheim.

Probst, M., Bosscher, R. (Eds.), 2001. Ontwikkelingen in de Psychomotorische Therapie [Developments in Psychomotor Therapy]. Cure & Care Publishers, Zeist.

Probst, M., Peuskens, J., 2010. Attitudes of Flemish physiotherapy students towards mental health and psychiatry. Physiotherapy 96, 44–51.

Probst, M., 2012. The International Organization of Physical Therapists working in Mental Health (IOPTMH). Mental Health Phys. Act. 5, 20–21.

Probst, M., Skjaerven, L., Parker, A., et al., 2015. Provisional definition of physiotherapy in mental health. IOPTMH Newsletter, 6 June 2015.

Reed, G.M., Spaulding, W.D., Bufka, L.F., 2009. The relevance of the international classification of functioning, disability and health (ICF) to mental disorders and their treatment. ALTER 3, 340–359.

Richardson, J., 2004. What patients expect from complementary therapy: a qualitative study. Am. J. Public Health 94, 1049–1053.

Roxendal, G., 1985. Body Awareness Therapy and the Body Awareness Scale, Treatment and Evaluation in Psychiatric Physiotherapy. Kompendietryckeriet, Kållered.

Saad, M., de Medeiros, R., 2012. Complementary therapies for the contemporary healthcare. Intech (Open access), Rijeka.

Schwank, A., Brunner, E., 2016. Attitudes towards psychiatry of physiotherapy students from German-speaking countries: an international comparison. Fisioterapia 38, 39.

Skjaerven, L.H., 2003. Basic Body Awareness Therapy. A Guide to Understanding, Therapy and Growth. Skjaerven LH, Bergen.

Stevenson, A., 2015. Oxford Dictionary of English, third ed. University Press, Oxford.

Stewart, A., Laasko, L., Connaughton, J., 2016. Attitudes of Queensland physiotherapists toward psychiatry. Fisioterapia 38, 5.

Ueberschlag, H., 1960. La kinesithérapie psychiatrique (French language) [physiotherapy in psychiatry]. Minerve (haut-Pyrénées). Hopital Psychiatrique de Lannemezan, p. 15.

Vancampfort, D., De Hert, M., Skjaerven, L.H., et al., 2012a. International Organization of Physical Therapy in Mental Health consensus on physical activity within multidisciplinary rehabilitation programmes for minimising cardio-metabolic risk in patients with schizophrenia. Disabil. Rehabil. 34, 1–12.

Vancampfort, D., Probst, M., Skjaerven, L., et al., 2012b. Systematic review of the benefits of physical therapy within a multidisciplinary care approach for people with schizophrenia. Phys. Ther. 92, 11–23.

Vroman, K., Arthanat, S., 2010. ICF and mental functions: applied to cross cultural case studies of schizophrenia. In: Stone, J.H., Blouin, M. (Eds.), International Encyclopedia of Rehabilitation. Retrieved from: http://cirrie.buffalo.edu/encyclopedia/en/article/308/.

World Health Organization (WHO), 2001. International Classification of Functioning, Disability, and Health. World Health Organization, Geneva.

WHO, 2005. Promoting mental health: concepts, emerging evidence, practice. Report of the World Health Organization, Department of Mental Health and substance abuse in collaboration with the Victorian Health Promotion Foundation and the University of Melbourne. World Health Organization, Geneva.

WHO, 2010. Global Recommendations on Physical Activity for Health. World Health Organization, Geneva.

Yucel, H., Acar, G., 2016. Levels of empathy among undergraduate physiotherapy students: a cross-sectional study at two universities in Istanbul. Pak. J. Med. Sci. 32, 85–90.

PSYCHOLOGICAL MODELS USED IN PHYSIOTHERAPY IN MENTAL HEALTH

2.1

FROM A BIOMEDICAL TO MORE BIOPSYCHOSOCIAL MODELS IN PHYSIOTHERAPY IN MENTAL HEALTH

GUNVOR GARD ▪ LIV HELVIK SKJAERVEN

SUMMARY

This chapter describes the development from a biomedical model towards more biopsychosocial models. Today, the relevance and importance of having a biopsychosocial perspective in physiotherapy is widely recognized. The biopsychosocial model can be the basis of such a perspective that it may also include cognitive behavioural principles, a focus on psychological factors and a behaviour-change process considering activity-related behaviour. We recommend that physiotherapists in mental health physiotherapy be aware of the importance of using such a model in their work, to promote, maintain and restore their patients' physical, psychological and social well-being. In the future, existential aspects may be included in the biopsychosocial model, because such aspects are increasingly important in our globalized world and because we need to integrate the voices of those from other cultures in mental health physiotherapy. It is important for physiotherapists to participate and have a voice in the ongoing discussion concerning which values are the basis for a biopsychosocial model in health care and how to develop the clinical work according to the model.

KEY POINTS

- The biopsychosocial perspective is a basic model to use for physiotherapists in mental health.
- It can be deepened by an increased focus on behaviour principles, the use of psychological factors and a behaviour-change process towards prioritized activity-related goals in clinical practice.

All therapies that are efficient in dealing with either somatic or psychological disorders are built upon a dualistic research paradigm. Modern medical care is based largely on a paradigm known as a *biomedical model* in which a 'gold standard' such as high-technology testing often guides clinical care. The biomedical model used in medicine has its roots in traditional Greek medicine, which is associated with Greek philosophy. Philosophical thinking in ancient Greece was abstract, systematic and governed by rationality and logic (Tamm, 1993). The world conception fostered by the philosophers was mainly dualistic, one that differentiated between spirit and matter, and mind and body. Hippocrates disengaged medicine from metaphysical ties. He had a scientific and objective view of diseases caused by biological factors. In 1637 Descartes published his opinion that Man consists of two separate entities—body and mind—linked to each other but qualitatively different.

The biomedical view has shown to be scientifically fruitful. It enabled studies of separate aspects of the human organism and reductionist mechanical models of the human body, and described its functions in exact quantifiable terms. The biomedical model is a disease model, reductionist in character and based on the assumption that disease is a pathological or mechanical dysfunction within the individual (Tamm, 1993). To have only a biomechanical perspective was soon shown to be insufficient in health care and a patient-centred perspective was developed, with an increased focus on patient–healthcare professional interaction (Illingworth, 2010; Hudon et al., 2012), which improved health outcomes in general (Dibbelt et al., 2009; Dillon, 2012).

The biopsychosocial perspective (Mead & Bower, 2000; Leplege et al., 2007) provides explanations for illness when no pathology is found. The International Classification of Functioning, Disability and Health (ICF) is a biopsychosocial model of health (Wadell & Burton, 2005) that explains both disease and illness as complex and dynamic processes where biological, emotional, cognitive and social factors interact (Wadell & Burton, 2005; Gatchel et al., 2007). The ICF classification consists of body functions and structures, activities and participation, as well as environmental factors which describe the influence of the context on the individual's functioning. All components interact in the process of functioning with a health condition. Participation represents the social perspective of functioning and is defined as being involved in a life situation. Restrictions on participation indicate the problems the individual may have in involvement in life situations (Fig. 1).

The relevance of the biopsychosocial model and of having a biopsychosocial perspective in physiotherapy is today widely recognized and used in different medical and physiotherapeutic areas, for example, concerning musculoskeletal pain problems and mental health (Nielson & Weir, 2001; Cornelius et al., 2011). According to the biopsychosocial model, assessment of an individual's health and rehabilitation potential involves measures at the social, psychological and biological levels (Cornelius et al., 2011). The biopsychosocial model can be used within physiotherapy to understand the complex biopsychosocial constructs of mental health problems. The ICF model is used internationally to categorize factors that can explain long-term disability due to mental disorders into groups: health-related, personal and external factors (Cornelius et al., 2011).

When working according to a biopsychosocial perspective as a physiotherapist, the interaction with the patient is a collaboration including clinical assessments, patient preferences and goals and professional knowledge (Jones et al., 2002). Each patient's rehabilitation needs have to be covered, together with their social, psychological and work-related needs. To consider psychological needs means, for example, to consider a patient's responsibility, opportunity to control, influence and participate in a physiotherapy treatment as well as considering motivational factors and self-efficacy (SBU, 2010; Gard, 2012). Salutogenic factors have also been identified as important resources for mental health. These factors have been defined as the experience of meaningfulness, comprehensiveness and the ability to cope with events

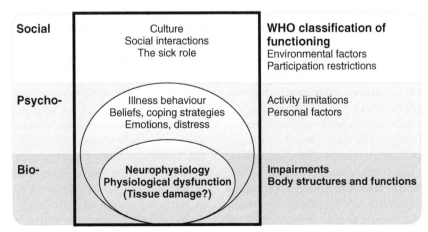

FIGURE 1 ■ The biopsychosocial model and the international classification by the World Health Organization (WHO) of body structures and functions, according to Wadell & Burton (2005).

in life (Flensborg-Madsen et al., 2006). Guidelines to manage musculoskeletal disorders and mental disorders recommend different self-reported health and work measures, using both professional assessment and patient self-report for the physiotherapist to use in order to understand and grasp a patient's situation from a broader perspective (Dagenais et al., 2010).

Today physical and psychological therapeutic modalities can be seen to be more or less integrated, as psychological factors are intertwined with physiological parameters and are suggested to operate within the same conceptual framework. In such an integrated perspective, mental health physiotherapy can be used to treat various disorders at multiple levels of functioning, and may be more effective in producing positive therapeutic outcomes than strategies solely reliant on biological or psychological approaches. The use of a biopsychosocial model is widely needed in mental health physiotherapy to promote, maintain and restore physical, psychological and social well-being, taking into account variations in individuals' health status, gender, cultures and worldview. This means that knowledge of behavioural medicine has to be included in mental health physiotherapy.

The social cognitive theory (Bandura, 2004) is an important psychological theory with relevance for physiotherapy in mental health. In our efforts to support our patients to achieve behavioural change, providing knowledge and information is not enough: it does not automatically lead to a change in behaviour. There must also be a focus on the individual's cognitive processes, such as thoughts, emotions and self-reflection, to facilitate learning and behaviour change (Bandura, 2004). An individual's beliefs regarding self-efficacy are important in social cognitive theory; they influence thoughts, cognitions, motivation, behaviour and actions (Bandura, 2004). Self-efficacy is an individual's belief in their own capacity to accomplish a task, and self-efficacy is positively related to success in obtaining a behaviour change (Bandura, 2004). The process of a successful behaviour change can be described as a clinical reasoning process with focus on a patient's prioritized activity-related behaviour. This is relevant for mental health physiotherapy, as a prioritized activity-related behaviour focuses on the patient's movements, thoughts and emotions that

are needed to perform a specific task and that are affected by both physical and social contexts (Elvén et al., 2015).

We will also acknowledge the importance of intentionality as a basis for actions and a successful behaviour change in life. Intentionality is focused within the psychological theory of reasoned action and is important in all clinical reasoning processes. Factors such as one's attitude toward a behaviour, one's subjective norms and perceived behavioural control are components that contribute to a strong intention (Ajzen, 2011). Attitude towards a behaviour is relevant because it is one's overall evaluation of a behaviour which includes beliefs about the consequences of the behaviour and an evaluation of the possible outcome. Acknowledging subjective norms is important today as we live in a multicultural society where different groups have different norms. The more favourable the attitude and subjective norm, and the greater the perceived behavioural control, the stronger is an individual's intention to perform a successful behaviour change (Clayton & Griffith, 2008).

Another theoretical model that is also important for physiotherapy in mental health concerns common therapeutic factors across therapies and mechanisms that can explain successful treatment outcomes in psychotherapy (Wampold, 2015). Formulating a goal in consensus with the patient, collecting treatment expectations and having good communication and collaboration with the patient are relevant common factors. In addition, to be genuine and empathetic, to confirm and develop an alliance with the patient and to try to understand the patient's culture, norms and beliefs are of great value for a positive treatment result (Wampold, 2015). The knowledge and awareness of these common factors are very relevant in mental health physiotherapy. To understand the evidence for the common factors, it is important to keep in mind that these factors are more than a set of therapeutic elements. They collectively shape a theoretical model about the mechanisms of change. The model emphasizes that the explanation given for an illness and the therapeutic actions must be acceptable to the patient. Acceptance is partly a function of consistency of the treatment with the patient's beliefs, particularly beliefs about how to cope with the effects of an illness. This suggests that evidence-based treatments that are culturally adapted will be more effective for members of the cultural group for which the adapted treatment is designed (Wampold, 2015). It is important to tailor and adapt physiotherapy treatments with regard to language and cultural aspects for the future because Europe is becoming increasingly multicultural.

In summary, we recommend that physiotherapists in mental health physiotherapy be aware of the importance of having a biopsychosocial model in their work and to use it to promote, maintain and restore their patients' physical, psychological and social well-being. For the future, existential aspects may be included in the biopsychosocial model, as such aspects are increasingly important in our globalized world and as we need to integrate the voices of people from other cultures in mental health physiotherapy. It is important for us as physiotherapists to participate and have a voice in the ongoing discussion concerning which values are the basis for a biopsychosocial model in health care and how to develop the clinical work according to the model.

REFERENCES

Ajzen, I., 2011. The theory of planned behavior: reactions and reflections. Psychol. Health 26 (9), 1113–1127.

Bandura, A., 2004. Health promotion by social cognitive means. Health Educ. Behav. 31 (2), 143–164.

Clayton, D.A., Griffith, C.J., 2008. Efficacy of an extended theory of planned behavior model for predicting caterers' hand hygiene practices. Int. J. Environ. Health Res. 18 (2), 83–98.

Cornelius, L.R., van der Klink, J.J., Groothoff, J.W., Brouwer, S., 2011. Prognostic factors of long-term disability due to mental disorders: a systematic review. J. Occup. Rehab. 21 (2), 259–274.

Dagenais, S., Tricco, A.C., Haldeman, S., 2010. Synthesis of recommendations for the assessment and management of low back pain from recent clinical practice guidelines. Spine 10 (6), 514–529.

Dibbelt, S., Schaidhammer, M., Fleischer, C., Greitemann, B., 2009. Patient–doctor interaction in rehabilitation: the relationship between perceived interaction quality and long-term treatment results. Patient Educ. Couns. 76, 328–335.

Dillon, P.J., 2012. Assessing the influence of patient participation in primary care medical interviews on recall of treatment recommendations. Health Commun. 27, 58–65.

Elvén, M., Hochwälder, J., Dean, E., Söderlund, A., 2015. A clinical reasoning model focused on clients' behavior change with reference to physiotherapists: its multiphase development and validation. Physiother. Theory Pract. 31 (4), 231–243.

Flensborg-Madsen, T., Ventegodt, S., Merrick, J., 2006. Sense of coherence and physical health. The emotional sense of coherence (SOC-E) was found to be the best-known predictor of physical health. Scientific World J. 6, 2147–2157.

Gard, G., 2012. Focus on psychological factors and body awareness in multimodal musculoskeletal pain rehabilitation. In: Bettany-Saltikov, J., Paz-Lourido, B. (Eds.), Physical Therapy Perspectives in the 21st Century—Challenges and Possibilities. InTech Open. <http://www.intechopen.com/books/physical-therapy-perspectives-in-the-21st-century-challenges-and-possibilities/>.

Gatchel, R.J., Peng, Y.B., Peters, M.L., et al., 2007. The biopsychosocial approach to chronic pain: scientific advances and future directions. Psychol. Bull. 133 (4), 581–624.

Hudon, C., Fortin, M., Haggerty, J., et al., 2012. Patient-centered care in chronic disease management: a thematic analysis of the literature in family medicine. Patient Educ. Couns. 88, 170–176.

Illingworth, R., 2010. What does "patient-centred" mean in relation to the consultation? Clin. Teach. 7, 116–120.

Jones, M., Edwards, I., Gifford, L., 2002. Conceptual models for implementing biopsychosocial theory in clinical practice. Man. Ther. 7 (1), 2–9.

Leplege, A., Gzil, F., Cammelli, M., et al., 2007. Person-centredness: conceptual and historical perspectives. Disabil. Rehabil. 29 (20-21), 1555–1565.

Mead, N., Bower, P., 2000. Patient-centredness: a conceptual framework and review of the empirical literature. Soc. Sci. Med. 51, 1087–1110.

Nielson, W., Weir, R., 2001. Biopsychosocial approaches to the treatment of chronic pain. Clin. J. Pain 17 (4), 114–127.

Tamm, M., 1993. Models of health and disease. Br. J. Med. Psychol. 66, 213–228.

The Swedish Council on Technology Assessment in Health Care, SBU, 2010. Rehabilitation for long-lasting pain conditions. A systematic literature review. SBU-report 198. ISBN 978-91-85413-34-8.

Wadell, G., Burton, A.K., 2005. Concepts of rehabilitation for the management of low back pain. Best Pract. Res. Clin. Rheumatol. 19, 655–670.

Wampold, B., 2015. How important are the common factors in psychotherapy? An update. World Psychiatry 14, 270–277.

2.2

PHENOMENOLOGY—A SOURCE OF INSPIRATION

ELINE THORNQUIST

SUMMARY

The purpose of this section is to stimulate an interest in phenomenology, because this philosophical tradition has the potential fruitfully to inform practice and documentation in physiotherapy. However, this task is not an easy one. Phenomenology is a rich and complex tradition, and what follows is a highly selective account of it.[1] I introduce first some basic concepts and tenets, after which I turn to Maurice Merleau-Ponty: the theorist who most systematically grounds human subjectivity in the body.

KEY TERMS

- Phenomenology
- Experiences
- Embodied subjects
- Practical agents
- Bodily habits
- Physiotherapy
- Clinical practice
- Research

LEARNING OBJECTIVES

- Give an account of the main differences between phenomenology and the empiricist/positivist tradition as regards views on perception and knowledge.

- Explain what Maurice Merleau-Ponty means by stating that the body is 'an ever-present guide' and that it has a double status.

- Account for some clinical implications of anchoring physiotherapy in a phenomenological framework.

BASIC CONCEPTS AND TENETS

Very briefly formulated, phenomenology is about the analysis of how experiences are given. Phenomenologists are interested in understanding the nature of experience: understanding how we come to know the world.

Phenomenology is often presented as a tradition that is concerned with the world as it appears for the subject. This statement has been much discussed, and is often misunderstood. The crucial point here is that experiences are viewed as subjective in the sense that only individual subjects can experience, and any fact has to be established by an active organization of the human consciousness.

Phenomenologists argue strongly against a view of perception as a basically receptive and mirroring process (cf. the concept *tabula rasa*).[2] Instead, they stress how human perception is influenced by our background, the situation at hand and the project we are involved in. Edmund Husserl—the founder of phenomenology—explored the complexity of human experience and emphasized that background and context are not sources of error or disturbing elements, but rather conditions of

---

[1]The best known phenomenologists are Edmund Husserl (1859–1938), Martin Heidegger (1889–1976) and Maurice Merleau-Ponty (1908–1961). It should be added that phenomenology is not a monolithic tradition; it has developed into different branches, which is why one often talks about the phenomenological 'movement'. For an overview, see Spiegelberg (1982).

[2]This concept stems from the empiricist/positivist tradition, a tradition that stands in sharp contrast to phenomenology. For further reading, see Hanson [1972].

our understanding. This is why many prefer to call phenomenology a *philosophy of constitution*. (For an accessible literature on this issue, see Hanson [1972], Langer [1989] and Zahavi [2003].) Husserl was particularly concerned with the impact of anticipations: how previous experiences and our own attitude come into play and 'colour' what we experience and apprehend. A main point here is that human beings do not live in a world of uninterpreted sensory impression, but in a world of meaningful objects and events, which appear to us not as raw sensory data, but already construed through experience, for example, a flower, a chair, a wedding, a car crash, a happy smile or a restrained posture.

Accordingly, phenomenologists have been central in furnishing critical arguments and objections to all kinds of documentation and research on human subjects which neglect the dimension of subjectivity and meaning. Moreover, they have called for greater respect for and sensitivity to the particular nature of human and sociocultural phenomena, and insisted on the importance of adjusting research approaches to the intrinsic nature of the object—the phenomenon. This principle is generally accepted today, although not always followed.

The Life-World and Taken-for-Grantedness

While earlier philosophical traditions, not least empiricism/positivism, operated with a distinct separation between everyday life and science, phenomenologists underscore the interconnections between the two domains.

The concept 'life-world' is frequently used in phenomenology, and it refers to the world as we immediately perceive it without conscious reflection. It refers to our taken-for-granted experiences. This concept is directly related to another central expression, 'being-in-the-world', which is written with hyphens to indicate our familiarity with and belonging to the world.

Phenomenologists emphasize that the life-world forms the basis upon which all other experiences, activities and learning take place. This applies to intellectual and abstract work, reasoning and research; not only to practical work. In general, they argue for the primacy of practical over reflective ways of being. We have 'a grip' on the world before we learn to know it verbally and cognitively, they claim. The subject in phenomenology is not a detached observer, but a practical agent inseparably bound up with the world. This brings us to Merleau-Ponty and his depiction of human beings as practical embodied agents.

BEYOND THE SILENT BODY AND THE SPEAKING MIND

To be a subject, according to Merleau-Ponty's philosophy, is identical to being in the world as embodied; it is *through* the body that we experience the world, learn about the world—have access to the world. The body is the very centre of all experience; 'an ever-present guide' (Merleau-Ponty, 1986). As human beings we are never—and can never be—cut off from our corporal situation; the *permanence* of the body is absolute. The *lived* body therefore is not an object akin to other physical objects in the world. I do not have a body as I have a house or a car; the body is not something I *possess*; it is something I *exist as*.

In other words, my body is not something additional to me, not an appendage to the subject, not something I can shed. It is what I am, Merleau-Ponty argues, which means that there is no perceived separation between body and self.

The body has, in other words, a double status; I *am* and I *have* a body. Each individual exists as subject and object simultaneously: as an embodied subject and a biological organism, a physical phenomenon subjected to gravity. This two-sidedness of the body means that I am always intertwined: a visible-seer, a tangible-toucher, etc. (Merleau-Ponty, 1986). The subject-status is, however, primary in the sense that it is as an experiencing and expressing embodied being that I go around doing my things, and I am still an experiencing body when gravity pulls on me as a material phenomenon, when I am in an upright position or lying, when I dance, go skiing or play. Consequently, the object-status of the 'lived' body is qualitatively different from the Cartesian body, which is solely physical matter.

It should be added here that phenomenology does not denigrate natural scientific knowledge at all; the point is to relocate it—to give such knowledge its due place within a new framework (Box 1). Once incarnate subjectivity is recognized, the premise is laid down for uniting that which for centuries has been separated: body and mind, nature and culture, sociality and individuality. Thereby the possibilities are opened for developing connections between biological and social processes, physical forces and universes of meaning.

In line with this, the body is regarded a conveyor of life and history and as therapists we get a new insight into the patient's world of experience and meaning. Verbal and bodily information and expressions are no longer seen as belonging to the separate worlds of *res cogitans* and *res extensa*, and thereby they can complement each other. Consequently, in clinical practice it is essential to compare patients' verbally expressed experiences with our observations and clinical findings, and to combine verbal and bodily dialogues.

Humans: Practical Agents

Merleau-Ponty portrays the body as a 'knower', stressing that knowledge is 'in the hands'; it is the body that understands (Merleau-Ponty, 1986). His examples are well known, and include typing, riding a bike, driving a car, etc., and he describes in detail how we become familiar with our surroundings through concrete actions, and how we learn to act without conscious planning and thinking.

Merleau-Ponty is constantly concerned with perception, and he accounts for perception as a living dialogue between the body-subject and its existential environment. Furthermore, *intentionality* is a basic concept in phenomenology. It comes from the Latin *intendere*, 'to stretch out or stretch for'. Intentionality refers to the outward directedness that characterizes our consciousness and our ways of being in the world; it is about a 'from–to structure'. While Husserl was primarily concerned with intentionality as a characteristic feature of our consciousness, in line with his cognitivist attitude more generally, Merleau-Ponty links intentionality consistently to our embodied existence. However, in recent years it has been recognized that Husserl became increasingly more interested in the body's role in our constitution of the world, see in particular the book often cited as *Ideas II* (Husserl, 1989).

What is typical for Merleau-Ponty is that he presents *motility* as 'basic intentionality' (Merleau-Ponty,

1986); 'to move one's body is to aim at things through it', he says, 'it is to allow oneself to respond to their call' (Merleau-Ponty, 1986). Furthermore, he stresses that 'Consciousness is in the first place not a matter of *I think that* but of *I can*' (Merleau-Ponty, 1986). The lived body is conceived of as an embodied consciousness that simultaneously engages, and is engaged in, the surrounding world. Consequently, physical space for humans becomes thereby *oriented* space.

In phenomenology it is underlined that I am 'always already' oriented in the world: 'I know what is up and down, heavy and light; I know what it is like to stumble and to regain balance, etc.', which means that the body's tacit knowledge is always prior to an objective awareness of things and events (cf. the concepts 'life-world' and 'being-in-the-world').

In the last two decades several scholars have emphasized that phenomenology can bring light to a number of aspects of experience that demonstrate the embodied nature of cognition, including basic perceptual processes (Gallagher, 2014). In a time with much interest in cognitive therapy, it is pertinent – not the least for physiotherapists – to learn more about the interrelationship between bodily experience and cognitive processes.

Interaction: Movements and Perception

Our embodiment affords us two basic modes of contact, actional and perceptual, and Merleau-Ponty elucidates how action and perception make up a unity; they are 'two facets of one and the same act' (Merleau-Ponty, 1986). He stresses that we respond through movements to the requirements of our surroundings, and things appear to us depending on our bodily capacities, accounting for how this is reflected at a very basic level. For instance, the fact that mountains are tall for us is a function of our embodied shape and motility. Moreover, habits come into the picture: foreigners who visit Norway for the first time and try to go skiing perceive the terrain as frightening, as steep, whereas those who are accustomed to skiing perceive the same terrain as rather flat. Things appear low and high, steep and flat, heavy and light in respect to what we master and are capable of doing, and in respect to how we can move and act bodily. There is a mutuality between what we are capable of doing and the manner in which we apprehend the world; a reciprocity between what we master and how the world appears to us that is of utmost importance for physiotherapists to understand. This means that our relation to the world is transformed as we acquire new skills and extend our repertoire of movement. Changing habits and movement repertoire therefore is not merely a question of changing our motor capacity; it involves us as people (Thornquist, 2012).

This is an insight that accords well with our clinical experiences, and it throws light on why it is often so difficult to change habits such as ways of standing, sitting, walking and relating to the surroundings. Change takes time; cf. the slogan 'Old habits die hard'.

Attention and Awareness

Most of the time our attention is directed away from the body and towards the environment or some project we are undertaking. This is exactly what the philosopher Leder refers to when he writes about 'the absent body' (Leder, 1990): under normal circumstances the body is not the object of my explicit attention; it is usually taken-for-granted, and represents a kind of tacit background. When we are caught up in involvement in a situation, our embodiment itself passes on in silence.

When we fall ill or have some kind of functional problem, our relation to the world and our own body is radically changed. Our taken-for-granted ways of acting and the unity between the body and self are disrupted. The body may be experienced as something outside my control, separated from my will and wishes, which may easily result in an observer-relationship to my body. I may even feel that I am at the body's mercy, and my sense of self may change (Leder, 1990; Toombs, 2001).

It is not only when we are ill that we observe ourselves. If a person differs from others, is fat among the slim, brown among the white or handicapped among the able, one quickly internalizes the gaze of others, and with idealized images of the human body everywhere these days, it is difficult not to observe ourselves and come away dissatisfied. Moreover, people suffering from traumatic experiences often establish a distance from their bodies as an integrated part of a general defence against negative and overwhelming feelings. The body emerges as an object which can be observed and manipulated, alien to the self. Against this background, it is often essential to help people to

BOX 2

'Experiences remain with us, not only as thought and conscious memories, but as part of our embodiment. We may consciously forget, but our body remembers what we have done, and what we have been exposed to; what we have experienced is expressed and imprinted in our bodies'.

rely on and accept their bodies by stimulating involvement, bodily anchoring and a feeling of mastery; i.e., to stimulate a sense of agency (Thornquist, 2012).

The Body as History and Memory

Recognizing our embodied existence has far-reaching implications for the understanding of human beings and social life in general. It means, for instance, that experiences cannot be obliterated. By recognizing incarnate subjectivity, it follows logically that human experiences can only be lived in and through the body, and that people cannot but express and convey their history bodily. Experiences remain with us, not only as thought and conscious memories, but as part of our embodiment. We may consciously forget, but our body remembers what we have done, and what we have been exposed to; what we have experienced is expressed and imprinted in our bodies (Box 2).

The process from illness-inducing conditions to manifesting illness may, however, be extremely complex (Mäkinen et al., 2006; Thornquist, 2006; 2012; Kirkengen 2010; Lanius et al., 2010). Adverse experiences may for instance be expressed as muscular tension, restricted breathing and hampered movements, or as muscular slackness, bodily resignation and apathy, and/or as hyperactivity and limitless behaviour. The people in question often suffer from several somatic and mental problems. It is therefore urgent not to interpret single observations and findings without context, but to recognize the body's ambiguity and take into account the interrelationship between local conditions and the general state of the body, and compare our findings with the patient's life experiences and social circumstances. The lived body is, in other words, a source of knowledge both for observers and for the persons themselves.

We all know that one and the same event may appear very different to a person. A divorce, for instance, may be experienced as a relief or it may be felt as a rejection that evokes bad memories which harm the person's health. Symptoms from a shoulder may be an integrated part of a reaction to long-standing stress, but they may also be caused by strain or an injury, and very often musculoskeletal problems are the result of a combination of factors.

Phenomenology encourages us to be sensitive and responsive to various kinds of bodily expressions and behaviour, in order to better understand the connections between life histories and illness histories.

Bodily dysfunctions and disorders may have a function in a psychological and social sense: they may represent protection against traumatic memories. A central challenge, then, is to turn around the vicious circle of bodily dysfunctions at the same time as it is essential to give the individual patient new and positive experiences so that s/he learns to rely on her/his body and become familiar with new ways of moving, acting and relating. In short, we must strive for a gradual change. The aim is to be able to go in and out of defence patterns and to be able to behave and adapt according to the situation.

I sum up by stating that anchoring physiotherapy in a phenomenological framework does not imply adhering to one specific physiotherapeutic approach. Instead, the ideal is individualization, and then all kinds of methods, means and tools can be employed. What is decisive is the way we use them and on which evaluation base.

REFERENCES

Gallagher, S., 2014. Phenomenology and embodied cognition. In: Shapiro, L. (Ed.), The Routledge handbook of embodied cognition. Routledge, London, pp. 9–18.

Hanson, N.R., 1972. Patterns of Discovery. Cambridge University Press, Cambridge.

Husserl, E., 1989. Ideas Pertaining to a Pure Phenomenology and to Phenomenological Philosophy, second ed. Kluwer, Dordrecht.

Kirkengen, A.L., 2010. The Lived Experience of Violence: How Abused Children Become Unhealthy Adults. Zeta Books, Bucharest.

Lanius, R.A., Vermetten, E., Pain, C. (Eds.), 2010. The Impact of Early Life Trauma on Health and Disease: The Hidden Epidemic. Cambridge University Press, Cambridge.

Langer, M.M., 1989. Merleau-Ponty's Phenomenology of Perception. MacMillan Press, London.

Leder, D., 1990. The Absent Body. The Chicago University Press, Chicago.

Mäkinen, T., Laaksonen, M., Lahelma, E., Rahkonen, O., 2006. Associations of childhood circumstances with physical and mental functioning in adulthood. Soc. Sci. Med. 62, 1831–1839.

Merleau-Ponty, M., 1986. The Phenomenology of Perception. Routledge & Kegan Paul, London.

Spiegelberg, H., 1982. The Phenomenological Movement: A Historical Introduction. Martinus Nijhoff, The Hague.

Thornquist, E., 2006. Face-to-face and hands-on: assumptions and assessments in the physiotherapy clinic. Med. Anthropol. 25, 65–97.

Thornquist, E., 2012. Movement and Interaction. The Sherborne Approach and Documentation. University Press, Oslo.

Toombs, K. (Ed.), 2001. Handbook of Phenomenology and Medicine. Kluwer Acedemic, Dordrecht.

Zahavi, D., 2003. Husserl's Phenomenology. Stanford University Press, Stanford.

2.3

PERSPECTIVES ON HUMAN MOVEMENT, THE PHENOMENON OF MOVEMENT QUALITY AND HOW TO PROMOTE MOVEMENT QUALITY THROUGH MOVEMENT AWARENESS AS PHYSIOTHERAPY IN MENTAL HEALTH

LIV HELVIK SKJAERVEN ■ GUNVOR GARD

SUMMARY

A perspective can be described as a mental view or a position from which something is considered or evaluated. In clinical practice the physiotherapist decides on the choice of perspective in any treatment modality, in description of the body, in the choice of exercises or movement and in what is communicated in dialogue with the patient. The perspective can be hidden or open, conscious or unconscious, and the expression of it can differ between what one describes in words and how one acts. However, the choice of perspective has impact on physiotherapy. To be conscious about what kind of perspective and knowledge experts in human movement use is important for the clinical approach to patients in mental health.

KEY POINTS

■ Perspectives on human movement and movement quality.

■ The phenomenon of movement quality.

■ The phenomenon and strategy of movement awareness learning.

■ The introduction of healthy movement quality aspects.

LEARNING OBJECTIVES

■ Gain a deeper understanding of a multidimensional perspective on human movement, the phenomenon of movement quality and its consequences for physiotherapy.

■ Gain insight into a methodology that is oriented towards healthy movement resources and a sense of coherence.

■ Understanding more of the phenomenon of movement awareness learning and the relationship between two phenomena: movement quality and movement awareness.

This short review describes some perspectives, terms and knowledge that have developed and deepened the understanding of the phenomenon of movement quality through the years. As movement quality is important in physiotherapy, the intention here is to direct attention to the richness and complexity of the phenomenon, through several perspectives.

HUMAN MOVEMENT—A CORE IN PHYSIOTHERAPY

Human movement and function are described as key components in physiotherapy (WCPT, 2017). Thus physiotherapeutic examination and evaluation tools of the patient's movement coordination are important to develop, maintain and restore optimal movement and function throughout the lifespan.

23

The development of scientific knowledge in physiotherapy has advanced significantly; however, research is mostly conducted within a biomedical paradigm (Wikström-Grotell & Eriksson, 2012). Physiotherapists are generally trained to attend to physical aspects, focusing on separate joints and limbs (Higgs et al., 2004). The vocabulary and working model used in physiotherapy have their roots in the tradition of physical training based on a biomedical perspective, even if a biopsychosocial perspective is commonly described in bachelor's degree programmes in physiotherapy. However, movement has seldom been studied from a psychosocial or existential perspective (Wikström-Grotell & Eriksson, 2012).

Concepts and Definitions

Defining basic concepts in physiotherapy is important (Wikström-Grotell & Eriksson, 2012). The role of concepts as basic elements in theory construction within the tradition of movement science has increasingly attracted attention within physiotherapy. Examining what kind of knowledge is used by experts in human movement in mental health and their own views on human movement is important for understanding how expert clinicians work and for reflecting on the practice (Jensen et al., 1999; Jensen, 2000). An editorial in *Advances in Physiotherapy* (Sundelin, 2009) focused on 'Challenging perspectives in physiotherapy', and points towards the need to broaden the scope of human movement. This is in line with the recommendation of Wikström-Grotell (2012).

In clinical practice, the physiotherapist decides on the perspective of the treatment modality, directing attention to a description of the body, exercises/movements and communication. The perspective can be hidden or open, conscious or unconscious. It can differ between what one expresses in words and what is actually implemented in the physiotherapist's action. The choice of perspective has an impact on the therapeutic meeting (Roxendal, 1985; Roxendal & Winberg, 2002).

Defining Awareness, Presence and Embodied Presence

A differentiation between a *concept* and a *phenomenon* is identified: a phenomenon is derived from the senses,

---

BOX 1
DICTIONARY DEFINITION OF A *CONCEPT* AND *PHENOMENON*

	Dictionary Definition
Concept	... an abstract idea; something conceived in the mind, a thought or an abstract idea (Merriam-Webster).
Phenomenon	... derived from the senses; an aspect known through the senses rather than by thought or intuition (Merriam-Webster)

---

while a concept is an abstract idea (Merriam-Webster). Accordingly, when promoting movement quality, the approach, and thus the vocabulary, is slightly different from the vocabulary used within the tradition of physical activity and physical training (Box 1).

Awareness, presence and embodiment are complex phenomena frequently referred to in physiotherapy. *Awareness* can be defined as an attentive, relaxed and alert presence (Brown & Ryan, 2003). The phenomenon includes variations from being unaware, subconsciously aware, partially aware or conscious of the body, a feeling, a thought, a movement of oneself. *Being aware* means continually monitoring the internal and external environments (Brown & Ryan, 2003). *Presence* is described as a state of being attentive and calmly aware of the experience of the present situation (Grotowski, 1996). *Embodied presence* is a bodily felt sense, a form of personal knowing that evokes understanding and fosters meaning (Todres, 2007).

PERSPECTIVES ON HUMAN MOVEMENT

Choice of Perspective

A perspective can be defined as an ordered view of one's own world, of what is taken for granted about the attributes of various objects, events and human nature (Rosberg, 2000). It can be described as a mental view or a position from which something is considered or evaluated (Merriam-Webster, 2014).

Illness and human suffering, especially in physiotherapy in mental health, cannot be understood from a biomedical perspective alone. Thus it is important to broaden the perspective of human movement within physiotherapy in mental health, including a health perspective (Antonovsky, 1987; Langeland, 2007).

Perspective on Health

The health perspective (Antonovsky, 1987) describes that a pathological orientation focuses on why people get sick, whereas a health orientation includes a focus on understanding the origin of health. Accordingly, to search for health has a different approach than a search for pathology. Thus the health continuum, including a span from pathology towards a focus on health, represents a shift in the therapeutic perspective on treatment, relating to the experience of connection, meaning and worthfullness, the *sense of coherence* (SOC). Consequently, the following questions arise: what is the nature of healthy movement and what are the elements and aspects of healthy movements?

Perspectives on Human Movement

In physiotherapy, movement and bodily function are seen as an integrated part of human action and interrelation. Turning to theory on motor science we see examples of different perspectives on human movement through different models, the Reflex Model, Hierarchic Model, Motor Program Model, Task Oriented Model, System Theory, Dynamic Theory, Ecologic Theory, etc. (Shumway-Cook & Woollacott, 2012). Within the history of medicine we have seen the development of the psychosomatic perspective, through the formation of psychosomatic medicine as a subspecialty, and the health professions (Alexander, 1950; Sivik & Theorell, 1995). In recent history we have become familiar with different perspectives—biomedical, psychosomatic, sociocultural, existential and phenomenological—as approaches to human movement, and more recently an existential perspective has been seen to be important for physiotherapy.

THE PHENOMENON OF MOVEMENT QUALITY

A Literature Review

Movement quality is a phenomenon frequently used by physiotherapists in oral language, written text and clinical practice. However, there exists little clarification of the phenomenon. A literature study was made, searching for elements and aspects of health included in the phenomenon of movement quality (Skjærven et al., 2008). By element (in cursiv) is meant a fundamental, essential or distinct constituent of an entity, an assumption or principles of a phenomenon; element is synonymous with component, factor or ingredient. By aspect (in cursiv) is meant an appearance, a feature, an expression (in the body); aspect is synonymous with characteristics, a quality (Merriam-Webster's Dictionary, 2014).

According to Prohl (1986), the phenomenon of movement quality includes objective-physical characteristics as well as subjective-psychological (aesthetical) characteristics of motor (internal) and movement (external) perception (Prohl, 1986), suggesting that the internal sensory-motor perception is expressed in the movement quality.

German expression psychology and psychiatric literature, which reveals indicators of psychopathological states as well as measurements of movement quality (Wallbott, 1985, 1989), defines movement quality as 'the way in which movements are done, relating to time and space'.

In the treatment of children with cerebral palsy, the development of assessment tools for movement quality is presented (Boyce et al., 1991, 1995; Bach et al., 1994; Gowland et al., 1995; Hickey & Ziviani, 1998; Thomas et al., 2001). In this context, movement quality includes alignment, stability, weight shift, coordination, movement fluency, grasp, target accuracy and dissociated movements as components in the description.

Considerable energy has been used in predicting neurologic outcomes in preterm infants with brain damage, considering their movement quality (Geerdink & Hopkins, 1993; Bos, 1998; Kakebeeke et al., 1998; Einspieler & Prechtl, 2005). Work has been done to describe the components of an integrated, organized appearance of movement fluency, variability, amplitude and elegance, as well as attainment of midline position, all presented as important in the assessment of movement quality.

Movement quality is a common term in the literature in the European Movement Tradition (Laban, 1960; Rederfern, 1965; Brooks, 1976; Bartennieff, 1980;

Johnson, 1983; Alon, 1990; Barlow, 1990; Feldenkrais, 1990), in actors' training (Chekhov, 1985; Stanislavski, 1992) and in modern dance (Laban, 1960; Rederfern, 1965; Bartennieff, 1980; Horosko, 1991). Core components in this literature are movement awareness, freeing of the breathing and postural alignment on the one hand and a variety of movement aspects/nuances on the other.

Za-Zen and tai chi are Eastern movement traditions brought to the Western world, and are presented as examples of the development of movement quality. Za-Zen meditation (Soto Zen) is a bodily form of mental training, practised through an upright, sitting position, aiming at a free breathing and a stable unified mind (Deshimaru, 1988; Suzuki, 1988). Tai chi chuan has roots in the Chinese movement tradition (martial arts), and aims to integrate slow, soft and unified movement coordinations with intentional, functional and existential aspects (Yang, J-M., 1991a, 1991b).

Fine art is described as an expression of true feelings (Langer, 1953), presented as a door-opener to a tacit knowledge when it comes to expression in human movement (Heidegger, 1996). It helps us see features, fundamental elements and aspects in posture and movement of which we were previously unaware (Heidegger, 1996). Fine art communicates a sense of movement nuances with extraordinarily delicate energy (Dewey, 1934). Historically, movement teachers and dancers have studied fine art and Greek sculptures (May, 1975, 1985; Chekhov, 1985) to deepen their understanding of human movement.

If the term *movement quality* is used merely in training from a neurophysiological perspective, stressing 'normal' movement and movement perfection, it can be criticized. This view represents a technique, and is a passive view of motor learning and promotion of movement quality (Ketelaar et al., 2001).

The phenomenon of movement quality has been frequently used by the French movement educator and psychotherapist Jacques Dropsy (Dropsy, 1987a, 1998). It has been clinically integrated in Basic Body Awareness Therapy, and further developed through research (Roxendal, 1985, 1987; Mattsson, 1998; Skjærven, 1999; Skatteboe, 2000; Gyllensten, 2001; Skjærven et al., 2003, 2004, 2008, 2010).

More recently, the phenomenon of movement quality is referred to in rheumatologic physiotherapy (Olsen & Skjærven, 2016), treatment of hip osteoarthritis (Strand et al., 2016) and in studies of back pain (Hodges et al., 2013).

HOW TO PROMOTE MOVEMENT QUALITY

Movement awareness is not given much attention in physical therapy and we are not taught its richness and how to use it. One major factor contributing to the lack of value put on this practical knowledge is probably because it has been difficult to make it explicit and articulate it (Higgs et al., 2004). A challenge for the physiotherapist is to learn reliable tools to identify the patient's needs and to acquire specific attitudes and skills for movement observation and guidance.

The phenomenon of movement awareness offers a specific focus on human movement and functions, and thus differs from body awareness, a more general phenomenon. The movement awareness is expressed in the body and can be observed through observing movement quality, as supported through phenomenological research (Skjærven et al., 2003, 2004, 2008, 2010).

It is important to foster reflective attention on how the person's movement awareness is expressed in their general movement quality, how it is observed and evaluated by the physiotherapist, and how it can be promoted and further developed as a therapeutic strategy. How the person, and the whole body, is coordinated, from the soles of the feet to the top of the head, as one human unit, challenges the physiotherapist when it comes to observation and treatment of the patient's movement habits and/or movement patterns. In order to evaluate and promote movement quality in physiotherapy, three 'maps' are suggested, being useful indicators for clinical implementation.

Map 1: The MQ-Model—Overview of Healthy Movement Elements and Aspects

A phenomenological study of the phenomenon of movement quality was conducted through in-depth interviews with 15 expert physiotherapists from neurologic physiotherapy, community health care and psychiatric/psychosomatic physiotherapy. The study revealed an essence of the phenomenon, presenting a multiperspective view, a biopsychosociocultural–existential perspective on human movement (Fig. 1) (Skjaerven et al., 2008).

Fig. 1 illustrates four perspectives, synthesized into the general term *movement quality*. Each of the four perspectives includes: (1) basic elements of movement quality, presented as preconditions to more functional movement quality, and (2) characteristics or aspects that are expressed in the movement. *Precondition* refers to fundamental elements that are important for the person to integrate in movement training to make the movement functional and practical. What is meant by 'characteristics' is an aspect of healthy movement or a particular quality experienced (by the patient) and observed (by the physiotherapist).

Fig. 1 represents a global impression of how the person moves, covering perspectives, preconditions and a range of movement characteristics. They are all interacting and interconnected processes that cannot be separated. The Movement Quality Model gives an overview of the essence of a whole. It is on this background that a description of movement quality is proposed: movement quality can be described as how postural balance, breathing and mental awareness are integrated and used in human movement and function; in other words, how (the way) the person moves in relation to space, time and energy, handling the internal as well as external environment. The Movement Quality Model can be used as a roadmap in clinical physiotherapy.

Map 2: Therapeutic Factors—an Overview

To transfer movement elements and aspects in such a way that the patient becomes aware and can use them in daily life is a challenge for the physiotherapist. Fig. 2 reveals therapeutic factors for promoting movement quality through: (1) the physiotherapist's embodied presence and their own movement awareness, (2) a platform for promoting movement quality and (3) therapeutic strategies (Skjærven et al., 2010).

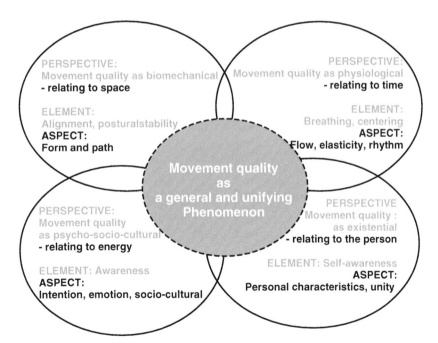

FIGURE 1 ▪ The modified Movement Quality Model (MQM) of 2017: Movement quality as interacting processes. *(Skjaerven et al., 2008. An Eye for Movement Quality: A Phenomenological Study of Movement Quality Reflecting a Group of Physiotherapist`s Understanding of the Phenomenon. Physiother. Theory Pract. 24 (1), 13-27. Reprinted by permission Taylor & Francis LLC)*

The physiotherapeutic guidance promoting movement quality is a support for the patient to find new movement patterns from within the body rather than imposing them upon the patient from outside. The therapeutic approach is not aiming at mechanical, mindless movements. Promoting movement awareness concerns bodily and mental processes, involving the whole person. Such an approach puts high demands on the therapist's own movement awareness. In order to be aware of the patient's reaction to the movement and where the patient is in the process, the physical therapist needs to be aware of how he/she communicates, also his/her own movements and the direction of more functional movement quality. Therefore it is important that the therapist personally becomes familiar with and develops their own movement awareness to provide appropriate guidance for their patients, as part of their professional development.

The physiotherapist is a role model, being a mirror for the patient, indicating how to develop the movement. This provides the patient with an internal image of the movement quality that is often difficult for the patient to find (Dropsy, 1987b). The therapist functions as a tacit communicator (Polanyi, 1983). Patient and physical therapist are exploring movements together; the therapist suggests the direction and the patient explores to find, develop and become conscious of it.

Map 3: the Movement Awareness Learning Cycle—a Process for Change

The Movement Awareness Learning Cycle introduces seven interrelated and overlapping steps to initiate a process of change in the movement quality (Fig. 3) (Skjærven et al., 2010).

Gaining a closer contact with the body is essential for developing movement quality, for the experience of well-being and health. It provides a basis for new ways of moving and insight into movement habits, compensations and how to recognize the more healthy and functional movement quality. Encouraging a state of movement exploration is important for stimulating the patient's curiosity and involvement. This leads towards new movement experiences of integrating new movement strategies, becoming consciously aware. Creating meaning and being able to translate movement experiences by integrating them into daily life early in therapy is important learning for patients. It empowers the patient's experience of mastery in everyday situations. Dialogue, conceptualization and reflection about the newly acquired movement quality and becoming aware, are important for insight and the process of change (Dewey, 1934). In the Movement Awareness Learning Cycle the therapist creates situations for the patient to explore, repeat and experience the movements by truly participating in them, and then to reflect and find words to

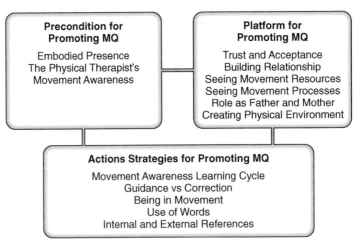

FIGURE 2 ■ Therapeutic factors promoting movement quality (MQ)—an overview. (Skjaerven et al., 2010. Reprinted from Phys. Ther. 2010;90(10):1479-1492 with permission of the American Physical Therapy Association. ©2010 American Physical Therapy Association.)

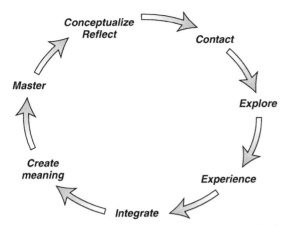

FIGURE 3 ■ The Movement Awareness Learning Cycle. *(Skjaerven et al., 2010. Reprinted from Phys. Ther. 2010;90(10): 1479-1492 with permission of the American Physical Therapy Association. ©2010 American Physical Therapy Association.)*

describe their experience of the new movement habits (Kolb, 1984).

EXPANDING THE PERSPECTIVES ON HUMAN MOVEMENT—SUMMING UP

Movement has been described as a 'missing component' or a 'blind spot' within physiotherapy (Jensen et al., 1999). This reveals a view that teaching functional activities and exercises can be so obvious for the physiotherapist that addressing movement itself is easily forgotten (Jensen et al., 1999). The capacity of the physiotherapist in mental health to fulfil their obligations depends on a number of factors, including the ability to recognize the broad scope of perspectives on human movement. These have consequence for physiotherapy, in movement observation and guidance, including not only pathologic but also a healthy perspective on human movement. The three maps presented are indicators for movement quality, expanding the perspective on human movement. To be conscious about the kinds of perspective and knowledge used by experts in human movement is considered important for the clinical approach to patients in mental health. However, further research is necessary for the future of the physiotherapy profession, especially in mental health.

REFERENCES

Alexander, F., 1950. Psychosomatic Medicine. Its Principles and Applications. W.W. Norton Company Inc. New York.

Alon, R., 1990. Mindful Spontaneity. Moving in Tune with Nature: Lessons in the Feldenkrais Method. Prism Press, Dorset, UK.

Antonovsky, A., 1987. Unraveling the Mystery of Health. How Well People Manage Stress and Stay Well. Jossey-Bass Publishers, San Fransisco.

Bach, T.M., Reddihough, D.S., Burgess, G., et al., 1994. Comparison of subjective and objective measures of movement performance in children with cerebral palsy. Dev. Med. Child Neurol. 36, 974–979.

Barlow, W., 1990. The Alexander Principle. How to Use Your Body Without Stress, second ed. Victor Gollancz, London, UK.

Bartennieff, I.L.D., 1980. Body Movement: Coping with the Environment. Gordon and Breach Science Publishers, New York.

Bos, A.F., 1998. Analysis of movement quality in preterm infants. Eur. J. Obstet. Gynecol. Reprod. Biol. 76 (1), 117–119.

Boyce, W.F., Gowland, C., Rosenbaum, P.L., et al., 1991. Measuring quality of movement in cerebral palsy: a review of instruments. Phys. Ther. 71 (11), 813–819.

Boyce, W.F., Gowland, C., Rosenbaum, P.L., et al., 1995. The Gross Motor Performance measure: validity and responsiveness of a measure of quality of movement. Phys. Ther. 75 (7), 603–613.

Brooks, C., 1976. Sensory Awareness. The Rediscovery of Experiencing, second ed. An Esalen Book, The Viking Press, Inc, New York, USA.

Brown, K.W., Ryan, R.M., 2003. The benefits of being present: mindfulness and its role in psychological well-being. J. Pers. Soc. Psychol. 84 (4), 822–848.

Chekov, M., 1985. Lessons for the Professional Actor. first ed. Performing Arts Journal Publications, New York.

Deshimaru, T., 1988. Samtal med en zenmästare (A. Blau, Trans.), second ed. Bokforlaget Åsak, Delsbo.

Dewey, J., 1934. Experience and Education. Collier Books, New York.

Dropsy, J., 1987a. Den harmoniska kroppen. En osynlig övning (The Harmonic Body. An Invisible Exercise). Natur och Kultur, Stockholm.

Dropsy, J., 1987b. Leva i sin kropp. Kroppslig uttryck och mänsklig kontakt (The Living Body. Bodily Expression and Human Contact) (I. Munck, Trans.). Natur och Kultur, Stockholm.

Dropsy, J., 1998. Human Expression—The Coordination of Mind and Body. In: Skjaerven, L.H. (Ed.), Quality of Movement—The Art and Health. Lectures on Philosophy, Theory and Practical Implications to Basic Body Awareness Therapy. Skjærven, Bergen, pp. 8–20.

Einspieler, C., Prechtl, H.F.R., 2005. Prechtl's assessment of general movements: a diagnostic tool for the functional assessment of the young nervous system. Ment. Retard. Dev. Disabil. Res. Rev. 11 (1), 61–67.

Feldenkrais, M., 1990. Awareness Through Movement: Health Exercises for Personal Growth, first ed 1972. Harper Collins, San Francisco.

Geerdink, J.J., Hopkins, B., 1993. Qualitative changes in general movements and their prognostic value in preterm infants. Eur. J. Pediatr. 152 (4), 362–367.

Gowland, C., Boyce, W., Wright, V., et al., 1995. Reliability of the Gross Motor Perfomance Measure. Phys. Ther. 75 (7), 597–602.

Grotowski, J., 1996. Barba, E. (Ed.), Towards a Poor Theatre, first published 1968 ed. Methuen Drama, London. Original edition, 1968.

Gyllensten, A.L., 2001. Basic Body Awareness Therapy. Doctoral dissertation, Lund University, Lund.

Heidegger, M., 1996. Being and Time (J. Stambaugh, Trans.). State University of New York Press, Albany, New York.

Hickey, A., Ziviani, J., 1998. A review of the Quality of Upper Extremities Skill Test (QUEST) for children with cerebral palsy. Phys. Occup. Ther. Pediatr. 18 (3-4), 123–135.

Higgs, J., Richardson, B., Dahlgren, M.A., 2004. Developing Practice Knowledge for Health Professionals. Butterworth-Heinemann, Edinburgh.

Hodges, P.W., Van Dillen, L.R., McGill, S., et al., 2013. State-of-the art approach to clinical rehabilitationof low back and pelvic pain: state of the art and science. Cholewicki, J., Hodges, P.W., Van Dieen, J.H. (Eds.). Churchill Linvingstone/ Elsevier, Edinburgh, pp. 243–309.

Horosko, M., 1991. Martha Graham. The Evolution of Her Dance Theory and Training 1926-1991. Chicago: a cappaella books. Chicago Review Press, Inc., USA.

Jensen, G.M., Gwyer, J., Hack, L.M., Shepard, K.F., 1999. Expertise in Physical Therapy Practice. Butterworth-Heinemann, USA.

Jensen, G.M., Gwyer, J., Shepard, K.F., Hack, L.M., 2000. Expert practice in physical therapy. Phys. Ther. 80, 28–43.

Johnson, D.H., 1983. Body: Recovering Our Sensual Wisdom. North Atlantic Books, Somatic Resources, California, USA.

Kakebeeke, T.H., von Siebenthal, K., Largo, R.H., 1998. Movement quality in preterm infants prior to term. Biol. Neonate 73 (3), 145–154.

Ketelaar, M., Vermeer, A., Hart, H., et al., 2001. Effects of a functional therapy program on motor abilities of children with cerebral palsy. Phys. Ther. 81 (9), 1534–1545.

Kolb, D.A., 1984. Experiential Learning. Experience as The Source of Learning and Development. Prentice-Hall, Inc, Englewood Cliffs, NY.

Laban, R., 1960. The Mastery of Movement. McDonald and Evans Ltd, London, UK.

Langeland, E., 2007. A Salutogenic Approach. Doctoral thesis, University of Bergen, Bergen.

Langer, S.K., 1953. Feeling and Form. A Theory of Art Developed from Philosophy in a New Key. Charles Scribner's Sons, New York.

Mattsson, M. (1998). Body Awareness Applications in Physiotherapy. Dissertation, Umeå University, Umeå.

May, R., 1975. The Courage to Create. W.W. Norton, New York.

May, R., 1985. My Quest For Beauty. Saybrook Publishing Company, New York.

Merriam-Webster, 2017. Merriam-Webster Dictionary. Merriam-Webster Inc. <https://www.merriam-webster-webster.com.>

Olsen, A., Skjærven, L.H., 2016. Patients suffering from rheumatic disease describing own experiences from participating in Basic Body Awareness Group Therapy: a qualitative pilot study. Physiother. Theory Pract. 32 (2), 98–106.

Polanyi, M., 1983. The Tacit Dimension. Peter Smith, New York.

Prohl, R. (1986). Some reflections on the phenomenon 'quality in (of) movement'. The Physical Education Teacher and Coach today, vol. 2. University of Heidelberg: Bundesinstitut für Sportwissenschaft, Forschungsberichte und Materialien.

Rederfern, B., 1965. Introducing Laban Art of Movement. MacDonald & Evans Ltd, London.

Rosberg, S. (2000). KROPP: Varande och Mening i ett Sjukgymnastisk perspektiv (Body: Being and Meaning in a Physical Therapy Perspective). Doctoral Dissertation, Göteborg Universitet, Göteborg.

Roxendal, G. (1985). Body Awareness Therapy and The Body Awareness Scale, Treatment and Evaluation in Psychiatric Physiotherapy. Doctoral dissertation, University of Göteborg and Psychiatric Department II, Lillhagen Hospital, Hisings Backa, Göteborg.

Roxendal, G., 1987. Body Awareness Scale; BAS med instruction, manual och rörelsestest och faktorer för delskalor. Studentlitteratur, Stockholm.

Roxendal, R., Winberg, A., 2002. Levande Människa. Natur och Kultur, Stockholm.

Shumway-Cook, A., Wollacott, M., 2012. Motor Control: Translating Research into Clinical Practice, fourth ed. WoltersKluwer/ Lippincott Williams & Wilkins, Philadelphia.

Siegel, D.J., 2007. The Mindful Brain. Reflection and Attunement in the Cultivation of Well-Being. W. W. Norton & Company, New York & London.

Sivik, T., Theorell, T., 1995. Psykosomatisk medisin. Studentlitteratur, Lund. (Psychosomatic Medicine).

Skatteboe, U.B., 2000. Basal kroppskjennskap og bevegelsesharmoni. Videreutvikling av undersøkelsesmetoden Body Awareness Rating Scale, BARS-Bevegelsesharmoni (Body Awareness Therapy and Movement Harmony. Further development of the Assessment Scale Body Awareness Rating Scale). Oslo: Høgskolen i Oslo, Avdeling for helsefag; No 12.

Skjærven, L.H., 1999. 'Å være seg selv—mer fullt og helt'. En tilnærming til Bevegelseskvalitet. En feltstudie av en bevegelsespraksis av bevegelsespedagog og psykoterapeut Jacques Dropsy. ('To be oneself—more fully'. An approach to Movement Quality. A Field study of the Movement Practice of the Movement Educator and Psychotherapist Jacques Dropsy). Master's Thesis, University of Bergen Bergen.

Skjærven, L.H., Gard, G., Kristoffersen, K., 2003. Basic elements and dimensions to quality of movement—a case study. J. Bodyw. Mov. Ther. 7 (4), 251–260.

Skjærven, L.H., Gard, G., Kristoffersen, K., 2004. Greek sculpture as a tool in understanding the phenomenon of movement quality. J. Bodyw. Mov. Ther. 8 (3), 227–236.

Skjaerven, L.H., Kristoffersen, K., Gard, G., 2008. An eye for movement quality: a phenomenological study of movement quality reflecting a group of physiotherapists' understanding of the phenomenon. Physiother. Theory Pract. 24 (1), 13–27.

Skjaerven, L.H., Kristoffersen, K., Gard, G., 2010. How can movement quality be promoted in clinical practice? A phenomenological study of physical therapist experts. Phys. Ther. 90 (10), 1479–1492.

Stanislavski, K., 1992. An Actor Prepares (E. R. Hapgood, Trans.), tenth ed. Methuen Drama, London, UK.

Strand, L.I., Olsen, A.I., Nygård, H., et al., 2016. Basic Body Awareness Therapy and patient education in hip osteoarthritis: a multiple case study. Eur. J. Physiother. doi:10.3109/21679169.2015.11 35982.

Sundelin, G., 2009. Challenging perspective in physiotherapy : editorial. Adv. Physiother. 11, 1.

Suzuki, S., 1988. Zen Mind, Beginner's Mind. Informal Talks on Zen Meditation and Practice. John Weatherhill, Inc, Tokyo.

Thomas, S., Buckon, C.E., Phillips, D.S., et al., 2001. Interobserver reliability of the Gross Motor Performance Measure: preliminary results. Dev. Med. Child Neurol. 43 (2), 97–102.

Todres, L., 2007. Embodied Enquiry. Phenomenological Touchstones for Research, Psychotherapy and Spirituality. Palgrave Macmillan, New York.

Wallbott, H., 1985. Hand movement quality: a neglected aspect of nonverbal behavior in clinical judgement and person perception. J. Clin. Psychol. 41, 345–359.

Wallbott, H.G. 1989. Movement Quality Changes in Psychopathological Disorders. Medical Sport Sciences (Med. Sport Sci.): Normalities and Abnormalities in Human Movement. Basel, Karger, 29, 128–146.

WCPT, 2017. Policy Statements: Description of Physical Therapy (WCPT). <http://www.wcpt.org/polocy/PS-descriptionPT.>

Wikström-Grotell, C., Eriksson, K., 2012. Movement as basic concept in physiotherapy—a human science approach. Physiother. Theory Pract. 28, 428–438.

Yang, J-W., 1991a. Advanced Yang Style T'ai Chi Chuan. Martial Application, vol. 2. Ymaa Publication Center, Yang's Martial Arts Association, Massachusetts.

Yang, J-W., 1991b. Advanced Yang Style T'ai Chi Chuan. T'ai Chi Theory and T'ai Chi Jing. Yamma Publication Center, Yang's Martial Arts Association, Massachusetts.

IMPROVING ADHERENCE TO PHYSIOTHERAPY IN MENTAL HEALTH SETTINGS: THE NEED FOR AUTONOMY, COMPETENCE AND SOCIAL RELATEDNESS

DAVY VANCAMPFORT ■ BRENDON STUBBS

SUMMARY

Physiotherapy has been shown to improve the health of people with mental health problems, yet treatment dropout poses an important challenge in this population. In this chapter we discuss how supporting three psychological needs: the need for autonomy (i.e., experiencing a sense of psychological freedom when engaging in an activity), competence (i.e., feeling effective in attaining desired outcomes) and relatedness (i.e., being socially connected) may improve adherence to physiotherapy in mental health settings. Fulfilling these psychological needs requires physiotherapists to be actively engaged with their patients, and that they take a patient-centred approach to the interaction.

KEY POINTS

- Physiotherapists should be aware of the range of possible cognitive, behavioural, organizational and practical barriers which may have an impact on a patient's adherence to physiotherapy.

- Autonomy supportive behaviours that physiotherapists can apply include eliciting and acknowledging patients' perspectives and emotions before making any recommendations, supporting patients' choices and initiatives, providing a rationale for advice given and providing a menu of options for change.

LEARNING OBJECTIVES

- Gain an understanding of the basic principles of autonomous-supportive environments.

THE NEED TO CONSIDER ADHERENCE

Recent reviews have concluded that physiotherapy may be of added value in the multidisciplinary treatment of many psychiatric conditions (Vancampfort et al., 2012a, 2013a, 2013b). However, high quality data from randomized controlled trials often indicate that the effect sizes of these physiotherapy interventions are moderate to small (Vancampfort et al., 2012a, 2012b, 2013a, 2013b; Scheewe et al., 2013). These small effect sizes may, in part, be related to nonadherence with the treatment, rather than poor treatment efficacy (Vancampfort et al., 2012b). Nonadherence is common in mental health settings and can be defined as the extent to which a person's behaviour does not correspond with agreed recommendations from a healthcare provider (World Health Organization, 2003). Within physiotherapy, the concept of adherence is multidimensional (Kolt et al., 2007) and could relate to attendance at appointments, correct performance of exercises or doing more or less than advised. Studies suggest that nonadherence with a physiotherapy regimen and exercise protocol could be as high as 90%, and may be particularly poor for unsupervised home exercise programmes (Vancampfort et al., 2012b). Given the potential impact of nonadherence on treatment outcomes, strategies which aim to optimize treatment adherence are required for clinical practice.

FACTORS CONTRIBUTING TO NONADHERENCE

Identification of barriers may help physiotherapists to identify patients at risk of nonadherence and suggest methods to reduce the impact of those barriers, thereby maximizing adherence. The factors which contribute to nonadherence are multifaceted. For example, patient-related factors such as low self-efficacy, depression, anxiety, poor social support and increased pain levels during exercise are strong predictors of poor treatment adherence in patients with severe mental illness (Vancampfort et al., 2012c, 2013c, 2014a; Soundy et al., 2014; Stubbs et al., 2014). Treatment-related factors include side effects of psychotropic medication such as fatigue, impaired coordination, nausea, dizziness, weight gain and lack of interest and support of healthcare providers (Vancampfort et al., 2012b; Soundy et al., 2014). Environmental factors including the lack of adequate exercise facilities and exercise equipment are also thought to influence patient adherence (Vancampfort et al., 2014b). Consequently, physiotherapists should be aware of the range of possible cognitive, behavioural, organizational and practical barriers that may have an impact on a patient's adherence to physiotherapy.

THE IMPORTANCE OF GAINING INSIGHT INTO REASONS WHY PATIENTS ARE ADHERING TO PHYSIOTHERAPY: THE VALUE OF THE SELF-DETERMINATION THEORY

A creative, flexible and individualized approach is necessary, and physiotherapists should be aware of a broad range of possible strategies which may help to optimize adherence. The self-determination theory (Deci & Ryan, 1985, 2000) is a flexible and individualized framework. It is increasingly being used to understand motivation and adherence and has its origins centred on the fulfilment of needs, self-actualization and the realization of human potential (Deci & Ryan, 1985, 2000). The self-determination theory may provide insight into reasons why patients with severe mental illness participate in physiotherapy-related interventions as it emphasizes the extent to which behaviours are relatively autonomous (i.e., the extent

to which behaviours originate from the self) versus relatively controlled (i.e., the extent to which behaviours are pressured or coerced by intrapsychic or interpersonal forces) (Deci & Ryan, 1985, 2000).

Specifically, the self-determination theory proposes motivation to be multidimensional and residing along a continuum of increasing autonomy. The regulation towards physiotherapy can be amotivated, extrinsically motivated or intrinsically motivated. At the lowest end of the continuum is amotivation, in which case patients lack the motivation to participate and follow the recommendations, either because they do not feel they achieve recommended targets or they do not see the value of the recommendations. Extrinsic motivation implies that a patient engages in the physiotherapy programme to achieve outcomes that are separable from the inherent goals of physiotherapy itself. Within extrinsic motivation there is a continuum of behavioural regulations, reflecting the degree of autonomy or self-integration. External regulation refers to exercising to avoid, for example, disappointing others (e.g., the physiotherapist, family or friends) or to obtain other-appreciation. While external regulation is associated with external pressures to engage in physiotherapy, introjected regulation refers to the imposition of pressures onto one's own functioning, for instance by buttressing one's engagement with feelings of guilt, self-criticism or contingent self-esteem (i.e., esteem based on the approval of others or on social comparisons). Both external and introjected regulation represent controlled types of motivation because in these cases patients are likely to feel pressured to follow physiotherapy. Conversely, within identified regulation the patient may follow physiotherapy more willingly even though it is not enjoyable. For instance, the patient will be engaged because the health outcomes are personally important (e.g., to improve mental health or physical fitness). The most autonomous form of the extrinsic motivation continuum is integrated regulation, within which following physiotherapy is consistent with other prevailing values, and recommendations have become prioritized within one's lifestyle. Identified and integrated types of regulation involve personal endorsement of the reason to engage in physiotherapy and, as a result, are more likely to be accompanied by feelings of choice and psychological freedom.

Finally, intrinsic motivation represents the most autonomous type of motivation and involves engaging in physiotherapy for its own sake, that is, because patients find the physiotherapy exercises offered to be challenging or enjoyable. The self-determination theory uses the term *internalization* to describe the process by which behaviours become relatively more autonomously regulated or valued over time (Deci & Ryan, 1985, 2000). Autonomous self-regulation is particularly important for health-related behaviours which are often targeted in physiotherapy because the more autonomously regulated a patient is towards a given behaviour, the greater effort, engagement, persistence and stability the patient is likely to evidence in that behaviour (Deci & Ryan, 1985, 2000). Research in patients with severe mental illnesses (Vancampfort et al., 2013d) has shown that there is good evidence for the principles of the self-determination theory in understanding, in particular, exercise behaviour, highlighting the importance of more autonomous forms of regulation in fostering participation in different kinds of aerobic and strength exercises.

HOW CAN ONE IMPLEMENT THE SELF-DETERMINATION THEORY PRINCIPLES INTO PHYSIOTHERAPEUTIC SETTINGS?

Given that more autonomous types of motivation are associated with higher attendance, understanding how to facilitate autonomous motivation is a clinical imperative. Therapeutic environments, or specific factors within therapeutic environments, that are referred to as *autonomous-supportive* have been found to promote adherence to therapy both by helping patients to maintain intrinsic motivation and facilitating internalization of extrinsic motivations. In practice, facilitating internalization of extrinsic motivations can take place in environments that support three psychological needs, that is, the need for autonomy (i.e., experiencing a sense of psychological freedom when engaging in physiotherapy), competence (i.e., feeling effective in attaining desired outcomes) and relatedness (i.e., being socially connected) (Deci & Ryan, 1985, 2000). Given the importance of need support in facilitating internalization, the self-determination

theory offers suggestions for specific strategies that may support one or more of these needs.

Autonomy-Support

In autonomy-supporting environments, pressure to engage in specific behaviours is minimized, and patients are encouraged to base their actions on their own reasons and values. Thus autonomy in behaviour is facilitated insofar as patients are helped to identify their own reasons for changing their behaviour and they do not feel pressured or manipulated towards certain outcomes. Autonomy-supportive behaviours that physiotherapists can apply include eliciting and acknowledging patients' perspectives and emotions before making any recommendations, supporting patients' choices and initiatives, providing a rationale for advice given, providing a menu of effective (i.e., evidence-based) options for changing, for example reducing sedentary behaviours, minimizing control and judgement, exploring how health behaviours are related to patients' aspirations in life, and using autonomy-supportive language (e.g., 'could' and 'choose' rather than 'should' and 'have to'). Motivational interviewing is one clinical method that has been used to good effect here and seems viable in physiotherapy settings (Ryan et al., 2011).

Competence-Support

Feelings of competence may be attained when patients with severe mental illnesses experience success during the treatment. Exercises need to be tailored to the capabilities of the patient, and sufficient instructions, practice and positive feedback are needed. Other competence-supporting strategies include identifying barriers together with the patient, skill building, problem solving and developing an action plan that is appropriately challenging. Goals within an action plan should therefore be explicit, achievable and challenging and they also need to be recorded. It may be useful to use SMART goals (i.e., an acronym for the five steps of specific, measurable, attainable, relevant and time-based goals). Also here, motivational interviewing techniques might facilitate feelings of competence (Ryan et al., 2011).

Relatedness-Support

Finally, relatedness-support includes providing unconditional positive regard (particularly in the face of failure to achieve desired goals), being empathic with patients' concerns and providing a consistently warm interpersonal environment. Thus a physiotherapist may support a patient's need for relatedness by expressing understanding about how difficult it can be to change a behaviour and by reflecting the patient's concerns about failure. Physiotherapists need to show enthusiasm and interest in their patients, both when pursuing change but also when refraining from change. They also need to consider the psychosocial barriers that may prevent participation, especially initially or when a patient is exposed to a new environment (e.g., a community-based environment) (Soundy et al., 2007). In addition to this, following an individual approach, physiotherapists should motivate their patients to be part of, for example, an exercise and physical activity group. This will foster an environment that supports autonomy and is able to provide access to, or reestablish, a more healthy identity, which is important in the recovery process (Soundy et al., 2012).

CONCLUSION

Support for the three psychological needs (autonomy, competence and relatedness) requires that physiotherapists are actively engaged with their patients, and that they take a patient-centred approach to the interaction. Eliciting and acknowledging the patient's perspective starts with active listening and includes reflections (e.g., brief summaries of the thoughts, emotions and plans the patient has about the health issue being addressed).

REFERENCES

Deci, E.L., Ryan, R.M., 1985. Intrinsic Motivation and Self-Determination in Human Behaviour. Plenum Press, New York, NY.

Deci, E.L., Ryan, R.M., 2000. The "what" and "why" of goal pursuits: human needs and the self-determination of behavior. Psychol. Inq. 11, 227–268.

Kolt, G.S., Brewer, B.W., Pizzari, T., et al., 2007. The sport injury rehabilitation adherence scale: a reliable scale for use in clinical physiotherapy. Physiotherapy 93 (1), 17–22.

Ryan, R.M., Lynch, M.F., Vansteenkiste, M., Deci, E.L., 2011. Motivation and autonomy in counseling, psychotherapy, and behavior change: a look at theory and practice. Couns. Psychol. 39, 193–260.

Soundy, A., Faulkner, G., Taylor, A., 2007. Exploring variability and perceptions of lifestyle physical activity among individuals with severe and enduring mental health problems: a qualitative study. J. Ment. Health 16, 493–503.

Soundy, A., Kingstone, T., Coffee, C., 2012. Understanding the psychosocial processes of physical activity for individuals with severe mental illness: a meta-ethnography. In: L'Abate (Ed.), Mental Illnesses—Evaluation, Treatments and Implications. In Tech, New York, NY. doi:10.5772/30120.

Soundy, A., Stubbs, B., Probst, M., et al., 2014. Barriers to and facilitators of physical activity among persons with schizophrenia: a survey of physical therapists. Psychiatr. Serv. 65, 693–696.

Scheewe, T.W., Backx, F.J., Takken, T., et al., 2013. Exercise therapy improves mental and physical health in schizophrenia: a randomised controlled trial. Acta Psychiatr. Scand. 127 (6), 464–473.

Stubbs, B., Eggermont, L., Soundy, A., et al., 2014. Barriers and facilitators to physical activity participation in community dwelling adults with dementia: a systematic review of physical activity correlates. Submitted for publication.

Vancampfort, D., Probst, M., Skjaerven, L., et al., 2012a. Systematic review of the benefits of physical therapy within a multidisciplinary care approach for people with schizophrenia. Phys. Ther. 92 (1), 11–23.

Vancampfort, D., De Hert, M., Skjaerven, L., et al., 2012b. International Organization of Physical Therapy in Mental Health consensus on physical activity within multidisciplinary rehabilitation programmes for minimising cardio-metabolic risk in patients with schizophrenia. Disabil. Rehabil. 34 (1), 1–12.

Vancampfort, D., Knapen, J., Probst, M., et al., 2012c. A systematic review of correlates of physical activity in patients with schizophrenia. Acta Psychiatr. Scand. 125 (5), 352–362.

Vancampfort, D., Vanderlinden, J., De Hert, M., et al., 2013a. A systematic review on physical therapy interventions for patients with binge eating disorder. Disabil. Rehabil. 35 (26), 2191–2196.

Vancampfort, D., Vanderlinden, J., De Hert, M., et al., 2013b. A systematic review of physical therapy interventions for patients with anorexia and bulimia nervosa. Disabil. Rehabil. 36 (8), 628–634.

Vancampfort, D., Correll, C., Probst, M., et al., 2013c. A review of physical activity correlates in patients with bipolar disorder. J. Affect. Disord. 145 (3), 285–291.

Vancampfort, D., De Hert, M., Vansteenkiste, M., et al., 2013d. The importance of self-determined motivation towards physical activity in patients with schizophrenia. Psychiatry Res. 210 (3), 812–818.

Vancampfort, D., Vanderlinden, J., Stubbs, B., et al., 2014a. Physical activity correlates in persons with binge eating disorder: a systematic review. Eur Eat Disord Rev 22, 1–8.

Vancampfort, D., De Hert, M., De Herdt, A., et al., 2014b. Associations between perceived neighbourhood environmental attributes and self-reported sitting time in patients with schizophrenia: a pilot study. Psychiatry Res. 215, 33–38.

World Health Organization, 2003. Adherence to long-term therapies - Evidence for action. World Health Organization, Geneva.

2.5

ACTIVEPHYSIO: ACCEPTANCE AND COMMITMENT THERAPY (ACT) FOR THE PHYSIOTHERAPIST IN THE AREA OF CHRONIC PAIN

GRACIELA ROVNER ■ MATTHEW D. SKINTA

*Moving from 'seeking to understand the reality of the world to seeking ways to **act** successfully in the world'*

(McCracken & Vowles, 2014, p. 185)

SUMMARY

Acceptance and commitment therapy (ACT) improves the patient's capacity to create a 'space' to *accept* chronic pain while responding in a creative and flexible way, instead of getting stuck in endless attempts to control it in order to reach a vital and meaningful life. The adaptation of ACT for the physiotherapist is the ACTivePhysio model, a patient centred and resource focused model, in which the course for rehabilitation will be set together with the patient's own life-values. The trained ACTivePhysio therapist will be able to use functional applied behaviour analysis in order to increase the patient's flexible and functional behaviours, rather than focusing on decreasing dysfunctional behaviours or symptoms. This chapter offers the understanding of the basic principles of ACTivePhysio, using the examples of three patient cases to model the implementation of ACTivePhysio in the area of chronic pain.

KEY POINTS

■ Mental and physical pain are not easily distinguished, subjectively or neurologically; however, in ACT and ACTivePhysio, mental and physical pain do not need to be distinguished to plan rehabilitation and improve wellness.

■ Patients with chronic pain often arrive for treatment focused on moving away from pain; the ACTivePhysio model will help them to move towards meaningful life directions, despite their pain.

■ Learning to become aware, open and active towards a fulfilled life will reduce the subjective experience of pain while increasing vitality.

■ An ACTivePhysio session incorporates this stance and thus can enhance the impact of the work with patients with chronic pain and mental issues.

LEARNING OBJECTIVES

1. You will understand how ACTivePhysio can improve your physiotherapeutic treatment skills while working with patients with chronic conditions (such as pain).

2. You will learn to identify and teach the skills necessary to the patient in order to implement the basis of ACTivePhysio in their life.

3. You will acquire a new tool—the ACTive Matrix—to guide your patients through the ACTivePhysio skills.

Differentiating between physical and mental pain makes pain difficult to understand. Even if the health system separates these types of pain, tissue pain and emotional pain seem to share similar neurological processes and mechanisms (Eisenberger, 2012). Evolutionarily, social rejection is probably the most painful experience we can face. As a young mammal our social attachment system shares the same pain system as physical pain, thus all 'hurting' has the same function: an alarm system that prompts us to seek help and connection (Panksepp, 1998). Furthermore, feeling understood (or not) activates neural systems related to social reward and pain (Morelli et al., 2014). Therefore when patients with chronic pain are stigmatized or considered to be complex or maladaptive, this social rejection will hurt. Neuroimaging has demonstrated that this social rejection has neuronal correlates with 'physical' pain (Novembre et al., 2015).

Acceptance and commitment therapy (ACT) (Hayes et al., 1999) suggests a compassionate and accepting approach to chronic pain. The adaptation of ACT for the physiotherapist is called *ACTivePhysio*. This model focuses on the patient's *healthy* functioning rather than the pathology and proposes a pragmatic agenda to achieve improvement in function when constant and long-lasting attempts to avoid, reduce or control symptoms (pain) are ineffective. ACTivePhysio sees the person in pain as a normal person with normal reactions to prolonged pain and does not differentiate whether this pain comes from a physical trauma or a psychological one. Pain is normal, functional and inevitable in life, but depending on how we respond to pain, we suffer more or less.

In taking the radical stance that the pain experienced by a patient with chronic pain is no different from any human suffering, we are breaking down a wall that often exists between providers and patients and removing judgement from the approach. ACT and ACTivePhysio acknowledge that each patient is the best expert on both how the pain has affected her or his life, and what would constitute a meaningful life worth living. The role of ACTivePhysio in this approach is to share tools that allow the patient to clarify and focus these values, providing practical tools from active physiotherapy, to aid in increasing movement, capacity and function in order to live a valued and vital life. Finally, this is not a stance that can merely be verbally described. Effective ACT-based rehabilitation requires training and supervision in ACTivePhysio to allow the physiotherapist to gain self-awareness about her or his own goals and values, and to acquire insight

into how common our own challenges are to those faced by our patients. This humanization is what allows us, as a therapist using ACTivePhysio, ultimately to infuse our work with skill, a sense of presence and compassion.

The ACTivePhysio model helps the physiotherapist to be aware and to understand how pain influences responses and behaviours, and proposes adopting an open attitude without trying to change the frequency or intensity of pain or judging the content of our thoughts (McCracken & Eccleston, 2003). This attitude stimulates the healthy resources of the individual and the capacity to open up, creating 'space' and a willingness to *accept* negative feelings, sensations or thoughts while responding in a creative and more flexible way, without getting stuck. The theoretical model underlying ACT and ACTivePhysio has been referred to as *psychological flexibility (PF)* (McCracken & Vowles, 2007; Kashdan & Rottenberg, 2010; McCracken & Morley, 2014).

The PF model is a set of six integrated component processes that apply with precision to a wide range of clinically relevant problems and issues of human functioning (Hayes et al., 1999). Fig. 1 (adapted from Hayes, 2004, p. 16; and from Strosahl et al., 2012) presents the six component processes mapped onto the three pillars of *openness*, *awareness* and *engagement*. Each of the component processes in Fig. 1 has been empirically developed and studied in the area of chronic pain (McCracken & Morley, 2014; McCracken & Vowles, 2014; Vowles et al., 2014a,b) and can be implemented in rehabilitation (Vowles et al., 2014b) by the physiotherapist trained in ACTivePhysio.

When applying ACTivePhysio, probably the most obvious pillar to start with is *engagement*. *Engagement* consists of identifying values and taking committed action for a more active life. *Values* are defined as freely chosen orientations for activities that bring meaning, importance or vitality to living, and *actions and commitment* are behaviours that encompass a flexible persistence oriented towards valued living. In other words: 'find your own motivation (values) and get moving (or committed to act)'. Patients with chronic pain have a different approach to their pain, and when they seek help, it is when they got 'hooked' on ineffective strategies or a vicious circle of pain and inactivity (and/or overdoing). For them, the central pillar of the model, *awareness*, is needed first. *Awareness* consists of two

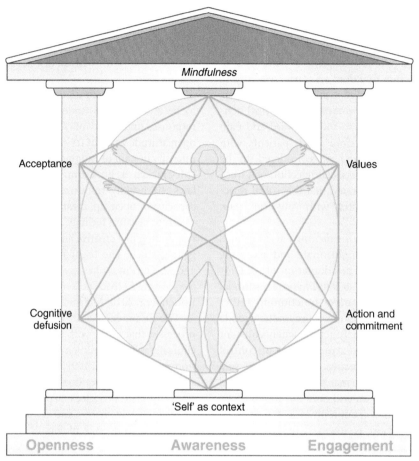

FIGURE 1 ■ The Psychological Flexibility (PF) model and the three pillars of Acceptance and commitment therapy (ACT). *(Adapted with permission, from Strosahl, Robinson & Gustavsson, 2013. Strosahl, K.D., Robinson, P. J., & Gustavsson, T., 2012. Brief Interventions for Radical Change: Principles and Practice of Focused Acceptance and Commitment Therapy. New Harbinger, Oakland, CA.).*

skills. The first, *mindfulness,* also called *'flexible awareness of the present',* is a purposeful, nonjudgemental, attending to present experiences, thoughts and sensations. *Self-as-context* is the capacity to differentiate between 'having' a thought and buying into all our thoughts. The realization that thoughts are always changing and are not accurate reflections of reality is grounding, and creates a common perspective for the patient and therapist to observe those thoughts without viewing them as real or requiring immediate action. On the left of the PF model is *openness.* Accepting and recognizing our life exactly as it is right at this moment has two components: *cognitive defusion,* which increases our awareness of how we treat our thoughts as reflections of reality, such as 'I can't change until the pain (or depression, anxiety, worry) stops', that make it harder to choose functional actions, and to be able to *accept* (Hayes et al., 2012). *Acceptance* is the willingness and capacity to choose to experience discomfort (pain, negative thoughts or difficult feelings), in the service of engaging with what is important in life. Despite having functional limitations or adversities, the patient is helped by ACT and ACTivePhysio to find a new way to relate to the pain and a flexible way to engage actively (McCracken et al., 2007), and to align their behaviour with personal values and goals (Brandtstädter & Rothermund, 2002) to create a meaningful and vital life.

Promoting pain acceptance decreases avoidance, anxiety, depression and medical consumption while increasing function and work capacity (McCracken et al., 1999, 2004). It has been demonstrated to be effective in lowering levels of psychological and physical disability, and in improving health, functioning (McCracken & Jones, 2012; McCracken et al., 2007) and quality of life (Butler & Ciarrochi, 2007; Elander et al., 2009; Wicksell et al., 2009).

ACT AND PHYSIOTHERAPY

ACT (pronounced as the word 'act') is an appropriate acronym and a good metaphor for physiotherapy because physiotherapists are experts in the science of movement and ACTivity. The main agenda for ACTivePhysio is to support the patient in increasing their physical capacity and function as well as stimulating their skills to respond flexibly to their situation.

If the patient has chronic and widespread pain, the training and activities must focus on regulating the nervous system (the brain and pain regulation system). This can be done by combining a well dosified and progressive physical activity programme (see for example Häkkinen et al., 2001; Valkeinen et al., 2004) with body/postural awareness training such as ACTiveBODY. The latter is important in order to readjust movement patterns if they have been modified by compensatory (or avoidant) movements. In this model, ACTive relaxation is included as an important component of rehabilitation for some patients if the aim is not to control or decrease the pain, but to regulate the nervous system and, thus, the pain mechanisms.

ACTiveBODY (see http://www.ACTinstitutet.se) is a protocol of rehabilitation activities implemented in the ACTivePhysio model. Based on modern neurophysiological research, it offers a combination of activities that the patient can choose together with the physiotherapist and that will be set up in the individual rehabilitation programme, even when delivered in a group. ACTiveBODY is a set of functional-adapted activities combining B (balance of strength), O (openness and flexibility) and D (dynamism), all of them used to find *Your way to move* and be active. Other simple activity programmes can be used, such as functional training, walking, taking the stairs instead of elevators, parking some blocks away, buying a desk

that allows working upright, combining with more intensive training such as Nordic walking; all of these, again, should be dosified in a way that regulates the nervous system and the pain mechanisms.

The Patient

ACTivePhysio is delivered in a group format for patients with chronic pain (groups comprise between six and nine patients). In this chapter, three examples of patients will be presented. These patients have undergone extensive prior examination, do not have a threatening condition (such as cancer) and generally have widespread pain (fibromyalgia) or neck pain after a whiplash trauma. They may have suffered other traumas, perhaps early in life, and suffer from post-traumatic stress disorder. They may also report psychological symptoms, although they do not have any condition that requires psychiatric inpatient treatment (psychotic or suicidal tendencies, or heavy misuse of drugs or alcohol). Many of them present with some kind of iatrogenic dependence on medicine (e.g., opiates), often prescribed by their doctors. It is normal for a person with long-standing pain to suffer when the healthcare system does not appear to understand them and refers to them as 'complex patients'. Imagine how you might feel if you were experiencing painful symptoms that your providers felt mystified by! According to ACT, there are no 'complex' persons or comorbid conditions; this is just one more person physically and mentally suffering, just like every one of us. They are not in need of stigmatization, they need new ways to frame and reframe their situation and fresh strategies for living a meaningful life, with or without pain.

Three Case Examples

Maria is 56 years old, and was diagnosed with fibromyalgia 10 years ago. She is overweight, limps and does not like to exercise (she said she actually hates physiotherapists!). She is in early retirement, and lives in a second-floor flat with her husband. On self-report measures she scored within normal limits on anxiety and depressive symptoms and has a good quality of life. She is very disappointed that the healthcare system is not helping her.

Noemi is 42 years old, married with two daughters (14 and 16 years old). She worked at a factory but has been on sick leave for 2 years owing to her widespread pain. She and her family like sports. She reported in the questionnaires having moderate anxiety and depressive symptoms and having a good quality of life. She expresses a strong wish to find new ways to handle her problems.

Raja is 28 years old, and emigrated as refugee from a country at war 12 years ago. She is married and has one child (6 years old). In addition to her traumatic experience during the war (her mother was raped in front of her) she has had two rear car accidents (3 and 6 years ago) and the pain in her neck related to whiplash trauma became widespread after the last accident. She reported high depressive and anxiety symptoms, and a low quality of life. She does not really know what she needs to do in order to feel better, and feels panic every now and then.

What they have in common is that their doctor, psychologist and physiotherapist in primary care told them that '*We cannot help you anymore, you need to learn to live with your pain, to accept it.*' They were then referred to the interprofessional pain rehabilitation programme.

The 'Interprofessional' Pain Rehabilitation Programme

When ACTivePhysio is used by an interprofessional team, the programme is called *ACTiveRehab*. This programme can run simultaneously with three to four different tracks of group rehabilitation, depending upon the patient's needs (see www.ACTinstitutet.se). ACtiveRehab can be delivered in 6–10 weeks and can be guided by an ACTivePhysio trained pain specialist physiotherapist and an ACT psychotherapist/psychologist (for a good psychotherapeutic guide, read Dahl, 2005). It is also important to collaborate with an ACT-informed medical doctor (because the need for medication decreases when the patient becomes more active and functional). It is also important to have access to a gym (or some weights, a TRX band, stairs, Pilates ball and a test bike), as well as the possibility of taking walks outside (if possible with Nordic walking poles) and a place to practise mindful stretching and relaxation (with mats and blankets).

Before You Start

ACT is truly patient centred and resource focused; the assessment is collaborative and will be directed by the patient's own values and what is important for her or him, and the values will set the course for rehabilitation. The trained ACTivePhysio therapist will also look for flexible and functional behaviours that the patient is capable of performing and that can be increased, rather than trying to decrease the undesired ones. This will fall in line with traditional applied functional behaviour analysis in stressing increasing functional and adaptive behaviours rather than just decreasing the dysfunctional ones (e.g., Cooper et al., 2007).

The physiotherapist should meet each patient individually for the initial assessment and present the rationale of the ACT programme, which aims to enhance quality of life and vitality (rather than targeting symptoms such as pain intensity). Patients who are willing to participate will sign an agreement and be allocated to the group that fits their needs according to their level of pain acceptance (Rovner et al., 2015). In this chapter we assume that our three patients are in the same group (while in reality they would probably not be allocated to the same group; see Rovner, 2014, for further discussion).

Matrix Overview

The three pillars (see Fig. 1) are used by us in practice and to train therapists; Fig. 2 demonstrates how they can be simplified by the Matrix, a clinical tool to be used with patients (for more examples on how to use the ACT-Matrix, see Polk & Schoendorf, 2014).

The values are placed in *quadrant I*, and in *quadrant IV* we define the actions/activities that will be used, according to these values; in other words: we will outline the *rehabilitation plan*. The *quadrants I* and *IV* represent the *towards moves* to a valued, vital and meaningful life. To the left, the Matrix shows the unwanted content and the *away moves*, or strategies used to avoid what we are not willing to accept (pain, ours or others' shortcomings, depression, etc.). This means that on quadrant II we will write what we wish to avoid (in our case it will be in the second column of Table 2, see later) and in quadrant III we will place the control agenda (Fig. 3).

The main process of sorting (discriminating) is the important part of the matrix. There is no wrong way

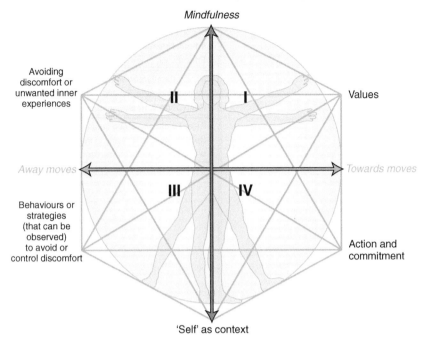

Mental or inner experiencing

Mindfulness

Avoiding
discomfort or
unwanted inner
experiences

Values

II   I

Away moves   Towards moves

III   IV

Behaviours or
strategies
(that can be
observed)
to avoid or
control discomfort

Action and
commitment

'Self' as context

Sensorial experiencing or observable activities

FIGURE 2 ■ The hexaflex and the Matrix (the X axis shows 'away and towards moves' and the Y axis differentiates mental or inner experiences from sensorial experiences or observable activities or strategies); in II what thoughts, fears, physical sensations are in our way to live up to our values; in III, which activities or behavioural strategies we use to handle these thoughts from Q II and in IV. The Matrix is a clinical and friendly application to use with the patients. In quadrant I we identify the values, in II what thoughts or fears are in our way that do not allow us to live up to our values, in III, which sensations or activities we use to handle the thoughts or fears, and in IV, which activities and strategies are 'towards' moves that will allow us to follow our values.

to sort, to discriminate, although we do avoid danger and depredation, and may avoid certain types of movement if the patient is injured or has been sick for a short time, with a functional problem. Flexibility means not being '*hooked*' by labelling any action or event as 'right' or 'wrong' when it is not functional; flexibility involves being attuned to what the situation requires and having access to a broad repertoire of functional and workable responses.

Assessment, Part 1: Values

The ACTivePhysio's first question will be: *What is important for you? What do you most value in life?*

Normally the automatic answer of the patient will be: '*to be pain-free!!*' In that case we add: *I mean overall in your life, what are the important things, people, what*

do you want to stand for or be remembered as? Another helpful illustration is that at times I will form my hands into a circle and as I move my hands out I say: '*Often when we are in pain, the energy and time we put towards being pain free begins to grow.*' I then begin to move my hands back together and say: '*every other part of our life begins to get pushed smaller and smaller… could you tell me what you would rather grow?*'

Noemi: (a bit surprised by the question) The most important for me is to be a good mum, I feel I have been too absent from my girls' activities. I also want to be a loving wife, this pain makes things a bit difficult and our intimate life… and of course I miss walking and running in the woods. Not moving makes me feel quite blue. I can tolerate pain while doing things, I just would like to know what can I do in order not to get worse.

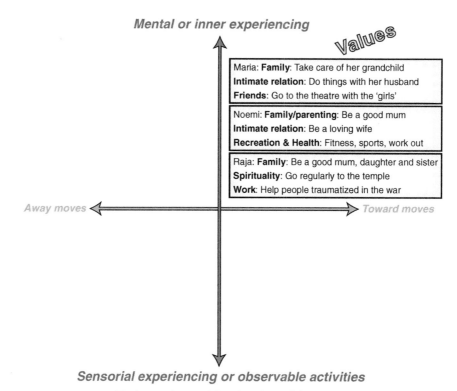

FIGURE 3 ■ The Matrix containing the values of the patients, in brief.

Noemi answered first and she was quite clear about what is important for her, and she could articulate her values in a few words. Not all the patients have this resource at hand and they may need more help to identify or clarify their values. Noemi could also easily discriminate the difference between doing important things and not doing them, and its consequences. According to her assessment she reported a high pain acceptance level (that is, she was not primarily driven by avoiding pain). Acceptance, as measured by the Chronic Pain Acceptance Questionnaire (CPAQ) (e.g., McCracken, 1998; McCracken et al., 2004; Vowles & McCracken, 2008), is an established index of functioning in chronic pain. In addition to strong correlations with a number of key measures of patient functioning, the CPAQ offers the advantage of evaluating adaptive functioning, as opposed to a focus strictly on measuring maladaptive functioning (e.g., pain-related distress, anxiety, 'catastrophizing'). It is validated in several languages and now even in a shorter form, the CPAQ-8. Noemi would probably benefit from a quite

intensive ACTiveREhab programme including education about the neurophysiology of widespread pain.

On the whiteboard the ACTivePhysio therapist draws two axes, X and Y. Beside the X positive they write 'towards moves' and beside the negative, 'away moves'. Thus the Y-axis differentiates between what we have in mind (the positive, Y+) and what we really do, our actions (Y−). Then they write 'values' in the first quadrant (X+; Y+) and 'Noemi: *Family*: be a good mum; *Intimate relations*: be a loving wife; and *Recreation & Health*: Fitness, sports, work out'. The question is then repeated to Maria and Raja, whose answers are shown in Fig. 3.

Assessment, Part 2: The Control Agenda

The ACTivePhysio's second question is: *What are the strategies you have used in the past?*

The patients are given a sheet showing Table 1 (but with far more rows to fill in), and after a short mindfulness exercise (to help them to focus and remember the pain strategies used) they will have 10–15 minutes to fill in this table.

| | | | TABLE 1 | | | |
| | | | Control Agenda | | | |

What I Did	Why? or In Order To...	Short-Term Results	Long-Term Results	Consequences or Comments	Is this working? Yes/No

Behaviourally speaking, our patients are learning to do a behavioural analysis; we call it the ABC of physiotherapy. The ABC means that they identify the **A**ntecedent of a behaviour (what triggers the behaviour), then they recognize their **B**ehaviour, and finally they become aware of the **C**onsequence. In other words, they learn how their choices and behaviours influence their life (more about the ABC can be found in Ramnerö & Törneke, 2008).

The same table is drawn on a page of a flipchart and filled out together with the patients, as shown in Table 2. The second column is very important (even if it seems ridiculously obvious), because when it is done, the patients realize how much focus and attention the pain has in their life and how controlling it does not seem to help. Then ask them to give a title to this agenda (for example: *The Control Agenda to decrease my pain*).

The agenda is used to reflect together with the patients in a nonjudgemental way. Most patients realize that most of these strategies listed in 'Doing the Control Agenda' generate a feeling of hopelessness, and at the same time they achieve a good feeling of 'being in the same boat'. It is important to reassure the patients that all the strategies they have tried are totally normal.

Assessment, Part 3: To Be or Not To Be, to Live Your Values or to Get Stuck in Avoidance and Control

Returning to the whiteboard with the Matrix that has values in **Quadrant I** (see Fig. 2), the therapist brings the sheet from the flipchart that has the Control Agenda on it. This is placed near the Matrix and the patients are asked whether *this agenda is a functional agenda in order for them to live according to their values*. Of course the answer is *NO!*

Quadrant II: Avoiding unwanted mental or inner experiences.

The patients agree that in the second column of the Control Agenda in Table 2 there are no 'life-values', '*other than something we do not want to experience and we must control: the pain!*' and they place this column in the quadrant of avoidance (see Fig. 3).

Quadrant III: Strategies used to avoid (the Control Agenda).

The rest of the Control Agenda is placed in *quadrant III* (Fig. 4), identifying the behaviours and strategies used to avoid and control the pain (e.g., eating sweets, drinking, looking endlessly on the internet for a cure, procrastinating, ruminating, etc.).

Individual questions may help each patient to recognize their own unique way in which they handle or cope with their situation. Ask: '*When you have pain, which one of these behaviours (or others) do you most often do?*'

Maria: I eat something sweet and watch TV in my room (not with my husband). Probably I will take an extra pill and rest.

Noemi: I do not give in! I go out and walk/run, ignoring and pushing through the pain, then the pain increases and I lie in bed for almost a week. I also yield to my children's and husband's requests.

Raja: I take an antidepressant and wonder 'why did I get in the car that day when I got in the crash?' and ruminate and then, if it is late, I get panicked and have negative thoughts. I go into my room in the dark and don't want to talk.

While they are answering, the ACTivePhysio therapist may complete the Control Agenda and then draw some arrows from quadrant II to quadrant III to show how these 'inner experiences' (in this case, pain) prompt these strategies/actions.

The patients are then asked: 'Does this behaviour help you get rid of the pain? Or does the pain eventually come back?' The answers are *no* and *yes*, so an arrow is drawn back to quadrant II, and then it can appear as a spiral or vicious circle back and forth.

TABLE 2
An Example of a 'Control Agenda'

What I Did	Why? or In Order To....	Short-Term Results	Long-Term Results	Consequences or Comments
Daytime rest	To control and decrease my pain	Yes, it helps during the day, but not during the night	I lie down so much that I lose strength and I cannot sleep at night	I get weaker and weaker and have no vitality, independently of how much I rest
Sick leave	To control and decrease my pain	Yes, at the beginning it was good and a bit relaxing	Not really, the pain came back to the same level	This had both economic consequences—I lost my position—and also feel isolated
Went to several doctors. Tried several meds	To control and decrease my pain, and to be able to sleep	New medicines always help in the short term	The side effects are horrible!	I just get confused, some doctors want to do surgery, others meds, others give me vitamins. Everything makes me more confused and now I am dependent on these meds
Surgery	To control and decrease my pain	Yes, at the beginning (for some patients) not at all for others	Increased pain and immobility	Now I have pain in areas I didn't have before. I feel weak and insecure when moving
Physiotherapy	To control and decrease my pain	Exercises increase the pain, body awareness and relaxation are nice but do not make any difference	I quit after a couple of weeks, so I do not know the long-term consequences, I guess even more and worse pain	I got more and more frustrated and sedentary. It is quite hopeless!
Massage	To control and decrease my pain	Nice, I sleep well that night	It lasts only 1 or 2 days... or over the weekend if the massage is on Friday and I can rest during the weekend	Too expensive, I do not have the money to afford it
Psychotherapy	To control and decrease my pain	Not at all, he made me feel that my pain was 'in my head', while my pain is in my body!!	I quit!	I felt angry and frustrated. Of course also ashamed. Besides, it is quite expensive!

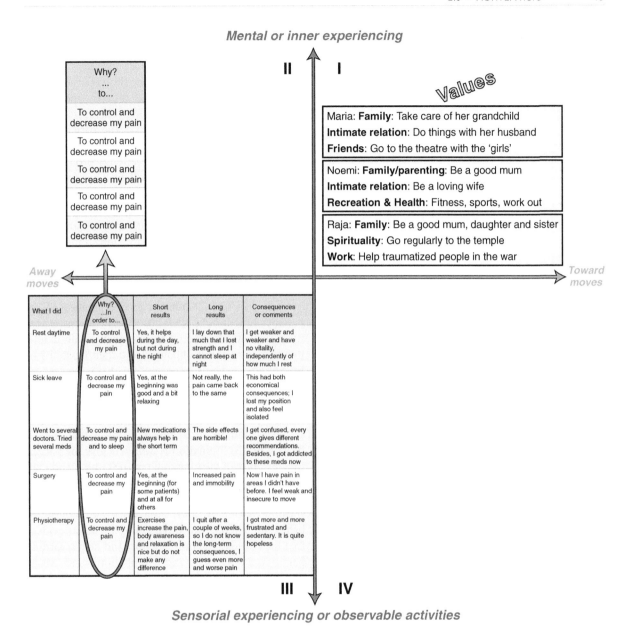

Mental or inner experiencing

II I

Why?
...
to...

| To control and decrease my pain |
| To control and decrease my pain |
| To control and decrease my pain |
| To control and decrease my pain |
| To control and decrease my pain |

Values

Maria: **Family**: Take care of her grandchild
Intimate relation: Do things with her husband
Friends: Go to the theatre with the 'girls'

Noemi: **Family/parenting**: Be a good mum
Intimate relation: Be a loving wife
Recreation & Health: Fitness, sports, work out

Raja: **Family**: Be a good mum, daughter and sister
Spirituality: Go regularly to the temple
Work: Help traumatized people in the war

Away moves ← → *Toward moves*

What I did	Why? ...In order to...	Short results	Long results	Consequences or comments
Rest daytime	To control and decrease my pain	Yes, it helps during the day, but not during the night	I lay down that much that I lost strength and I cannot sleep at night	I get weaker and weaker and have no vitality, independently of how much I rest
Sick leave	To control and decrease my pain	Yes, at the beginning was good and a bit relaxing	Not really, the pain came back to the same	This had both economical consequences; I lost my position and also feel isolated
Went to several doctors. Tried several meds	To control and decrease my pain and to sleep	New medications always help in the short term	The side effects are horrible!	I get confused, every one gives different recommendations. Besides, I got addicted to these meds now
Surgery	To control and decrease my pain	Yes, at the beginning (for some patients) and at all for others	Increased pain and immobility	Now I have pain in areas I didn't have before. I feel weak and insecure to move
Physiotherapy	To control and decrease my pain	Exercises increase the pain, body awareness and relaxation is nice but do not make any difference	I quit after a couple of weeks, so I do not know the long-term consequences, I guess even more and worse pain	I got more and more frustrated and sedentary. It is quite hopeless

III ↓ IV

Sensorial experiencing or observable activities

FIGURE 4 ■ The Control Agenda can be placed in quadrant III because it describes the behaviours and strategies used to avoid discomfort. However, the second column (Why? Or in order to?) explains what we are avoiding and goes in quadrant II.

At this point the patients realize that they have been stuck for a long time, struggling with pain in a kind of autopilot behaviour and not in contact with what really matters in their life. This insight normally leads them to feel hopeless but, because the right side of the Matrix still lists their values, they are starting to see that there is more than being stuck and feeling hopeless. This is what in ACT is called 'creative hopelessness' (Hayes et al., 2012), whereby the hopelessness leads to a deep, emotional connection to the unworkability of old behaviours, prompting creativity and flexibility towards trying something new.

The Rehab-Plan: From Creative Hopelessness into Values in ACTion

At this point we have called attention to the right side of the Matrix and begun building motivation to work on actions that can help the patients to live according to their values, and to do what matters, independent of thoughts, emotions or sensations (Box 1).

Quadrant IV: ACTions and commitments: the ACTiveRehab plan (Fig. 5).

Committed ACTion leads us to live and behave according to our values, step-by-step, and in this case it will also be the *rehabilitation plan*. The ACTivePhysio's rehabilitation plan is based on the evidence of what is most effective for thriving with chronic pain (explained in the ACTiveBODY model), where the focus is to help the patient to increase their physical capacity and function *as well as* increasing their knowledge about chronic pain. This second part is essential because understanding pain mechanisms can decrease the patient's fear and the risk of catastrophic thinking, which may be one of the most powerful threats to the nervous system, in turn triggering more pain. The ACTivePhysio therapist has to be very knowledgeable, up-to-date and an excellent teacher in order to transmit the neurophysiology of pain to patients and help them to understand why and for how long it may hurt after starting rehabilitation. Effective psychoeducation allows both the physiotherapist and the patient to navigate the experience of pain, but alone it will not produce long-lasting changes.

Quadrant IV can also be presented and further developed in a table of ACTions and commitments guided by values (Table 3) and the general question to open this fruitful discussion could be: What would you need to do (differently) in order to live your values? How do we move towards them?

In Table 3 we share Maria's answers. Each column is explored value by value and is divided into different tasks. At this point, Maria is asked what she thinks she needs to do in order to accomplish each task. The patient often needs more support and ideas with the third column, which is why they should have already participated in the course and didactic module of ACTiveRehab offered by the physiotherapist. For the fourth column, the therapist asks the patient which activities she or he likes to do, in order to choose activities, for example from the ACTiveBODY protocol, that are attractive and easy for the patient. The progression of the rehabilitation is, at the beginning, a task for the physiotherapist, but should always be developed in collaboration with the patient, and eventually the patient will learn to do the progressions him/herself.

The ACTive Matrix Explained

The ACTive Matrix would then be completed for each individual in turn; it offers a good evaluation of the patient's functioning, their challenges (the issues that the patient avoids or fears), the way they usually handle them (their methods of control and their flexibility or inflexibility), what is important for them, their values and source of motivation for change and what the patient can do to take steps to live a valued life.

The next step will be to fill in quadrants III and IV, the away and towards moves, because that mental process of discrimination is what will give the patient the flexibility of creating different responses, and map a departure from the autopilot of the control agenda.

The assessment in ACT is looking for flexibility (healthy resources) and more workable patterns of behaviour. Among our three examples, it was evident that Raja needed the most support and help regarding her trauma history (and rumination) and Maria needed some help with the usual way she handled and denied emotions. Noemi could be managed by a behaviourally informed and knowledgeable physiotherapist, and a patient like Noemi would do well with more knowledge and understanding. Her 'over-doing' *per se* is not a problem; it can be a good resource if used wisely and with acceptance.

CONCLUSION

ACTive physiotherapy has a total focus in function and workability. These goals require a focus on the function of a behaviour—that is, what it brings into our

---

BOX 1

Through ACT and the practice of the Matrix, patients realize that our thoughts, emotions and sensations are like clouds in the sky, but we really only need to be aware that the blue sky is still there and that we are keeping in contact with it, with our values and meaning in life, and that is what is meant by being mindful, being present in what matters.

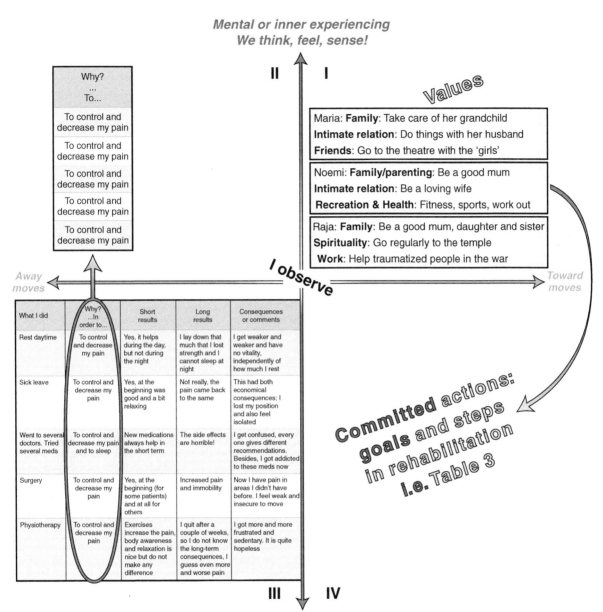

FIGURE 5 ⬛ The Matrix and the observer (Self-as-context) observing and discriminating all the quadrants—not *being* the quadrants!

TABLE 3

ACTions: Quadrant IV Expanded With Detailed 'ACTions and Commitments' Into a (Rehab) Plan

Value	I Will Do... (Task)	I Need to Be Able to... (Goals)	Baseline Sub-Max Test Grip Test Strength Test	Rehabilitation Plan Goal Sub-Max Test Goal Grip Test Goal Strength Test
Take care of my grandchild	Pick him up from nursery	Walk five blocks back and forth.	One block (100 m) and then needs to sit down and rest for 5 minutes	Days 1–3: 20 m back and forth from home. Days 4–6: two times, 1 minute rest. Increase this progression. Add Nordic poles
	To bring him home	Climb two stairs carrying him	Can do two stairs but slowly, with high heart rate and no balance when carrying	Days 1–3: one stair before breakfast and one before lunch Days 4–6: add one before dinner Days 7–9: two stairs three times before meals
	Changing diapers	Bending forwards Lifting 12 kg	Can bend X° Can lift X kg/lb; no good lifting technique	Flexibility training: three different yoga-stretch programmes of 10 minutes each to alternate after each exercise Functional strength-lifting technique
Activities with my husband	Riding the bike on Sundays	Ride 45 minutes	Can ride 15 minutes slowly and need to rest. At normal speed tolerates 5 minutes. Back to normal heart rate: 4 minutes	Every third day cycle (2 hours after a meal) starting with 10 minutes slow and then short intervals of 1 minute at normal speed (followed by 1 minute slow). Starting with two intervals and increasing by two intervals each time. Then increasing time at normal speed, etc.

life and what values we move closer towards—as opposed to the abstract goals that our patients sometimes share, such as pain-free movement or returning to a life as it was lived in the past. In other words, an ACT physiotherapist may use a wide variety of standard active model techniques to increase physical capacity and regulate or restore the nervous system, as the unique contribution of ACT is not *what* we do (within the realm of evidence-based care with a provider knowledgeable about the neuroanatomy of pain), but rather *why* we do it and *how*.

REFERENCES

Brandtstädter, J., Rothermund, K., 2002. The life-course dynamics of goal pursuit and goal adjustment: a two-process framework. Dev. Rev. 22 (1), 117–150.

Butler, J., Ciarrochi, J., 2007. Psychological acceptance and quality of life in the elderly. Qual. Life Res. 16 (4), 607–615. doi:10.1007/s11136-006-9149-1.

Cooper, J.O., Heron, T.E., Heward, W.L., 2007. Applied Behavior Analysis, second ed. Pearson/Merrill-Prentice Hall, Upper Saddle River, NJ.

Dahl, J., 2005. Acceptance and Commitment Therapy for Chronic Pain. Context Press, Reno.

Eisenberger, N.I., 2012. The neural bases of social pain: evidence for shared representations with physical pain. Psychosom. Med. 74 (2), 126–135. doi:10.1097/PSY.0b013e3182464dd1.

Elander, J., Robinson, G., Mitchell, K., Morris, J., 2009. An assessment of the relative influence of pain coping, negative thoughts about pain, and pain acceptance on health-related quality of life among people with hemophilia. Pain 145 (1-2), 169–175.

Häkkinen, A., Häkkinen, K., Hannonen, P., Alen, M., 2001. Strength training induced adaptations in neuromuscular function of premenopausal women with fibromyalgia: comparison with healthy women. Ann. Rheum. Dis. 60 (1), 21–26.

Hayes, S.C., 2004. Acceptance and Commitment Therapy and the new behavior therapies: mindfulness, acceptance and relationship. In: Hayes, S.C., Follette, V.M., Linehan, M. (Eds.), Mindfulness and Acceptance: Expanding the Cognitive-Behavioral Tradition. Guilford Press, New York, pp. 1–29.

Hayes, S.C., Strosahl, K., Wilson, K.G., 1999. Acceptance and Commitment Therapy: An Experiential Approach to Behavior Change. Guilford Press, New York.

Hayes, S.C., Strosahl, K., Wilson, K.G., 2012. Acceptance and Commitment Therapy: The Process and Practice of Mindful Change, second ed. Guilford Press, New York.

Kashdan, T.B., Rottenberg, J., 2010. Psychological flexibility as a fundamental aspect of health. Clin. Psychol. Rev. 30 (7), 865–878. doi:10.1016/j.cpr.2010.03.001.

McCracken, L.M., 1998. Learning to live with the pain: acceptance of pain predicts adjustment in persons with chronic pain. Pain 74 (1), 21–27. doi:S0304-3959(97)00146-2 [pii].

McCracken, L.M., Eccleston, C., 2003. Coping or acceptance: what to do about chronic pain? Pain 105 (1-2), 197–204.

McCracken, L.M., Jones, R., 2012. Treatment for chronic pain for adults in the seventh and eighth decades of life: a preliminary study of Acceptance and Commitment Therapy (ACT). Pain Med. 13 (7), 860–867. doi:10.1111/j.1526-4637.2012.01407.x.

McCracken, L.M., Morley, S., 2014. The psychological flexibility model: a basis for integration and progress in psychological approaches to chronic pain management. J. Pain 15 (3), 221–234. doi:10.1016/j.jpain.2013.10.014.

McCracken, L.M., Vowles, K.E., 2007. Psychological flexibility and traditional pain management strategies in relation to patient functioning with chronic pain: an examination of a revised instrument. J. Pain 8 (9), 700–707. doi:10.1016/j.jpain.2007.04.008.

McCracken, L.M., Vowles, K.E., 2014. Acceptance and commitment therapy and mindfulness for chronic pain: model, process, and progress. Am. Psychol. 69 (2), 178–187. doi:10.1037/a0035623.

McCracken, L.M., Spertus, I.L., Janeck, A.S., et al., 1999. Behavioral dimensions of adjustment in persons with chronic pain: pain-related anxiety and acceptance. Pain 80 (1-2), 283–289.

McCracken, L.M., Carson, J.W., Eccleston, C., Keefe, F.J., 2004. Acceptance and change in the context of chronic pain. Pain 109 (1-2), 4–7.

McCracken, L.M., Gauntlett-Gilbert, J., Vowles, K.E., 2007. The role of mindfulness in a contextual cognitive-behavioral analysis of chronic pain-related suffering and disability. Pain 131 (1-2), 63–69.

Morelli, S.A., Torre, J.B., Eisenberger, N.I., 2014. The neural bases of feeling understood and not understood. Soc. Cogn. Affect. Neurosci. 9 (12), 1890–1896. doi:10.1093/scan/nst191.

Novembre, G., Zanon, M., Silani, G., 2015. Empathy for social exclusion involves the sensory-discriminative component of pain: a within-subject fMRI study. Soc. Cogn. Affect. Neurosci. 10 (2), 153–164. doi:10.1093/scan/nsu038.

Panksepp, J., 1998. Affective Neuroscience: The Foundations of Human and Animal Emotions. Oxford University Press, Oxford.

Polk, K.L., Schoendorf, B., 2014. The ACT Matrix : A New Approach to Building Psychological Flexibility Across Settings and Populations. New Harbinger Publications, Inc, Oakland, CA.

Ramnerö, J., Törneke, N., 2008. The ABCs of Human Behavior: Behavioral Principles for the Practicing Clinician. New Harbinger Publications, Oakland, CA.

Rovner, G. S., 2014. Indicators for behavioral pain rehabilitation: impact and predictive value on assessment, patient selection, treatment and outcome. Doctoral Dissertation, Department of Clinical Neuroscience and Rehabilitation, Institute of Neuroscience and Physiology, Sahlgrenska Academy at University of Gothenburg, Gothenburg, Sweden. <https://gupea.ub.gu.se/handle/2077/35446.>

Rovner, G.S., Vowles, K.E., Gerdle, B., Gillanders, D., 2015. Latent class analysis of the Short and Long Forms of the Chronic Pain Acceptance Questionnaire: further examination of patient subgroups. J. Pain 16 (11), 1095–1105. doi:10.1016/j.jpain.2015.07.007.

Strosahl, K., Gustavsson, T., Robinson, P.A., 2012. Brief Interventions for Radical Behavior Change: Principles and Practice of Focused Acceptance and Commitment Therapy. New Harbinger Publications, Oakland, CA.

Valkeinen, H., Alen, M., Hannonen, P., et al., 2004. Changes in knee extension and flexion force, EMG and functional capacity during strength training in older females with fibromyalgia and healthy controls. Rheumatology (Oxford) 43 (2), 225–228. doi:10.1093/rheumatology/keh027.

Vowles, K.E., McCracken, L.M., 2008. Acceptance and values-based action in chronic pain: a study of treatment effectiveness and process. J. Consult. Clin. Psychol. 76 (3), 397–407.

Vowles, K.E., Sowden, G., Ashworth, J., 2014a. A comprehensive examination of the model underlying acceptance and commitment therapy for chronic pain. Behav. Ther. 45 (3), 390–401. doi:10.1016/j.beth.2013.12.009.

Vowles, K.E., Witkiewitz, K., Sowden, G., Ashworth, J., 2014b. Acceptance and commitment therapy for chronic pain: evidence of mediation and clinically significant change following an abbreviated interdisciplinary program of rehabilitation. J. Pain 15 (1), 101–113. doi:10.1016/j.jpain.2013.10.002.

Wicksell, R.K., Melin, L., Lekander, M., Olsson, G.L., 2009. Evaluating the effectiveness of exposure and acceptance strategies to improve functioning and quality of life in longstanding pediatric pain—A randomized controlled trial. Pain 141 (3), 248–257.

Section 3 METHODOLOGIES WITHIN PHYSIOTHERAPY IN MENTAL HEALTH AND PSYCHIATRY

3.1 NORWEGIAN PSYCHOMOTOR PHYSIOTHERAPY, A BRIEF INTRODUCTION

KIRSTEN EKERHOLT ▪ ANNE GRETLAND

SUMMARY

This chapter outlines the historical background and core features of Norwegian psychomotor physiotherapy (NPMP). This physiotherapeutic approach has its origins in the clinical work carried out by the Norwegian physiotherapist (PT) Aadel Bülow-Hansen and psychiatrist Trygve Braatøy in the late 1940s. NPMP conceptualizes a reciprocal relationship between bodily phenomena such as restrictions of movement, muscular tension and autonomous (dys)function on one hand, and regulation and restriction of emotions on the other. Respiration is ascribed a vital role in the regulation of emotions, and as such it has been of special interest in the examination of the body as well as guiding the PT during treatment. The overall aim for the therapeutic process is the development of perception and contact with signals and reactions in the body, and thereby experiencing and understanding the connection between the body and emotions, experiencing oneself as an embodied identity.

KEY POINTS

▪ Norwegian Psychomotor Physiotherapy is based upon knowledge of the interactions and mutual relationships among biological, physical, psychological and social aspects in human beings.

▪ Local complaints and symptoms are seen in the context of the body as a whole and the bodily function and dysfunction relative to the patient's life experiences and current situation.

▪ Muscular tension, breathing and emotions are interdependent factors, mutually influencing each other.

▪ Reported core aspects in the patient's recovery processes are formulated as "narratives of awakening", i.e. becoming present in the world and in their lives.

LEARNING OBJECTIVES

This chapter intends to give the reader a brief introduction to the following items:

▪ The historical background for NPMP.
▪ The core features of NPMP.
▪ Theoretical frames of references in NPMP.
▪ The clinical examination in NPMP.
▪ Therapeutic aims in NPMP.
▪ Patients' experiences with NPMP.
▪ Quantitative body examinations derived from NPMP.
▪ Education in NPMP: From being an apprentice to achieving a Master's degree.

HISTORICAL BACKGROUND

Norwegian Psychomotor Physiotherapy (NPMP) has its origins in clinical work carried out by physiotherapist (PT) Aadel Bülow-Hansen and psychiatrist Trygve Braatøy from 1947 until the sudden death of Braatøy in 1953. Bülow-Hansen had worked with patients with orthopaedic problems for 20 years when she met Braatøy, who was specialized in psychoanalysis (Bülow-Hansen, 1982; Thornquist & Bunkan, 1991). Together,

Bülow-Hansen and Braatøy developed a physiothera-peutic method to complement the psychoanalytic treatment of neurotic patients. They saw muscular tensions, breathing and emotions as interdependent factors mutually influencing one another, and their physiotherapeutic approach aimed at helping the patient to recognize and change habitual muscular tensions involved in the regulation and inhibition of emotional experiences (Thornquist & Bunkan, 1991; Heller, 2007).

The idea of the body and emotions being closely related, as described by Braatøy (1947, 1948a, 1948b) was new and strange to professionals at that time. Nevertheless, the practice-based theory explained why patients could react emotionally in physiotherapy, and paved the way for the evolution of a specific physio-therapeutic approach. From initially being regarded as a way of treating neurotic patients, NPMP now has a wide range of usage in every part of the health service, including psychiatric hospitals and outpatient clinics.

As the method has developed, it has gradually evolved into an independent physiotherapeutic approach, originally called the *Braatøy–Bülow-Hansen therapy* or just *Aadel Bülow-Hansen's physiotherapy* (Øvreberg & Andersen, 2003). However, the official designation used in Norwegian legal documents and in official health care since 1973 is *psychomotor physio-therapy*. To distinguish this specific physiotherapeutic tradition from relaxing therapies called *psychomotor therapy* throughout Europe, the term now used inter-nationally is *Norwegian psychomotor physiotherapy* (Bunkan, 2010).

CORE FEATURES OF NPMP

Patients who come to NPMP have usually suffered from their ailments for a long time (Breitve et al., 2010) and many patients need long-lasting therapeutic processes. Muscular tension is often imbued with emotional difficulties and with past and current demanding life experiences. Whatever problem the patient presents, the psychomotor PT does not look for symptoms and clinical signs in the traditional biomedical sense. Local clinical signs must be put into the context of the body as a whole and the bodily func-tion and dysfunctions should be assessed relative to the patient's life experiences and current situation

(Thornquist & Bunkan, 1991; Øvreberg & Andersen, 2003; Thornquist, 2006).

NPMP consists of practice-driven comprehension of the body, its functions and dysfunctions, and a specialized practical mode of assessing and treating patients, derived from experience. The main tradi-tional sources additional to Braatøy's writings are the experience-based books of Bunkan (1982), Thorn-quist & Bunkan (1991 [original edition 1986]) and Øvreberg & Andersen (2003 [original edition 1986]). NPMP conceptualizes a reciprocal relationship between bodily phenomena such as restrictions of movement, muscular tension and autonomous (dys)functions on one hand, and regulation and restriction of emotions on the other. Respiration is ascribed a vital role in the regulation of emotions, and as such it has been a focus of attention in the physical examination of the body, as well as guiding the PT during treatment. This means that tension, restricted breathing and various forms of bodily patterns and habits may all have a role in protecting the person from painful memories and emotions. The effect of loosening up may therefore be harmful and can evoke memories and emotional conflicts, leading to a strengthening of bodily imbal-ances and dysfunctional habits (Thornquist, 2010). In such cases, the PT will emphasize exercises which are intended to increase the patient's feeling of stability and control (Bunkan, 2010).

The NPMP therapeutic approach is adapted indi-vidually to the patient and can consist of both stabiliz-ing and relaxing elements, combining massage, exercises and movements. The treatment is always adjusted according to the patient's reactions. Conse-quently, NPMP is not a standardized treatment, but a readjustment process that involves the whole body, in fact the whole person (Bunkan, 2010).

THEORETICAL FRAMES OF REFERENCE IN NPMP

Theoretical frames influence what is regarded as clini-cally relevant information, as well as the interpretation of signs and words, and how the patient's problems are defined as 'something to act on' by the professional (Thornquist, 1995). Originally, Bülow-Hansen's physi-otherapeutic techniques and her intuition, combined with Braatøy's psychoanalytic knowledge of and interest in the somatic aspect in psychiatry, created this therapeutic approach (Bunkan, 1982). From the mid-1970s, the theoretical development of NPMP mainly followed the psychoanalytical heritage handed down by Braatøy (Bülow-Hansen, 1982; Bunkan, 1982; Monsen, 1989). In assessing function, Thornquist (2006) found that the PTs were first and foremost emotionally and individually oriented, and not concerned with the socially and culturally informed and informing body. Symptoms and the state of the body were interpreted in the context of the body as an expression and regulator of the person's emotional life; as a kind of mirror of yesterday's life. The PT distinguished between function and dysfunction (i.e., between desirable and undesirable conditions), on the basis of the interrelationship between local physical conditions and the general state of the body, and by comparing the patient's verbal and bodily expressions (Thornquist, 2006).

From the 1990s, Merleau-Ponty's phenomenology of perception (1986) has been a vital reflective source for researchers in the field of NPMP (Thornquist, 1990, 1991, 2001a, 2001b, 2006, 2012; Ekerholt & Bergland, 2004, 2006, 2008; Gretland, 2007; Øien et al., 2007; Dragesund & Råheim, 2008; Øien et al., 2009; Sviland, et al., 2012; 2014). Following Merleau-Ponty's theory, NPMP researchers and therapists have emphasized the embodied nature of human subjects, maintaining that the body is social by nature. Perceiving human beings as embodied social agents open to experience has also led psychomotor PTs to empirically based social science research illuminating relationships between objective social conditions and events and various forms of embodiment and agency, as well as health problems (Thornquist, 1991, 1995, 2001a, 2001b, 2006; Gretland, 2007). As human subjects, individuals incorporate habitual ways of movement and perception—i.e., sensomotor schemes on how to comport oneself in a concrete social world—using implicit or silent knowledge on how to interact with others to ensure social bondings (Bourdieu, 1990; Stern, 2004).

Braatøy (1937) and Bülow-Hansen (in Isdahl & Thornquist, 1983) were primarily concerned with the traumatic effects of being forced to restrain oneself and stay quiet—hampering one's ability to release muscular tensions. 'They must learn to speak up!'

Bülow-Hansen said about her patients (Isdahl & Thornquist, 1983). Conceiving muscular tensions as a kind of sociomoral agency incorporated by need in repressive relationships, a patient's participation in an active collaboration between equal partners is set as a vital guideline for the entire treatment in NPMP (Thornquist & Bunkan, 1991). In recent years, the scope has widened. Knowledge of neurotic tensions deriving from oppressive relationships is of course still relevant, but it is augmented with knowledge of how neglect, as well as abuse and violence, can affect an individual's development and their physical and mental health (Lanius et al., 2010).

Theoretical elaborations of the social nature of the body and its clinical relevance for understanding health problems, and research studies of clinical practice in NPMP, have highlighted the relational aspects of clinical work, as well as its relevance to the patient's health and participation in society.

Theories of infant development (Stern, 1985; Bråten, 2007) have also informed studies of clinical practice in NPMP (Gretland, 2007; Thornquist, 2012), because they suggest that bodily contact and interaction are the earliest experiences and primary levels of contact, paving the way for preverbal intersubjectivity, and from preverbal to verbal intersubjectivity.

CLINICAL EXAMINATION

Trial-Treatment: a Dynamic, Intersubjective Perception of Body Relationships

In NPMP, the original clinical examination is termed a *trial-treatment* owing to its interactive and dynamic aspects. In this clinical examination, both parties contribute to an evolution of information on the patient's problems, their resources and their ability to change. Whether the main communicative channel is verbal or bodily interaction, the trial-treatment can be seen as a semistructured dialogue, allowing both parties to participate in a creative process open to intersubjectivity at several levels (Thornquist, 1990, 2006). The diagnostic enterprise in NPMP includes the entire body and the examination is characterized by the therapist's engaging in exploration as well as merging action, experiences and conversation, directed at stimulating the patient's bodily awareness (Thornquist, 1991). The patient's experiences are seen as potential bodily matters that could be discussed and observed throughout the examination. The patient's statements about tension or their experiences of being 'stiff', 'tense' and 'trapped' in their bodies are followed up both in the conversation and in the clinical examination. Thus there is continuity between the different elements of the examination and between the patient's verbal and bodily messages and expressions. The therapist's practice should be of a searching and contextualized nature, and patients are encouraged to do things in different ways, to experience differences and nuances and, in doing so, to become more aware of their habitual patterns; that is, to learn something about themselves (Thornquist, 2006).

The trial treatment is divided into several sections (Box 1). The patient is examined in various bodily positions (standing, sitting, lying both supine and prone on the treatment table and then standing again). The examination ends up with a concluding talk on the experiences they had during the session. The PT and the patient usually also consider whether the patient should continue with the NPMP or not. If yes, they will discuss which aims they consider reasonable for the therapeutic process.

During all subassessments, the PT observes the patient's movements, spontaneous ones as well as those performed under instruction, and also the body's posture, respiration, autonomic and motor reactions. The PT assesses the patient's flexibility, stability and how the patient yields to or resists gravity. The PT palpates the skin and muscles all over the patient's body, all the time focusing on the interplay between respiration, muscular tension and movements (Thornquist, 1990). During the examination, the PT raises questions verbally, as well as through the hands. The exchanges between the PT and the patient are mainly grounded in the latter's immediate bodily reactions, often used as a starting point for short verbal dialogues. 'Can you let your head slide gently forwards?', 'Do you feel you are holding back?', 'Do you normally feel you have difficulty in freeing your head?' Such questions give the PT an insight into how the patient usually uses their body, and whether they are aware of what is happening in their body (Thornquist, 1990). With their hands, the PT can feel whether the patient lets tension go or holds back, and can even gently invite the patient to exceed the initial range of movement so the responses to these challenges to the spontaneous limits can be observed. The PT can directly call the patient's attention to their bodily potentials, such as letting go of tension, and ask them to follow impulses to move, to express themselves, etc. The patient's responses to and experiences of a gentle play on their limits supply important information to the PT about the patient's potential for change, while the PT focuses on the interplay between respiration, muscular conditions, posture and movement responses (Thornquist & Bunkan, 1991).

Most of the time, the patient and the PT are close to each other, the PT using hands-on techniques. Thus interaction is embedded in the clinical encounter, and is dependent on the perception of signs through various senses, including vision and hearing, as well as the sense of touch and pressure, movement and position (Thornquist, 2006). Bülow-Hansen emphasized the importance of the PT being sensitive to the patient's reactions, to see, listen, and—last, but not least—feel. 'What PTs must train is their intuition', she claimed, rejecting measurements of bodily phenomena as sources of relevant information (Øvreberg & Andersen, 2003). The trial treatment is a sort of schematic progress; both the examination and the treatment plan should be adjusted to the actual situation and the patient's precondition (Box 2; Thornquist & Bunkan, 1991).

BOX 1

A SCHEMATIC PRESENTATION OF THE TRIAL TREATMENT

Introduction to Norwegian psychomotor physiotherapy (NPMP)
Information on medical and social history
Comprehensive examination of the whole body:
  Standing position
  Sitting position
  Lying supine position
  Lying prone position
  Standing position
Concluding talk, sharing experiences from the trial treatment
Clinical reasoning, involving patient and physiotherapist:
  Would NPMP be relevant for this patient?
  If yes, what would be the therapist–patient goal agreement?

BOX 2
THE FIRST ENCOUNTER BETWEEN AMY AND THE PSYCHOMOTOR
PHYSIOTHERAPIST

Amy (45) has had health problems from her childhood. Today her main problem is sleeplessness, weakness and numbness in her hands and arms. She has extensive stiffness in the back, neck and shoulders, and her blood pressure is too high. Her job is demanding, and there have been serious problems in her family lately.

When we enter the situation, the physiotherapist (PT) and Amy have talked for about 10 minutes, and they have nearly finished the body examination in the standing position. Then the PT wants to see how Amy reacts to her attempting to move Amy—first by nudging her pelvis gently forward, to check Amy's ability and response to being moved passively. No or little movement can be observed. The PT then wants to move Amy's arm:

PT: 'I'll try to move your arm, try to let it go.'
A: [closes her eyes] 'It's not easy.'
PT: 'No, it's not easy?' [She goes on, Amy keeps her eyes closed]
A: 'No' [smiles a little, as PT lets her arm down]
PT: [placing one hand on Amy's shoulder, and the other on her back, she pulls the shoulder gently backwards. The PT's movement rotates Amy's

whole body; the shoulder seems to be fixed to the body. 'Let's do the same on the other side.'
A: [smiles] 'I would like to keep control.'
PT: 'You want to keep control?'
A: 'Yes, I really like to keep control! Yes, that's familiar to me.' [Amy is still smiling]

This passage illustrates how both the PT and the patient seem to be focusing on a common project, and they seem to share a sense of Amy resisting the PT's attempts to move her body and her arms. Amy verbalizes her resistance as a need for control, adding that she recognizes herself—as a person who wants to have control in other situations, as well. There is a movement in her attribution of meaning—from the situated bodily signs, to a generalized feeling of personal traits.

The text is drawn from a transcription of a video recorded during the first meeting between a patient and a PT specializing in NPMP. The recording is part of a research project approved by the Regional Committee for medical and healthcare research. The participants have signed an agreement on informed consent.

THERAPEUTIC AIMS

Treatment is aimed at the body, and everything the therapist does is based upon an understanding of the body as an integrated physical–psychological phenomenon. The basis for NPMP is the whole person and the key is the body. First and foremost, it is the patient's ability to adjust, which can be understood as the person's possibility for change, which is the main focus in NPMP (Thornquist & Bunkan, 1991).

The overall aim may be defined as the development of perception and contact with signals and reactions in the body, thereby experiencing and understanding the connection between the body and feelings, experiencing oneself as having an embodied identity (Thornquist & Bunkan, 1991). The theoretical reorientation described previously has allowed an extension of therapeutic issues in NPMP. From originally being restricted to the enhancement of bodily and emotional functioning ('free stretching, free respiration, free feelings'), the understanding of the connection between bodily functioning and social life has increased. Therapeutic aims may then be related to issues such as bringing nuances

to bodily functioning in time and space, to sense, respect and mark personal borders, to be confident with and be able to express feelings and to mentalize one's experiences (Gretland, 2007, 2009; Sternberg & Bohen, 2009; Thornquist, 2010; Biguet, 2012; Ekerholt et al., 2014). Allowing room for emotions is important in NPMP. Rejection of emotions may be exactly what the patient has experienced earlier, resulting in their problems. Gaining contact with one's emotions and being able to express them can be a vital element in the therapeutic process. The prerequisite is, however, that the attitude of the PT is one of acceptance of that to which the patient is relating (Thornquist & Bunkan, 1991; Ekerholt & Bergland, 2006, 2008).

PATIENTS' EXPERIENCES

Several studies over the last 25 years have explored patients' experiences in NPMP (Thornquist, 1990, 1991, 2001a, 2001b, 2006, 2012; Ekerholt & Bergland, 2004, 2006, 2008; Gretland, 2007; Øien et al., 2007; Dragesund & Råheim, 2008; Øien et al., 2009, 2011; Ekerholt, 2011; Sviland et al., 2012; 2014). These research projects have shown good consistency in their findings, regarding both the patients' satisfaction as well as which aspects of the therapy the patients considered to be most important.

■ **Becoming familiar with the body**

The core aspect in the patients' recovery processes was to become familiar with their bodies, sensing in a more differentiated way and increasing the feeling of being present in their bodies. Becoming aware of and managing to perceive tension vaguely grew into the beginning of an indeterminate experience 'that something is there'. Perceiving tension is a prerequisite to changing restricted moving and breathing patterns, it was also the beginning of the ability to get in contact with one's own emotions.

■ **Searching for meaning**

The patients became better acquainted with bodily reactions and emotional awareness through the therapeutic process, which involved a search for meaning. The patients learned to view the body as an expression of and as a conveyer of their own lives and history, thus superseding the often-accepted model of separation between the body and human experience. The patients' understanding of earlier life experiences became clearer and the patients started to view past events differently.

■ **Sense of identity**

The patients learned to interpret bodily reactions and bodily symptoms and to connect these reactions to relational dimensions and habitual ways of acting. By acquiring a sense of embodiment, which means that cognition is situated in the body and that their lived experiences could give access to implicit, embodied knowledge, the patients' sense of identity seemed to emerge, and they became more secure about themselves and the surroundings. The feeling of being a narrating and acting person may correspond with what can be referred to as recognizing one's own 'personality'.

■ **The unity of body and mind**

The integration of interpretation, narration, communication and self-understanding was an important part in the interpretation process for the patients. The therapeutic process was described as a change towards experiencing body and mind as more of a unity. They were 'moving back into the body'. The change was formulated as a narrative of awakening. The process of awakening was a powerful experience of being present in the world and in their lives: 'Perhaps the most important change was feeling better towards myself. Then I could turn outwards towards others.'

QUANTITATIVE BODY EXAMINATIONS DERIVED FROM NPMP

From the original body examination (i.e., the trial treatment in NPMP), four main quantitative body examinations have been developed: the resource oriented body examination (ROBE), the comprehensive body examination (CBE), the global physiotherapeutic muscle examination (GPM) and the global physiotherapy examination (GPE-52) (Bunkan et al., 2002, 2004). The purpose of the development of these examinations was to fulfil the need to obtain information concerning the patient's potential for improvement and to define the appropriate level of intervention. The intention was also to quantify the outcome of physiotherapy and to study body features in groups of patients (Heløe et al., 1980; Sundsvold et al., 1982; Bunkan et al., 1999, 2001; Kvåle et al., 2001; Friis et al., 2002, 2012; Meurle-Hallberg et al., 2004; Meurle-Hallberg & Armelius, 2006; Kvåle et al., 2008, 2010; Breitve et al., 2010).

EDUCATION: FROM BEING AN APPRENTICE TO ACHIEVING A MASTER'S DEGREE

Education in NPMP was administered by the Association of Norwegian Physiotherapists from 1960 to 1994. Training in NPMP was primarily oriented towards method, providing extensive instruction in specific examination and treatment methods. This, in turn, instilled confidence and security in the students as the therapists learned about tools which are useful in dealing with patients suffering from complex ailments such as myalgia, dorsalgia and so on (Thornquist,

2006). Clinical training and practical supervision may be helpful to students who are learning how to act in certain situations and to handle problems in ways that do not provoke insecurity. However, the programme neither encouraged the critical reflection that is commonplace in academic traditions (Thornquist, 2006), nor provided the qualifications required by today's professionals.

Since 1994, education in NPMP has been included in postgraduate education in psychosomatic and psychiatric physiotherapy at Oslo University College of Applied Sciences. Today, education in NPMP is offered at Oslo and Akershus University College of Applied Sciences, and at UiT, the Arctic University of Norway (Tromsø). Education to the level of a master's degree is required for recognition in the practice of NPMP in Norway.

REFERENCES

Biguet, G., 2012. Psykomotorisk fysioterapi—grundläggande principer, potentialer og utmaningar (NPMP—principles, potentials and challenges). In: Biguet, G., Keskinen Rosenquist, R., Berg, A.L. (Eds.), Att Förstå Kroppens Budskap—Sjukgymnastiska Perspektiv (Understanding the Meaning of the Body—Physiotherapeutic Perspectives). Studentlitteratur, Lund.

Bourdieu, P., 1990. The Logic of Practice. Oxford Polity Press, Cambridge.

Braatøy, T., 1937. Sorger Og Sinnslidelser (Sorrows and Mental Illness). Cappelen, Oslo.

Braatøy, T., 1947. De Nervøse Sinn. (Anxious Minds). Cappelen, Oslo.

Braatøy, T., 1948a. Psykologi contra anatomi ved sykegymnastisk behandling av armnevrose ol. Del I: bevegelse, affekt og holdning (Psychology versus anatomy in physiotherapy for arm neurosis etc. Part I: movement, affects and posture). Nord. Med. 39, 923–930.

Braatøy, T., 1948b. Psykologi contra anatomi ved sykegymnastisk behandling av armnevroser o.l. Del II. Respirasjon, affekt og ord (Psychology versus anatomy in physiotherapy for arm neurosis etc. Part II: respiration, affect and words). Nord. Med. 38, 971–976.

Bråten, S. (Ed.), 2007. On Being Moved: from Mirror Neurons to Empathy. John Benjamins Publishing Company, Amsterdam.

Breitve, M.H., Hynninen, M.J., Kvåle, A., 2010. The effect of psychomotor physical therapy on subjective health complaints and psychological symptoms. Physiother. Res. Int. 15 (4), 212–221.

Bülow-Hansen, A., 1982. Psykomotorisk fysioterapi (Psychomotor physiotherapy). In: Bunkan, B.H., Radøy, L., Thornquist, E. (Eds.), Psykomotorisk Behandling. Festskrift Til Aadel Bülow-Hansen. (Psychomotor Treatment. Memorial Volume to Aadel Bülow-Hansen). Norwegian University Press, Oslo, pp. 15–21.

Bunkan, B.H., 1982. Den psykomotoriske tradisjon (The psychomotor tradition). In: Bunkan, B.H., Radøy, L., Thornquist, E. (Eds.), Psykomotorisk Behandling. Festskrift til Aadel Bülow-Hansen (Psychomotor Treatment. Memorial Volume to Aadel Bülow-Hansen). Norwegian University Press, Oslo, pp. 22–29.

Bunkan, B.H., Opjordsmoen, S., Moen, O., et al., 1999. What are the basic dimensions of respiration? A psychometric evaluation of the Comprehensive Body Examination. II. Nord Psychiatry 53, 361–369.

Bunkan, B.H., Ljunggren, A.L., Opjordsmoen, S., et al., 2001. What are the basic dimensions of movement? A psychometric evaluation of the Comprehensive Body Examination. III. Nord Psychiatry 53, 33–40.

Bunkan, B.H., Moen, O., Opjordsmoen, S., et al., 2002. Interrater reliability of the Comprehensive Body Examination. Physiother. Theory Pract. 18, 121–129.

Bunkan, B.H., Ljunggren, A.L., Opjordsmoen, S., et al., 2004. Development of body examinations—an overview. Fysioterapeuten nr 10, pp. 22–28.

Bunkan, B.H., 2010. A comprehensive physiotherapy. In: Ekerholt, K. (Ed.), Aspects of Psychiatric and Psychosomatic Physiotherapy. Oslo University College, Oslo, HiO report, no 3 pp. 5–10.

Dragesund, T., Råheim, M., 2008. Norwegian psychomotor physiotherapy and patients with chronic pain: patients' perspective on body awareness. Physiother. Theory Pract. 24 (4), 243–254.

Ekerholt, K., 2011. Awareness of breathing as a way to enhance the sense of coherence: patients' experiences in psychomotor physiotherapy. Body Movem. D. Physiot. 6 (2), 103–115.

Ekerholt, K., Bergland, A., 2004. The first encounter with Norwegian Psychomotor Physiotherapy. Scand. J. Public Health 32, 403–410.

Ekerholt, K., Bergland, A., 2006. Massage as interaction and a source of information. Adv. Physio. 8, 137–144.

Ekerholt, K., Bergland, A., 2008. Breathing: a sign of life and a unique area for reflection and action. Phys. Ther. 88, 832–840.

Ekerholt, K., Schau, G., Mathismoen, K.M., Bergland, A., 2014. Body awareness—a vital aspect in mentalization: experiences from concurrent and reciprocal therapies. Physiother. Theory Pract. Early Online: 1–7 2014, Inc. <http://informahealthcare.com/ptp.> ISSN: 0959–3985 (print), 1532–5040 (electronic).

Friis, S., Bunkan, B.H., Opjordsmoen, S., et al., 2002. The Comprehensive Body Examination (CBE): from global impressions to specific sub-scales. Adv. Physiot. 4, 161–168.

Friis, S., Kvåle, A., Opjordsmoen, S., Bunkan, B.H., 2012. The Global Body Examination (GBE). A useful instrument for evaluation of respiration. Adv. Physiot. 14 (4), 146–154.

Gretland, A., 2007. Den Relasjonelle Kroppen. (The Relational Body). Fagbokforlaget, Bergen.

Gretland, A., 2009. Psykomotorisk fysioterapi som støttende behandling – et eksempel (Norwegian Psychomotor Physiotherapy as a supportive therapy—a clinical example). In: Ekerholt, K. (Ed.), Festskrift til Berit Heir Bunkan (Memorial Volume to Berit Heir Bunkan), HiO report, 10. Oslo University College, Oslo, pp. 45–59.

Heller, M.C., 2007. The golden age of body psychotherapy in Oslo. I: from gymnastics to psychoanalysis. Body Movem. D. Physiot. 2 (1), 5–16.

Heløe, B., Heiberg, A.N., Krogstad, B.S., 1980. A multiprofessional study of patients with myofascial pain-dysfunction syndrome, I. Acta Odontol. Scand. 38 (2), 109–117.

Isdahl, P.J., Thornquist, E., 1983. Kroppen mellom hendene. Intervju med Aadel Bülow-Hansen (The body between her hands. Interview with Aadel Bülow-Hansen). (Journal of the Norwegian Psychological Association) Tidsskrift for norsk psykologforening 20, 273–275.

Kvåle, A., Bunkan, B.H., Ljunggren, A.E., et al., 2010. Sammenligning av to undersøkelsesmetoder innen psykomotorisk tradisjon: GFM-52 og DOK (Comparison of two clinical assessments in the Norwegian Psychomotor Physiotherapy: GFM and DOK). Fysioterapeuten 2, 24–32.

Kvåle, A., Ellertsen, B., Skouen, J.S., 2001. Relationships between physical findings (GPE-78) and psychological profiles (MMPI-2) in patients with long-lasting musculoskeletal pain. Nord. J. Psychiatry 55, 177–184.

Kvåle, A., Wilhelmsen, K., Fiske, H.A., 2008. Physical findings in patients with dizziness undergoing a group exercise programme. Physiother. Res. Int. 13 (3), 162–175.

Lanius, R.A., Vermetten, E., Pain, C. (Eds.), 2010. The Impact of Early Life Trauma on Health and Disease. The Hidden Epidemic. Cambridge University Press, Cambridge.

Meurle-Hallberg, K., Armelius, K., 2006. Associations between physical and psychological problems in a group of patients with stress-related behaviour and somatoform disorders. Physiother Theory Pract. 22 (1), 17–31.

Meurle-Hallberg, K., Armelius, B.A., von Koch, L., 2004. Body patterns in patients with psychosomatic, musculoskeletal and schizophrenic disorders: psychometric properties and clinical relevance of Resource Oriented Body Examination (ROBE II). Adv. Physiot. 6, 130–142.

Merleau-Ponty, M., 1986. Phenomenology of Perception. Routledge et Kegan Paul, London.

Monsen, K., 1989. Psykodynamisk Kroppsterapi (Psychodynamic Body Treatment). Tano, Oslo.

Øien, A.M., Iversen, S., Stensland, P., 2007. Narratives of embodied experiences—therapy processes in Norwegian psychomotor physiotherapy. Adv. Physiot. 9, 31–39.

Øien, A.M., Råheim, M., Iversen, S., Steihaug, S., 2009. Self-perception as embodied knowledge-changing processes for patients with chronic pain. Adv. Physiot. 11 (3), 121–129.

Øien, A.M., Steihaug, S., Iversen, S., Råheim, M., 2011. Communication as negotiation process in long-term physiotherapy: a qualitative study. Scand. J. Caring Sci. 2 (5), 53–61.

Øvreberg, G., Andersen, T. (2003 [original edition 1986]). Aadel Bülow-Hansens Fysioterapi (The Physiotherapy of Aadel Bülow-Hansen). Compendium forlag, Skarnes.

Stern, D., 1985. The Interpersonal World of the Infant: A View from Psychoanalysis and Development Psychology. W.W. Norton.

Stern, D.N., 2004. The Present Moment in Psychotherapy and Everyday Life. Karnac Books, London.

Sternberg, S., Bohen, R., 2009. Fysioterapeutisk intervention ved personlighedsforstyrrelser. In: Ekerholt, K. (Ed.), Festskrift til Berit Heir Bunkan (Memorial Volume to Berit Heir Bunkan). HiO report, 10. Oslo University College, Oslo, pp. 239–245.

Sundsvold, M.Ø., Vaglum, P., Denstad, K., 1982. Global Fysioterapeutisk Muskelundersøkelse (Global Physiotherapeutic Assessment). Eget forlag, Oslo.

Sviland, R., Martinsen, K., Råheim, M., 2014. To be held and to hold one's own: narratives of embodied transformation in the treatment of long lasting musculoskeletal problems. Med. Health Care Philos. 17, 609–624.

Sviland, R., Råheim, M., Martinsen, K., 2012. Touched in sensation—moved by respiration. Embodied narrative identity—a treatment process. Scand. J. Caring Sci. 26, 811–819.

Thornquist, E., 1990. Communication: what happens during the first encounter between patient and physiotherapist? Scand. J. Prim. Health Care 8, 133–138.

Thornquist, E., 1991. Body communication is a continuous process. The first encounter between patient and physiotherapist. Scand. J. Prim. Health Care 9, 191–194.

Thornquist, E., 1995. Musculoskeletal suffering: diagnosis and a variant view. Sociol. Health Illn. 17 (2), 166–192.

Thornquist, E., 2001a. Diagnostics in physiotherapy—process, patterns and perspectives. Part I. Adv. Physiot. 3, 140–150.

Thornquist, E., 2001b. Diagnostics in physiotherapy—process, patterns and perspectives. Part II. Adv. Physiot. 3, 151–162.

Thornquist, E., 2006. Face-to-face and hands-on: assumptions and assessments in the physiotherapy clinic. Med. Anthropol. 251, 65–97.

Thornquist, E., 2010. Psychomotor physiotherapy—principles, perspectives and potentials. In: Ekerholt, K. (Ed.), Aspects of Psychiatric and Psychosomatic Physiotherapy. HiO report 3. Oslo University College, Oslo, pp. 203–217.

Thornquist, E., 2012. Movement and Interaction. The Sherborne Approach and Documentation. Norwegian University Press, Oslo.

Thornquist, E., Bunkan, B.H., 1991 [original edition 1986]. What Is Psychomotor Therapy? Norwegian University Press, Oslo.

3.2

BASIC BODY AWARENESS THERAPY (BBAT): A MOVEMENT AWARENESS LEARNING MODALITY IN PHYSIOTHERAPY, PROMOTING MOVEMENT QUALITY

LIV HELVIK SKJAERVEN ■ MONICA MATTSSON

SUMMARY

Basic Body Awareness Therapy (BBAT) is a physiotherapeutic movement awareness learning programme directed towards daily life movement coordination and function. It is well known for its strategy of promoting movement quality, well-being and health, through the multiperspective movement awareness approach. The physiotherapist acts as a guide, bridging the therapy situation with everyday life and the patient's needs. BBAT is designed to involve the patient, in order to allow transfer of the learning to home, work and daily functioning. The physiotherapist has a reflective talk with the patient on the movement experiences to enhance learning and insight. The modality provides reliable and valid assessment tools and structured, evidence-based strategies for individual and group therapeutic settings for use in mental health and psychiatry, including preventive health care and health promotion. The movement principles are increasingly being implemented in somatic health care, including rheumatology and for patients with hip arthroses.

KEY POINTS

■ Describing and promoting movement quality.

■ Therapeutic factors promoting movement awareness.

■ Movement awareness learning cycle.

LEARNING OBJECTIVES

■ Knowledge of therapeutic factors promoting movement quality through a movement awareness approach in physiotherapy.

■ Knowledge of a vocabulary describing movement quality and movement awareness.

■ Knowledge of the interacting processes communicating movement awareness in physiotherapy.

INTRODUCTION

Long-lasting musculoskeletal disorders and mental health problems are leading causes of sick leave worldwide (WHO, 2015). To meet the needs of the patient, physiotherapists offer a wide range of approaches with a focus on human movement and function. One of the treatment modalities is Basic Body Awareness Therapy (BBAT), a systematically developed approach directed towards the patient's functional movement quality.

BBAT is a physiotherapeutic movement awareness learning programme, offering a structured treatment programme and reliable and valid assessment tools: the Body Awareness Scale—MQ-E (Hedlund et al., 2016) and Body Awareness Rating Scale—Movement Quality and Experience (BARS-MQE) (Skjaerven et al., 2015). The structured treatment programme refers to the organization and transference of therapeutic components implemented in the treatment process, promoting more functional movement quality through the movement awareness learning programme.

When the movement principles of BBAT are implemented in physiotherapy, presence in and awareness of movement are core aspects of the therapy. The approach is person-centred and aims towards promoting health and learning coping strategies for daily use. To enhance the contact with 'the self', the physiotherapist arranges situations that focus on basic movement principles, incorporating physical, physiological, psychological, relational and existential components into the therapy. BBAT has been shown to be applicable in many and varied clinical settings, and is particularly known for its movement quality approach. Today, it is offered by physiotherapists in mental health and somatic institutions, in community health care, in health promotion and in preventive health care, especially in the northern part of Europe. Over the last 15 years BBAT has been implemented in several countries and continents. The movement principles, knowledge and competence in BBAT are being increasingly incorporated into somatic health care, including rheumatology (Olsen & Skjaerven, 2016) and for patients with hip arthroses (Strand et al., 2016).

CLINICAL HYPOTHESIS

The World Health Organization (WHO, 2015) has documented an increase in the prevalence of long-lasting musculoskeletal and mental health problems. Physiotherapists are reporting from clinical practice that people with multifactorial suffering have a lack of contact with themselves, their physical body, emotions, boundaries, the external environment and/or relationship to others, with consequences for daily function, habits and health (Skjaerven et al., 2010).

BBAT is based on the clinical hypothesis of 'the threefold contact problem', problems in human beings caused by a lack of contact with their own physical body, internal physiological and mental processes and with the external environment, including the relationship with others (Dropsy, 1973; 1984, 1998a, 1998b). This lack of contact may lead to dysfunctional movements and reduced functioning in daily life. On that basis, BBAT includes a multifaceted perspective in its training programme: biomechanical, physiological, psychosociocultural and existential perspectives (Dropsy, 1973). Thus it takes into account that the person is affected by physical, existential and relational aspects of functioning and existence in everyday movement and life (Thörnborg & Mattsson, 2009). The aim of BBAT is to improve the person's self-awareness of the body and its movement coordination, and to mobilize their resources for health through movement.

EVERYDAY MOVEMENTS—CORE MOVEMENTS FOR DAILY USE

BBAT includes movement coordination, situations and approaches designed to involve the patient personally during the period of treatment, to enhance the transference to their life situation (Skjærven & Sundal, 2016). The BBAT movements represent an extract of everyday movements: lying, sitting, standing, walking, relational movements, use of the voice and massage (touch), a span of movement coordination. The movements are simple, small, soft, rhythmical and applicable to the daily variations of movements.

BBAT is developed to foster more functional movement quality and habits, aiming for the patient to come into contact with, gain insight in and learn more functional movement strategies. Embodied and mindful presence, awareness and movement quality represent keys in the therapeutic approach (Gyllensten et al., 2010; Skjaerven et al., 2010). The modality aims to increase the coordination between mind and body through sensory motor awareness and perception. Implementing more mindful movements influences the patient's movement quality, a phenomenon that is observable and thus possible for the physiotherapist to describe, assess and promote in a structured therapeutic way.

The therapy situation does not require equipment other than a floor, a mat and a chair. The patient is invited to wear clothes that allow them to move and breathe freely, being comfortable and at ease. The approach is user-friendly because the patient can keep their normal clothes on and the therapist is qualified in movement analysis, being trained to be sensitive to movement quality. The physiotherapist acts as a guide, bridging the therapy situation with everyday life and needs. A treatment contract is developed in dialogue with the patient, focusing on how the movement principles can be adjusted and practised at home, at work, etc. Use of a diary is a concrete and helpful tool to strengthen the learning process and influences the therapeutic outcome (Skjærven, 2013).

AWARENESS, BODY AWARENESS AND MOVEMENT AWARENESS

In recent years, physical therapists and researchers have paid more attention to phenomena such as

BOX 1
DEFINITION OF AWARENESS, BODY AWARENESS AND MOVEMENT AWARENESS

PHENOMENON	DEFINITION
Awareness	Can be defined as an attentive, relaxed and alert presence, not analogous with concentration. Awareness is a relative phenomenon, and being aware means continually monitoring internal sensations and the external environment, providing heightened sensitivity to experiences (Brown & Ryan, 2003)
Body awareness	Can be described as the sensitivity to bodily signals, being aware of bodily states and identifying subtle bodily reactions to internal and environmental conditions (Ginzburg et al., 2014)
Movement awareness	Can be described as a sensitivity to movement nuances, becoming aware of one's own movement coordination, and how movements are performed in relation to space, time and energy, identifying subtle movement reactions in relation to internal, environmental and relational conditions (Skjærven et al., 2015)

awareness, body awareness and movement awareness (Box 1).

Awareness is derived from human consciousness that encompasses both awareness and attention (Brown & Ryan, 2003). Awareness can be defined as an attentive, relaxed and alert presence, not analogous with concentration. It is possible to be aware of stimuli without making them the centre of attention. Awareness is a relative phenomenon, and being aware means continually monitoring internal sensations and the external environment, providing heightened sensitivity to experiences (Brown & Ryan, 2003).

Body awareness is a frequently used term in the literature (Mehling et al., 2011; Ginzburg et al., 2014). Mehling describes body awareness involving an attentional focus on and awareness of internal body sensations, defining it as the subjective, phenomenological aspect of proprioception and interoception that enters conscious awareness, modifiable by mental processes including attention, interpretation, appraisal, beliefs, memories, conditioning, attitudes and affect (Mehling et al., 2011). It is further described as the sensitivity to bodily signals, being aware of bodily states and identifying subtle bodily reactions to internal and environmental conditions (Ginzburg et al., 2014).

Historically, Roxendal developed the first Body Awareness Scale (BAS) (Roxendal, 1985, 1987). This was followed by Skatteboe's development of the Body Awareness Rating Scale (BARS) (Skatteboe et al., 1989; Skatteboe, 2000), Mattsson's and Gyllensten's applications of body awareness in physiotherapy (Mattsson, 1998; Gyllensten, 2001) and studies of the phenomenon of movement quality by Skjaerven (Skjaerven 1999, Skjaerven et al 2003, 2004, 2008, 2010).

In BBAT, the focus is particularly directed towards *movement awareness* and the sensitivity to *how* the movements are performed and experienced (Skjaerven et al., 2008). Movement awareness can be described as a sensitivity to movement nuances, becoming aware of one's own movement coordination, and how movements are performed in relation to space, time and energy, identifying subtle movement reactions in relation to internal, environmental and relational conditions. Movement that takes place without listening to, or becoming aware of, the way it is being carried out is described as mechanical (Alon, 1990).

MOVEMENT QUALITY IN BBAT

Movement quality (MQ) is a common term in physiotherapy. The phenomenon of MQ has been frequently used in BBAT, directing attention to how the movements are performed, observed by the physiotherapist and experienced by the patient. MQ can be described as 'the way in which movements are, in relation to space, time and energy'. The Movement Quality Model presents an overview of perspectives, movement elements and aspects identified in the phenomenon, altogether described as a general or an umbrella phenomenon, that is used as a roadmap for clinical implementation (Skjærven, 1999; Skjærven et al., 2003, 2004; 2008).

Postural balance, free breathing and mental awareness are identified as fundamental elements for gaining more functional MQ. It is how these three elements of balance, free breathing and mental awareness are integrated into the general movement coordination that adds quality, in general, to the movement coordination. According to Dropsy (Skjærven, 1999; 2002), 'it is the mind that gives the quality to the movement'.

Movement aspects, such as flow, elasticity, rhythm and intentionality, and also emotional, cultural and personal characteristics are observable and clinically used to improve functional movement coordination. Functional MQ is described as being balanced, free, centred, rhythmic, synchronous and unified. Dysfunctional movement quality is described as its opposite: unstable, mechanical, stiff, unrhythmical and lacking unity (Skjærven et al., 2008). Accordingly, a movement vocabulary for clinical use is available as a support for communication within the movement awareness domain (Skjaerven et al., 2007; Skjærven et al., 2008).

THERAPEUTIC FACTORS AND MOVEMENT PEDAGOGY

To promote MQ according to BBAT, the physiotherapist needs knowledge, skills and competence to communicate with the patient, team, family, etc., implementing a movement awareness approach

(Skjaerven et al., 2010). BBAT offers a set of therapeutic factors and a movement pedagogy for therapeutic use in transferring such perspectives, elements and aspects into individual and group physiotherapy. Therapeutic factors related to the promotion of MQ have been structured as: (1) *preconditions* for promoting MQ; (2) the *platform* and (3) the *strategy* for promoting MQ (Skjaerven et al., 2010).

The preconditions for promoting MQ point to the physiotherapist's own embodied movement awareness (Gyllensten et al., 2010; Skjaerven et al., 2010). The therapist's embodied presence and movement awareness are important for the quality and effectiveness of therapy, and for developing the physiotherapist's sensitivity to a broader view of movement and of the movement nuances. *Embodied presence* brings the possibility of closeness and familiarity between mind and body and of the coordination between the two. It is an expanded attention where being and knowing meet. Presence is different from knowledge that creates abstract explanations and is less easily brought into practice. Through presence the therapist focuses attention on the patient and on what is going on in that moment. When mentally and physically present, the therapist makes him/herself available to the patient; doing so has a positive treatment effect (Todres, 2007).

The platform for promoting MQ includes especially factors concerning the physiotherapist's preparation for the therapy and for creating a therapeutic atmosphere, being aware of physical, mental and relational processes during therapy. It is well known that the therapist–patient encounter is important for therapy and learning. The physiotherapist's genuineness, acceptance, trust and empathetic understanding are basic facilitators for learning. With increased awareness of the way in which the therapeutic process is perceived by the patient, the therapist increases the likelihood of significant learning. It is important to provide the patient with opportunities to experience learning situations that give rise to trust and acceptance. This form of therapy and learning differs markedly from an evaluative and technical approach. The physiotherapist is also in charge of providing a clear, developmental direction during therapy.

The strategies for promoting MQ include concrete actions for the movement awareness training and learning, such as the implementation of the Movement

Awareness Learning Cycle by supporting the patient to 'get it', meaning to become aware of old and new habits, of compensations as well as more healthy aspects (Skjaerven et al., 2010). Stepwise, the physiotherapist guides the patient to: (1) make contact with the body, (2) explore and experience the movement, (3) integrate the basic elements and aspects into the movements, (4) become familiar with and master the movements and (5) conceptualize and reflect upon the movement experiences. Presence is the hidden agent of help, in all forms of therapy (Yalom, 1995). Presence, awareness, embodiment and MQ represent keys in the therapeutic approach in BBAT. The physiotherapist guides the person to be involved in the here-and-now situation, obtaining self-experience and insight, performing very simple movements to rediscover more functional and useful ways of moving and acting in daily life.

An experiential learning model fosters practical learning based on insight into the use of principles, and therefore the ability to adapt to a variety of clinical situations (Dewey, 1934; Kolb, 1984; Duesund, 1995). Theory of movement pedagogy describes three types of movement teaching/learning: (1) learning about movement, (2) learning through movement and (3) learning by 'being in' movement (Dewey, 1934; Arnold, 1973; Skjærven et al., 2010) (Box 2). Learning about

movement is achieved by teaching movement as an academic subject, as in teaching the theory of human movement. Learning through movement is accomplished by teaching physical activities to stimulate specific goals. Learning by 'being in' movement means being in contact with what is 'going on', here and now.

The emphasis is on learning by being present, by experiencing and gaining insight in movement development as a process that is experienced and becomes integrated in the person. This type of teaching/learning is valuable in arousing the curiosity about how to change movement habits and improve self-awareness. 'Being in' movement requires a present state of the mind, 'being in' the here and now. Presence is an integral factor in the training of all movements (Skjærven et al., 2003; 2010).

BBAT can be implemented in traditional physiotherapy as a whole treatment concept or through the use of basic movement principles. As a consequence of its wide-ranging applicability, the BBAT literature describes its richness of perspectives, therapeutic factors and movement pedagogy.

Group Therapeutic Factors

BBAT is also intended to promote the ability to deal with personal and social relationships. Group therapy, in smaller or larger groups (up to 20 people), is therefore provided in addition to individual physiotherapy. In general, group therapeutic factors are a part of BBAT-groups, as in all models of group psychotherapy, and are consciously used by physiotherapists (Friis et al., 1989; Skatteboe et al., 1989; Leirvåg et al., 2010). According to Yalom, the most valuable factors are: (1) therapeutic attitude, (2) instillation of hope, (3) universality, (4) altruism, (5) interpersonal learning, (6) group cohesion and (7) existential factors with a focus on being present. Used with knowledge and good sense these factors are useful and practical elements to enhance the effect of physiotherapy (Friis et al., 1989; Skatteboe et al., 1989; Yalom, 1995; Leirvåg et al., 2010).

WHO CAN BENEFIT FROM BBAT?

Research has demonstrated that persons suffering from anxiety, depression and posttraumatic diseases have good results with BBAT (Danielsson, 2015;

BOX 2
THREE WAYS OF MOVEMENT LEARNING (ARNOLD, 1973)

WAYS OF MOVEMENT LEARNING	DESCRIPTIONS OF THE THREE WAYS OF LEARNING
Learning **about** *movement*	Learning *about* movement is achieved by teaching movement as an academic subject, as in teaching the theory of human movement
Learning **through** *movement*	Learning *through* movement is accomplished by teaching physical activities to stimulate specific goals
Learning **by** being **in** *movement*	Learning by *being in* movement means being in contact with what is 'going on', here and now.

Danielsson & Rosberg, 2015; Madsen et al., 2016). The studies reveal that participants become more aware of their bodies as a means to connect to themselves and to life, becoming more attuned to inner sensations and emotions, as well as to other people. Symptoms related to depression are reduced, resulting in improved motivation towards behavioural changes. A significant effect of treatment was reported and is described as a perceptual opening towards oneself and others, and towards more functional coping strategies in daily life (Danielsson & Rosberg, 2015; Johnsen & Råheim, 2010). Structured movement awareness training and learning, organized by the patient themselves, was described as necessary for gaining an effect.

Studies of the effectiveness of BBAT in treatment of persons diagnosed with schizophrenia showed more functional movement quality, better body image and less anxiety (Gyllensten et al., 2003; 2009), as well as stronger affect regulation and sense of greater well-being, vitality and interest (Hedlund & Gyllensten, 2013; Hedlund, 2014). Furthermore, BBAT has been shown to increase the ability to accept and tolerate more unpleasant experiences, coping with anxiety and promoting a sense of coherence. Improved body awareness and strengthened presence were reported to stimulate increased physical activity, safety and concentration (Skatteboe, 1991; Roxendal, 1985). Other studies with a qualitative research design support these findings (Hedlund & Gyllensten, 2010, 2013).

How patients suffering from eating disorders relate to their body and their body image is of special importance. Research has been conducted to search for relationships between the physiotherapist's observation of movement quality and the patient's report of movement experience, where BBAT was the main approach (Catalan-Matamoros, 2007; Thörnborg & Mattsson, 2009; Catalan-Matamoros et al., 2011). The results indicated that BBAT was useful in establishing a more realistic body image (Thörnborg & Mattsson, 2009).

BBAT has been implemented in physiotherapy for women with chronic pelvic pain (Mattsson et al., 1997; 1998; 2000) and has been used in the study of factors enhancing motivation (Grahn et al., 2000; Mannerkorpi & Gard, 2003; Fjellman-Wiklund et al., 2004). Studies including patients diagnosed with fibromyalgia indicate positive experiences from the embodied

learning process. By exploring new movement strategies, health-related quality of life and effectiveness of treatment were promoted. It was reported that when new movement principles became integrated, the patient learned how to reestablish a release and change the pattern of activity (Mannerkorpi & Gard, 2003; Gard, 2005).

After 1 year of follow-up physiotherapy for patients with long-lasting chronic pain where BBAT was included, it was found that physiotherapeutic assessment, focusing on movement quality, was a useful measure of body awareness. Such a measurement was important for gaining an overview of patient need and as a basis for an effective rehabilitation programme (Bergström et al., 2014).

BBAT Group Therapy as the main component in the treatment programme of people suffering from borderline personality disorder is reported in two studies (Skatteboe et al., 1989; Leirvåg et al., 2010). The participating patients improved significantly in: (1) functioning, (2) symptoms and (3) interpersonal problems. The magnitude of change in functioning and symptoms was significantly higher in the BBAT group when compared with therapeutic talk alone (Leirvåg et al., 2010). Movement group therapy, implemented in community-based physiotherapy, for patients with long-lasting pain, indicated more functional MQ, improved self-efficacy and relief of pain (Klingberg-Olsson et al., 2000).

BBAT is not directed specifically towards physical activity and training. However, clinical experience shows that patients can take up more demanding physical activity when they learn how to trust their bodies and when a sense of movement quality is established.

HISTORICAL ROOTS

BBAT was originally inspired by the French movement educator and psychotherapist Dropsy (Dropsy, 1973; 1984, 1998b). The Swedish physiotherapist Dr. Gertrud Roxendal introduced the approach into physiotherapy in Sweden and Norway at the end of the 1970s (Roxendal, 1985). In the last 30 years quality improvement, professional development and research have been initiated from the International Association of Teachers in Basic Body Awareness Therapy (IATBBAT)

(Skatteboe et al., 1989; Skatteboe, 1990; Mattsson, 1998; Skjærven, 1999; Gyllensten, 2001). BBAT was recognized in physiotherapy in Norway and Sweden in the late 1980s.

Background Influences

Building on basic knowledge within physiotherapy, BBAT additionally is influenced by theories of existential philosophy and psychology, and phenomenology, as well as aspects from movement science, also being inspired from Western and Eastern awareness traditions. BBAT draws upon Western philosophy (Buber, 1957; Merleau-Ponty, 1962; Pearls et al., 1973; Husserl, 1977). Seeing the body as a centre of human qualities such as perception, thoughts and feelings characterizes the perceptual processes as belonging to the body. Perception is seen as the prereflective background for any analytical thought. Particular emphasis is placed on the opportunity for the individual to learn through an increased ability to become aware, perceive and experience. Every practical experience is a physical interaction with the world and every practical understanding involves states of consciousness as well as states in the body (Merleau-Ponty, 1962; Skjaerven, 2008).

Study of the phenomenon of MQ made it possible to identify movement aspects from modern dance (Laban, 1960; Rederfern, 1965; Johnson, 1983; Horosko, 1991; Daly, 1995) and actors' training (Chekhov, 1985; Stanislavski, 1992; Grotowski, 1996) that have influenced BBAT. Gaining awareness in how to move is described as the gateway to movement learning (Alon, 1990). The theory and practice of movement awareness therapies have developed over more than 100 years (Jones, 1976; Johnson, 1983; Barlow, 1990; Feldenkrais, 1990). From the Eastern tradition, BBAT is slightly inspired by aspects from Za Zen meditation and tai chi (Suzuki, 1988; Yang, J-M., 1991a, 1991b).

QUALIFICATION

BBAT is for physiotherapists who aim to qualify in promoting human movement from a multiperspective approach. This provides the therapist with knowledge, skills and a general competence to practise basic movement principles with a multiperspective view, especially designed for the 'multifactorial suffering'.

BBAT is established within the curriculum in several of the Nordic physiotherapy BA study programmes, lately also at MA and PhD level. It is most often taught within the Association of Physiotherapy as a postgraduate course, but is also offered as private study programmes. It takes about 2 years to reach clinical competence. Several hundred physiotherapists have gained such qualification.

Western Norway Univeristy of Applied Sciences, has for 14 years offered an International postgraduate study programme, Basic Body Awareness Methodology (60 study points) for English-speaking physiotherapists, involving part-time study over 2 years. Around 120 physiotherapists, from 16 countries and three continents, have graduated during the period to gain clinical competence.

FOCUSING A NEED IN SOCIETY

BBAT, as a physiotherapeutic approach, was developed within Scandinavian physiotherapy in mental health and is increasingly attracting international interest. There is a professional need for physiotherapy approaches to meet the documented increase of people suffering from long-lasting multiperspective musculoskeletal and mental health problems within the cultural diversity in society. There is also a need to further develop structured, evidence-based approaches within the movement awareness domain in physiotherapy.

BBAT is clinically reported to be cost-effective, involves the patient and provides practical skills and insight for use in daily life. There is an increasing evidence base and wide clinical use. The outcome of physiotherapy needs, however, to be further studied. BBAT's movement principles and therapeutic strategies are simple and user-friendly, with a structured group approach and concrete focus on functional and health-promoting factors in movement awareness learning. This is of specific value in transferring knowledge from therapist to patient.

BBAT is known for its well-developed criteria for observing movement quality, and for having a vocabulary and criteria for describing, analysing, scoring, guiding and being in dialogue with the patient. It is, however, important to underline that BBAT cannot be implemented in physiotherapy for all kinds of musculoskeletal problems, and it is not for everyone.

A physiotherapeutic evaluation and clinical reasoning are basic to all clinical choices. There is still a need for further critical evaluation, research and clinical review, as well as opinion from society and from the patient's point of view in relation to BBAT.

REFERENCES

Alon, R., 1990. Mindful Spontaniety. Moving in Tune with Nature: Lessons in the Feldenkrais Method. Prism Press, Dorset, UK.

Arnold, P.J., 1973. Education and the concept of movement. Bull. Phys. Educ. IX 13–22.

Barlow, W., 1990. The Alexander Principle. How to Use Your Body Without Stress, second ed. Victor Gollancz, London, UK.

Bergström, M., Ejelöv, M., Mattsson, M., Stålnacke, B.M., 2014. One-year follow-up of body awareness and perceived health after participating in a multimodal pain rehabilitation programme—a pilot. Eur. J. Physiother. 16 (4), 246–254.

Brown, K.W., Ryan, R.M., 2003. The benefits of being present: mindfulness and its role in psychological well-being. J. Pers. Soc. Psychol. 84 (4), 822–848.

Buber, M., 1957. Pointing the Way. Harper and Row, New York.

Catalan-Matamoros, D., 2007. Physical Therapy in Mental health: Effectiveness of a Physiotherapeutic Intervention in Eating Disorders. Doctoral Thesis, Malaga University.

Catalan-Matamoros, D., Helvik-Skjaerven, L., Labajos-Manzanares, M.T., et al., 2011. A pilot study on the effect of Basic Body Awareness Therapy in patients with eating disorders: a randomized controlled trial. Clin. Rehabil. 25 (7), 617–626.

Chekhov, M., 1985. Lessons for the Professional Actor, first ed. Performing Arts Journal Publications, New York.

Daly, A., 1995. Done Into Dance. Isadora Duncan in America. Indiana University Press, Bloomington and Indianapolis.

Danielsson, L., 2015. Moved by Movement. A Person-Centered Approach to Physical Therapy in the Treatment of Major Depression. Doctoral thesis, Gøteborg University, Gøteborg.

Danielsson, L., Rosberg, S., 2015. Opening toward life: experiences of basic body awareness therapy in persons with major depression. Int. J. Qual. Stud. Health Well-being 10, 27069.

Dewey, J., 1934. Experience and Education. Collier Books, New York.

Dropsy, J., 1973. Vivre dans son Corps. Expression Corporelle et Relations Humaines (Living in your Body. Bodily Expression and Human Contact). Epi S.A, Paris.

Dropsy, J., 1984. Le Corps Bien Accordé—Un exercice Invisible (The Harmonic Body—An Invisible Exercise). Desclée De Brouwer, Paris.

Dropsy, J., 1998a. Body attunement—the conditions for body use. In: Skjaerven, L.H. (Ed.), Quality of Movement—the Art and Health. Lectures on Philosophy, Theory and Practical Implications to Basic Body Awareness Therapy. Skjærven, Bergen, pp. 21–34.

Dropsy, J., 1998b. Human expression—the coordination of mind and body. In: Skjaerven, L.H. (Ed.), Quality of Movement—the Art and Health. Lectures on Philosophy, Theory and Practical Implications to Basic Body Awareness Therapy. Skjærven, Bergen, pp. 8–20.

Duesund, L., 1995. Kropp, Kunnskap og Selvoppfatning (Body, Knowledge and Self-Experience). Universitetsforlaget, Oslo.

Feldenkrais, M., 1990. Awareness Through Movement: Health Exercises for Personal Growth, first ed. 1972. First HarperCollins, San Francisco.

Fjellman-Wiklund, A., Grip, H., Andersson, H., et al., 2004. EMG trapezius muscle activity pattern in string players: Part II – Influences of basic body awareness therapy on the violin playing technique. Int. J. Ind. Ergon. 33 (4), 357–367.

Friis, S., Skatteboe, U.B., Hope, M.K., Vaglum, P., 1989. Body awareness group therapy for patients with personality disorders. 2. Evaluation of the Body Awareness Rating Scale. Psychother. Psychosom. 51, 18–24.

Gard, G., 2005. Body awareness therapy for patients with fibromyalgia and chronic pain. Disabil. Rehabil. 27 (12), 725–728.

Ginzburg, K., Tsur, N., Barak-Nahum, A., Defrin, R., 2014. Body awareness: differentiating between sensitivity to and monitoring of bodily signals. J. Behav. Med. 37 (3), 564–575.

Grahn, B., Ekdahl, C., Borgquist, L., 2000. Motivation as a predictor of changes in quality of life and working ability in multidiscplinary rehabilitation. Disabil. Rehabil. 22 (15), 639–653.

Grotowski, J., 1996. Towards a Poor Theatre, first ed. published 1968. Methuen Drama, London.

Gyllensten, A.L., 2001. Basic Body Awareness Therapy. Doctoral Dissertation, Lund University, Lund.

Gyllensten, A.L., Hansson, L., Ekdahl, C., 2003. Outcome of Basic Body Awareness Therapy. A randomised controlled study of patients in psychiatric outpatient care. Adv. Physiother. 5, 179–190.

Gyllensten, A.L., Ekdahl, C., Hansson, L., 2009. Long-term effect of Basic Body Awareness Therapy in psychiatric outpatient care. A randomized controlled study. Adv. Physiother. 11, 2–12.

Gyllensten, A.L., Skar, L., Miller, M., Gard, G., 2010. Embodied identity—a deeper understanding of body awareness. Physiother. Theory Pract. 26 (7), 439–446.

Hedlund, L., Gyllensten, A.L., 2010. The experiences of basic body awareness therapy in patients with schizophrenia. J. Bodyw. Mov. Ther. 14 (3), 245–254.

Hedlund, L., Gyllensten, A.L., 2013. The physiotherapists' experience of Basic Body Awareness Therapy in patients with schizophrenia and schizophrenia spectrum disorders. J. Bodyw. Mov. Ther. 17 (2), 169–176.

Hedlund, L., 2014. Basal Kroppskänndeom och Psykomotorisk Function hos Personer med Allvarlig Psykisk Sjukdom. Doctoral Thesis, Lund University, Lund.

Hedlund, L., Gyllensten, A.L., Waldegren, T., Hansson, L., 2016. The reliability and validity of Body Awareness Scale movement quality and experience in persons with severe mental illness. Physiother. Theory Pract. 32 (4), 296–306.

Horosko, M., 1991. Martha Graham. The Evolution of Her Dance Theory and Training 1926–1991. A Cappella book. Chicago Review Press, Inc, Chicago, USA.

Husserl, E., 1977. Phenomenological Psychology. The Hague, Nijhoff.

Johnsen, R.W., Råheim, M., 2010. Feeling more in balance and grounded in one's own body and life. Focus group interviews on experiences with basic body awareness therapy in psychiatric healthcare. Adv. Physiother. 12, 166–174.

Johnson, D.H., 1983. Body: Recovering Our Sensual Wisdom. North Atlantic Books, California, USA. Somatic Resources.

Jones, F.P., 1976. Body Awareness in Action. A Study of the Alexander Technique. Schocken Books, New York.

Klingberg-Olsson, K., Lundgren, M., Lindström, I., 2000. 'Våga välja vad jag vill'—Basal Kroppskänndom och samtal i grupp—ett samarbetsprojekt mellan sjukgymnast och psykolog. Nordisk Fysioterapi 4, 133–142.

Kolb, D.A., 1984. Experiential Learning. Experience as the Source of Learning and Development. Prentice-Hall, Inc., Englewood Cliffs, New Jersey.

Laban, R., 1960. The Mastery of Movement. McDonald and Evans Ltd, London.

Leirvåg, H., Pedersen, G., Karterud, S., 2010. Long-term continuation treatment after short-term day treatment of female patients with severe personality disorders: Body Awareness Group Therapy versus Psychodynamic Group Therapy. Nord. J. Psychiatry 64 (3), 153–157.

Madsen, T.S., Carlsson, J., Nordbrandt, M., Jensen, J.A., 2016. Refugee experiences of individual basic body awareness therapy and the level of transference into daily life. An interview study. J. Bodyw. Mov. Ther. 20, 243–251.

Mannerkorpi, K., Gard, G., 2003. Physiotherapy group treatment for patients with fibromyalgia—an embodied learning process. Disabil. Rehabil. 25, 1372–1380.

Mattsson, M., Dahlgren, L., Mattsson, B., Armelius, K., 1997. Body Awareness Therapy with sexually abused women. Part 1: Description of treatment modality. J. Bodyw. Mov. Ther. 1, 280–288.

Mattsson, M., 1998. Body Awareness Applications in Physiotherapy. Dissertation, Umeå University, Umeå.

Mattsson, M., Wikman, M., Dahlgren, B., et al., 1998. Body awareness therapy with sexually abused women. Part 2: Evaluation of body awareness in a group setting. J. Bodyw. Mov. Ther. 2 (1), 38–45.

Mattsson, M., Wikman, M., Dahlgren, L., Mattsson, B., 2000. Physiotherapy as empowerment—treating women with chronic pelvis pain. Advances in Physiotherapy 2, 125–143.

Mehling, W.E., Wrubel, J., Daubenmier, J.J., et al., 2011. Body Awareness: a phenomenological inquiry into the common ground of mind-body therapies. Philos. Ethics Humanit. Med. 6, 6.

Merleau-Ponty, M., 1962. Phenomenology of Perception. Routledge & Kegan Paul Ltd, London.

Olsen, A.L., Skjaerven, L.H., 2016. Patients suffering from rheumatic disease describing own experiences from participating in Basic Body Awareness Group Therapy: a qualitative pilot study. Physiother. Theory Pract. 32 (2), 98–106.

Pearls, F., Hefferline, R., Goodman, P., 1973. Gestalt Therapy, Excitement and Growth in the Human Personality. Penguin Books, London.

Rederfern, B., 1965. Introducing Laban Art of Movement. MacDonald & Evans Ltd, London.

Roxendal, G., 1985. Body Awareness Therapy and the Body Awareness Scale, Treatment and Evaluation in Psychiatric Physiotherapy. Doctoral degree, University of Göteborg and Psychiatric Department II, Lillhagen Hospital, Hisings Backa, Göteborg.

Roxendal, G., 1987. Body Awareness Scale; BAS med instruction, manual och rörelsestest och faktorer för delskalor. Studentlitteratur, Stockholm.

Skatteboe, U.B., Friis, S., Hope, M.K., Vaglum, P., 1989. Body Awareness Group Therapy for Patients with Personality Disorders. 1. Description of the therapeutic method. Psychother. Psychosom. 51 (1), 11–17.

Skatteboe, U., 1990. Å være i samspill. En kroppsorientert gruppeterapi for pasienter med kroniske nevroser og personlighetsforstyrrelser (Being in relation. a bodyoriented group therapy for patients with chronic nevrosis and personality disorders). MSc, Statens Spesiallærerhøgskole Oslo. Hosle, Norway.

Skatteboe, U.B., 2000. Basal kroppskjennskap og bevegelsesharmoni. Videreutvikling av undersøkelsesmetoden Body Awareness Rating Scale, BARS-Bevegelsesharmoni (Body Awareness Therapy and Movement Harmony. Further development of the Assessment Scale Body Awareness Rating Scale). Oslo: Høgskolen i Oslo, Avdeling for helsefag; No 12.

Skjærven, L.H., 1999. 'Å være seg selv—mer fullt og helt'. En tilnærming til BEVEGELSESKVALITET. En feltstudie av en bevegelsespraksis av bevegelsespedagog og psykoterapeut Jacques Dropsy ('To be oneself – more fully'. An approach to movement quality. A Field study of the movement practice of the movement educator and Psychotherapist Jacques Dropsy). Masters Thesis, University of Bergen, Bergen.

Skjærven, L.H., (Ed.). 2002. Quality of Movement—the Art and Health. Lectures on Philosophy, Theory and Practical Implications to Basic Body Awareness Therapy. Bergen.

Skjærven, L.H., Gard, G., Kristoffersen, K., 2003. Basic elements and dimensions to quality of movement—a case study. J. Bodyw. Mov. Ther. 7 (4), 251–260.

Skjærven, L.H., Gard, G., Kristoffersen, K., 2004. Greek sculpture as a tool in understanding the phenomenon of movement quality. J. Bodyw. Mov. Ther. 8 (3), 227–236.

Skjaerven, L., Kristoffersen, K., Gard, G., 2007. A Movement Vocabulary for Use in Training Movement Quality. Paper presented at the World Confederation of Physical Therapy, WCPT, Vancouver, Canada.

Skjærven, L.H., Kristoffersen, K., Gard, G., 2008. An eye for movement quality: a phenomenological study of movement quality reflecting a group of physiotherapists' understanding of the phenomenon. Physiother. Theory Pract. 24 (1), 13–27.

Skjaerven, L.H., Kristoffersen, K., Gard, G., 2010. How can movement quality be promoted in clinical practice? A phenomenological study of physical therapist experts. Phys. Ther. 90 (10), 1479–1492.

Skjærven, L.H., 2013. Basic Body Awareness Therapy—Promoting Movement Quality and Health for Daily Life. Documentary and Tutorial films. Basic Body Awareness Methodology (BBAM). Bergen, Norway.

Skjaerven, L.H., Gard, G., Sundal, M.A., Strand, L.I., 2015. Reliability and validity of the Body Awareness Rating Scale (BARS), an observational assessment tool of movement quality. Eur. J. Physiother. 19–28.

Skjærven, L.H., Sundal, M.A., 2016. Basic Body Awareness Therapy—Movement awareness, everyday movement and health promotion in physiotherapy. Fysioterapeuten 4, 42–44.

Stanislavski, K., 1992. An Actor Prepares. (E.R. Hapgood, Trans.), 10th ed. Methuen Drama, London, UK.

Strand, L.I., Olsen, A.L., Nygård, H., et al., 2016. Basic Body Awareness Therapy and patient education in hip osteoarthritis: a multiple case study. Eur. J. Physiother. 18, 116–125.

Suzuki, S., 1988. Zen Mind, Beginner's Mind. Informal talks on Zen meditation and practice. John Weatherhill, Inc, Tokyo.

Thörnborg, U., Mattsson, M., 2009. Rating body awareness in persons suffering from eating disorders—a cross-sectional study. Advances in Physiotherapy 12, 1–11.

Todres, L., 2007. Embodied Enquire. Phenomenological Touchstones for Research, Psychotherapy and Spirituality. Palgrave Macmillan, New York.

WHO, 2013. A European policy framework supporting action across government and society for health and well-being: Proceedings of regional Committee for Europe. WHO Europe, Copenhagen.

Yalom, I., 1995. The Theory and Practice of Group Psychotherapy, third ed. BasicBooks, New York.

Yang, Jwing-Ming, 1991a. Advanced Yang Style T'ai Chi Chuan. Martial Application, vol. 2. Ymaa Publication Center, Yang's Martial Arts Association, Massachusetts.

Yang, Jwing-Ming, 1991b. Advanced Yang Style T'ai Chi Chuan. T'ai Chi Theory and T'ai Chi Jing. Yamma Publication Center. Yang's Martial Arts Association, Massachusetts.

3.3

PSYCHOMOTOR THERAPY OR PHYSIOTHERAPY IN MENTAL HEALTH FOR PATIENTS WITH PSYCHIATRIC PROBLEMS

MICHEL PROBST ▪ TINE VAN DAMME ▪ DAVY VANCAMPFORT

SUMMARY

This chapter proposes a framework for physiotherapists working in mental health and psychiatry using three different approaches: a developmental and physical health-related approach, a psychosocial and physiopsychological approach and a psychotherapeutic physiotherapy approach. This framework is based on evidence-based research and clinical practice. Originally this framework was conceived by physiotherapists working with patients with severe psychiatric disorders in a residential treatment programme. Owing to the socialization of care, these ideas were translated for physiotherapists working in general mental health care.

KEY POINTS

- Considering a physiotherapy framework for treating severe psychiatric disorders.
- Group psychotherapy in residential psychiatric treatment is a worth-full strategy.
- The focus of the physiotherapy approach was on the physical and mental health, lifestyle and quality of life of patients with severe mental illness.

LEARNING OBJECTIVES

- Gaining a deeper understanding of the use of physical activity as a psychosocial and psychotherapeutic physiotherapy approach.
- Describe why ideas deduced from psychotherapy is a more value for physiotherapy in psychiatry.

- Improve the physical and mental health, lifestyle and quality of life of patients with severe mental illnesses.
- Include ideas on psychotherapy to offer more effective physiotherapy interventions.
- Think outside the well-known physiotherapy box and discover new ideas.

INTRODUCTION

In Belgium, psychomotor therapy or physiotherapy in mental health has been a specific domain within the field of physiotherapy since 1965.

Psychomotor therapy is defined as a method of treatment based on a holistic view of the human being that is derived from the unity of body and mind. Assessments (observation and/or evaluation) are essential to achieving concrete psychosocial objectives methodically. Psychomotor therapy uses movement, body awareness and a wide range of movement activities to optimize movement behaviour as well as the cognitive, affective and relational aspects of psychomotor functioning (i.e., the relationships between physical movements and cognitive and social affective aspects). Consequently, the approach to this type of therapy integrates the physical, cognitive and emotional aspects of functioning in relation to the capacity of being and acting in a psychosocial context in order to achieve clearly defined goals in consultation with the patient (Probst et al., 2010).

Psychomotor therapy is considered an important standard supplemental treatment to biomedical treatment for patients with mental health problems in all residential centres ($n = 33$) in the Dutch-speaking part of Belgium. In addition, psychomotor therapy is also currently included in primary health care.

Physiotherapists in mental health care distinguish themselves from other specializations in physiotherapy because they aim to achieve positive therapeutic results regarding the patient's mental health problems (depression, anxiety, schizophrenia, autism, eating disorders, etc.), by systematically using (adapted) body experiences and physical activities, movement, sensory awareness and sports. During these activities, the emphasis is placed on the interests and capabilities of individuals with limiting conditions. Today, physiotherapy in mental health is focused on the prevention, treatment and rehabilitation of people with light, mild and severe mental health problems in residential, community and primary health care. Both individual as well as group approaches are offered.

HISTORY

In 1962 the graduate education programme for the study of physiotherapy at the KU Leuven (Catholic University of Leuven) was updated. At that time, Professor Denayer, the Dean of the department, underlined the importance of including physiotherapy for persons with physical disabilities as well as persons with mental health problems. For that era, these ideas were innovative.

These ideas resulted from the approach of Simon (1929) and Meyer (1977, 1983) and also from the approach used in the Netherlands (Probst & Bosscher, 2001), who were trendsetters for a more active approach towards patients with mental illness. These ideas were adapted to the Belgian context by Professor Pierloot and Professor Vancoppenolle (Pierloot, 1968; Pierloot & Van Coppenolle, 1981). Initially, the term *movement therapy* was used.

The biopsychosocial model of Engel, which incorporates biological, psychological and social elements, had an important influence on the psychomotor therapy approach in mental health. Gradually, the attention changed from physical activity (*mens sana in corpore sano*) to how people move in relation to their environment and how they use physical activity in

their tasks, activities and responsibilities. The main idea was the interaction between physical activity and the mind. The topic pertained to a therapeutic working approach to the body in movement for children and adults. Attention was given to cognitions, emotions, perception, awareness and social and contextual factors. Therefore the term *psychomotor therapy* (PMT) was preferred; this name change accommodated the notion that PMT encompasses 'movement' or 'physical activity' in a strict sense (Probst et al., 2010; Probst and Simons, 2008).

THE CORNERSTONES OF PHYSIOTHERAPY IN MENTAL HEALTH

Although physical activity has somatic effects (on the morphological, muscular, cardiorespiratory, metabolic and motor levels), PMT is still mainly considered a psychosocial treatment. The relationship between the patient and the psychomotor therapist is a central aspect. The experiences during PMT and the responses that emerge through these experiences function as a dynamic power of change (Probst et al., 2010). This notion can be embedded in several psychotherapeutic approaches. However, the term *psychomotor* progressed independently and has been adapted in various countries. The (dis)similarities regarding the term *psychomotor* must be understood in the context of the divergent cultural histories of the different countries. Today, the term *psychomotor therapy* or *physiotherapy* in mental health refers to a developmental and health-related approach, a psychosocial approach and a psychotherapeutic physiotherapy approach.

Developmental and Health-Related Approach

The developmental approach includes the identification, observation and treatment of individuals with developmental disabilities, including individuals with intellectual disabilities. In agreement with the cornerstone of psychomotor therapy, namely the unity between body and mind, the general starting point is the strong and continuous interaction between the different developmental domains (motor, cognitive and social-affective). For instance, the absence of proficient motor ability may have an impact on opportunities for social development or influence the development of self-esteem. Consequently, this approach is mainly directed towards supporting and aiding an individual's (psycho)motor development, while accounting for the complex and continuous interactions between different developmental domains. Within this approach, diagnostic assessment through standardized motor assessment instruments and qualitative observations is predominant. Moreover, interventions aiming to improve fine and gross motor skills, writing skills, body coordination, hand–eye coordination, balance and time and space perception are being implemented.

In addition to the functional recovery of motor impairment and disability in the field of mental health disorders, the physical health-related approach aims to improve global physical health. Specifically, the use of physical activity in the therapeutic environment focuses on enabling good physical condition and maintaining good physical health in people with mental health problems. Similar to the developmental approach, other factors are considered, for example, the fact that people with mental health problems are more susceptible to inactivity and are at risk of a sedentary lifestyle. Moreover, it is well established that the use of psychotropic drugs can result in the development of metabolic syndrome, obesity, osteoporosis and cardiovascular disease.

The health-related approach is consistent with recent recommendations from national and international policy makers. The World Health Organization (WHO) drew attention to 'physical inactivity' as one of the most common and persistent contributors to poor health worldwide.

In 2012 the theme of the World Physical Therapy Day (of the World Confederation for Physical Therapy) was 'Movement for Health: Fit for Life'. Emphasis was also placed on noncommunicable diseases and the importance of physical activity across the lifespan to promote the health, wellness and fitness of global populations regardless of their age.

In recent years, many efforts have been made to improve the physical health and lifestyle of patients with severe mental illness (i.e., major depression, schizophrenia and bipolar disorders). Physical diseases in this group of patients contribute to premature death, with over 20 years lost compared with the general population. Moreover, these diseases constitute a serious threat to their quality of life. Physical therapists along with medical doctors are well placed to work on improving physical health. In addition, physical inactivity is not only present in patients with mental health problems; each year, 2 million people die from inactivity worldwide (WHO, 2002).

Furthermore, it is important to promote physical activity during childhood because inactive children and adolescents stay inactive when they grow up (Vanreusel, 2009). In contrast, several studies have indicated that children with good motor skills are more likely to become fit adolescents (Barnett et al., 2008) and to maintain adequate fitness levels into adulthood (Stodden et al., 2009). However, it is well established that co-occurring motor problems are highly prevalent in children and adolescents with mental health problems (Van Damme et al., 2015). Consequently, because motor ability is an important determinant of physical activity, these children are at risk of being less physically active and developing an inactive lifestyle.

The consequences of physical inactivity in mental health are very serious; it is therefore important to promote physical activity. Although campaigns promoting physical activity exist, most of them fail. One of the possible reasons for this failure is that these campaigns do not underline the importance of tailoring physical activity to each person's individual abilities. The isolation and fewer social contacts of individuals with mental health problems may lead to an inability to reach these people and therefore present an additional challenge to these types of campaign within the field of mental health. Furthermore, the surplus value of the consequences of physical activity with regard to quality of life is often not mentioned. It is important to bear in mind (and live in adherence to these values) that individuals should stay active throughout their daily life. In this way, they can enjoy the present and establish solid foundations for the coming years. Those who do not continue to exercise lose independence and will not maximize their potential in life. If individuals have problems that might affect how they exercise, they should receive advice from a physical therapist. The old Latin quote 'mens sana, in corpore sano' still applies. The literature offers different guidelines (Box 1), but it is important to integrate and adapt these guidelines to the context of a person with mental health problems.

BOX 1
CANADIAN GUIDELINES FOR
PHYSICAL ACTIVITY

FOR CHILDREN (5–11 YEARS) AND
ADOLESCENTS (12–17 YEARS) THE FOLLOWING
IS ADVISED:

- daily moderate- to vigorous-intensity physical activity for at least 60 minutes;
- additionally, vigorous-intensity activities at least 3 days per week;
- activities that strengthen muscle and bone at least 3 days per week.

FOR ADULTS (18–65 YEARS OLD):

- at least 150 minutes of moderate- to vigorous-intensity aerobic physical activity per week, in sessions of 10 minutes or more;
- in addition, engaging in muscle- and bone-strengthening activities that use major muscle groups at least 2 days per week.

For both age groups, the rule of more physical activity providing greater health benefits applies, see http://www.csep.ca/en/guidelines/get-the-guideline.

Psychosocial-Oriented and Psychophysiological Approaches

In the psychosocial-oriented approach, the emphasis lies mainly on the acquisition of mental and physical proficiencies related to the body in motion and on supporting personal development to enhance an individual's ability to function independently in society.

The activities aim at learning, acquiring, training and/or practising psychomotor, sensomotor, perceptual, cognitive, social and emotional proficiencies. More concretely, the following aspects are highlighted: attention, interaction with materials, recognition of stimuli, suppression of passivity, altering of behaviour, goal-oriented working, enhancing attention on others, improving social proficiency, learning to collaborate, learning to cope with emotionality, learning to accept responsibilities and being able to put oneself in someone else's place.

Other elementary proficiencies are stressed, such as relaxation education, relaxation skills, stress management, breathing techniques, psychomotor and sensory skills, and also cognitive, expression and social skills. Through exercises, patients acquire a broader perspective and can experience their own abilities.

Moreover, learning the basic rules of communication is also integrated.

The psychophysiological approach involves the use of physical activity to influence mental health problems, for instance depression and anxiety.

Many investigations have reported the occurrence of beneficial mental health effects as a consequence of participation in physical activity. Physical activity is believed to have a positive influence on mental well-being, self-esteem, mood and executive functioning. Through these effects, a downward spiral leading to dejection may be stopped. Well-balanced and regularly executed endurance activities (walking, biking, jogging, swimming), power training (fitness training) and mindfulness-derived exercises augment physical and mental resilience, improve the quality of sleep, enhance self-confidence, energy level, endurance level and relaxation and, in general, decrease physical complaints. At the very least, physical activity seems to be equally effective as the classic approach of medication and supportive contact. This type of intervention is based on research in the field of exercise, sport psychology and psychomotor therapy.

Because an increase in physical fitness is not necessarily accompanied by an improvement in physical self-concept, therapists need to focus not only on training effects but also on enhancing strategies for improving physical self-concept.

Psychotherapeutic-Oriented Physiotherapy Approach

A less common approach is the psychotherapeutic-oriented physiotherapy approach. The motor domain is employed as a gateway to ameliorating the social affective functioning of an individual. Within this approach, the physiotherapist creates a setting that favours the initiation and development of a process in the patient using specific working methods that aim to help patients access their inner workings.

By offering activities related to the theme of 'body in motion', individuals are invited to venture outside their comfort zone, experience new things and become more in touch with their inner self. This allows them to gain better insight into their own performance.

Patients are invited to participate, individually or in groups, in a wide range of physical activities and movements. In participating actively, patients experience many emotions (depressive feelings, fear, guilt, anger, stress, feelings of unease, estrangement and dissatisfaction) and negative thoughts (intrusion, obsession, morbid preoccupations, worry).

Patients with mental health problems are confronted with their behaviour (i.e., impulses, lack of abilities) or cognitive symptoms (i.e., derealisation, lack of concentration). In some cases, however, patients do not experience these emotions or symptoms at all. Throughout physiotherapy interventions, an alternative perspective on experiences can be proposed. Experiencing the notion that an alternative may exist will trigger new emotions and experiences, and a discrepancy between reality and the patient's perception of their reality will emerge. Consequently, it is important to note that it is not the physical activity itself but the patient's experiences and inner perception that plays the central role. The following themes are taken into consideration: being aware of body and movement, expressing and regulating emotions, augmenting tolerance for frustration, refraining from impulsive behaviour, improving reality orientation, improving social interaction, learning to define limits, strengthening self-confidence, improving body perception and self-perception, dealing with fear of failure, developing self-reflection, exploring actual emotional and social life and providing better insight into one's consciousness through inter- and intrapsychic conflicts.

The careful guidance and encouragement of the physiotherapist and the opportunity to experience feelings in a safe environment allow the patient to develop behaviour that he or she would not have developed otherwise. The underlying problems are not necessarily resolved, but the therapist tries to improve the patient's management of their problems. The patient shares their behaviour, feelings and thoughts with the therapist initially, and eventually with their peers. More emphasis is placed on experiences and how reactions to these experiences function as a dynamic source of power.

In this approach, a rationale for applying psychological models (e.g., cognitive behavioural therapy, acceptance and commitment therapy) is offered as a tool to strengthen physiotherapy interventions in children, adolescents, adults and the elderly. Currently, cognitive behavioural therapy is recommended in a wide variety of disorders (chronic low back pain, eating disorders, etc.). Although physiotherapists are not trained in cognitive behavioural therapy, clinical practice reveals that some effective and appropriate cognitive behavioural strategies can be implemented in a patient's physiotherapy treatment. Therefore additional and adapted training in cognitive behavioural therapy for physiotherapists is necessary to provide effective interventions.

In addition to the cognitive behavioural therapy treatment approach, different modalities such as relaxation, mindfulness-oriented exercises, cognitive functional training, graded exercise therapy and adaptive pacing therapy for children and adults are integrated into this treatment.

REFERENCES

Barnett, L.M., Van Beurden, E., Morgan, P.J., et al., 2008. Does childhood motor skill proficiency predict adolescent fitness? Med. Sci. Sports Exerc. 40, 2137–2144.

Meyer, A., 1977. The philosophy of occupational therapy. Reprinted from the Archives of Occupational Therapy, Volume 1, pp. 1–10, 1922. Am. J. Occup. Ther. 31, 639–642.

Meyer, A., 1983. The philosophy of Occup Ther Ment Health. Occup. Ther. Ment. Health 2 (3), 79–86.

Pierloot, R., 1968. Algemene Grondslagen van de Bewegingstherapie in de Psychiatrie. Fonteyn, Leuven.

Pierloot, R., Van Coppenolle, H., 1981. Grondslagen van de Psychomotorische Therapie. Lochem, De Tijdstroom.

Probst, M., Bosscher, R.J. (Eds.), 2001. Ontwikkelingen in de Psychomotorische Therapie (Developments in Psychomotor Therapy.) Cure & Care Publishers, Zeist, pp. 37–50.

Probst, M., Knapen, J., Poot, G., Vancampfort, D., 2010. Psychomotor therapy and psychiatry: what's in a name? Open Complement Med. J. 2, 105–113.

Probst, M., Simons, J., 2008. Psychomotorische therapie in Vlaanderen: voorstel tot beroepsprofiel en functieomschrijving (Psychomotor therapy in Flanders: Proposition of a Functional Description.) In: Simons, J. (Ed.), Actuele Themata uit de Psychomotorische Therapie. Acco, Leuven, pp. 11–46.

Simon, H., 1929. Aktivere Krankenbehandlung in der Irrenanstalt (Active Treatment in a Residential Center.) W. de Gruyter, Berlin.

Stodden, D., Langendorfer, S., Roberton, M.A., 2009. The association between motor skill competence and physical fitness in young adults. Res. Q. Exerc. Sport 80, 223–229.

Van Damme, T., Simons, J., Sabbe, B., van West, D., 2015. Motor abilities of children and adolescents with a psychiatric condition: a systematic literature review. World J. Psychiatry 5 (3), 315–329.

Vanreusel, B., Meulders, B., 2007. Sedentary lifes styles and physical (in-)activity in youth, a social risk perspective. In: Brettschneider, W., Naul, R. (Eds.), Obesity in Europe: young people's physical activity and sedentary life styles. Peter Lang, Frankfurt am Main, pp. 119–133.

World Health Organisation, 2002. The World Health report 2002. Reducing risks, promoting healthy life. WHO, Geneva.

3.4

PRESCRIBING PHYSICAL ACTIVITY IN MENTAL HEALTHCARE SETTINGS

DAVY VANCAMPFORT ■ ANDREW SOUNDY ■ BRENDON STUBBS

SUMMARY

Physiotherapists are ideally placed to promote the health and well-being of people with severe mental illnesses through physical activity prescription. In this chapter we describe how physiotherapists can motivate people with severe mental illness, starting from the 5A model (assess, advise, agree, assist, arrange). The 5A model of behaviour change and counselling has been shown to increase healthy behaviours, positively influence mediators of behavioural change, increase communication skills about health behaviour change and to improve patient outcomes.

KEY POINTS

■ When trying to motivate people with severe mental illness, psychosocial factors such as readiness for change and self-efficacy should be assessed.

■ Counselling of people with severe mental illness should be tailored to the individual patient's stage of change.

■ With shared decision-making and active listening, physiotherapists should agree with their patients on a set of SMART (specific, measurable, attainable, relevant, time-based) goals.

■ Physiotherapists should arrange for follow-up assessment, feedback and social support.

LEARNING OBJECTIVES

■ Understand how the 5A model of behaviour change and counselling can be implemented in daily clinical physiotherapy practice.

■ Understand why physiotherapists are ideally placed to motivate people with severe mental illness towards an active lifestyle.

PHYSIOTHERAPISTS HAVE A CENTRAL ROLE IN PROMOTING PHYSICAL ACTIVITY IN MENTAL HEALTHCARE SETTINGS

The universal aim of physiotherapy is to maximize human movement potential within the spheres of promotion, prevention, treatment and rehabilitation (World Confederation for Physical Therapy, 2007). This predominantly includes providing services for individuals whose function and movement are impaired or threatened by disease, injury or environmental factors. Furthermore, physiotherapy involves the interaction between the physiotherapist, patient, other health professionals, families, caregivers and wider community in a process where movement potential is assessed and goals are agreed upon (Probst, 2012). According to the position statement of the World Confederation for Physical Therapy (2007), physiotherapists may be concerned in a variety of settings with any of the following purposes:

■ promoting the health and well-being of individuals, emphasizing the importance of physical activity and exercise,

■ preventing impairments, activity limitations, participatory restrictions and disabilities in individuals at risk of altered movement behaviours due to health or medical-related factors, socioeconomic stressors, environmental factors and lifestyle factors,

■ providing interventions/treatment to restore integrity of body systems essential to movement, maximize function and recuperation, minimize incapacity, and enhance the quality of life, independent living and workability in individuals and groups of individuals with altered movement behaviours resulting from impairments, activity limitations, participatory restrictions and disabilities,

- modifying environmental, home and work access and barriers to ensure full participation in one's normal and expected societal roles.

Thus it is clear that physiotherapists are healthcare professionals specialized in human movement and its relationship with health. Additionally, physiotherapists are trained to prescribe safe physical activity, even among high-risk patients. This makes physiotherapists ideal for promoting safe and healthy physical activity in people with a severe mental illness.

In a recent survey of physiotherapists from over 30 countries working with severely mentally ill patients (Stubbs et al., 2014a), respondents reported that one of their most important roles is to act as a bridge between physical and mental health issues. In particular, respondents felt that they have an important role in the promotion of lifestyle physical activity and in overseeing the delivery of structured exercise in this population.

THE BENEFITS OF PHYSICAL ACTIVITY AND EXERCISE PRESCRIPTION IN PEOPLE WITH SEVERE MENTAL ILLNESS

The physical and mental health benefits of regular physical activity in people with severe mental illnesses are well documented. Numerous studies have articulated the need to promote an active lifestyle in the management of the physical and mental health in this population. Trials of physical activity as a treatment modality for depression has demonstrated that physical activity is as effective as antidepressants or psychotherapy for mild to moderate anxiety and depression (Cooney et al., 2013). For more severe mental illnesses (such as schizophrenia), physical activity has been found to be an important complementary therapy ameliorating the physical as well as mental health of these patients (Gorczynski & Faulkner, 2010;

Vancampfort et al., 2012a, 2014a; Rosenbaum et al., 2014). Structured physical activity is also effective in improving behavioural functioning among those with eating disorders (Vancampfort et al., 2013a,b). Next to this, physical activity is known to promote mental health in various ways (e.g., by internal factors such as increased self-efficacy and decreased stress, and external factors such as increased social contact) (Scully et al., 1998; Eime et al., 2013). The international guidelines for promoting physical and mental health recommend an accumulation each week of a minimum of 150 minutes of exercise at moderate intensity or a minimum of 75 minutes at vigorous intensity, in bouts of at least 10 minutes, 3 to 5 days per week (Vancampfort et al., 2012b). Nevertheless, only a minority of persons with severe mental illness are physically active at a level compatible with these proposed health recommendations (Soundy et al., 2014a). Therefore (1) a more conservative approach to the intensity of prescription and (2) consideration of a structured or supported environment initially, have been recommended previously for persons with severe mental illness (Skrinar, 2003).

GENERAL PRINCIPLES OF PHYSICAL ACTIVITY COUNSELLING

A lack of motivation to undertake physical activity has been identified as a primary reason for physical inactivity or sedentary behaviour, including reports from individuals with severe mental illness (Ussher et al., 2007), mental health physiotherapists (Soundy et al., 2014b) and other healthcare professionals (McKibbin et al., 2014). Further to this, individuals often report being ambivalent about changing their physical activity behaviour (Soundy et al., 2007). Given the complex interplay of both physical and mental health related barriers for being physically active in individuals with severe mental illness, it is important that physical activity counselling is adopted by trained mental health physiotherapists. It should be considered a key aspect of their role. The 5A model (assess, advise, agree, assist, arrange) of behaviour change and counselling has been shown to increase healthy behaviours, to positively influence mediators of behavioural change, to increase communication skills about health behaviour change and to improve patients' outcomes

(Glasgow et al., 2004; Beaulac et al., 2011; Orrow et al., 2012). The 5A model is a well-established model that can be utilized in physiotherapy practice. In the next paragraphs, we give a brief overview of the most important principles.

Assess

Assessing a patient's current physical activity level is complex. Eliciting the frequency, intensity and duration of physical activity from patients is important in determining if they meet the minimum health recommendations. In order to achieve this, mental health physiotherapists will need to consider the type, intensity and duration of physical activity patients are participating in and be aware of the broad range of activities (e.g., lifestyle physical activity and/or work-related physical activity) that can be included outside structured physical activity programmes. Thus it is important that mental health physiotherapists understand these activities in order to tailor recommendations to patients' preferences. Physical activity can be assessed through objective and self-reported measures, although the choice of tool requires important consideration. Objective monitoring devices such as pedometers and accelerometers have been used in people with a severe mental illness; however, with poor rates of compliance resulting in limited valid data (Jerome et al., 2009). Older age, current employment, tertiary education, nonsmoking and high level of self-reported health have all been found to be associated with higher compliance with accelerometer protocols in the general population (Lee et al., 2013). Given that many people with a severe mental illness are unemployed, have a lower education level, smoke and show worse health perceptions, compliance with such devices is likely to be suboptimal. Self-report questionnaires provide a feasible, cost-effective alternative to objective measures, with varying levels of agreement and correlation with objective measures (Warren et al., 2010). Self-report tools may, however, lack precision, may not detail the different domains of physical activity (frequency, intensity and type) or may be influenced by a recall bias (Soundy et al., 2014a). Recently, a comprehensive review of the selection, use and psychometric properties of physical activity measures used in studies evaluating physical activity in people with severe mental illness was

conducted, highlighting methodological limitations in the few studies reporting validity coefficients for self-report questionnaires (Soundy et al., 2014a). The heterogeneity in the instruments also highlights a lack of agreement between researchers studying physical activity and mental illness as to the most appropriate questionnaire for use in this particular population (Soundy et al., 2014a). Well-utilized questionnaires in the general population are likely to be the most appropriate (e.g., the International Physical Activity Questionnaire; Craig et al., 2003), however, the validation of such tools in individuals with severe mental illness is often not without methodological weaknesses. To date, no population-specific tool has been devised that incorporates the complex and unique challenges faced by people with mental illness.

Psychosocial factors, such as readiness for change, social support and self-efficacy (i.e., patients' self-confidence that they can change behaviour) must also be assessed because all these factors are known to be associated with physical activity participation in people with severe mental illness (Vancampfort et al., 2012c, 2013c; Soundy et al., 2014b). In the same way, physiotherapists are encouraged to assess the patient's willingness to involve family or friends in order to increase physical activity (Vancampfort et al., 2012c, 2013c; Soundy et al., 2014b). Finally, the physiotherapist must determine if there are medical conditions that require diagnostic evaluation or modified management before the patient can safely initiate or increase physical activity (Vancampfort et al., 2012c, 2013c; Soundy et al., 2014b).

Advise

Advice should, at a minimum, be focused on the potential benefits of being physically active, the physical activity recommendations incorporating FITT-principles (frequency, intensity, type and time) and potential barriers, facilitators and risks. Previous research in people with severe mental illnesses (Gorczynski et al., 2010; Vancampfort et al., 2014b) demonstrated that advice should vary at different stages of change. One framework that might assist physiotherapists in categorizing a person's readiness to change their behaviour is the transtheoretical model of change (Prochaska & DiClemente, 1983; Prochaska & Marcus, 1994).The transtheoretical model of change includes five stages. In the first stage, the precontemplation phase, individuals are physically inactive and are not thinking about becoming more active within the next 6 months. During the second stage, the contemplation stage, individuals think about becoming more active within the next 6 months. In these stages physiotherapists can provide their patients with information on the benefits of physical activity that are tailored to the individual and based on gradually achieving the current physical activity guidelines (e.g., that physical activity can be accumulated during the course of the day). In the third stage, the preparation stage, individuals are engaging in some physical activity. Patients in the preparation stage could, for example, be advised to develop plans using SMART goals (an acronym for the five attributes of specific, measurable, attainable, relevant and time-based goals) to increase their physical activity to the recommended levels. This could be supplemented by taking advantage of social and recreational programming offered in the community (Gorczynski et al., 2010). In the penultimate stage, the action stage, individuals have been regularly active for less than 6 months while the last stage, the maintenance stage, is characterized by an individual having sustained regular physical activity for more than 6 months. Patients in the action and maintenance stages could be encouraged to think about relapse prevention and put in place strategies to overcome relapses in regular physical activity.

Agree

With shared decision making and active listening, physiotherapists can agree with their patients on a set of SMART goals. Physiotherapists should determine what steps the patient is willing to take to increase physical activity and should endorse the patient's plans, if appropriate. Understanding the best steps to take for each stage of the transtheoretical model of behaviour change (Prochaska & DiClemente, 1983; Prochaska & Marcus, 1994) can help physiotherapists facilitate change.

Assist

Changing physical activity behaviours is challenging. However, physical activity counselling that is patient-centred and nonjudgmental, respects patient autonomy, incorporates patient preferences and motivations,

takes into account the competences of the individual and uses processes of change is most likely to be successful (Gorczynski et al., 2010; Vancampfort et al., 2013d). Counselling in people with severe mental illness should therefore be tailored to the individual patient's stage of change (Gorczynski et al., 2010; Vancampfort et al., 2014b).

Arrange

Physiotherapists should arrange for follow-up assessment, informative feedback and social support. Follow-up is associated with better maintenance of behaviour change. It can take the form of a follow-up appointment, brief telephone call or online contact. SMART goals should be reviewed to build to the recommended activity levels for mental and physical health benefits and to cope with barriers while continued activity is reinforced. Providing social support is a significant part of the physiotherapist's role (Soundy et al., 2014c). There are different types of functional social support physiotherapists can offer: (1) emotional support (i.e., communication that meets an individual's emotional or affective needs), (2) esteem support (i.e., communication that bolsters an individual's self-esteem or beliefs in their ability to handle barriers), (3) informational support (i.e., communication that provides useful or required information to make decisions in challenging situations) and (4) looking for tangible support (i.e., any practical assistance provided by others) (Soundy et al., 2014c). Further consideration of an individual's previous identity associated with physical activity and sport may provide a physiotherapist with ideas of what groups the individual may like to be part of. This is important since a positive athletic identity can have a very positive impact on individuals' mental health (Soundy et al., 2012).

THE NEED TO UNLOCK THE POTENTIAL OF PHYSIOTHERAPISTS IN MENTAL HEALTHCARE SETTINGS

There is an ongoing debate regarding the integration of physical activity counsellors without a physiotherapy background into general practice (Verhagen & Engbers, 2009). There has been some research that has investigated the role of such counsellors, but this has had little success. For example, Chalder et al. (2012) investigated the influence of a physical activity programme by such counsellors among people with depression and demonstrated no effect on depressive symptoms or reduction of antidepressant use. The same group of researchers made the bold conclusion that advice and encouragement to increase physical activity is not an effective strategy for reducing symptoms of depression. Whilst such studies have not yet been replicated among people with severe mental illness, this study only serves to exemplify that people with depression and severe mental illness have a great difficulty in breaking unhealthy behaviours and adopting newer healthier ones. Regrettably, this appears to be a common misunderstanding among researchers, clinicians and policy makers. Until multidisciplinary teams take into account the unique challenges faced by people with severe mental illness and offer individualized social support, patient outcomes are unlikely to change. Physiotherapists are particularly skilled and knowledgeable in the unique challenges regarding the barriers to and facilitation of physical activity in people with severe mental illness (Soundy et al., 2014b). They are poised to promote comprehensive physical activity interventions to patients for the prevention and management of chronic disease given their breadth and depth of expertise in injury management and prevention. They have expertise in the evaluation and management of medical conditions affecting lifestyle physical activity and sports. A third competency, the promotion of lifestyle physical activity and sports for the prevention of chronic disease, is perhaps the most important competency, and is clearly the domain in which physiotherapists are likely to have the greatest health impact within mental healthcare settings. Since physiotherapists have an in-depth understanding of the physical and mental health needs of people with severe mental illness (Stubbs et al., 2014a), they are ideally placed to lead such research and implementation in clinical practice. Physiotherapy-led research to improve physical activity and health outcomes among people with severe mental illness is urgently needed (Stubbs et al., 2014b).

CONCLUSION

Because of their role, training, experience, position within the multidisciplinary team and possibility to act as a bridge between the hospital and the community environment, physiotherapists are ideally placed to promote the health and well-being of people with severe mental illnesses through physical activity prescription. Policymakers and other caregivers should become aware of the potential of physiotherapists in promoting safe and healthy physical activity.

REFERENCES

Beaulac, J., Carlson, A., Jamie Boyd, R., 2011. Counseling on physical activity to promote mental health: practical guidelines for family physicians. Can. Fam. Physician 57 (4), 399–401.

Chalder, M., Wiles, N.J., Campbell, J., et al., 2012. Facilitated physical activity as a treatment for depressed adults: randomised controlled trial. Br. Med. J. 344, e2758.

Cooney, G.M., Dwan, K., Greig, C.A., et al., 2013. Exercise for depression. Cochrane Database Syst. Rev. (9), CD004366.

Craig, C.L., Marshall, A.L., Sjöström, M., et al., 2003. International physical activity questionnaire: 12-country reliability and validity. Med. Sci. Sports Exerc. 35, 1381–1395.

Eime, R.M., Young, J.A., Harvey, J.T., et al., 2013. A systematic review of the psychological and social benefits of participation in sport for adults: informing development of a conceptual model of health through sport. Int. J. Behav. Nutr. Phys. Act. 10, 135.

Glasgow, R., Goldstein, M., Ockene, J., Pronk, N., 2004. Translating what we have learned into practice: principles and hypotheses for interventions addressing multiple behaviors in primary care. Am. J. Prev. Med. 8, 88–101.

Gorczynski, P., Faulkner, G., 2010. Exercise therapy for schizophrenia. Cochrane Database Syst. Rev. (5), CD004412, pub2.

Gorczynski, P., Faulkner, G., Greening, S., Cohn, T., 2010. Exploring the construct validity of the transtheoretical model to structure physical activity interventions for individuals with serious mental illness. Psychiatr. Rehabil. J. 34 (1), 61–64.

Jerome, G.J., Rohm Young, D., Dalcin, A., et al., 2009. Physical activity levels of persons with mental illness attending psychiatric rehabilitation programs. Schizophr. Res. 108, 252–257.

Lee, P.H., Macfarlane, D.J., Lam, T., 2013. Factors associated with participant compliance in studies using accelerometers. Gait Posture 38, 912–917.

McKibbin, C.L., Kitchen, K.A., Wykes, T.L., Lee, A.A., 2014. Barriers and facilitators of a healthy lifestyle among persons with serious and persistent mental illness: perspectives of community mental health providers. Community Ment. Health J. 50 (5), 566–576.

Orrow, G., Kinmonth, A.L., Sanderson, S., Sutton, S., 2012. Effectiveness of physical activity promotion based in primary care: systematic review and meta-analysis of randomised controlled trials. Br. Med. J. 344, e1389.

Probst, M., 2012. The International Organization of Physical Therapists working in Mental Health (IOPTMH). Ment. Health Phys. Act. 5, 20–21.

Prochaska, J.O., DiClemente, C.C., 1983. Stages and processes of self-change of smoking: towards an integrative model of change. J. Consult. Clin. Psychol. 51, 390–395.

Prochaska, J.O., Marcus, B.H., 1994. The transtheoretical model: applications to exercise. In: Dishman, R.K. (Ed.), Advances in Exercise Adherence. Human Kinetics, Champaign, IL, pp. 161–180.

Rosenbaum, S., Tiedemann, A., Sherrington, C., et al., 2014. Physical activity interventions for people with mental illness: a systematic review and meta-analysis. J. Clin. Psychiatry 75 (9), 964–974.

Scully, D., Kremer, J., Meade, M.M., et al., 1998. Physical exercise and psychological well being: a critical review. Br. J. Sports Med. 32 (2), 111–120.

Skrinar, G.S., 2003. Chapter 47 mental illness. In: Durstine, J.L., Moore, G.E. (Eds.), ACSM's Exercise Management for Person With Chronic Diseases and Disabilities, second ed. Human Kinetics, Champaign, IL, USA.

Soundy, A., Faulkner, G., Taylor, A., 2007. Exploring the variability and perception of lifestyle physical activity among individuals with severe and enduring mental health problems: a qualitative study. J. Ment. Health 16, 493–503.

Soundy, A., Kingstone, T., Coffee, P., 2012. Understanding the psychosocial process of physical activity for individuals with severe mental illness: a meta-ethnography. In: L'Abate, L. (Ed.), Mental illnesses – Evaluation, Treatment and Implications. InTech.

Soundy, A., Roskell, C., Stubbs, B., Vancampfort, D., 2014a. Selection, use and psychometric properties of physical activity measures to assess individuals with severe mental illness: a narrative synthesis. Arch. Psychiatr. Nurs. 28, 135–151.

Soundy, A., Stubbs, B., Probst, M., et al., 2014b. Barriers to and facilitators of physical activity among persons with schizophrenia: a survey of physical therapists. Psychiatr. Serv. 65 (5), 693–696.

Soundy, A., Freeman, P., Stubbs, B., et al., 2014c. The value of social support to encourage people with schizophrenia to engage in physical activity: an international insight from specialist mental health physiotherapists. J. Ment. Health 23 (5), 256–260.

Stubbs, B., Soundy, A., Probst, M., et al., 2014a. Understanding the role of physiotherapists in schizophrenia: an international perspective from members of the International Organisation of Physical Therapists in Mental Health (IOPTMH). J. Ment. Health 23 (3), 125–129.

Stubbs, B., Probst, M., Soundy, A., et al., 2014b. Physiotherapists can help implement physical activity programmes in clinical practice. Br. J. Psychiatry 204 (2), 164.

Ussher, M., Stanbury, L., Cheeseman, V., Faulkner, G., 2007. Physical activity preferences and perceived barriers to activity among those with severe mental illness. Psychiatr. Serv. 58, 405–408.

Vancampfort, D., Probst, M., Skjaerven, L., et al., 2012a. Systematic review of the benefits of physical therapy within a multidisciplinary care approach for people with schizophrenia. Phys. Ther. 92 (1), 11–23.

Vancampfort, D., De Hert, M., Skjaerven, L., et al., 2012b. International Organization of Physical Therapy in Mental Health consensus on physical activity within multidisciplinary rehabilitation programmes for minimising cardio-metabolic risk in patients with schizophrenia. Disabil. Rehabil. 34 (1), 1–12.

Vancampfort, D., Knapen, J., Probst, M., et al., 2012c. A systematic review of correlates of physical activity in patients with schizophrenia. Acta Psychiatr. Scand. 125 (5), 352–362.

Vancampfort, D., Vanderlinden, J., De Hert, M., et al., 2013a. A systematic review on physical therapy interventions for patients with binge eating disorder. Disabil. Rehabil. 35 (26), 2191–2196.

Vancampfort, D., Vanderlinden, J., De Hert, M., et al., 2013b. A systematic review of physical therapy interventions for patients with anorexia and bulimia nervosa. Disabil. Rehabil. 36 (8), 628–634.

Vancampfort, D., Correll, C., Probst, M., et al., 2013c. A review of physical activity correlates in patients with bipolar disorder. J. Affect. Disord. 145 (3), 285–291.

Vancampfort, D., De Hert, M., Vansteenkiste, M., et al., 2013d. The importance of self-determined motivation towards physical activity in patients with schizophrenia. Psychiatry Res. 210 (3), 812–818.

Vancampfort, D., Probst, M., De Hert, M., et al., 2014a. Neurobiological effects of physical exercise in schizophrenia: a systematic review. Disabil. Rehabil. 36 (21), 1749–1754.

Vancampfort, D., De Hert, M., Vansteenkiste, M., et al., 2014b. Self-determination and stage of readiness to change physical activity behaviour in schizophrenia: a multicentre study. Ment. Health Phys. Act. 7 (3), 171–176.

Verhagen, E., Engbers, L., 2009. The physical therapist's role in physical activity promotion. Br. J. Sports Med. 43, 99–101.

Warren, J.M., Ekelund, U., Besson, H., et al., 2010. Assessment of physical activity—a review of methodologies with reference to epidemiological research: a report of the exercise physiology section of the European Association of Cardiovascular Prevention and Rehabilitation. Eur. J. Cardiovasc. Prev. Rehabil. 17 (2), 127–139.

World Confederation for Physical Therapy, 2007. Position Statement. Description of Physical Therapy. World Confederation for Physical Therapy, London.

3.5 RELAXATION THERAPY

TINE VAN DAMME

SUMMARY

In this contribution, the concept and applications of relaxation therapy (RT) are outlined. This chapter commences with the rationale for employing RT within the context of mental health care. We continue by elaborating on both the stress response and its physiological antithesis, the relaxation response. Some relaxation techniques that have made a major contribution to the field of RT are discussed. In addition, studies regarding the efficacy of these techniques in relation to mental health care are briefly addressed. Lastly, some attention is paid to assessment, evaluation and compliance in the field of RT.

KEY POINTS

- Relaxation therapy is an umbrella term for a number of techniques promoting stress and anxiety reduction.
- Relaxation therapy is a valued therapeutic approach that embraces the relationship between body and mind.
- A variety of techniques can be employed to elicit a relaxation response.
- Increasing evidence indicates that relaxation therapy is an effective treatment and has multiple applications within the field of mental health care.

LEARNING OBJECTIVES

- Concept of relaxation therapy and stress in mental health care.
- Description of the major relaxation techniques.
- Tips for assessment and compliance.

RATIONALE

The term *relaxation therapy* (RT) is used to describe a number of techniques promoting stress and anxiety reduction by means of decreasing tension throughout the body and creating a peaceful state of mind. It is a valued therapeutic approach commonly used in mental health care. As RT embraces the relationship between body and mind and as stress often manifests itself in physical symptoms, it is not unusual for a physiotherapist to apply relaxation training as a treatment approach.

RT is often discussed in relation to the concept of stress. The term *stress* is well integrated in society, but we have come to view stress as a negative experience. Moreover, public awareness of the adverse effects of stress has never been higher. However, stress is inherent to life, as it emerges whenever events occur that require an adjustment or solution. The body reacts to this challenge by activating the sympathetic nervous system, which results in a fight-or-flight reaction. A distinction should be made between stress that is harmful (distress) and positive stress. Distress arises when there is an imbalance between the demands of daily life and the capacity to cope with these requests. The presence of distress affects different functional areas, resulting in a range of physical, emotional, cognitive and social complaints (such as headache, unstable mood, attention problems, social withdrawal, etc.).

The relationship between distress and a variety of mental health problems is well recognized. Stress-related diseases are known to be a major contributor to mental illness. Conversely, individuals with a psychiatric condition or mental health problems are especially vulnerable to the negative effects of stress. Consequently, RT is an obvious choice of treatment. It can enable a person to regulate their tension levels, enhance feelings of control and increase body awareness, with the definitive goal of improving the quality of life. Teaching RT to a patient may have several advantages. First, it is a safe and inexpensive treatment. Second, it is a nonpharmacological approach, thus no side effects will emerge. Third, when mastered, RT can be used outside the therapeutic setting to help individuals overcome stressful situations and return to a focused calm state on their own.

THE STRESS RESPONSE AND THE RELAXATION RESPONSE

The term *stress* was first introduced by Selye (1956), who demonstrated that when a body is subjected to a challenging stimulus, a characteristic response occurs. Selye conceptualized this stress response (the system whereby the body copes with stress) and described the physiology of stress in his stress model, namely the general adaptation syndrome. In this model, he described three stages of the stress response: the alarm stage, the resistance stage and the exhaustion stage. The stress response was regarded as the result of the autonomic release of hormones and chemicals whose purpose is to create the appropriate physiological changes.

However, Selye's focus was on the physiological aspects, and his conclusions are no longer in agreement with current ideas on stress. Nowadays the stress response is considered to represent the ultimate intertwining of physiology and psychology. It is well recognized that many aspects might influence and/or mediate this relationship. However, two aspects, namely coping and perception, have repeatedly been identified as major contributors. Within this context, stress is defined as 'a perceptual phenomenon arising from a comparison between the demand on the person and the ability to cope' (Payne & Donaghy, 2010). Consequently, an imbalance gives rise to the experience of stress and to the stress response (Payne & Donaghy, 2010). Since the level and impact of stress is related to the way an individual perceives and interprets stimuli, as well as to how an individual is able to handle certain

situations, it is not surprising that stress is a highly individual and variable concept.

The relaxation response was described by Benson et al. (1974) and can be considered to be the physiological antithesis of the stress response, namely a physiological state characterized by a decreased activation of the sympathetic nervous system. The relaxation response is regarded as a state, rather than a specific technique. However, this state does not appear spontaneously, but can be elicited by using many different body-mind techniques, including relaxation techniques, breath awareness, meditation and yoga. The essential component of relaxation response-inducing techniques is to break the chain of everyday thinking, creating a sense of 'quieting' the mind and body (Park et al., 2013).

RELAXATION TECHNIQUES

A wide variety of relaxation techniques has been developed, but the common basis of all these techniques is eliciting the relaxation response. Inducing a state of relaxation is possible in different ways; some methods focus mainly on the body, whereas others put emphasis on the mental processes. Although each technique has its merits, the choice of a certain relaxation technique should always be considered with care and targeted to the client's strengths, difficulties, needs and interests.

The scope of this contribution is limited to the main relaxation techniques that have made a major contribution to the field of RT. Research concerning the effectiveness of these methods in mental health care is briefly discussed.

Breathing

Breathing is directly related to the system that controls physiological arousal. Moreover, the respiratory system is strongly influenced by an individual's emotional state. Therefore breathing techniques can be very useful to induce a relaxation response. Paying attention to breathing is a feature of almost every relaxation technique. Although breathing exercises can be used as a sole intervention, it is rarely applied in this way. Various breathing techniques or routines have been proposed, including deep and slow breathing, respiratory retraining, breathing meditation, breathing awareness, abdominal breathing, etc. An advantage of these techniques is that they are easily learned and can be carried out anywhere.

Progressive Relaxation Training

Progressive relaxation training (PRT) originates in the work of Jacobson (1939), a pioneer in the field of the physiologically oriented approach of RT. He proposed that relaxation of musculature results in a calming influence on the whole organism, including the mind. By creating and releasing tension in the muscles, one can learn to recognize different levels of tension and how to release that tension. As the original procedure is time consuming, clinical practice shifted from Jacobson's initial method to more practical training procedures. To date, several modifications of this technique have been developed. The procedure of PRT (see Appendix A), developed by Bernstein & Borkovec (1973) is probably the best-known and most widely applied modification.

The progressive relaxation literature consistently affirms the clinical efficacy of PRT for several disorders, including insomnia, depression, anxiety disorders, posttraumatic stress disorder, aggression and schizophrenia (Carlson & Hoyle, 1993; Vaughan et al., 1994; Echeberua et al., 1996; Morin et al., 1999; Nickel et al., 2005; Conrad & Roth, 2007; Jorm et al., 2008; Manzoni et al., 2008; Vancampfort et al., 2013).

Autogenic Training

Autogenic training (AT) is an approach derived from self-hypnosis and was developed by the German psychiatrist J.H. Schultz. By repeated concentration on specific autosuggestions, a meditative state and psychological relaxation is achieved, which is accompanied by physical relaxation (Schultz, 1979). The autosuggestions, also referred to as *formulas*, are based on passive concentration on bodily perceptions (see Appendix B). The term *autogenic* refers to the central principle of AT, which indicates the notion that relaxation is self-induced and emphasizes the importance of the responsibility of the patient.

Systematic reviews indicate that AT reduces stress and anxiety and is effective in the treatment of anxiety disorders, mild-to-moderate depression, psychosomatic disorders and functional sleep disorders (Kanji & Ernst, 2000; Stetter & Kupper, 2002). However, these results should be interpreted carefully, as the authors warn about many methodological shortcomings. Goldbeck & Schmid (2003) investigated the effect of autogenic relaxation training in children and adolescents with mild to moderate behavioural and/or emotional problems. They

concluded that AT results in a reduction of stress and psychosomatic complaints and has clinically relevant effects on internalizing and externalizing problems.

Mindfulness

As the purpose of mindfulness (MFN) is teaching individuals to accept and cope with the inevitable stress of daily life, MFN can be viewed as a more general approach, perhaps even a way of life. Kabat-Zinn (2003), a notable contributor to the field, defined MFN as 'moment-by-moment nonjudgemental awareness'. Several mindfulness-based therapies have been developed. The mindfulness-based stress reduction programme seeks to help individuals to manage stress and distress associated with illness. Another programme, mindfulness-based cognitive therapy, was originally designed as a preventative intervention for patients with a major depression in periods of remission. Over the years, MFN has become increasingly popular, resulting in numerous applications and tailored interventions for a range of psychiatric disorders, including autism, eating disorders, substance abuse, psychosis, etc.

Research on MFN supports the idea that cultivating greater attention, awareness and acceptance through meditation practice is associated with lower levels of psychological distress, including less anxiety, depression, anger and worry (Greeson, 2009). As mindfulness-based therapies are built on a strong research tradition, numerous studies have examined the effectiveness. We refer to the review of Keng et al. (2011) for a comprehensive overview.

ASSESSMENT, EVALUATION AND COMPLIANCE

As with any other form of therapy, assessment and evaluation have an important role. Not only is assessment vital to identify symptoms and complaints, it is needed to evaluate whether an intervention is effective. Also, perhaps even more important, assessment is essential to increase compliance. For instance, a client who practises every day, but does not experience progress, will quickly lose motivation. Apart from the wide variety of available standardized questionnaires, some other tools can be employed. For instance, a visual analogue scale is useful to evaluate the perceived tension level of a client. Furthermore, it is recommended to use a diary, in which clients can record their daily practice, their successes and failures and register their complaints and/or symptoms. Although a diary might serve as a powerful motivator for clients, it also provides important information for the therapist.

Owing to the need to train and practise relaxation techniques, most of the time, progress is not immediately perceived. Therefore it is recommended that a therapist radiates a strong and firm belief in the effectiveness of RT. Moreover, it is important that a therapist provides an optimistic, but also a realistic picture of what can be expected in terms of achievement and progress. Lastly, it is recommended that the therapist,

together with the patient, examines—a priori—personal reasons for potential dropout or barriers. Consequently, listing potential problems together with their possible solutions, might improve compliance.

CONCLUSION

RT is a valued approach in mental health care. Numerous relaxation techniques have been developed with similar goals of addressing stress-related issues. Despite many methodological shortcomings, increasing evidence indicates that RT is an effective treatment and has multiple applications in psychiatric populations.

REFLECTIVE QUESTIONS

- Why is RT a valued approach within mental health care?
- Why can we consider the stress response and the relaxation response to be an ultimate intertwining between physiology and psychology?
- Do you know any relaxation techniques that have made a major contribution to the field of RT?

REFERENCES

Benson, H., Beary, J.F., Carol, M.P., 1974. The relaxation response. Psychiatry 37 (1), 37–46.

Bernstein, D.A., Borkovec, T., 1973. Progressive Relaxation Training. A manual for the Helping Professions. Research Press Company, New York.

Carlson, C.R., Hoyle, R.H., 1993. Efficacy of abbreviated progressive muscle relaxation training: a quantitative review of behavioral medicine research. J. Consult. Clin. Psychol. 61 (6), 1059–1067.

Conrad, A., Roth, W.T., 2007. Muscle relaxation therapy for anxiety disorders: it works but how? J. Anxiety Disord. 21 (3), 243–264.

Echeberua, E., de Corral, P., Sarasua, B., Zubizarreta, I., 1996. Treatment of acute posttraumatic stress disorder in rape victims: an experimental study. J. Anxiety Disord. 10 (3), 185–199.

Goldbeck, L., Schmid, K., 2003. Effectiveness of Autogenic Relaxation Training on children and adolescents with behavioral and emotional problems. J. Am. Acad. Child Adolesc. Psychiatry 42 (9), 1046–1054.

Greeson, J.M., 2009. Mindfulness research update: 2008. Complement. Health Pract. Rev. 14 (1), 10–18.

Jacobson, E., 1939. Progressive Relaxation. University Press, Chicago.

Jorm, A.F., Morgan, A.J., Hetrick, S.E., 2008. Relaxation for depression. Cochrane Database Syst. Rev. (4), Art. No. CD007142.

Kabat-Zinn, J., 2003. Mindfulness-based interventions in context: past, present and future. Clin. Psychol. Sci. Pract. 10 (2), 144–156.

Kanji, N., Ernst, E., 2000. Autogenic training for stress and anxiety: a systematic review. Complement. Ther. Med. 8 (2), 106–110.

Keng, S.L., Smoski, M.J., Robins, C.J., 2011. Effects of mindfulness on psychological health: a review of empirical studies. Clin. Psychol. Rev. 31 (6), 1041–1056.

Manzoni, G.M., Pagnini, F., Castelnuovo, G., Molinari, E., 2008. Relaxation training for anxiety: a ten-years systematic review with meta-analysis. BMC Psychiatry 8 (1), 41.

Morin, C.M., Hauri, P.J., Espie, C.A., et al., 1999. Nonpharmacologic treatment of chronic insomnia. An American Academy of Sleep Medicine review. Sleep 22 (8), 1134–1156.

Nickel, C., Lahmann, C., Tritt, K., et al., 2005. Stressed aggressive adolescents benefit from progressive muscle relaxation: a random, prospective, controlled trial. Stress Health 21 (3), 169–175.

Park, E.R., Traeger, L., Vranceanu, A.M., et al., 2013. The development of a patient-centered program based on the relaxation response: the Relaxation Response Resiliency Program (3RP). Psychosomatics 54 (2), 165–174.

Payne, R.A., Donaghy, M., 2010. Relaxation techniques: A Practical Handbook for the Health Care Professional. Elsevier Health Sciences, London.

Selye, H., 1956. The Stress of Life. McGraw-Hill, New York.

Schultz, J.H., 1979. Das Autogene Training. Konzentrative Selbstentspannung. Thieme, Stuttgart.

Stetter, F., Kupper, S., 2002. Autogenic training: a meta-analysis of clinical outcome studies. Appl. Psychophysiol. Biofeedback 27 (1), 45–98.

Vancampfort, D., Correll, C.U., Scheewe, T.W., et al., 2013. Progressive muscle relaxation in persons with schizophrenia: a systematic review of randomized controlled trials. Clin. Rehabil. 27 (4), 291–298.

Vaughan, K., Armstrong, M.S., Gold, R., et al., 1994. A trial of eye movement desensitization compared to image habituation training and applied muscle relaxation in post-traumatic stress disorder. J. Behav. Ther. Exp. Psychiatry 25 (4), 283–291.

Appendix A

PROCEDURE OF PROGRESSIVE RELAXATION TRAINING

	Initial Procedure With 16 Muscle Groups	
	Muscle Groups	**Method of Tensing**
1	Dominant hand and forearm	Make a tight fist while allowing upper arm to remain relaxed
2	Dominant upper arm	Press elbow down against chair
3	Nondominant hand and forearm	Same as dominant
4	Nondominant upper arm	Same as dominant
5	Forehead	Raise eyebrows as high as possible
6	Upper cheeks and nose	Squint eyes and wrinkle nose
7	Lower face	Clench teeth and pull back corners of mouth
8	Neck	Counter pose muscles by trying to raise and lower chin simultaneously
9	Chest, shoulders and upper back	Take a deep breath; hold it and pull shoulder blades together
10	Abdomen	Counter pose muscles by trying to push stomach out and pull it simultaneously
11	Dominant upper leg	Counter pose large muscle on top of leg against two smaller ones underneath
12	Dominant calf	Point toes towards head
13	Dominant foot	Point toes downward, turn foot in and curl toes gently
14	Nondominant upper leg	Same as dominant
15	Nondominant calf	Same as dominant
16	Nondominant foot	Same as dominant

	Shorter Procedure Combining Muscle Groups
	Combining Muscle Groups
1	Dominant hand, forearm and upper arm
2	Nondominant hand, forearm and upper arm
3	All facial muscles
4	Neck
5	Chest, shoulders, upper chest and abdomen
6	Dominant upper leg, calf and foot
7	Nondominant upper leg, calf and foot

	Final Procedure Combining Muscle Groups
	Combining Muscle Groups
1	Both arms and both hands
2	Face and neck
3	Chest, shoulders, back and abdomen
4	Both legs and both feet

Appendix B

PROCEDURE OF AUTOGENIC TRAINING

Basic Exercises		
	Formula	Repetition
Heaviness experience	My right arm is heavy	6 times
	I am very quiet	Once
	My left arm is heavy	6 times
	I am very quiet	Once
	My right leg is heavy	6 times
	I am very quiet	Once
	My left leg is heavy	6 times
	I am very quiet	Once
	Both my arms and legs are heavy	6 times
	I am very quiet	Once
Warmth experience	My right arm is pleasantly warm	6 times
	I am very quiet	Once
	My left arm is pleasantly warm	6 times
	I am very quiet	Once
	My right leg is pleasantly warm	6 times
	I am very quiet	Once
	My left leg is pleasantly warm	6 times
	I am very quiet	Once
	Both my arms and legs are warm	6 times
	I am at peace	Once
Regulation of the heart	My heart is beating calmly and regularly	6 times
	I am very quiet	Once
Regulation of breathing	The breathing is calm. It breaths me	6 times
	I am at peace	Once
Regulation of visceral organs	Sun rays are streaming and warm (Concentrating on solar plexus)	6 times
	I am quiet	Once
Regulation of the head	My forehead is cool	6 times
	I am at peace	Once
Taking back	Make fists; bend arms; breathe deeply; open eyes	

3.6

THE ADDED VALUE OF BIOFEEDBACK FOR THE PSYCHOSOMATIC PHYSIOTHERAPIST

EVELINE C. KEMPENAAR ▪ DANIELLE M. MATTO

SUMMARY

Biofeedback is an objective measurement tool in physiotherapy. Additionally, it can be used as a treatment modality. It is often seen that people with physical complaints are not aware of current muscle tension. While using biofeedback, patients will be more aware of their tension and in this way, they can alternate the tension. This will increase body awareness and self-regulation. In this chapter, biofeedback, biofeedback assessment and training are explained. Finally, several treatment modalities are explained.

KEY POINTS

- Biofeedback is an objective method used to measure physical parameters (muscle tension, respiration, heart rate, skin conductance).
- Biofeedback increases body awareness and self-regulation.
- During treatment, it is important to determine the patient's stress profile and to perform a psychophysiological assessment.

LEARNING OBJECTIVES

- Understand how can you implement biofeedback therapy in your physiotherapy treatment.
- Describe the relationship between body and mind, while using biofeedback.

INTRODUCTION

Within the field of physical therapy, the use of therapeutic interventions is becoming more and more objective. Determining the effect of an intervention (e.g., by means of a questionnaire) makes this possible. Actual measurement of the change in body signals is another method used to determine the therapeutic effect. This can be realized using biofeedback.

Biofeedback is a method in which body signals are measured. The most commonly used measurements are muscle tension, respiration, heart rate, skin conductance and hand temperature. Biofeedback works as a 'psychophysiological mirror' by providing the patient and the therapist with direct information on the condition of the autonomic nervous system.

Providing the patient with immediate feedback, the effect of a thought, an attitude or emotion on the body becomes clearer. The patient will learn that they have a real influence on the cause of the complaint. This stimulates the process of body awareness and internal self-regulation. By inviting the patient to engage actively in the therapy, they will take more responsibility for their health and become more self-reliant.

As biofeedback gives information about the possible cause of the patient's symptoms, it will be easier for the therapist to determine what kind of counselling or intervention is the best choice in the treatment plan. Nevertheless, it remains a creative process to determine the best treatment plan for the patient with their specific array of symptoms. Biofeedback can also be used to test the effect of an intervention. Consequently, if an intervention is not the correct choice for the specific patient, the therapist will learn at an early stage and may change to a different approach.

In recent decades, developments in computer engineering have made great progress. This has had a positive influence on the field of biofeedback. Measuring equipment is smaller and easier to use nowadays, and an increasing number of psychophysiological applications have been developed for tablets and smartphones. This has increased the accessibility of biofeedback, for both the therapist and the patient. By using apps and small measuring devices, home practising with biofeedback has become possible and more fun.

In this chapter we offer a brief definition of biofeedback, followed by some examples of how to use biofeedback in the field of psychosomatic physical therapy.

DEFINITION OF BIOFEEDBACK

The first definition of biofeedback dates from 1973: 'Biofeedback can be defined as the use of monitoring instruments (usually electrical) to detect and amplify internal physiological processes within the body, in order to make this ordinarily unavailable internal information available to the individual and literally feed it back to him in some form' (Birk, 1973). In this definition, the emphasis is on the process of measuring of body signals. In 1999 this definition was revised due to the realization that biofeedback was used much more widely: as part of a total treatment and in combination with other techniques.

Biofeedback was seen as 'applied psychophysiology', which led to the following definition: 'Applied psychophysiology includes a group of interventions and evaluation methods with the exclusive or primary intentions of understanding and effecting changes that help humans move toward and maintain healthier psychophysiological functioning. The group of interventions use all forms of biofeedback, relaxation methods, breathing methods, cognitive behavioural therapies, patient education, behavioural changes, meditative techniques and imagery techniques'(Schwartz, 1999a,b).

Biofeedback can be seen as a process of operant conditioning. Showing the body signal on screen, for example as a line graph, provides insight into the way the body signal behaves under the current circumstances. An example of this is muscle tension. To teach a patient to write with a relaxed shoulder, the biofeedback device gives a warning, such as a tone, as soon as the muscle tension in the shoulder rises above the threshold. Another possibility is to give a reward (e.g., pleasant music) if the muscle tension stays below the threshold.

ASSESSMENT AND TRAINING WITH BIOFEEDBACK

Biofeedback Assessment

In this case, the measured signals are visible only to the therapist. A good example is the biofeedback *stress profile*, also called *psychophysiological assessment*. Muscle tension of both shoulders (upper trapezius muscles), respiration, heart rate, skin conductance and hand temperature are measured simultaneously under various conditions. The test starts with a baseline measurement for a few minutes, in which the patient is measured while reading a magazine. This is followed by a relaxation period of 2 minutes. Then a stressor is introduced, for instance a short mental task, such as a 1-minute mathematics test. After the stressor, the patient is asked to relax again. The assessment contains a series of stressor-relax intervals, in order to test the ability of the patient to switch between mental activity and relaxation. After the psychophysiological assessment, the measured values are compared with normal values. During relaxation, the patient should have a normal breathing pattern and breathing rate, normal resting values of the heart rate, relaxed shoulder muscles and dry, warm hands. During the stressor the stress system may respond, but in the period of relaxation after the stressor, the body signals should return to resting values (Khazan, 2013). It is interesting that the response to stress is very individual. Some patients respond with increased muscle tone, while others get cold hands or change to a more rapid and shallow breathing pattern. There are also individual differences between patients as to their ability to relax after a stressor. Some patients keep tensing their shoulders, others might continue worrying during the relaxation phase about a bad performance on the mental task, leading to a continued reactivity in skin conductance.

In summary, the psychophysiological assessment provides insight into the basic tension of the patient, their specific stress response and ability to relax after stress. This information is important in determining the most useful interventions in the treatment plan. In addition, discussing the findings with the patient is an excellent tool to provide them with information about psychophysiology and to discuss the how learning relaxation can mean better recovery after stress. In our experience, this is a very important stage in therapy because it makes the patient aware of stress reactions, which is the first step in the process of change (Gevirtz, 2007).

Biofeedback Training

When the treatment plan has been made, biofeedback can be used in various ways to achieve the treatment goals. There is a long list of applications in which biofeedback has been proven effective. In 2002 the efficacy of biofeedback training was investigated by Don Moss and Jay Gunkelman. This led to the publication of a review article, in which the various biofeedback applications were described with reference to the scientific studies, demonstrating efficacy (Yucha & Montgomery, 2008). Another source of information about biofeedback applications can be found in the book, *Biofeedback, a practitioner's guide* (Schwartz & Andrasik, 2003). Here we give an overview of biofeedback training applications that are useful for physiotherapists who work in the field of mental health.

Lowering Muscle Tension With Electromyography Feedback

In electromyography (EMG), training the muscle tension is displayed to the patient on a monitor. The first reaction is often the remark, 'I can see what I'm doing!', which naturally leads to spontaneous exploration with different postures and strategies to influence muscle tension. Even without direct coaching from the therapist, feedback in this exploration phase can itself lead to a normalization of muscle tension. When the therapist asks what the patient did to normalize muscle tension, often the surprising answer is, 'I lowered my shoulders.'

If the patient does not succeed in influencing their muscle tension in the desired way, an additional instruction can be given, such as, 'make the shoulders heavy' or 'tense the muscles even more to then let them go' (Jacobson–Progressive Muscle Relaxation). Another application of biofeedback for increased muscle tone is learning to reduce muscle tension in different

postures and under different conditions, such as standing, bending and walking. It is also interesting to look at the recovery of a muscle after a number of repeated movements. After a movement sequence, if a number of muscles are measured simultaneously, it is possible to discover unnecessary cocontraction. Direct EMG feedback also helps the patient to follow the instructions more easily. Often within one session of EMG feedback it is possible to achieve body awareness and the first steps of internal self-regulation (Cram, 2011).

Demonstrating the Interaction of Mind and Body

Depending on the individual stress response (measured during the psychophysiological assessment) biofeedback training can be done in different ways; for example, using the body signal that gave an extremely strong response during the stressor or one that had problems returning to the resting value after the stressor. In the example of the patient who kept worrying during the relaxation phase about his bad performance on the mental task, this response results in a continued reactivity in skin conductance. By showing skin conductance results on screen, the patient becomes immediately aware of how the mind influences the body because they can instantly see the effect of their emotional state on screen. Then, with the help of the therapist, the patient can learn which strategy helps to lower skin conductance, for example, ceasing any critical 'self-talk' or focusing on relaxation and letting go of disturbing thoughts.

Biofeedback as Part of a Specific Treatment Protocol

There are several treatment protocols in which biofeedback training is an essential part.

Examples are:

- Teaching hand warming with biofeedback as part of the treatment protocol for training patients with hypertension how to lower their blood pressure,
- Measuring respiration with biofeedback in order to teach patients with dysfunctional breathing patterns how to lower respiration rate and extend an expiratory pause,
- Using biofeedback to teach patients with migraines how to attain voluntary control over the level of vasodilation and vasoconstriction in the area of the arteria temporalis.

In summary, providing the patient with information about body signals by displaying this information on the screen invites the patient to start exploring strategies to get voluntary control over their body signals. In addition, with feedback it is easier for a patient to follow a specific instruction, as the effect of that instruction is immediately visible. The patient is also more aware of the influence of thoughts and emotions on the body and learns which strategies work best for relaxation. This facilitates the process of body awareness, which is an important first step in the process of change.

Measuring the Effect of an Intervention With Biofeedback

Finally, biofeedback is used as a method for measuring the effect of a treatment or intervention. It is possible to measure the effect of the treatment by performing another psychophysiological assessment at the end of the series of treatment sessions. Another possibility is to use biofeedback measurement to evaluate the effect of interventions that are used in psychological therapy. This can help in the process of objectifying treatment effects.

THE PSYCHOSOMATIC PHYSIOTHERAPIST AS BIOFEEDBACK TRAINER

There are a number of things that the physiotherapist will need to learn before biofeedback can be successfully applied. First, it is important that the therapist acts as a supportive and creative coach: being involved in the treatment, intervening at the right time and being able to wait and let the process of awareness and learning happen at its own pace. Furthermore, it is important that the physiotherapist feels capable to work with the biofeedback hardware and software. If this is not the case, the patient–therapist relationship will be negatively affected by frustration of the therapist about the failure of the equipment or will create confusion in the patient because of incorrect measurements. Proper training in biofeedback is therefore necessary. Finally, it is important that the therapist learns to take the right steps in biofeedback training. Showing the patient their specific psychophysiological response to stress and teaching body awareness is the first step.

Then the biofeedback can be used to teach internal self-regulation. To facilitate the process of internal self-regulation, the therapist needs an active and engaged attitude. The last element is necessary to motivate the patient to apply the learned strategies to influence their body signals in daily life without the use of biofeedback equipment. This can start in relatively simple situations, such as relaxing during a break, and then expand to more difficult situations, such as staying calm during a difficult or stressful conversation.

EXAMPLES OF BIOFEEEDBACK APPLICATIONS IN PSYCHOSOMATIC PHYSICAL THERAPY

Tension Headache

Patients with tension headaches are often referred to a psychosomatic physiotherapist. The obvious treatment protocol is to focus on teaching the patient to relax the muscles of neck and shoulders. However, tension headaches can be caused by several factors. Performing a biofeedback assessment would be a good way to reveal the exact cause of the headaches. Fig. 1 shows the biofeedback assessment of a patient referred because of tension headaches. It is remarkable that there is no increased tension in the trapezius muscles.

Looking for increased tension in other muscles, the therapist performed an additional EMG measurement of the masseter, temporalis and frontalis muscles. These muscles are known to be a possible cause of tension headaches. With this patient, no increased muscle tension was found in these muscles. There was, however, another remarkable finding: the skin conductance (a measure of reaction/emotion) had very high values and maintained increased values during the relaxation phase. This indicated that the patient was aroused all the time. When discussing this finding with the patient, he recognized this fact and said that he felt alert all the time, seeing and hearing everything. The best treatment plan would be to focus on teaching the patient to be less alert instead of teaching muscle relaxation. Possible ways to achieve this are mindfulness and body awareness exercises. However, in a large group of patients who have tension headache, increased tension is found in the neck, shoulders or facial muscles (Nestoriuc et al., 2008). These patients will benefit

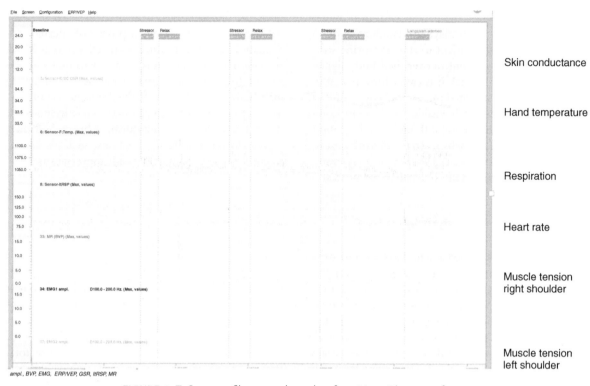

FIGURE 1 ■ Stress profile screen shot taken from Nexus Biotrace software.

from EMG training and muscle relaxation exercises, such as progressive muscle relaxation. In another patient, the headache was caused by a special EMG pattern: the trapezius muscles tensed when inhaling and relaxed when exhaling. The EMG pattern followed the breathing pattern. This biofeedback stress profile is an indication of a dysfunctional breathing pattern, where the patient is not using the diaphragm, but is instead using the trapezius muscles and often also the sternocleidomastoid and scalenus muscles to facilitate the breathing process. The headache is caused by a continued stretching of the attachment of the linea nuchea. For such patients, it makes sense to teach an effortless diaphragmatic breathing pattern.

Musculoskeletal Problems

Learning to reduce muscle tension is good training for all patients with recurrent neck–shoulder pain and temporomandibular dysfunction. In addition to the biofeedback stress profile, additional EMG research is necessary with these patients. An example is the so-called *Sella protocol* (Sella, 1996). In this short test the patient is asked to tense the tested muscle to peak value for 9 seconds and then fully relax the muscle for 9 seconds. This is repeated five times. This test shows whether the tested muscle is able to quickly switch between contraction and relaxation. A tensed muscle has difficulty performing this test because the muscle is not able to reach the same peak values and has difficulty fully relaxing after being tensed. Another test is to measure the EMG of multiple muscles simultaneously in order to look for cocontraction. After the EMG test phase, the therapist starts with the actual EMG training. It is important to ask the patient if they know what the triggers are for EMG tension and combine this information in the EMG training. It is remarkable how fast EMG training works. The patient learns very quickly to relax the trained muscles and to feel muscle tension, even without the use of an EMG device. This improved body awareness tells the patient at an early stage that the muscle is starting to tense, so the patient can then relax the muscle.

BIOFEEDBACK TREATMENT OF PATIENTS WITH MEDICALLY UNEXPLAINED SYMPTOMS

The possibilities of biofeedback were nicely demonstrated in a research project by Katsamanis and Lehrer. Katsamanis works in the field of psychosomatic therapy. He used biofeedback with patients that had medically unexplained symptoms (Katsamanis et al., 2011) testing this group for the added value of a psychophysiological approach using biofeedback. The study consisted of a standardized protocol of 10 sessions of biofeedback training. In the first session, a stress profile was performed and the patients received information and instruction on the most abnormal parameter of the test. Then the patients received EMG training, heart-rate biofeedback training and temperature biofeedback training, combined with autogenic training. It appeared that the psychophysiological approach had a clear added value. This was reflected in improved mood, reduced symptoms and improved functioning of the patients. A striking feature of this study was the compliance to the therapy: there were no dropouts. In general, these patients are not as open to psychological counselling because they often have the belief that there is something wrong in the body. Biofeedback training appeared to be more relevant because working with psychophysiological measurements helped this group of patients to make the link between emotion and the body, thus making it easier for the psychosomatic physiotherapist to negotiate this issue with the patients.

REFERENCES

Birk, L. (Ed.), 1973. Biofeedback: Behavioral Medicine. Grune & Stratton, New York.

Cram, J.R., 2011. Cram's Introduction to Surface Electromyography, second ed. Jones and Barlett Publishers, Sudbury, Canada.

Gevirtz, R.N., 2007. Psychophysiological perpectives on stress-related and anxiety disorders. In: Lehrer, P.M., Woolfolk, R.L., Sime, W.E. (Eds.), Principles and Practice of Stress Management, 3rd ed. pp. 209–226.

Katsamanis, M., Lehrer, P.M., Escobar, J.I., et al., 2011. Psychophysiologic treatment for patients with medically unexplained symptoms: a randomized controlled trial. Psychosomatics 52, 218–229.

Khazan, I.Z., 2013. The Clinical Handbook of Biofeedback a Step-By-Step Guide for Training and Practice With Mindfulness. John Wiley & Sons Ltd, Chichester, UK.

Nestoriuc, Y., Martin, A., Rief, W., Andrasik, F., 2008. Biofeedback treatment for headache disorders: a comprehensive efficacy review. Appl. Psychophysiol. Biofeedback 33, 125–140.

Schwartz, M.S., 1999a. What is applied psychophysiology? Towards a definition. Appl. Psychophysiol. Biofeedback 24, 3–10.

Schwartz, M.S., 1999b. Responses to comments and closer to the definition of applied psychophysiology. Appl. Psychophysiol. Biofeedback 24, 43–54.

Schwartz, M.S., Andrasik, F., 2003. Biofeedback: A Practitioner's Guide. Guilford Press, New York.

Sella, G.E., 1996. Neuromuscular Testing With Surface EMG. GENMED, Wheeling, West Virginia.

Yucha, C., Montgomery, D. (2008). Evidence-based practice in biofeedback and neurofeedback. Association for Applied Psychophysiology & Biofeedback, AAPB. <http://www.aapb.org.>

3.7
GROUP THERAPEUTIC FACTORS FOR USE IN PHYSIOTHERAPY IN MENTAL HEALTH: A CORE IN GROUP PHYSIOTHERAPY

LIV HELVIK SKJAERVEN ▪ ANNE REITAN PARKER ▪ MONICA MATTSSON

SUMMARY

Group therapy as a medical and psychological treatment has existed for more than 100 years. Different kinds of group therapy have developed within physiotherapy in the last 50 years. It is predominantly within the speciality of physiotherapy in mental health that group therapy has been developed and used. Being a skilled physiotherapist requires more than collecting patients in a group. The physiotherapist gains competence from qualifying in implementing group therapeutic factors to promote group awareness and an atmosphere for interpersonal learning.

KEY POINTS

- Group therapeutic factors.
- History of group therapy.
- Group physiotherapy.

LEARNING OBJECTIVES

- Gain a good understanding of group leadership and group processes.
- Gain a greater understanding of group therapeutic factors.
- Gain insight into the historical development of group therapies.
- Knowledge on the integration of group therapeutic factors particularly into BBAT.

Group therapy as a medical and psychological treatment has existed since the turn of the twentieth century (Pratt, 1908) and many group therapies have been developed for people suffering from mental health problems. A form of self-experience in so-called *encounter groups* was developed in the USA in the period before and after the Second World War (Alexander, 1932; Moreno, 1944; Pearls et al., 1973; Schutz, 1973). Health professionals' interest in group therapy for mental health conditions has continued to grow. In Scandinavia, interest in group physiotherapy has been increasing and developing since the 1970s (Urdal, 1975; Roxendal, 1985; Skatteboe, 1991).

The foundation of group therapy is based on theories of interpersonal relationships. According to these theories, the patient's symptoms are a manifestation of disturbed relationships with important 'others' early in life, with problems from early childhood and adolescence being repeated later in life, in a new environment (Yalom, 1989).

Fairbairn is among the earliest theorists who emphasized the importance of interrelationships as basic factors in human development (Fairbairn, 1952). In a group, participants are expected to interrelate and work together. During the sessions, situations will arise that highlight problems and provide opportunities for solving conflicts and dealing with triggers that arise in the group relationship. When a disturbance has taken place while interrelating with other people, it becomes natural to solve the problem within a similar framework. To quote Sullivan: '*It takes people to make people sick, and it takes people to make people well again'* (Sullivan, 1953).

Irvin Yalom, professor of psychiatry, School of Medicine, Stanford University, USA, has published several books and papers on group therapy, proposing core therapeutic factors that are demonstrated to be effective in all models of the method (Yalom, 1980, 1983, 1989, 1995), see Box 1.

These factors are reported to be common for all therapeutic approaches that include basic, universal mechanisms connected to the process of change. The following seven factors have been developed and elaborated by Yalom and are considered important for the positive development of a group:

1. *Instillation of hope* is an important factor underlining the correlation between positive results and the high degree of expectation from therapy. This factor is important for people's improvement—sharing optimism with each other—and also for the therapist's belief in his or herself. Mobilizing hope in the group members is vital. When new and old group members function together, old members become vectors to instil hope in the newer members.

2. *Universality* refers to the patients' sense of loneliness, which is reinforced by their social isolation. This leads to low self-esteem, making it impossible to come close to others. Being in group therapy fosters a sense of group connectedness, of 'being in the same boat', reducing the feeling of being different from others and being alone.

3. *Altruism* is defined as 'love of your neighbour and consideration of other people'. Patients often have a deep sense of having nothing of value to give others. A group format enables patients to give each other support, hope and new thoughts, and to share insights and new problem-solving ideas. Such acts promote a sense of having something valuable to share with others.

4. *Interpersonal learning* in a group setting, working through transference and elaborated emotional experiences, is considered the most important group factor. In the theory of interrelationship, the group is seen as a microcosm, working in the 'here and now'. Learning from interaction in situations of varying difficulty that arise in the group, balances the group as a whole and fosters trust. It leads, in turn, to a gradual recognition of disturbed relationships, and the development of more functional relationships through learning from each other.

5. *Group cohesion* encompasses patients' relationships with all members in the group. Accordingly, group membership, acceptance and approval of the others in the group are important. Three aspects that stimulate a developing sense of group cohesion are: (1) being accepted by other members in the group, (2) recognizing characteristics of oneself in others and (3) having the possibility to turn to other members for help and reflection.

6. *Existential factors*, that is questions concerning life and death, human freedom, responsibility and isolation, allow the meaning of life to be elaborated. Gradually, each group participant learns to relate to that part of themselves that may be experienced as a personal threat to one's world view, moral system and existence.

7. *Catharsis* in this context does not mean the process of exposing one's emotional problems, but rather the unexpected discovery that others have problems similar to one's own. Catharsis as a strong emotional expression is not considered an effective therapeutic factor. In this kind of group therapy, it is the effective sharing of the

---

BOX 1

OVERVIEW OF GROUP THERAPEUTIC FACTORS (Yalom, 1995)

NO	GROUP THERAPEUTIC FACTORS
1	Installation of hope
2	Universality
3	Altruism
4	Interpersonal learning
5	Group cohesion
6	Existential factors
7	Catharsis

inner world of experiences that is considered to be important. Therefore the group leader becomes a model for others in the group, an important consideration to make when expressing how to handle one's own feelings.

During the last decades, self-psychology has exerted considerable influence on psychotherapy (Karterud & Stone, 2003). The self-psychological approach has been shown to be particularly fruitful when applied to group situations led by physiotherapists who have an integrated understanding of therapeutic processes (Skatteboe, 2005).

GROUP THERAPY WITHIN PHYSIOTHERAPY

Group therapy within physiotherapy has a long tradition. It has been used within psychiatric and psychosomatic physiotherapy for 40–50 years, and implemented in mental health care, rehabilitation, health promotion and preventive health care. Patients have been recruited either from individual physiotherapy or referred directly for 'movement groups'.

Many traditions are reflected in movement groups, such as Norwegian psychomotor physiotherapy, the Belgian psychomotor tradition, physical training, relaxation programmes, body awareness programmes, dance and other kinds of movement activities. Movement groups led by a physiotherapist are considered to be an important resource in psychiatric institutions (Bunkan, 2008).

Historically in the Nordic countries, group-based interventions have been clinically integrated into Basic Body Awareness Therapy (BBAT) for more than 30 years. Since the mid-1980s, group therapy theory and practice has been a core subject in BBAT education, and have been taught in the bachelor programme of physiotherapy and in postgraduate BBAT courses by the Norwegian Physiotherapy Association. Accordingly, physiotherapists have had the opportunity to achieve competence in group physiotherapy for many years.

Group physiotherapy has been developed particularly for BBAT. A group format that pays attention to human communication, relational movements, use of the voice to promote communication and includes massage and touch has the potential to become a very powerful and effective therapy. The tradition developed within BBAT draws upon inspiration from group dynamics, psychodrama, improvisations, actor training and approaches in encounter groups (Dropsy, 1973, 1984). Examples of the theoretical foundation can be seen in the works of Pratt, Alexander, Morena, Fairbain, Schutz, Pearls, Bion and Kohut (Karterud, 1989, 1998). These pioneers have been of great importance for psychiatric and psychosomatic physiotherapy (Friis et al., 1989; Skatteboe et al., 1989; Skatteboe, 2005; Leirvåg et al., 2010).

Basic Body Awareness movement group therapy is reported as having a positive outcome in two studies where it was the main component of the treatment programme for people suffering from borderline personality disorder (Skatteboe et al., 1989; Leirvåg et al., 2010). The patients included in the studies improved significantly in (1) functioning, (2) symptoms and (3) interpersonal problems. The magnitude of change in functioning and symptoms was significantly higher in the BBAT group compared with therapeutic talk alone (Leirvåg et al., 2010). Movement group therapy, implemented in community-based physiotherapy for patients with long-lasting pain, indicates more functional movement quality, improved self-efficacy and relief of pain (Klingberg-Olsson et al., 2000).

COMPETENCY IN GROUP PHYSIOTHERAPY

Being a skilled group physiotherapist requires more than 'collecting' patients in a group. To enable learning from group processes, the group physiotherapist needs to create and promote a 'good enough' group awareness and group atmosphere (Karterud & Stone, 2003). Taking on group leadership requires knowledge of therapeutic strategies and the capacity to handle both the individual in the group and the whole group. Regular supervision from a professional group therapist in leading groups is a means for the physiotherapist to gain the necessary skills and competence.

Whether working in an institution or in community mental health care, a key factor for the outcome is the integration of group physiotherapy into the rest of the teamwork. It is therefore of the greatest value if the other health workers can participate in the movement groups. The aim of the physiotherapist is to introduce the patient to a world of bodily movements, reawakening their interest in being physically active along with others. Moving together with another person is of significant importance, and provides a shared experience of moving and being.

It is an important and often challenging role for the physiotherapist to motivate other staff to take part in group physiotherapy. To begin with, it can be difficult to persuade and convince other team members of the benefits and value of participation in groups and why movement groups are important. Inviting team members to join the groups is one way of providing insight into the effects of the movement group and the therapeutic effect from it. To see other health professions taking part has an effect on the patients' motivation to enrol and remain in the group. The mutual sharing of experiences made in the group brings much needed personal and professional support for the physiotherapist. The role of the other team members can be that of cotherapists with shared responsibility for running the group or just being participant observers (Mattsson, 1998).

COMPOSITION OF THE INPATIENT GROUP

Different approaches are used in group therapy in mental health care (as well as in other health care) (Yalom, 1983). In discussion with the ward staff, the physiotherapist decides how to build the group: whether to choose an open or a closed group, two different configurations that are implemented in other physiotherapy settings. A closed group is where patients join without new patients entering during a given time. An open group means that patients leave when they are discharged from the hospital and new patients enter on admission or when they are able to join the group therapy. The open group model is often used within physiotherapy in mental health where there is high turnover. Group physiotherapy is also offered in outpatient care, running over a long period.

Rapid patient turnover, or sudden drop-outs, present a major problem in a physiotherapy group-therapy programme. If the therapist is to develop group stability, Yalom suggests having group meetings as frequently as possible. A group that meets daily at an inpatient department ward has a changing membership, but there will be carry-over of members from one meeting to another to provide some measure of group stability (Yalom, 1983). This carry-over phenomenon from people more familiar with the group therapy to newcomers may also be true within therapeutic movement groups (Skatteboe, 1991).

GROUP THERAPEUTIC FACTORS: SUMMING UP

This contribution focuses on group therapeutic factors for use in group physiotherapy where human movement and function and movement awareness provide a gateway to promote movement quality. Group therapeutic factors are particularly developed and implemented within BBAT. The physiotherapist's self-knowledge as a group leader plays a role in every aspect of therapy. The inability of the physiotherapist to perceive counter-transference reactions, or recognize personal distortions and their own blind spots, all limit the effectiveness of the physiotherapist. Such issues are not addressed in this chapter, but they do, however, play a central role in the relationship between patient and therapist.

REFERENCES

Alexander, F., 1932. The Use of the Self. Dutton, New York.

Bunkan, B.H., 2008. Kropp, Respirasjon og Kroppsbilde. Teori og Helsefremmende Behandling. (Body, Respiration and Body Image. Theory and Health Promoting Treatment), 4utg. ed. Gyllendal Akademisk, Oslo.

Dropsy, J., 1973. Vivre dans son Corps. Expression Corporelle et Relations Humaines (Living in your Body—Bodily Expression and Human Contact). Epi S.A, Paris.

Dropsy, J., 1984. Le Corps bien Accordé—un Exercice invisible (The harmonic body—an Invisible Exercise). Desclée De Brouwer, Paris.

Fairbairn, W.R., 1952. Psychoanalystic Studies of the Personality. Tavinstock, London.

Friis, S., Skatteboe, U.B., Hope, M.K., Vaglum, P., 1989. Body awareness group therapy for patients with personality disorders. 2. Evaluation of the Body Awareness Rating Scale. Psychother. Psychosom. 51, 18–24.

Karterud, S., 1989. Group Processes in Therapeutic Communities. Otto Falch as, Oslo.

Karterud, S., 1998. The group self, empathy, intersubjectivity and hermenutics: a group analytic perspective. In: Harwood, N.H., Pines, M. (Eds.), Self Experiences in Group. Intersubjectivity and Psychological Pathways to Human Understanding. Jessica Kingsley Publishers Ltd, London, pp. 83–97.

Karterud, S., Stone, W.N., 2003. The group self: a neglected aspect of group psychotherapy. Group Analysis 36 (1), 7–22.

Klingberg-Olsson, K., Lundgren, M., Lindström, I., 2000. Våga välja vad jag vill"—Basal kroppskänndom och samtal i grupp—ett samarbetsprojekt mellan sjukgymnast och psykolog. Nordisk Fysioterapi 4, 133–142.

Leirvåg, H., Pedersen, G., Karterud, S., 2010. Long-term continuation treatment after short-term day treatment of female patients with severe personality disorders: Body Awareness Group Therapy versus Psychodynamic Group Therapy. Nord. J. Psychiatry 64 (3), 153–157.

Mattsson, M., 1998. Body Awareness Applications in Physiotherapy. (Dissertation). Umeå University, Umeå.

Moreno, J.L., 1944. Spontaneity Test and Spontaneity Training. Psychodrama Monograph 4. Beacon House, New York.

Pearls, F., Hefferline, R., Goodman, P., 1973. Gestalt Therapy, Excitement and Growth in the Human Personality. Penguin Books, London.

Pratt, J., 1908. Results obtained in the treatment of pulmonary tuberculosis by the class method. Br. Med. J. 2, 1070–1071.

Roxendal, G., 1985. Body Awareness Therapy and the Body Awareness Scale, Treatment and Evaluation in Psychiatric Physiotherapy. (Doctoral degree). University of Göteborg and Psychiatric Department II, Lillhagen Hospital, Hisings Backa, Göteborg.

Schutz, W.C., 1973. Elements of Encounter. Jou Press, Big Sur. Joy Press: Big Sur, California.

Skatteboe, U.B., 1991. Terapeutiske faktorer i gruppebehandling (Therapeutic factors in group treatment). Fysioterapeuten (Journal of Norwegian Physiotherapy) 58, 24–30.

Skatteboe, U.B., 2005. Basic body awareness therapy and movement harmony. Development of the Assessment Method Body Awareness Rating Scale (BARS). Oslo University College, Oslo, p. 157.

Skatteboe, U.B., Friis, S., Hope, M.K., Vaglum, P., 1989. Body awareness group therapy for patients with personality disorders. 1. Description of the therapeutic method. Psychother. Psychosom. 51 (1), 11–17.

Sullivan, H.S., 1953. The Collected Work of Harry Stack Sullivan. Norton, New York.

Urdal, B., 1975. Å lede en gruppe: refleksjoner omkring ledelse affekter og kropp/sjel problematikk i en gruppedynamisk sammenheng. Fysioterapeuten 42, 167–169.

Yalom, I.D., 1989. Group Psychotherapy. Basic Books, New York.

Yalom, I.D., 1995. The Theory and Practice of Group Psychotherapy, third ed. Basic Books, New York.

Yalom, I.D., 1980. Existential Psychotherapy. Basic Books, Inc., Publishers, New York.

Yalom, I.D., 1983. Inpatient Group Psychotherapy. Basic Books, New York.

OBSERVATION AND EVALUATION TOOLS

4.1

OBSERVATION AND EVALUATION TOOLS WITHIN PHYSIOTHERAPY IN MENTAL HEALTH

MICHEL PROBST

SUMMARY

Observation and evaluation are two important aspects in physiotherapy. Firstly, observation allows the therapist to gain insight into the current disorders of the patient. Secondly, evaluation gives the patient and therapist information about treatment progress. In this chapter, several observation and evaluation tools will be discussed. Tools developed both within and outside the field of physiotherapy will be discussed and explained.

KEY POINTS

- Observation and evaluation tools for physiotherapy in mental health.
- The use of observation and evaluation tools is essential for the physiotherapy intervention.
- 'Measuring is knowing'.
- Gain a deeper understanding in observation and evaluation tools within physiotherapy in mental health.

LEARNING OBJECTIVES

- To become more familiar with different observation and evaluation tools.
- To understand that physiotherapy interventions can be improved by using tools appropriated from other disciplines.
- To consider the standardization, reliability and validity of testing.

INTRODUCTION

In this section, the editors have collected different observation and evaluation tools that are used in the fields of mental health and psychiatry. A distinction is made between the tools conceived within the field of physiotherapy in mental health and others frequently used in mental health that have been developed outside the field of physiotherapy, but that have applications within the discipline.

Observation is a way of gathering relevant information by observing the behaviour or physical characteristics of an individual in a specific setting. An observation is a neutral and strictly objective picture of what is observed without the imposition of judgements, interpretation or opinion of the observer. In theory, the possibilities of observation are limitless, but often it can be impossible to observe everything. Therefore observation is defined as an intensive, goal-oriented and systematic (therapeutic) activity. It can be thought of as perception combined with a critical attitude. Observation is an essential element of the physiotherapist's skills when working in mental health. In general, observations should be brief, focused and designed to provide information about a topic relevant to the observer that has been clearly defined in advance. Observations give the physiotherapist important information about a patient's performance and provide guidance for the design of the physiotherapy treatment.

The advantages of observation are that data are collected where and when an activity is occurring. The observation does not rely on people's willingness or ability to provide information. Observation allows the physiotherapist to observe behaviours and interactions directly. One disadvantage of the observation methodology is the susceptibility of the observer to bias. Additionally, observation is time-consuming and does not give information about the reasons for specific (movement) behaviours. In direct observation, the Hawthorne effect (i.e., the fact that subjects perform better when they know they are being observed) can influence the objectivity of the observations. Indirect observation may reduce this influence.

Evaluation is a methodological area that is closely related to, but distinguishable from observation and has different meanings. One of the definitions of evaluation is the systematic acquisition of useful information provided by the person themself concerning a specific and relevant domain, for instance by answering a questionnaire about pain, body image, physical activity or body awareness. In contrast to observation, evaluation emphasizes the importance of self-observation or self-description. Evaluation is an act of observing and appraising oneself. In this meaning, the basis of evaluation is self-knowledge and self-experience. It is a self-description of the client without the interpretation of the therapist. The crucial question is whether the client is able to understand and answer the various statements or questions presented. Because of the subjectivity of the answers, the reliability of patient self-evaluation can be called into question.

Evaluation can also provide useful feedback in between two periods or at the end of a period of time or treatment. Both evaluation strategies can influence decision making about the physiotherapy approach.

This chapter looks at the different observation and evaluation tools frequently used in physiotherapy in mental health. In the first part, different physiotherapists describe tools they themselves have developed. In the second part tools developed outside the field of physiotherapy are described and explained: 'four-dimensional symptom questionnaires', 'self-concept questionnaires', 'physical activity and exercise questionnaires' and 'motor assessment tools'. Although these tools have not been developed within the field of physiotherapy, they have an interface with physiotherapy in mental health.

4.1.1 The Louvain Observation Scales for Objectives in Psychomotor Therapy

JOHAN SIMONS

The development of the Louvain Observation Scales for Objectives in Psychomotor Therapy (LOFOPT) was based on the premise that the observation method should give information about those aspects that are directly related to the goals. This observation tool provides data about disturbed features of the personality in movement situations that could be corrected in therapy.

In the first stage, 213 therapeutic objectives were inventoried. Via cluster analysis, these objectives were reduced to, and named in, nine categories of goals that are important to psychiatric patients: improving emotional relations; self-confidence; activity; relaxation; movement control; focusing on the situation; movement expressivity; verbal communication and social regulation ability. In the second phase these objectives were made operational as observation items. Thus the behavioral characteristic was first specified and defined through the consensus of experts. For each item on the LOFOPT a 7-point scale was established, from -3 to $+3$, indicating at one end an excessively disturbed behaviour and at the other end the opposite and equally disturbed behaviour. The disturbed behaviour of patients with psychiatric illness can therefore be presented as an excess or as a lack. The zero score corresponds to nondisturbed behaviour with regard to the item observed.

The LOFOPT can be considered to be objective and reliable (Simons, 1987; Van Coppenolle et al., 1989).

REFERENCES

Simons, J., 1987. Psychomotor observation in psychiatry. Construction and evaluation of an objective directed observation method. Doctoral dissertation. KU Leuven, Leuven.

Van Coppenolle, H., Simons, J., Pierloot, R., et al., 1989. The Louvain observation scales for objectives in Psychomotor therapy. Adap Phys Act Q 6, 145–153.

4.1.2   Exercise and Eating Disorder Questionnaire

MARIT DANIELSEN

The Exercise and Eating Disorder (EED) questionnaire (Danielsen et al., 2015) is a short, validated self-report questionnaire. It was developed to cover a broad perspective on attitudes towards compulsive exercise in eating disorders. It is a clinically derived questionnaire measuring attitudes towards compulsive exercise in patients with eating disorders and is intended for use in clinical settings (Danielsen et al., 2015).

The EED consists of 19 statements with a four-factor structure and a six-point response scale from zero to five (never, rarely, sometimes, often, usually and always) (Box 1). The scale is reversed for statements with positive meaning. Items 4, 5, 6, 7, 8, 9, 10, 11, 12 and 13 are scored from never = 0 to always = 5; Items 1, 2, 3, 14, 15, 16, 17, 18 and 19 from always = 0 to never = 5.

The global score and subscale scores are based on mean values. Higher scores indicate greater compulsivity and unhealthy exercise. The subscales cover clinically relevant issues:

1. Compulsive exercise (being physically active to avoid dealing with negative emotions; if not active: it feels wrong, I don't eat, I can't relax, I get a bad conscience, my body feels big or nasty; I listen to my body). The subscale consists of item 6, 8, 9, 10, 11, 12, 13 and 19.
2. Positive and healthy exercise (enjoy being physically active; physically active to be healthy; like to exercise with other people; items 1, 2 and 3).
3. Awareness of body signals (I notice when: I feel fit/am in shape, when I get tired, thirsty or hungry; items 14, 15, 16, 17 and 18).

4. Exercise for weight and shape reasons (active in order to be thin, burn calories and for appearance reasons; item 4, 5 and 7).

The EED has been shown to have satisfactory psychometric properties. In the validation study, EED discriminated significantly ($p < .001$) between patients and controls on global scale, subscales and all single items showed good internal consistency (Cronbach's alpha .90 in global scale) and a satisfactory test-retest stability (Pearson's correlation factor = .86 on global score) (Danielsen et al., 2015). The subscale on compulsive exercise showed the strongest correlation with eating disorder symptomatology (r (441) = 0.70, $p < .01$).

The EED included three questions investigating the frequency, intensity and duration of exercise, all of which have been validated and used elsewhere (Kurtze et al., 2008; Danielsen et al., 2012).

The EED measures changes in attitudes towards compulsive exercise and the impact on outcome at follow-up in female adult hospitalized patients with eating disorders (Danielsen et al., 2016).

During the study, the EED global score was used to predict body mass index at outcome and follow-up, and the subscale on compulsive exercise was used as a predictor variable in the analyses using EDI-2 as the main outcome measure.

To estimate the severity of the scores on the EED questionnaire the following classification is proposed:

▪ no symptom of compulsive exercise: global score below 1.8,

BOX 1
EXERCISE AND EATING DISORDER QUESTIONNAIRE

		Never	Rarely	Sometimes	Often	Usually	Always
1	I enjoy being physically active.						
2	I like to exercise with other people.						
3	I am physically active to be healthy (see item 1).						
4	I am physically active to become thin.						
5	I am physically active to burn calories I've eaten.						
6	I am physically active to avoid dealing with negative emotions.						
7	I am physically active for appearance reasons.						
8	It feels wrong if I can't be active every day.						
9	If I haven't been physically active, I don't eat.						
10	If I haven't been physically active, I can't relax.						
11	If I haven't been physically active, I get a bad conscience.						
12	If I haven't been physically active, my body feels big.						
13	If I haven't been physically active, my body feels disgusting.						
14	I notice when I feel fit/in shape.						
15	I notice when I get tired.						
16	I notice when I get thirsty.						
17	I notice when I get hungry.						
18	I notice physical pain.						
19	I listen to my body.						

- low severity of compulsive exercise: global score from 1.8 to 2.4,
- moderate severity of compulsive exercise: global score from 2.4 to 3.2,
- high severity of compulsive exercise: global score above 3.2.

Increased severity is associated with increasing exercise frequency and intensity, and eating disorder symptoms.

The original questionnaire was developed in Norway at the Nord Trøndelag Hospital Trust, department of psychiatry by a physiotherapist working at the Regional Unit for Eating Disorders. The questionnaire was translated to English by M. Danielson and D. Reas

following the current translation principles. The use of the questionnaire is free of charge.

REFERENCES

Danielsen, M., Bjornelv, S., Rø, Ø., 2015. Validation of the exercise and eating disorders questionnaire. Int. J. Eat. Disord. 48, 983–993.

Danielsen, M., Bratberg, G.H., Rø, Ø., 2012. A pilot study of a new assessment of physical activity in eating disorder patients. Eat. Weight Disord. 17, e70–e77.

Danielsen, M., Rø, Ø., Romild, U., Bjørnelv, S., 2016. Impact of female adult eating disorder inpatients' attitudes to compulsive exercise on outcome at discharge and follow-up. J. Eat. Disord. 4, 7.

Kurtze, N., Rangul, V., Hustvedt, B.E., Flanders, W.D., 2008. Reliability and validity of self-reported physical activity in the Nord-Trondelag Health Study: HUNT 1. Scand. J. Public Health 36, 52–61.

4.1.3   Physical Activity and Unrest Test

MICHEL PROBST

This new experimental questionnaire, developed by Probst (2003) at the University of Leuven (KU Leuven), was designed for the assessment of physical activity and unrest in individuals with eating disorders. The Physical Activity and Unrest Test (PAUT) (Box 1) contains 15 items and each item is scored on a four-point scale (1–4; never = 1, sometimes = 2, usually = 3 and always = 4). The total score is the sum of the 15 items and may range from 15 to 60. Factor analysis with varimax rotation revealed two factors with an eigenvalue greater than one. Factor one was named urge to move and exercise (items 1, 2, 4, 6, 9, 10 and 14) and factor two, restlessness

and unrest (items, 3, 5, 7, 8, 11, 12, 13 and 15). The internal consistency of the PAUT was examined using Cronbach's alpha. The Cronbach's alpha coefficient was .93 for the clinical subjects and .80 for the nonclinical group. Comparison between eating disorder patients and nonclinical subjects showed different significance on the total score, subscales as item level (except for item 8). In contradiction to the control group, the eating disorder group showed a positive, moderate but significant relation between the questionnaire and body experiences variables. Clinical subjects scored significantly higher than nonclinical subjects on both questionnaires.

BOX 1
PHYSICAL ACTIVITY AND UNREST TEST

Name:

Date:

Birth date: Weight: Height:

		Never	Sometimes	Usually	Always
01.	Sitting still is very difficult for me.				
02.	I feel agitated.				
03.	After eating, I have the urge to be physically active.				
04.	I am very active during the day.				
05.	I feel guilty when I don't do exercise every day.				
06.	When I am not doing anything, I feel tense.				
07.	When participating in sports or other physical activities, I want to surpass my achievements.				
08.	I feel a need for bodily movement.				
09.	I consider resting a waste of time.				
10.	I continually want something to do.				
11.	I force myself to exercise, even when I don't feel like it.				
12.	I exercise in order to burn calories.				
13.	I can only relax after having sufficiently exercised.				
14.	I feel the need to be busy doing something.				
15.	I prefer standing up to sitting down.				

Within the clinical group, no significant difference was found between the patients with Anorexia Nervosa (AN) and Bulimia Nervosa (BN) (Probst, 2003; Ferri et al., 2009; Neefs & Probst, 2015).

REFERENCES

Ferri, I., Carraro, A., Probst, M., 2009. Hyperactivity in eating disorder patients. Unpublished master's thesis, Padua: University of Padua.

Neefs, M., Probst, M., 2015. Physical activity and unrest in patients with eating disorders. Master's thesis. KU Leuven, Leuven.

Probst, M., 2003. Assessment of hyperactivity and excessive exercise in eating disorders. Paper presented at the European Council on Eating Disorders in Budapest, 12 September 2003.

Probst, M., 2003. Hyperactivity the unknown enemy in exercise therapy. Proceedings XIth European Congress of sport psychology. Fepsac-CR-rom, Copenhagen.

4.1.4 The Global Physiotherapy Examination (GPE-52)

ALICE KVÅLE

The Global Physiotherapy Examination (GPE) is based on the construct from Norwegian psychomotor physiotherapy that the body reacts to both physical and psychological strain over time, affecting flexibility and the ability to relax, muscle tension, respiration and posture (Sundsvold & Vaglum, 1985; Bunkan & Thornquist, 1990). The method was developed by Sundsvold in the 1970s and 1980s, in which time several versions existed (Sundsvold et al., 1982). Based on results from confirmatory factor analysis in the early 2000s, a shorter version with 52 tests was developed, without hampering either the reliability or validity of the method (Kvåle et al., 2002, 2003a,b). The GPE-52 version consists of 52 well-defined and standardized items within five domains: posture, respiration, movement, muscle and skin, which cover 13 subdomains, each with four items. The 52 items are scored according to deviation from a predefined standard, 0 (see Box 1 and illustration). For an experienced physiotherapist, the complete examination takes about 30 minutes to carry out and the method has been found useful for physiotherapists working in pain clinics and/or with psychosomatic patients, particularly in Scandinavian countries. The single items give localized somatic information, whereas the absolute sum-scores within the subdomains and main domains give an impression of degree and site of the problems.

Research indicates high GPE-scores for patients with extensive problems, physically as well as psychologically (Kvåle et al., 2001, 2008) and total GPE-52 sum-scores are around 34 (SD 6.4) in healthy subjects ($n = 104$), versus 47 (SD 8.0) in patients with long-lasting musculoskeletal pain ($n = 247$) (Kvåle et al., 2003c). Responsiveness to important change has been examined in patients with long-lasting musculoskeletal problems. Although all main domains demonstrated sensitivity to change, only the main domains respiration and movement, especially in the subdomain of flexibility, demonstrated responsiveness (Kvåle et al., 2005). The domain of muscle showed some degree of responsiveness, but more in patients with localized pain than in patients with widespread pain.

BOX 1

ILLUSTRATION AND SCORING OF THE SUB-DOMAIN FLEXIBILITY IN THE GPE-52

The sub-domain Flexibility has four tests, and information is obtained about flexibility and degree of muscle tension, as well as the ability to voluntarily relax in the spine, trunk and shoulder region. When the cervical and lumbar spine is evaluated, the patient has a supported forward flexed position (buttocks towards a wall) and the physiotherapist starts a passive rhythmical movement where the force of gravity is exploited. Resistance is evaluated through the handling, and degree of flexibility through the observation of self-movement that is being set off.

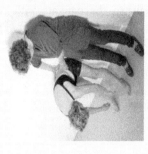

Movement Flexibility (4 tests)	Scoring Scale −2	−1	0	+1	+2	Procedure
1. Shoulder retraction resistance	Very yielding, limp and floppy resistance	Slightly yielding and limp (too little resistance)	Soft and living resistance when the shoulder is pulled slowly back	Slightly increased and tardy resistance	Very increased and tardy resistance	
2. Lumbo-sacral flexibility	Very limp and floppy self-movement	Slightly limp and floppy self-movement	Soft, free, living self-movement. Movement spreads from the lumbar region to the atlanto-occipital joint	Slightly reduced and restricted self-movement	Very restricted and reduced self-movement. No movement spreads through the spine	

3. Head-nod flexibility	Very limp and 'loose-jointed' self-movement	Slightly limp and 'loose-jointed' self-movement	Soft, free, living self-movement of the cervical spine	Slightly reduced and restricted self-movement	Very restricted and reduced self-movement
4. Head rotation resistance	Very yielding and limp (no resistance)	Slightly yielding and limp (too little resistance)	Soft and living resistance when head is passively rotated	Slightly increased and tardy resistance	Very increased and tardy resistance

Head will be sideways rotated. Resistance will be evaluated.

REFERENCES

Bunkan, B.H., Thornquist, E., 1990. Psychomotor therapy: an approach to the evaluation and treatment of psychosomatic disorders. In: Hegna, T., Sveram, M. (Eds.), International Perspectives in Physical Therapy. 5: Psychological and Psychosomatic Problems, vol. 5. Churchill Livingstone, London, pp. 45–74.

Kvåle, A., Ellertsen, B., Skouen, J.S., 2001. Relationships between physical findings (GPE-78) and psychological profiles (MMPI-2) in patients with long-lasting musculoskeletal pain. Nord. J. Psychiatry 55 (3), 177–184.

Kvåle, A., Johnsen, T.B., Ljunggren, A.E., 2002. Examination of Respiration in patients with long-lasting musculoskeletal pain: reliability and validity. Adv. Physiother. 4 (4), 169–181.

Kvåle, A., Johnsen, T.B., Ljunggren, A.E., 2003a. Examination of Movement in patients with long-lasting musculoskeletal pain: reliability and validity. Physiother. Res. Int. 8 (1), 36–52.

Kvåle, A., Ljunggren, A.E., Johnsen, T.B., 2003b. Palpation of muscle and skin. Is this a reliable and valid procedure in assessment of patients with long-lasting musculoskeletal pain? Adv. Physiother. 5, 122–136.

Kvåle, A., Skouen, J.S., Ljunggren, A.E., 2003c. Discriminative validity of the Global Physiotherapy Examination-52 in patients with long-lasting musculoskeletal pain versus healthy persons. J. Musculoskelet. Pain 11 (3), 23–36.

Kvåle, A., Skouen, J.S., Ljunggren, A.E., 2005. Sensitivity to change and responsiveness of the Global Physiotherapy Examination (GPE-52) in patients with long-lasting musculoskeletal pain. Phys. Ther. 85 (8), 712–726.

Kvåle, A., Wilhelmsen, K., Fiske, H.A., 2008. Physical findings in patients with dizziness undergoing a group exercise programme. Physiother. Res. Int. 13 (3), 162–175.

Sundsvold, M.Ø., Vaglum, P., 1985. Muscular pains and psychopathology: evaluation by the GPM method. In: Michel, T.H. (Ed.), International Perspectives in Physical Therapy. 1: Pain, vol. 1. Churchill Livingstone, London, pp. 18–47.

Sundsvold, M.Ø., Vaglum, P., Denstad, K., 1982. Global Fysioterapeutisk Muskelundersøkelse. [The Global Physiotherapeutic Muscle Examination]. Private Oslo: Private Publishing Company.

4.1.5   The Global Body Examination

ALICE KVÅLE

Several examination methods have been developed from the Norwegian Psychomotor Physiotherapy tradition regarding the documentation of where and to what degree physical aberrations have occurred throughout the body. These findings may inform treatment (Sundsvold et al., 1982; Thornquist, 1994). The two most commonly used methods are the Global Physiotherapy Examination (Sundsvold et al., 1982; Sundsvold & Vaglum, 1985; Kvåle, 2003) and the Comprehensive Body Examination (Bunkan, 2003). Both methods can be used to examine patients with long-term musculoskeletal disorders and/or with psychological complaints, in a global and systematic way. It was decided to further develop the methods into one new Global Body Examination (GBE) method by selecting the most informative and discriminative items. This has recently been achieved and four separate articles have been published for each of the main domains in the GBE: posture (Kvåle et al., 2010), respiration (Friis et al., 2012), movement (Kvåle et al., 2011) and palpation (Kvåle et al., 2013).

The new GBE has in total 53 items: posture with three subscales and nine items, respiration with three subscales and 16 items, movement with two subscales and 12 items and palpation with one subscale for muscle and one for skin totalling 16 items. The items are scored according to a predefined standard. Deviations from 0 indicate degree of aberration, either negative or positive, as, for example, findings can be too flexible or too constrained. Absolute scores can be added to a sum-score for each subscale or main domain. All main domains and subscales discriminate significantly between healthy persons and patients and to some extent also between patients with localized pain, patients with widespread pain and patients hospitalized with psychoses (Kvåle et al., 2010, 2011, 2013; Friis et al., 2012).

REFERENCES

Bunkan, B.H., 2003. Den Omfattende Kroppsundersøkelsen (DOK)—The Comprehensive Body Examination (CBE). Gyldendal Akademisk, Oslo.

Friis, S., Kvåle, A., Opjordsmoen, S., Bunkan, B.H., 2012. The Global Body Examination (GBE). A useful instrument for evaluation of respiration. Adv. Physiother. 14 (4), 146–154.

Kvåle, A., 2003. Measurement properties of a Global Physiotherapy Examination in patients with long-lasting musculoskeletal pain. Section of Physiotherapy Science, Department of Public Health and Primary Health Care, Faculty of Medicine, University of Bergen.

Kvåle, A., Bunkan, B.H., Opjordsmoen, S., Friis, S., 2011. Development of the movement domain in the Global Body Examination. Physiother. Theory Pract. 28 (1), 41–49.

Kvåle, A., Bunkan, B.H., Opjordsmoen, S., Friis, S., 2013. Development of the palpation domain for muscle and skin in the Global Body Examination. J. Musculoskelet. Pain 21 (1), 9–18.

Kvåle, A., Bunkan, B.H., Opjordsmoen, S., et al., 2010. Development of the Posture domain in the Global Body Examination (GBE). Adv. Physiother. 12 (3), 157–165.

Sundsvold, M.Ø., Vaglum, P., 1985. Muscular pains and psychopathology: evaluation by the GPM method. In: Michel, T.H. (Ed.), International Perspectives in Physical Therapy 1: Pain. Churchill Livingstone, London, pp. 18–47.

Sundsvold, M.Ø., Vaglum, P., Denstad, K., 1982. Global Fysioterapeutisk Muskelundersøkelse. [The Global Physiotherapeutic Muscle Examination]. Private Publishing Company, Oslo.

Thornquist, E., 1994. Varieties of functional assessment in physiotherapy. Scand. J. Prim. Health Care 12 (1), 44–50.

4.1.6 Body Awareness Rating Questionnaire (BARQ)

TOVE DRAGESUND

SUMMARY

Body Awareness Rating Questionnaire (BARQ) is a self-administered questionnaire aiming to capture the phenomenon of body awareness. BARQ will be further developed using Rasch analysis (RUMM 2030) before it will be recommended for clinical use.

LEARNING OBJECTIVES

- Understand the concept of body awareness.
- Be able to explain measurement properties of the BARQ.
- Be able to define Rasch analysis in one sentence.

Body awareness is an essential concept addressed in Norwegian Psychomotor Physiotherapy (NPMP) (Øvreberg & Andersen, 1986; Kvåle & Ljunggren, 2007). The term is described somewhat differently in different fields (Mehling et al., 2009).

The BARQ is a self-administered questionnaire, aiming to capture the phenomenon of body awareness as it is understood in NPMP.

Physiotherapists specializing in NPMP, patients with long-lasting musculoskeletal pain and healthy persons participated in the development of the questionnaire (Dragesund & Råheim, 2008; Dragesund et al., 2010; 2012).

Initially a pool of items reflecting aspects of body awareness was developed. Exploratory factor analysis (EFA) of the items demonstrated four factors: function, mood, feelings and awareness. Test-retest reliability of the factors (subscales) was examined by calculating relative (ICC 2,1) and absolute reliability (S_w), and construct validity by testing hypothesis using Pearson (r) or Spearman rank (r_s) correlation. The ability to discriminate between patients and healthy people was examined using a receiver operating characteristic (ROC) curve. Responsiveness to important change was examined by one-way repeated measures analysis of variance (ANOVA), relating change scores of BARQ subscales to the Patient Global Impression of Change (PGIC) categories.

The three subscales function, feelings and awareness, had satisfactory test-retest reliability, construct and discriminative validity, while function and awareness also demonstrated evaluative ability. The subscale Mood lacks evidence for satisfactory measurement properties.

BARQ will be further developed using Rasch analysis (RUMM 2030) before it will be recommended for clinical use.

REFERENCES

Dragesund, T., Ljunggren, A.E., Kvåle, A., Strand, L.I., 2010. Body Awareness Rating Questionnaire. Development of a self-administered questionnaire for patients with long-lasting musculoskeletal and psychosomatic disorders. Adv. Physiother. 12 (2), 87–94.

Dragesund, T., Råheim, M., 2008. Norwegian Psychomotor Physiotherapy and patients with chronic pain. Patients' perspective on body awareness. Physiother. Theory Pract. 24 (4), 243–254.

Dragesund, T., Råheim, M., Strand, L.I., 2012. Body Awareness Rating Questionnaire. Measurement properties. Physiother. Theory Pract. 28 (7), 515–528.

Kvåle, A., Ljunggren, A.E., 2007. Body awareness therapies. In: Schmidt, R.F., Willis, W.D. (Eds.), Encyclopedia of Pain. Springer Verlag, Berlin, pp. 167–169.

Mehling, W.E., Daubenmier, G.J., Price, C.J., et al., 2009. Body awareness: construct and self-report measures. PLoS ONE 4 (5), 1–6. <http://www.plosone.org>

Øvreberg, G., Andersen, T., 1986. Aadel Bülow-Hansens Fysioterapi: En Metode til Omstilling og Frigjøring av Respirasjon. Øvreberg, Harstad.

4.1.7   The Body Awareness Scale Movement Quality and Experience (BAS MQ-E)

AMANDA LUNDVIK GYLLENSTEN

The Body Awareness Scale Movement Quality and Experiences (BAS MQ-E) is an assessment for use in mental health physiotherapy (Gyllensten & Mattsson, 2011, 2015). It can be used to plan treatment in collaboration with the patient and to evaluate the treatment outcome. It can also be used to communicate with the patient and communicate and assess the resources/assets and the difficulties of the patient in team conferences. The BAS MQ-E consists of a movement test, a short questionnaire and a short qualitative interview. This gives information about what the physiotherapist observes when the patient moves, the patient's own views of how the body is functioning in everyday life and a qualitative part about the experience of doing the movements. The BAS MQ-E is inspired by the Body Awareness Scale (BAS), the BAS–Health (Roxendal, 1985, 1993) and the International Classification of Function (ICF) (WHO, 2014).

■ **The movement test** is structured and consists of everyday movements. The movements assess balance, stability, coordination, breathing and ability to relate to one's own body and to another person. The scale ranges from health and vitality to severe movement difficulties/inability to perform the movement. Factor analysis has revealed three factors: (1) stability in function, (2) coordination and breathing and (3) relation and awareness (Sundén et al., 2016).

■ **The questionnaire** consists of nine questions about the experience of the body as a whole, symptoms of pain, muscle tension, ability to perform daily activities, exercise habits, relationship to appearance and breathing. It also includes a focus on motivation to change and coping strategies.

■ **The qualitative interview** focuses the patient's experiences of stability, movement coordination, breathing, the experience of moving up from the floor and the ability to be present. The patient performs five movements and during the test tells about their experiences doing them.

The BAS MQ-E has been validated for patients with musculoskeletal pain (hip osteoarthritis), schizophrenia, affective disorders and for healthy adults (Sundén et al., 2013, 2016). The interrater reliability is acceptable and the BAS MQ-E can discriminate between patients with musculoskeletal pain, patients with psychiatric problems and healthy adults (Sundén et al., 2016).

The interrater reliability and the concurrent validity of BAS MQ-E have also been investigated in a sample of people with severe mental illness. The concurrent validity and the relationships between neurological soft signs, alexithymia, fatigue, anxiety and mastery were studied. Sixty-two people with severe mental illness participated in the study. The results showed a satisfactory interrater reliability and a concurrent validity with neurological soft signs, especially cognitive- and perceptual-based signs. There were also associations between BAS MQ-E and physical fatigue and alexithymia.

The scores of BAS MQ-E were generally higher for people with schizophrenia compared with people with other diagnoses within the schizophrenia spectrum disorders and bipolar disorders (Hedlund et al., 2016).

REFERENCES

Gyllensten, A., Mattsson, M., 2011. Manual Body Awareness Scale Movement Quality and Experience, BAS MQ-E. (BAS Rörelsekvalitet och Kroppsupplevelse) Lund, Sweden.

Gyllensten, A., Mattsson, M., 2015. Manual Body Awareness Scale Movement Quality and Experience, BAS MQ-E. Revised (BAS Rörelsekvalitet och Kroppsupplevelse) Umeå, Sweden.

Hedlund, L., 2014. Basic Body Awareness Therapy and psychomotor function in persons with severe psychiatric disorders. Dissertation. Department of Health Sciences, Faculty of Medicine. Lund University, Sweden.

Roxendal, G., 1985. Body Awareness Therapy and the Body Awareness Scale, Treatment and Evaluation in Psychiatric Physiotherapy. Dissertation, Gothenburg University; Sweden.

Roxendal, G., 1993. Body Awareness Scale With Body Awareness Scale Health. Studentlitteratur, Lund.

Sundén, A., Ekdahl, C., Horstman, V., Gyllensten, A.L., 2016. Analyzing movements development and evaluation of the Body Awareness Scale Movement Quality (BAS MQ). Physiother. Res. Int. 21 (2), 70–76.

Sundén, A., Ekdahl, C., Magnusson, P.S., et al., 2013. Physical function and self-efficacy—Important aspects of health-related quality of life in individuals with hip osteoarthritis. Eur. J. Physiother. 15 (3), 151–159.

WHO (World Health Organization), 2014. International Classification of Functioning, Disability and Health (ICF). Available from http://www.who.int/classifications/icf/en/.

4.1.8 Body Awareness Rating Scale–Movement Quality and Experience (BARS-MQE)

LIV HELVIK SKJAERVEN ■ GUNVOR GARD ■ MARY-ANNE SUNDAL ■ LIV INGER STRAND

SUMMARY

The Body Awareness Rating Scale–Movement Quality and Experience (BARS-MQE) is used to evaluate movement quality in patients with long-term musculoskeletal disorders and mental health problems. The BARS-MQ is an important tool because of its multi-perspective view on movement, for its broad scope of daily-life movements and for being an indicator of health and self-efficacy. It consists of two parts: first, the physiotherapist's observation of movement quality, and second, the patient's immediate description of the movement experience. The healthy movement aspects are of the utmost importance. The BARS-MQE is well structured regarding criteria for observation, movement guidance and communication with the patient. The examination situation also functions as a communication platform, encouraging the patient's attention and adjustment of movement quality. The BARS-MQE is widely used in somatic and preventative health care. A study of the BARS-MQE's internal consistency, intertester and test-retest reliability, and construct validity shows highly satisfactory measurement properties.

KEY POINTS

■ The BARS-MQE is a movement quality evaluation tool.

■ It involves a phenomenological interview on direct movement experience.

■ It is a process-orientated evaluation tool for movement quality.

LEARNING OBJECTIVES

■ Develop a deeper understanding of physiotherapeutic observations of movement quality.

■ Develop a deeper understanding of physiotherapeutic interviews regarding the patient's immediate description of movement experience.

■ Develop a deeper understanding of an evaluation tool that focuses on how movement awareness is expressed in the movement quality and how it can be observed by the physiotherapist and described by the patient.

INTRODUCTION

The Body Awareness Rating Scale–Movement Quality and Experience (BARS-MQE) is a physiotherapeutic evaluation tool for patients suffering from long-term musculoskeletal disorders and mental health problems. It was developed in the late 1980s in Norway (Friis et al., 1989; Skatteboe et al., 1989; Skatteboe, 1990). BARS has its roots in Basic Body Awareness Therapy (BBAT) (Dropsy, 1973, 1984, 1998a,b; Roxendal, 1985) and focuses on how the patient's movement awareness is expressed in their general movement quality (Skjaerven et al., 2003). The physiotherapist evaluates the quality of the patient's general movement coordination, compensation and healthy movement resources and, in addition, records the patient's descriptions of their own movement experiences (Skjaerven et al., 2008). BARS-MQE functions as a basis for therapeutic intervention and assessment of therapeutic effect.

BARS-MQE has roots in the psychiatric field and was developed by Skatteboe and Friis (Friis et al., 1989; Skatteboe et al., 1989), further developed by Skatteboe (Skatteboe, 2005) and Skjaerven (Skjaerven, 1999; Skjaerven et al., 2003, 2004, 2008, 2010, 2015), and most recently developed by Skjaerven & Sundal. Based on factor analysis (Friis et al., 1989; Skatteboe et al., 1989; Skatteboe, 1990) the BARS-MQE consists of two parts: (1) the physiotherapist's evaluation of the patient's movement quality and (2) a phenomenological interview on the patient's immediate description of the movement experience. The patient's general movement quality is observed, described, evaluated and scored by the physiotherapist according to the way the movements are performed in relation to space, time and energy. The interview sequence opens with the physiotherapist's question: 'How was this movement for you? Can you describe your experiences from it?'

BARS-MQE–12 Movement Coordinations

The BARS-MQE consists of 12 movements including lying, sitting, standing, relational movement and walking and thus mirrors movement coordinations used in everyday life. It discriminates between pathology and health (Fig. 1) (Skjaerven et al., 2015). The patient wears clothes that allow them to move freely in and the movements are simple and soft.

The physiotherapist creates the therapeutic atmosphere for the meeting with regard to physical, psychological and relational perspectives. The patient is provided with oral and written information of the movement awareness focus, and invited to be 'present' in the movement. The therapist guides verbally and through their own movements supports the patient to come into contact with, explore and perform the movement (Box 1) (Skjaerven et al., 2010, 2015).

The evaluation requires an open floor space, a mat and a chair. The physiotherapist acts as a guide. The approach is user-friendly because the patient can keep their clothes on and the therapist is qualified in movement analysis and is sensitive to movement quality.

BARS-MQE–Scale Structure

The BARS-MQE has an ordinal scale, ranging from 1–7, where 1 is the most pathological, dysfunctional movement quality and 7 is the most healthy and functional movement quality (Box 2). The sum score ranges from 12 to 84 (Skjaerven et al., 2015).

The middle point on the scale is 4.0 where the movement quality changes from being stiff and staccato (3.5 on the scale) to being stable, free and unified (4.0 on the scale) (Box 3). This shift in quality is observed when breathing and awareness starts to be integrated into the movement. The scale includes half (0.5) scores to make it more sensitive and clinically useful (Skjaerven et al., 2015).

The BARS-MQE includes structured criteria for assessing movement quality (Skjaerven et al., 2003, 2004, 2008). It is considered a resource if in the evaluation situation the patient expresses, orally and/or bodily, the ability to change.

The physiotherapist assesses movement quality according to operationalized criteria in the BARS-MQE (Skjaerven et al., 2015). Each movement is given about 10 repetitions in order to explore and perform it thoroughly. The optimal movement quality is scored by the therapist. The BARS-MQ takes about 40 minutes in total.

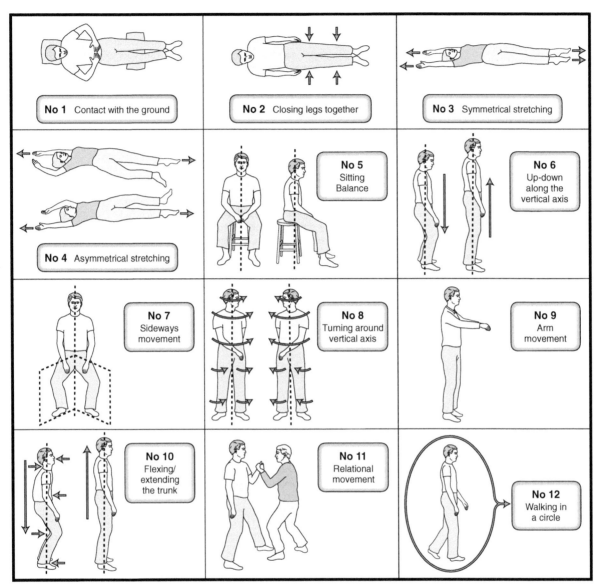

FIGURE 1 ■ Overview of the 12 movement coordinations in BARS-MQE (*Skjaerven et al., 2010*).

COMMUNICATING BARS-MQE FINDINGS

The physiotherapist is in charge of communicating the findings from the BARS-MQE to the patient, to colleagues, the medical doctor and the healthcare team. The BARS-MQE can be a strong motivating factor for many patients. During the clinical talk, the physiotherapist strives to transmit information to the patient, underlining the movement resources.

RELIABILITY AND VALIDITY

Several pilot studies of intertester reliability have been performed without being published (Skatteboe, 2005) and there has been one study on validity (Sundal, 2007). A study of the BARS's internal consistency,

BARS-MQE: EXAMPLE OF MOVEMENT GUIDANCE–MOVEMENTS 7 AND 8
(SKJAERVEN ET AL., 2015)

No 7:
Sideways movement

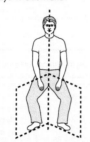

Stand with your feet further apart. Contact the ground and the vertical axis. Flex your knees and hips as if to sit on a high stool. Find a position where your knees are free, open and flexible without support from your arms. Move sideways, shifting the weight from the left to the right foot, search to keep a firm contact with the vertical axis. Keep your legs flexible and elastic to allow them to 'absorb' the movement when continuing the sideways movement searching for a flow and continuity in the movement.

No 8:
Turning around the vertical axis

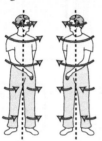

Stand with your feet underneath your hips, arms loose by your side. Contact the vertical axis with all joints free, allowing your breathing to find its own rhythm. Search from the centre of your body to maintain contact with your whole body. Start turning from left to right and right to left in a continuous movement, around the vertical axis. The movement involves the whole body from head to toe. Aim for all parts of the body to start and end at the same time: head, trunk, pelvis, knees and ankles. The movements are not separate, but synchronous. Continue at a comfortable pace, searching for flow and continuity in the movement.

BARS-MQE CRITERIA FOR SCORING (AN EXAMPLE): 5.0, 4.0, 3.0
(SKJAERVEN ET AL., 2015)

Scoring	Description of Scoring 5.0, 4.0 and 3.0
Moderate functional MQ: Score: 5.0	The vertical axis is moderately well balanced, stable, firm and free. Movement characteristics: moderate functional form, flow, elasticity and rhythm; moderate clarity in the intention and direction of the movements. The amount of energy expressed is moderately appropriate to the task. There are moderate signs of movement originating from the centre of the trunk. The movements are characterized by a moderate and variable amount of unity and integration. The movements in the person as a whole are characterized by moderate unity and integration. They express moderate movement harmony.
Some functional MQ: Score: 4.0	The vertical axis has some balance, stability, firmness and freedom. Movement characteristics: some glimpses of functional form, flow, elasticity and rhythm; some glimpses of intention and direction of the movements. The amount of energy expressed in the movement is somewhat appropriate to the task. There are some signs of movement originating from the centre of the trunk. The movements in the person as a whole are characterized by some glimpses of unity and integration. They express some movement harmony.
Weak functional MQ: Score: 3.0	The vertical axis has an uncertain balance, little stability, firmness or freedom. Movement characteristics: somewhat dysfunctional in form, somewhat mechanical, staccato, stiff, arrhythmical and lifeless. The movements are characterized by some weakness in the intention and direction. The amount of energy in the movement is more discordant with the task, being smaller and more closed or larger and more open or having too much or too little energy. The movements originate more from the periphery than from the centre of the trunk. The movements are characterized by weak unity and integration. They express weak movement harmony.

BOX 3
BARS-MQE, THE 1–7 MQ-SCORES (SKJAERVEN ET AL., 2015)

No	BARS-MQE Scores (Overview)
1	Dysfunctional MQ
2	Mostly dysfunctional MQ
3	Weak functional MQ
4	Some functional MQ
5	Moderate functional MQ
6	Good functional MQ
7	Very good functional MQ

intertester reliability, test-retest reliability and construct validity has been conducted, with highly satisfactory measurement properties (Skjaerven et al., 2015). Movement quality assessed by BARS-MQE shows it to be an indicator of health in patients with long-term musculoskeletal and mental health problems. It is used in multiple clinical settings, most recently in projects including hip osteoarthritis and scoliosis.

REFERENCES

Dropsy, J., 1973. Vivre dans son Corps. Expression Corporelle et Relations Humaines (Living in Your Body—Bodily Expression and Human Contact). Epi SA, Paris.

Dropsy, J., 1984. Le Corps Bien Accordé—un Exercice Invisible (The Harmonic Body—an Invisible Exercise). Desclée De Brouwer, Paris.

Dropsy, J., 1998a. Body attunement—the conditions for body use. In: Skjaerven, L.H. (Ed.), Quality of Movement – the Art and Health. Lectures on Philosophy, Theory and Practical Implications to Basic Body Awareness Therapy. Skjaerven, Bergen, pp. 21–34.

Dropsy, J., 1998b. Human expression—the coordination of mind and body. In: Skjaerven, L.H. (Ed.), Quality of Movement - the Art and Health. Lectures on Philosophy, Theory and Practical Implications to Basic Body Awareness Therapy. Skjaerven, Bergen, pp. 8–20.

Friis, S., Skatteboe, U.B., Hope, M.K., Vaglum, P., 1989. Body Awareness Group Therapy for patients with personality disorders. 2. Evaluation of the Body Awareness Rating Scale. Psychother. Psychosom. 51, 18–24.

Moe-Nilsen, N., 2016. Movement quality within a physiotherapy perspective years after scoliosis surgery. A descriptive cross-sectional study using Body Awareness Rating Scale – Movement Quality (BARS-MQ), Master in Health Sciences Physiotherapy. Department of Global Public Health and Primary Care, University of Bergen.

Roxendal, G., 1985. Body Awareness Therapy and The Body Awareness Scale, Treatment and Evaluation in Psychiatric Physiotherapy. (Doctoral degree), University of Göteborg and Psychiatric Department II, Lillhagen Hospital, Hisings Backa, Göteborg.

Skatteboe, U.-B., 1990. Å være i samspill. En kroppsorientert gruppeterapi for pasienter med kroniske nevroser og personlighetsforstyrrelser. (Being in interrelation. A Body-oriented Group Therapy for Patients with Chronic Nevrosis and Personality Disorders). (MSc) Statens spesiallærerhøgskole, Bærum, Oslo. (now University of Oslo).

Skatteboe, U.B., 2005. Basic Body Awareness Therapy and Movement Harmony. Development of the Assessment Method Body Awareness Rating Scale (BARS). (pp. 157). Oslo University College, Oslo.

Skatteboe, U.B., Friis, S., Hope, M.K., Vaglum, P., 1989. Body Awareness Group therapy for patients with personality disorders. 1. Description of the therapeutic method. Psychother. Psychosom. 51 (1), 11–17.

Skjaerven, L.H., 1999. 'Å vaere seg selv—mer fullt og helt'. En tilnaerming til Bevegelseskvalitet. En feltstudie av en bevegelsespraksis av bevegelsespedagog og psykoterapeut Jacques Dropsy. To be oneself - more fully'. An approach to Movement Quality. A Field study of the Movement Practice of the Movement Educator and Psychotherapist Jacques Dropsy (Master Degree Master Thesis), University of Bergen Bergen.

Skjaerven, L.H., Gard, G., Kristoffersen, K., 2003. Basic elements and dimensions to quality of movement—a case study. J. Bodyw. Mov. Ther. 7 (4), 251–260.

Skjaerven, L.H., Gard, G., Kristoffersen, K., 2004. Greek sculpture as a tool in understanding the phenomenon of movement quality. J. Bodyw. Mov. Ther. 8 (3), 227–236.

Skjaerven, L.H., Gard, G., Sundal, M.A., Strand, L.I., 2015. Reliability and Validity of the Body Awareness Rating Scale (BARS), an observational assessment tool of movement quality. Eur. J. Physiother. 17, 19–28.

Skjaerven, L.H., Kristoffersen, K., Gard, G., 2008. An eye for movement quality: a phenomenological study of movement quality reflecting a group of physiotherapists' understanding of the phenomenon. Physiother. Theory Pract. 24 (1), 13–27.

Skjaerven, L.H., Kristoffersen, K., Gard, G., 2010. How can movement quality be promoted in clinical practice? A phenomenological study of physical therapist experts. Phys. Ther. 90 (10), 1479–1492.

Sundal, M., 2007. Bevegelseskvalitet—Et Uttrykk for Helse og Velvaere? (Movement Quality—An Expression of Health and Wellbeing?) (MSc), University of Bergen, Bergen.

4.1.9   'ABC'–The Awareness Body Chart: A New Tool Assessing Body Awareness

URSULA DANNER

To encounter the limitations of questionnaires (reading and interpretation problems; the predefined concept), many healthcare professionals use anatomical maps, body charts or drawings in their communications, but without the use of standardized scoring tools. To overcome this shortcoming, the Awareness Body Chart (ABC), a self-reporting assessment tool for the evaluation of body awareness by colouring the different areas from the top of the head to the feet, was developed.

The ABC form consists of simple drawings of the female (Fig. 1) and male bodies from both front and back. The division in 51 regions was done according to anatomical structures. Depending on the intensity of their perception, subjects use different coloured pencils to express their awareness of the different body regions. The different colours correspond to the level of awareness in accordance to Pöhlmann et al. (2009). The following colours were used: orange = I can perceive with much detail ('*kann ich mit vielen Details*

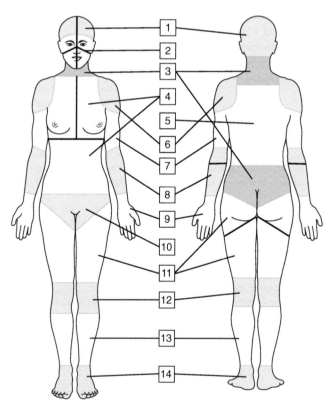

FIGURE 1 ▪ Illustration of the 51 regions and 14 body parts on the female body chart. *1,* Cranium; *2,* face; *3,* cervical/lumbar region; *4,* chest/abdomen; *5,* back; *6,* shoulder; *7,* upper arm; *8,* lower arm/elbow; *9,* hand; *10,* genital area; *11,* thigh/hip; *12,* knee; *13,* lower leg; *14,* foot.

wahrnehmen'), yellow = I can perceive distinctly (*'kann ich deutlich wahrnehmen'*), green = I can perceive (*'kann ich wahrnehmen'*), blue = I can perceive indistinctly (*'kann ich undeutlich wahrnehmen'*), black = I cannot perceive (*'kann ich nicht wahrnehmen'*). To quantify the information, every region of the body was coded as an extra item and the data of the colours were transcribed: orange (5); yellow (4); green (3); blue (2) and black (1). Additionally, a red felt-tip pen could be used to indicate the localities of possible pain awareness and the pain intensity could be marked on a pain scale ranging from 0 to 100.

The ABC has good proven psychometric properties with high internal consistency, a high retest reliability and high construct validity, and is therefore a valid tool in clinical practice as well as for further research projects. The newly developed ABC is an easy-to-use, low-cost tool. It is noninvasive, independent of verbal skills and almost every person can use it. It can be used in the clinical setting and in the broad field of research.

REFERENCES

Pöhlmann, K., Berger, S., Von Arnim, A., Joraschky, P., 2009. Der Kurze Fragebogen zur Eigenwahrnehmung des Körpers (KEKS): Entwicklung und Validierung. In: Joraschky, P., Loew, T., Röhricht, F. (Eds.), Körpererleben und Körperbild. Ein Handbuch zur Diagnostik. Schattauer, Stuttgart.

4.1.10 The Body Attitude Test

MICHEL PROBST

The Body Attitude Test (BAT; Probst et al. 1995) measures the subjective body experience and attitudes towards one's body. The scale was originally developed by a team of physiotherapists. The authors developed the scale for female patients suffering from eating disorders, but the questionnaire can also be used for other disorders as well as for men (Probst et al., 2008b). The questionnaire is also used in patients with muscle dysmorphobia (Babusa & Tury, 2012), women undergoing adjuvant breast cancer therapy (Biglia et al., 2010) and dancers (Hidayah & Bariah, 2011).

The Body Attitude Test consists of 20 items scored on a six-point scale. With the exception of the negatively scored items (4 and 9), items are scored from always (5) to never (0). The maximum score is 100, and the higher the score is, the greater the level of deviation and difficulties.

The psychometric characteristics of the BAT have been tested and demonstrated satisfactory levels of reliability and validity (Probst et al., 1995, 1997 & 2008a,b).

Previous repeated analysis yielded a stable four-factor structure: (1) negative appreciation of body size (factor 1: items 3, 5, 6, 10, 11, 13, and 16); (2) lack of familiarity with one's own body (factor 2: items 2, 4, 9, 12, 14, 17, and 19); (3) general dissatisfaction (factor 3: items 1, 7, 8, and 18); and (4) a rest factor (items 15 & 20) (Probst et al., 1995).

The BAT demonstrated satisfactory levels of internal reliability (internal consistency, Cronbach's alpha = 0.93) for both a group of non-clinical subjects and subjects with eating disorders. The factor-total correlations of the subscales range from 0.88 to 0.90. The short-term test-retest reliability (one-week interval) measured by female high school and university students and patients with eating disorders ranged from r= 0.87- 0.92 for the total score and from r= 0.72 to r= 0.95 (all p<0.01) for the subscales (Probst et al., 1995; Carano et al., 2006).

The BAT has shown good convergent validity with existing body experience-related questionnaires (Eating disorder Inventory subscale drive for thinness, body dissatisfaction; Body Shape Questionnaire; Body image questionnaire; Body Uneasiness Test; Dresdner Körperbildfragebogen (DKB-35) psychopathological phenomena and complaints (Symptom Check List, Beck Depression Inventory, Borderline syndrome index, Dissociation questionnaire, Rosenberg Self-esteem) and eating disorder-related questionnaires

(Eating disorder evaluation scale; Eating Disorder Diagnostic Scale; Eating Disorder Inventory (Probst et al, 1997; Probst et al., 1998; Favaro et al., 1997, Brytek & Rogoza, 2016; Krabbenborg et al.,2012; Danielsen & Rø, 2012) and personality traits (Schok, 1994). In binge eating disorders (BED), a global assessment was associated with BAT (Vancampfort et al., 2014)

The critical score (cut-off score) that determines the distinction between patients and non-clinical subjects was established at 36 using Shrout and Fleiss' model (1981). The BAT has a sensitivity of .69 and a specificity of .80. The positive predictive value has been established at .75, and the negative predictive value at .80. Persons with a score above 36 have a negative attitude towards their body (Probst et al., 1995).

The responses of patients with eating disorders (N=1312) to each of the subscales differed significantly from those of individuals in the community (n=1724). The total BAT score differentiates between the community sample and Weight Watchers and between eating disorder patients and Weight Watchers on subscales 1 and 2 (Probst 1995).

A comparison of the three types of eating disorders (anorexia nervosa restricting type and purging type and bulimia nervosa) showed that patients with the restricting type of anorexia nervosa obtain the lowest scores and patients with bulimia nervosa the highest. The BAT differentiates between types of eating disorder.

A review of the application of the BAT from an international perspective concluded that there was a universal congruence in BAT scores. The variance in the total BAT score in different populations was consistent with the original sample. A cut-off score of 36 seems to be a good universal convention (Pelsmaekers et al., 2016). The BAT differentiated significantly between BED with and without alexithymia (Carano et al., 2006)

A comparison of the scores between age categories showed no significant differences. Age did not interact with BAT scores. A positive linear relationship exists between the BAT and the BMI. Scores on the BAT increase as BMI increases. The BMI was shown to be the best predictor of BAT scores after ½ and 1 year of therapy (Probst et al., 1995; Devacht & Vandereycken, 1998). Subscale 2 of the BAT has shown a significant

relation with the VAS-quality of life in patients with eating disorders (Thörnborg et al., 2005).

The BAT is a good predictor of dissociative experiences and global therapy outcomes (Vanderlinden et al., 1995). A differentiation between patients with and without self-injurious behaviour can also be made by the BAT (Claes et al., 2003). Research shows that the BAT also differentiates between patients, students and women with fertility problems (Devacht & Vandereycken, 1998). Positive relationships between the BAT and the schema domains of Young (disconnection, impaired autonomy, improved links, other directives and overvigiliance), personal opinions and evaluative concerns of perfectionism were found (Boone et al., 2013).

The BAT can be used as a follow-up instrument to evaluate progress in treatment (Probst et al., 1999; Geerdens et al., 2013; Ruwaard et al.,2013; Catalan et al., 2011).

Normative data for patients from 14 years old with eating disorders and female non-clinical subjects are presented in Table 1. Normative data for males can be found in Probst et al. (2008).

The first version of the BAT was originally drafted in Dutch (Van Coppenolle et al., 1984). The questionnaire is now available in different languages without copyright costs. The Spanish (Gila et al., 1999), Hungarian (Tury et al., 2000), Japanese (Kashiima et al, 2003), Polish (Brytek & Probst, 2014), Italian (Santonastoso et al., 1995), and Norwegian (Danielsen et al., 2012), and the Czech (Uher et al., 2004) versions of the BAT are validated.

The questionnaire is also available by the author in Chinese, Danish, Estonian, French, Finnish, German (Probst et al, 1990), Portuguese, and Swedish.

Users of this questionnaire must analyze the answers prior to drawing conclusions. Some (eating disorders) subjects have the tendency to skew answers in a certain direction regardless of the content of the stimulus (i.e., response style). For instance, in the assenting response style, all items are positively scored regardless of the content. An abnormal response style refers to the presence of atypical and unusual scores, and the extreme response style, to extreme categories. Other subjects deliberately attempt to guide the answer in a certain direction (misleading answers, i.e., false good; false bad; social desirability) or with a non-verbal message ('cry for help').

	TABLE 1		

Normative Data and Descriptive Characteristics of Belgian Female Patients With Anorexia Nervosa, Bulimia Nervosa and Female Non-Clinical Subjects for the Body Attitude Test (Mean, Standard Deviations and Percentile Distributions for the Total Score)

	Anorexia Nervosa	Bulimia Nervosa	Female Control Subjects
N	813	419	1724
Age (year)	22.20 (±7.20)	23.90 (±6.90)	17.90 (±3.40)
BMI (kg/m^2)	14.88 (±1.71)	21.91 (±4.33)	20.37 (±2.78)
BAT total score	52.08 (±19.82)	62.61 (±19.37)	27.39 (±15.97)
P10	25	34	10
P25	37	50	16
P50	53	65	24
P75	67	78	34
P90	79	86	51

BOX 1
BODY—ATTITUDE - TEST (BAT)

		Always	Usually	Often	Sometimes	Rarely	Never
1	When I compare myself with my peers' bodies, I'm dissatisfied with my own						
2	My body appears to be a numb thing						
3	My hips seem too broad to me						
4	I feel comfortable within my own body						
5	I have a strong desire to be thinner						
6	I think my breasts are too large						
7	I'm inclined to hide my body (e.g. by loose clothing)						
8	When I look at myself in the mirror, I'm dissatisfied with my own body						
9	It's easy for me to relax physically						
10	I think I'm too thick						
11	I feel my body as a burden						
12	My body appears as if it is not mine						
13	Some parts of my body look swollen						
14	My body is a threat for me						
15	My bodily appearance is very important to me						
16	My belly looks as if I am pregnant						
17	I feel tense in my body						
18	I envy others for their physical appearance						
19	There are things going on in my body that frighten me						
20	I am observing my appearance in the mirror						

REFERENCES

Babusa, B., Túry, F., 2012. Muscle dysmorphia in Hungarian noncompetitive male bodybuilders. Eat. Weight Disord. 17 (1), e49–e53. doi:10.1007/BF03325327.

Biglia, N., Moggio, G., Peano, E., et al., 2010. Effects of Surgical and Adjuvant Therapies for Breast Cancer on Sexuality, Cognitive Functions, and Body Weight. Journal of Sexual Medicine 7, 1891–1900. doi:10.1111/j.1743-6109.2010.01725.x.

Boone, L., Braet, C., Vandereycken, W., Claes, L., 2013. Are maladaptive schema domains and perfectionism related to body image concerns in eating disorder patients? European Eating Disorders Review 21 (1), 45–51. doi:10.1002/erv.2175.

Brytek-Matera, A., Probst, M., 2014. Psychometric properties of the Polish version of the Body Attitude Test. Archives of Psychiatry and Psychotherapy 1, 39–46. doi:10.12740/APP/21445.

Carano, A., De Berardis, D., Gambi, F., et al., 2006. Alexithymia and body image in adult outpatients with binge eating disorder. International Journal of Eating Disorders 39 (4), 332–340. doi:10.1002/eat.20238.

Catalan-Matamoros, D., Helvik-Skjaerven, L., Labajos-Manzanares, M.T., et al., 2011. A pilot study on the effect of Basic Body Awareness Therapy in patients with eating disorders: a randomized controlled trial. Clin. Rehabil. 25 (7), 617–626. doi:10.1177/0269215510394223.

Claes, L., Vandereycken, W., Vertommen, H., 2003. Eating-disordered patients with and without self-injurious behaviors: A comparison of psychopathological features. European Eating Disorders Review 11, 379–396.

Czeglédi, E., Urbán, R., Csizmadia, P., 2010. A testkép mérése: A testi attitüdök tesztjének (Body Attitude Test) pszichometriai vizsgálata. Magyar Pszichológiai Szemle 65 (3), 431–461.

Danielsen, M., Rø, Ø., 2012. Changes in body image during inpatient treatment for eating disorders predict outcome. Eat. Disord. 20 (4), 261–275. doi:10.1080/10640266.2012.689205.

Devacht, I., Vandereycken, W., 1998. Het verband tussen eetproblemen en vruchtbaarheids-problemen. KU Leuven, Psychodiagnostiek, unpublished masterthesis.

Exterkate, C., Vriesendorp, P., de Jong, C., 2009. Body attitudes in patients with eating disorders at presentation and completion of intensive outpatient day treatment. Eating Behavior 10 (1), 16–21. doi:10.1016/j.eatbeh.2008.10.002.

Favaro, A., Gigli, G., Miotto, P., Santonastaso, P., 1997. Validita del questionario di Ben Tovim & Walker per attegiamenti verso il corpo. Bollettino di Psicologia Applicata 221, 39–47.

Fernandez, F., Turon, V., 1998. Trastornos de la alimentacion. Masson, Barcelona.

Geerdens, C., Vanderlinden, J., Pieters, G., et al., 2013. Missing Data in Long-term Follow-up of Patients with Eating Disorders Using the Body Attitude Test. European Eating Disorders Review 21, 224–229. doi:10.1002/erv.2205.

Gila, A., Castro, J., Gomez, M., et al., 1999. The Body Attitude Test: validation of the spanish version. Eating & Weight Disorders 4, 175–178. doi.org/10.1007/BF03339733.

Hidayah, G.N., Bariah, A.S., 2011. Eating Attitude, Body Image, Body Composition and Dieting Behaviour ainong Dancers. Asian Journal of Clinical Nutrition 3 (3), 92–102.

Kashiima, A., et al., 2003. Japanese Version of the Body Attitude Test: its reliability and validity. Psychiatry Clin. Neurosci. 57, 511–516. doi:10.1046/j.1440-1819.2003.01156.x.

Krabbenborg, M., Danner, U., Larsen, J., et al., 2012. The Eating Disorder Diagnostic Scale: Psychometric Features Within a Clinical Population and a Cut-off Point to Differentiate Clinical Patients from Healthy Controls. European. Eating. Disorders Review 20, 315–320. doi:10.1002/erv.1144.

Miotto, P., De Coppi, M., Frezza, M., et al., 2003. Eating disorders and aggressiveness among adolescents. Acta Psychiatr. Scand. 108 (3), 183–189. doi:10.1034/j.1600-0447.2003.00121.x.

Pelsmaekers, M., Nackaerts, J., Probst, M., 2016. The Body Attitude Test in an international perspective. Unpublished masterthesis Leuven (Belgium): KU Leuven.

Probst, M., Pieters, G., Vanderlinden, J., 2008a. Evaluation of body experience questionnaire in eating disorders and non-clinical subjects. International Journal of Eating Disorders 41, 657–665.

Probst, M., Pieters, G., Vanderlinden, J., 2008b. Body experience assessment in non-clinical male and female subjects. Eat. Weight Disord. 14 (1), doi:10.1007/BF03354623.

Probst, M., Van Coppenolle, H., Vandereycken, W., 1997. Further experience with the Body Attitude Test. Eating & Weight Disorders 2, 100–104. doi:10.1007/BF03339956.

Probst, M., Van Coppenolle, H., Vandereycken, W., Meermann, R., 1990. Zur Evaluation der Körperbild-Wahrnehmung bei Patienten mit Anorexia Nervosa. Psychiatr. Prax. 17, 115–120.

Probst, M., Vandereycken, W., Van Coppenolle, H., Vanderlinden, J., 1995. Body Attitude Test for patients with an eating disorder: psychometric characteristics of a new questionnaire. Eating disorders: The Journal of Treatment and Prevention 3, 133–145. doi.org/10.1080/10640269508249156.

Probst, M., Vandereycken, W., Van Coppenolle, H., Pieters, G., 1998a. Body size estimation using video distortion on a life-size screen and psychological variables in restricting anorexia nervosa patients. J. Psychosom. Res. 44 (3/4), 451–456.

Probst, M., Vandereycken, W., Van Coppenolle, H., Pieters, G., 1999. Body experience in eating disorders before and after treatment: a follow up study. European Psychiatry 14, 333–340. doi:10.1016/S0924-9338(99)00159-5.

Probst, M., Vandereycken, W., Vanderlinden, J., Van Coppenolle, H., 1998b. The significance of body size estimation in eating disorders: its relationship with physiological and psychological variables. International Journal of Eating Disorders 24, 167–174.

Raudsnik, L., Probst, M., 2013. Body experience and psychological quality of life in Estonian Females. KU Leuven, Rehabilitation Sciences, unpublished masterthesis KU Leuven, Belgium.

Ruwaard, J., Lange, A., Broeksteeg, J., et al., 2013. Online Cognitive–Behavioural Treatment of Bulimic Symptoms: A Randomized Controlled Trial. Clin. Psychol. Psychother. 20, 308–318. doi:10.1002/cpp.1767.

Santonastoso, P., Favaro, A., Ferrara, S., et al., 1995. Confronto degli atteggiamenti corporei di un gruppo di pazienti con disturbi dell'alimentazione con un campione di studentesse: validazione italiana del Body Attitudes Test. Rivista Sperimentale di Freniatria 69, 423–436.

Shrout, P.E., Fleiss, J.L., 1981. Reliability and case detection. In: Wing, J.K. (Ed.), What is a Case? The Problem of Definition in Psychiatric Community Surveys. Grant McIntyre, London, pp. 125–137.

Stok, M.L., 1994. Comorbiditeit bij eetstoornissen. Universiteit Utrecht: Gezondheidspsychologie.

Thörnborg, U., Nordholm, L., Wallström, A., Svantesson, U., 2005. Quality of life assessment for patients with eating disorders. Eat. Weight Disord. 10 (3), e56–e60.

Tury, F., Szabo, P., 2000. Disorders of eating behaviour anorexia and bulimia nervosa psychiatry on the turn of the millennium series. Medicina publishing, Budapest.

Uher, R., Pavlová, B., Papežová, H., et al., 2004. Vztah k vlastnimu tělu a somatoformni disociace u poruch příjmu potravy. Czechoslovensá Psychologie 48, 385–396.

Van Coppenolle, H., Vandereycken, W., Pierloot, R., Depreitere, L., 1984. Constructie van een vragenlijst over de lichaamsbeleving bij anorexia nervosa. Bewegen en Hulpverlening 1, 42–60. (Translation in: Van Coppenolle, H., Probst, M., Vandereycken, W., Goris, M., & Meermann, R. (1990). Construction of a Questionnaire on the body experience of anorexia nervosa. In H. Remschmidt, M. Schmidt (Eds.). *Anorexia nervosa* (pp. 103-123). Hogrefe: Stuttgart.).

Vancampfort, D., Probst, M., Adriaens, A., et al., 2014. Clinical correlates of global functioning in obese treatment seeking persons with binge eating disorder. Psychiatrica Danubina 26, 256–260.

Vanderlinden, J., Vandereycken, W., Probst, M., 1995. Dissociative Symptoms in eating disorders: a follow up study. European Eating Disorders Review 3, 174–184. doi:10.1002/erv.2400030306.

4.2 NONPHYSIOTHERAPEUTIC OBSERVATION AND EVALUATION TOOLS

4.2.1 Four-Dimensional Symptom Questionnaire (4DSQ)

MICHEL PROBST

INTRODUCTION

The Four-Dimensional Symptom Questionnaire (4DSQ) was originally a Dutch self-rating questionnaire measuring four dimensions of common psychopathology: distress, depression, anxiety and somatization. It was developed in general practice. The principal aim of the 4DSQ is to distinguish between stress-related syndromes (denoted as 'stress', 'burnout', 'nervous breakdown' or in Dutch 'overspanning' or 'surmenage') and psychiatric disorders (e.g., depression and anxiety disorders) (Terluin, 1996). To improve treatment results, early detection and appropriate therapy are essential. Therefore the use of the 4DSQ can be helpful for physiotherapists in detecting possible mental problems (van der Horst, 2008).

THE SCALES

The Distress Scale

The distress scale measures nonspecific symptoms of psychopathology, ranging from worrying and irritability to fatigue and demoralization. As a general nonspecific component, distress is always part of the symptomatology of anxiety and depressive disorders, in which case distress accompanies specific symptoms of anxiety or depression. Distress alone, or in combination with somatization, is characteristic of uncomplicated stress-related syndromes that are commonly encountered in general practice. The distress score is associated with any psychosocial diagnosis as established by general practitioners (GPs) in general practice patients (Terluin et al., 2004, 2006). This is covered in questions 17, 19, 20, 22, 25, 26, 29, 31, 32, 36, 37, 38, 39, 41, 47 and 48.

The Depression Scale

The depression scale measures severe anhedonia and depressive thoughts, including suicidal ideation—symptoms that are characteristic of depressive disorders. The depression score indicates the probability of having a major depressive disorder. This is covered in questions: 28, 30, 33, 34, 35 and 46.

The Anxiety Scale

The anxiety scale measures free-floating anxiety, panic and phobic anxiety, symptoms that are specific to the anxiety disorders. The anxiety score indicates the probability of having one or more anxiety disorders. This is covered in questions 18, 21, 23, 24, 27, 40, 42, 43, 44, 45, 49 and 50.

The Somatization Scale

The somatization scale measures a range of common physical symptoms known to be related to distress or psychopathology. Examples are headache, palpitations, nausea and muscle aches. Moderate levels of somatization commonly accompany psychological distress that is not necessarily pathological. High levels of somatization reflect pathological–psychological mechanisms such as 'sensitization', illness attributes and health anxiety. The somatization score is associated with the GP's suspicion of a psychosocial background in patients presenting with physical symptoms. This is covered in questions 1–16.

QUESTIONNAIRE ITEMS

The questionnaire contains 50 items (see Box 1) that query the previous 7 days. Each item has five answer options in which the patient has to choose: 'no', 'sometimes', 'regularly', 'often', 'very often' or 'constantly'. Afterwards, each item is scored by 0, 1 or 2. Zero points are given for answer option 'no'. One point is given for 'sometimes' and two points are given for items scored as 'frequently', 'often' or 'always'. Finally, the scores of the different items, which together represent one subscale, are added up. All items can be divided into four subscales: distress (16 items, score range 0–32), depression (6 items, score range 0–12), anxiety (12 items, score range 0–24) and somatization (16 items, score range 0–32) (Terluin, 1996). A score of zero is given when items on the questionnaire were not filled in. In addition, when more than two items were missing on the distress, anxiety and somatization scale, and more than one item was missing on the depression scale, the whole questionnaire was excluded (Terluin & Duijsens, 2007). The 4DSQ is available on the internet free of charge.

RELIABILITY AND VALIDITY

The reliability of the 4DSQ in a GP population was measured as good (Egberink et al., 2014). Therefore

TABLE 1			

Cut–Off Scores for the Different 4DSQ Subscales (Terluin & Duijsens, 2007; Terluin et al., 2014)

	Low Score	Moderately Elevated Score	Highly Elevated Score
Distress	0–10	11–20	21–32
Depression	0–2	3–5	6–12
Anxiety	0–4	4–10	10–24
Somatization	0–10	11–20	21–32

internal consistency was calculated for each subscale using Cronbach's alpha (distress: .94, depression: .94, anxiety: .88 and somatization .84) (Terluin, 1996). The test-retest reliability was also determined and varied from 0.89 to 0.94 between the different subscales (Terluin, 1998). Criteria validity and construct validity were measured as sufficient (Egberink, et al., 2005).

To interpret the results of the 4DSQ, Terluin proposed some cut-off scores for each subscale (Table 1).

This study has shown that the 4DSQ is a reliable questionnaire for use in private physiotherapy practices. Mental health problems in physiotherapy patients seem to occur in different severities. Therefore the questionnaire can be used as a helpful and easy instrument in private physiotherapy practices to detect psychological symptoms ranging from normal stress-related symptoms to more severe psychiatric problems, such as depression, anxiety and somatization. Based on the results of the questionnaire, the physiotherapist can adapt their treatment to the specific needs of the patient. In case of highly elevated scores, referral can be made.

The 4DSQ is already translated from Dutch into German, English, Polish, Turkish and French and is freely available for noncommercial use, for instance in clinical practice and research. For more information see http://www.emgo.nl/quality-of-our-research/research-tools/4dsq.

BOX 1
FOUR-DIMENSIONAL SYMPTOM QUESTIONNAIRE (4DSQ)

The following is a list of questions about various complaints and symptoms you may have. Each question refers to the complaints and symptoms that you had **in the past week (the past 7 days, including today)**. Complaints you had before then, but no longer had during the past week, do not count.

Please indicate for each complaint how often you noticed that you had it in the past week by putting an 'X' in the box under the answer that is most appropriate.

	No	Sometimes	Regularly	Often	Very Often or Constantly
During the past week, did you suffer from:					
1. Dizziness or feeling light-headed?	☐	☐	☐	☐	☐
2. Painful muscles?	☐	☐	☐	☐	☐
3. Fainting?	☐	☐	☐	☐	☐
4. Neck pain?	☐	☐	☐	☐	☐
5. Back pain?	☐	☐	☐	☐	☐
6. Excessive sweating?	☐	☐	☐	☐	☐
7. Palpitations?	☐	☐	☐	☐	☐
8. Headache?	☐	☐	☐	☐	☐
9. A bloated feeling in the abdomen?	☐	☐	☐	☐	☐
10. Blurred vision or spots in front of your eyes?	☐	☐	☐	☐	☐
11. Shortness of breath?	☐	☐	☐	☐	☐
12. Nausea or an upset stomach?	☐	☐	☐	☐	☐
During the past week, did you suffer from:					
13. Pain in the abdomen or stomach area?	☐	☐	☐	☐	☐
14. Tingling in the fingers?	☐	☐	☐	☐	☐
15. Pressure or a tight feeling in the chest?	☐	☐	☐	☐	☐
16. Pain in the chest?	☐	☐	☐	☐	☐
17. Feeling down or depressed?	☐	☐	☐	☐	☐
18. Sudden fright for no reason?	☐	☐	☐	☐	☐
19. Worry?	☐	☐	☐	☐	☐
20. Disturbed sleep?	☐	☐	☐	☐	☐
21. A vague feeling of fear?	☐	☐	☐	☐	☐
22. Lack of energy?	☐	☐	☐	☐	☐
23. Trembling when with other people?	☐	☐	☐	☐	☐
24. Anxiety or panic attacks?	☐	☐	☐	☐	☐
During the past week, did you feel:					
25. Tense?	☐	☐	☐	☐	☐
26. Easily irritated?	☐	☐	☐	☐	☐
27. Frightened?	☐	☐	☐	☐	☐

BOX 1

FOUR-DIMENSIONAL SYMPTOM QUESTIONNAIRE (4DSQ)—CONT'D

	No	Sometimes	Regularly	Often	Very Often or Constantly
During the past week, did you feel:					
28. That everything is meaningless?	☐	☐	☐	☐	☐
29. That you just can't do anything anymore?	☐	☐	☐	☐	☐
30. That life is not worthwhile?	☐	☐	☐	☐	☐
31. That you can no longer take any interest in the people and things around you?	☐	☐	☐	☐	☐
32. That you can't cope anymore?	☐	☐	☐	☐	☐
33. That you would be better off if you were dead?	☐	☐	☐	☐	☐
34. That you can't enjoy anything anymore?	☐	☐	☐	☐	☐
35. That there is no escape from your situation?	☐	☐	☐	☐	☐
36. That you can't face it anymore?	☐	☐	☐	☐	☐
During the past week, did you:					
37. No longer feel like doing anything?	☐	☐	☐	☐	☐
38. Have difficulty in thinking clearly?	☐	☐	☐	☐	☐
39. Have difficulty in getting to sleep?	☐	☐	☐	☐	☐
40. Have any fear of going out of the house alone?	☐	☐	☐	☐	☐
During the past week:					
41. Did you easily become emotional?	☐	☐	☐	☐	☐
42. Were you afraid of anything when there was really no need for you to be afraid? *(for instance animals, heights, small rooms)*	☐	☐	☐	☐	☐
43. Were you afraid to travel on buses, streetcars/trams, subways or trains?	☐	☐	☐	☐	☐
44. Were you afraid of becoming embarrassed when with other people?	☐	☐	☐	☐	☐
45. Did you ever feel as if you were being threatened by unknown danger?	☐	☐	☐	☐	☐
46. Did you ever think 'I wish I was dead'?	☐	☐	☐	☐	☐
47. Did you ever have fleeting images of any upsetting event(s) that you have experienced?	☐	☐	☐	☐	☐
48. Did you ever have to do your best to put aside thoughts about any upsetting event(s)?	☐	☐	☐	☐	☐
49. Did you have to avoid certain places because they frightened you?	☐	☐	☐	☐	☐
50. Did you have to repeat some actions a number of times before you could do something else?	☐	☐	☐	☐	☐

REFERENCES

Egberink, I.J.L., Vermeulen, C.S.M., Frima, R.M., 2014. COTAN beoordeling 2005, Vierdimensionale klachtenlijst, 4DKL, [COTAN review 2005, Four-Dimensional Symptom Questionnaire, 4DSQ]. <www.cotandocumentatie.nl.>

Terluin, B., 1996. De Vierdimensionale Klachtenlijst (4DKL). Een vragenlijst voor het meten van distress, depressie, angst en somatisatie. Huisarts Wet. 39 (12), 538–547.

Terluin, B., 1998. Wat meet de Vierdimensionale Klachtenlijst (4DKL) in vergelijking met enkele bekende klachtenlijsten? Tijdschr. Gezondheidswet. 76, 435–441.

Terluin, B., Duijsens, I., 2007. Handleiding van de Vierdimensionale Klachtenlijst. <http//www.datec.nl/4DKL.>

Terluin, B., van Marwijk, H., Adèr, H.J., et al., 2006. The Four-Dimensional Symptom Questionnaire (4DSQ): a validation study of a multidimensional self-report questionnaire to assess distress, depression, anxiety and somatisation. BMC Psychiatry 6, 34.

Terluin, B., Oosterbaan, D.B., Brouwers, E.P., et al., 2014. To what extent does the anxiety scale of the Four-Dimensional Symptom Questionnaire (4DSQ) detect specific types of anxiety disorder in primary care? A psychometric study. BMC Psychiatry 14 (1), 121.

Terluin, B., Van Rhenen, W., Schaufeli, W.B., De Haan, M., 2004. The Four-Dimensional Symptom Questionnaire (4DSQ): measuring distress and other mental health problems in a working population. Work Stress 18, 187–207.

van der Horst, M., 2008. The prognostic value of the four-dimensional symptom questionnaire (4DSQ) in the presence of mental disorders in physiotherapy practice. Ned Tijdschr Fysiother 2005 115, 106–111. <http://www.icppmh.org/conferences.html.>

4.2.2 Self-Concept and the Physical Self-Concept

MICHEL PROBST

Marsh's self-description questionnaire (SDQ) is based on a transtheoretical, multifaceted and hierarchical model. The SDQ is a multidimensionality-sensitive tool for measuring self-concept. The SDQ-I has been developed for preadolescents (Marsh, 1998), the SDQ-II for adolescents (Marsh, 1990) and the SDQ-III for late adolescents and adults (Marsh & O'Neill, 1984).

The SDQ-III is a 136-item self-report questionnaire that comprises 13 scales, assessing four areas of academic self-concept (verbal, mathematic, problem-solving and general academic), eight areas of nonacademic self-concept (physical ability, physical appearance, peer relations–same sex, peer relations–opposite sex, parent relations, emotional stability, honesty, trustworthiness and spiritual values) and a general self-scale derived from the Rosenberg self-esteem scale (Rosenberg, 1965). The total score has also been retained because it is an apparently definable indicator of general self-concept. Each of the 13 SDQ-III scales is inferred on the basis of the responses to 10 or 12 items, half of which are negatively worded to disrupt acquiescence response biases. Subjects evaluated their response on an 8-point scale where the response options vary from 1 (definitely false) to 8 (definitely true). The SDQ-III is reliable and valid and used worldwide.

Simons and Simons (2002) proposed a short version consisting of 65 items, five items for each of the scales.

REFERENCES

Marsh, H., 1998. The Self-Description Questionnaire I: SDQ Manual and Research Monograph. Psychological Corporation, San Antonio.

Marsh, H.W., 1990. A multidimensional, hierarchical model of self-concept: theoretical and empirical justification. Educ. Psychol. Rev. 2 (2), 77–172.

Marsh, H.W., O'Neill, R., 1984. Self-Description Questionnaire III (SDQ III): the construct validity of multidimensional self-concept ratings by late-adolescents. J. Educ. Meas. 21, 153–174.

Rosenberg, M., 1965. Society and the Adolescent Self-Image. Princeton University Press, Princeton, NJ.

Simons, J., Simons, J., 2002. De constructive van een verkorte vragenlijst voor het evalueren van het zelfbeeld bij Vlaamse Adolescenten. Diagnostiekwijzer 5 (2), 62–71.

4.2.3 Physical Self-Description Questionnaire

MICHEL PROBST

INTRODUCTION

The Physical Self-Description Questionnaire (PSDQ) scales reflect some of Marsh's original self-description questionnaire (see Section 4.2.2). The PSDQ consists of nine specific components of physical self-description (strength, body fat, activity, endurance and fitness, sport competence, coordination, health, appearance and flexibility), a global physical scale and a global self-esteem scale. Each of the 70 PSDQ items is a simple declarative statement, and individuals respond on a six-point true-or-false scale. The PSDQ is designed for adolescents, but is also appropriate for older participants.

THE PHYSICAL SELF-DESCRIPTION QUESTIONNAIRE

PSDQ research has demonstrated (a) good reliability (median coefficient alpha of .92) across the 11 scales (Marsh et al., 1994a,b); (b) good test–retest stability over the short-term (median $r = .83$ over 3 months) and longer-term (median $r = .69$ over 14 months; Marsh, 1994a); (c) a well-defined, replicable factor structure as shown by confirmatory factor analysis (CFA) (Marsh, 1994a,b); (d) a factor structure that is invariant over gender, as shown by multiple-group CFA (Marsh et al., 1994a); (e) convergent and discriminant validity (Marsh et al., 1994a); (f) convergent and discriminant validity as shown by PSDQ relationships with external criteria (e.g., measurements of body composition, physical activity, endurance, strength and flexibility; see Marsh, 1994a, Marsh & Yeung, 1997); and (g) applicability

for participants aged 12 to 18 years (or older) and for elite athletes and nonathletes (Marsh & Yeung, 1997). In summary, the PSDQ is a psychometrically strong instrument.

THE PSDQ-S

Marsh et al. (2010) presented a short form of the PSDQ (PSDQ-S). This short form balances brevity and psychometric quality in relation to established guidelines for evaluating short forms with the construct validity approach that is the basis of PSDQ research. Based on the PSDQ normative archive, 40 of 70 items were selected and evaluated in new cross-validation samples. Reliabilities for the 40 PSDQ-S items were consistently high. The authors concluded that the strong support for the psychometric properties and construct validity of the widely used PSDQ instrument generalizes very well to the PSDQ-S.

REFERENCES

Marsh, H.W., Richards, G., Johnson, S., et al., 1994a. Physical self-description questionnaire: psychometric properties and a multi-trait-multimethod analysis of relations to existing instruments. J. Sport Exerc. Psychol. 16, 270–305.

Marsh, H.W., Redmayne, R.S., 1994b. A Multidimensional physical self-concept and its relations to multiple components of physical fitness. J. Sport Exerc. Psychol. 16, 43–55.

Marsh, H.W., Yeung, A.S., 1997. Casual effects of academic self-concept on academic achievement: structural equation models of longitudinal data. J. Educ. Psych. 189, 41–54.

Marsh, H.W., Martin, A.J., Jackson, S., 2010. Introducing a short version of the physical self-description questionnaire: new strategies, short-form evaluative criteria, and applications of factor analyses. J. Sport Exerc. Psychol. 32, 438–482.

4.2.4   Physical Self-Perception Profile

MICHEL PROBST

INTRODUCTION

The Physical Self-Perception Profile (PSPP) (Fox, 1990; Fox & Corbin, 1989; Fox, 2000) is a 30-item inventory that consists of four specific scales (physical condition, sport competence, physical strength and attractive body) and one general (physical self-worth) factor. The PSPP uses a nonstandard response format, in which each item consists of a matched pair of statements, one negative and one positive (e.g., 'some people feel that they are not very good when it comes to sports' but 'others feel that they are really good at just about every sport'). Each item consists of two contrasting descriptions, and respondents are asked which description is most like them and whether the description they select is 'sort of true of me' or 'really true of me'. Responses are scored on a scale of 1–4, with 1 representing a 'really true of me' response to the negative statement and 4 representing a 'really true of me' response to the positive statement.

THE PSPP

The PSPP consists of five six-item scales of sport (perceived sport competence), body (perceived bodily attractiveness), strength (perceived physical strength and muscular development), condition (perceived level of physical conditioning and exercise) and physical self-worth. Fox (1990) recommended that the 10-item Rosenberg Self-Esteem Scale (Rosenberg, 1965) be used alongside the PSPP to provide a global measure.

Fox (1990) reported factor analyses indicating that each item loads most highly on the factor that it is designed to measure and that individual scale reliabilities are between .80 and .90.

The PSPP research demonstrates (a) good reliability (coefficient alpha of .80–.95; Fox, 1990; Sonstroem et al., 1992); (b) good test–retest stability over the short term (r-values of .74–.89; Fox, 1990); (c)

a well-defined, replicable factor structure, as shown by confirmatory factor analysis (CFA) (Fox & Corbin, 1989; Sonstroem et al., 1994); (d) convergent and discriminant validity in studies showing PSPP relationships with external criteria, such as exercise behaviors, mental adjustment variables and health complaints (Fox & Corbin, 1989) and (e) applicability for an older-adult population (Sonstroem et al., 1994).

A version of the PSPP for children and adolescents has been developed and validated—the Children and Youth Physical Self-Perception Profile (CY-PSPP; Whitehead, 1995; Eklund et al., 1997).

The PSPP and the CY-PSPP are established instruments that have been translated into several languages and have been used with a range of populations. However, the format and the high correlations among factors in both instruments may limit their usefulness in some settings.

REFERENCES

Eklund, R.C., Whitehead, J.R., Welk, G.J., 1997. Validity of the children and youth physical self-perception profile: a confirmatory factor analysis. Res. Q. Exerc. Sport 68 (3), 249–256.

Fox, K.R., Corbin, C.B., 1989. The Physical Self-Perception Profile: development and preliminary validation. J. Sport Exerc. Psychol. 11, 408–430.

Fox, K.R., 1990. The Physical Self-Perception Profile Manual. Northern Illinois University, Dekalb, IL.

Fox, K.R., 2000. Self-esteem, self perception and exercise. Int. J. Sport Psychol. 21, 228–240.

Rosenberg, M., 1965. Society and the Adolescent Self-Image. Princeton University Press, Princeton, NJ.

Sonstroem, R.J., Speliotis, E.D., Fava, J.L., 1992. Perceived physical competence in adults: an examination of the Physical Self-Perception Profile. J. Sport Exerc. Psychol. 14 (2).

Sonstroem, R.J., Harlow, L.L., Josephs, L., 1994. Exercise and self-esteem: validity of model expansion and exercise associations. J. Sport Exerc. Psychol. 16, 29–42.

Whitehead, J.R., 1995. A study of children's physical self-perceptions using an adapted physical self-perception profile questionnaire. Pediatric Exerc. Sci. 7, 132–151.

4.2.5   Physical Self-Inventory

MICHEL PROBST

The Physical Self-Inventory (PSI) is a French adaptation of the PSPP that was originally developed for use with Francophone adults (Ninot et al., 2000). The authors used a 6-point Likert response scale. Next, the authors replaced the PSPP global physical items with items from the SDQ physical scale and the PSPP global self-esteem items with items from Coopersmith (1967). The final PSI consists of 25 items measuring six PSC factors (four specific and two global, as with the PSPP) and has satisfactory psychometric properties that have been confirmed. The questionnaire is available on request from the author.

Maïano and coworkers (2008) subsequently constructed a short form of the PSI for use with adolescents. This version included 18 items, rated on a 6-point Likert scale (from 1 = not at all, to 6 = entirely), and aiming to assess six a priori subscales (GSW = global self-worth; PSW = physical self-worth; PC = physical condition; SC = sport competence; PA = physical attractiveness; PS = physical strength). The questionnaire is available free of charge to researchers.

A very short form of a 12-item inventory (PSI-VSF, two items per scale) had good psychometric properties (Maiano et al. 2009, 2011, 2015a,b). Maïano and coworkers also noted that PSI-SF responses showed very high test–retest stability. Comparison of the PSI-SF and PSI-VSF demonstrated that the measurement model, mean structure, structural parameters and criterion-related validity were equivalent across samples and versions.

REFERENCES

Coopersmith, S., 1967. The Antecedents of Self-Esteem. W.H. Freeman, San Francisco.

Maïano, C., Morin, A.J.S., Ninot, G., et al., 2008. A short and very short form of the physical self-inventory for adolescents: development and factor validity. Psychol. Sport Exerc. 9, 830–847.

Maïano, C., Bégarie, J., Morin, A.J.S., Ninot, G., 2009. Assessment of physical self-concept in adolescents with intellectual disability: content and factor validity of the very short form of the Physical Self-Inventory. J. Autism Dev. Disord. 39, 775–787.

Maïano, C., Morin, A.J.S., Bégarie, J., Ninot, G., 2011. The intellectual disability version of the very short form of the physical self-inventory (PSI-VS-ID): cross-validation and measurement invariance across gender, weight, age and intellectual disability level. Res. Dev. Disabil. 32, 1652–1662.

Maïano, C., Morin, A.J.S., Mascret, N., 2015a. Psychometric properties of the short form of the physical self-description questionnaire in a French adolescent sample. Body Image 12, 89–97.

Maiano, C., Morin, A., Probst, M., 2015b. Cross-linguistic validity of the French and Dutch versions of the Very Short form of the Physical Self-Inventory among adolescents. Body Image 15, 35–39.

Ninot, G., Delignières, D., Fortes, M., 2000. L'évaluation de l'estime de soi dans le domaine corporel. Sci. Techn. Act. Phys. Sportives 53, 35–48.

4.2.6   Rosenberg Self-Esteem Scale

MICHEL PROBST

The Rosenberg Self-Esteem scale (Rosenberg, 1965) is a unidimensional scale. It is a widely used self-esteem measure assessing positive and negative attitudes regarding self-worth and global self-esteem. The scale consists of 10 items with five positive and five negative items and uses a 4-point Likert scale format ranging from 'strongly agree' to 'strongly disagree' (strongly agree = 1; agree = 2; disagree = 3; strongly disagree = 4). The negative items are reverse scored. Lower rating indicates more positive self-esteem. The scale may be used without explicit permission. Different versions are used in terms of the order of the items and the scoring system.

REFERENCES

Rosenberg, M., 1965. Society and the Adolescent Self-Image. Princeton University Press, Princeton, NJ.

4.2.7   Physical Activity and Exercise Questionnaires

MICHEL PROBST

THE INTERNATIONAL PHYSICAL ACTIVITY QUESTIONNAIRE

The International Physical Activity Questionnaire (IPAQ) short version (van der Ploeg et al., 2010) considers a 7-day recall period, identifying physical activity (PA) undertaken in the morning, afternoon and evening. Data from the IPAQ is summarized according to minutes of walking, moderate PA (e.g., activities that make one breathe somewhat harder than normal, such as carrying light loads, cycling at a regular pace or easy swimming), and vigorous PA (e.g., activities that make you breathe much harder than normal, such as heavy lifting, digging, aerobics or fast cycling) per week. Previous research (Faulkner et al., 2006; Vancampfort et al., 2016) has identified that the IPAQ is a reliable and valid surveillance tool to assess levels of PA in people with severe mental illness.

THE SIMPLE PHYSICAL ACTIVITY QUESTIONNAIRE

The Simple Physical Activity Questionnaire (SIMPAQ) (Rosenbaum & Ward, 2016) is a physical activity measurement tool designed to be used as a structured interview. Completion of the SIMPAQ should take between 3 and 8 minutes and can be administered by clinicians or researchers. The SIMPAQ is structured to start with details about time in bed, sedentary time (including napping during the day), and structured exercise, and progresses to incidental or nonstructured physical activity. The SIMPAQ does not aim to specify or discriminate activities based on intensity, but rather groups activities into either walking, exercise/sport or incidental/other categories. SIMPAQ has been structured to provide a snapshot of a 24-hour period that is representative of the previous week. The SIMPAQ is currently being translated into many languages (Dutch, French, German, Spanish, Portuguese, Farsi and most Scandinavian languages). A validation study in over 25 centres in 15 countries (including both developed and low- to middle-income countries)

comparing the data obtained via SIMPAQ to objective accelerometer-based measurements, is ongoing at the time of writing and involves patients with a range of psychiatric diagnoses treated in both inpatient and outpatient settings. The English-language version of SIMPAQ is currently freely available from the project website (www.simpaq.org), with versions in other languages being added as they are finalized. Once validation is complete, the SIMPAQ will hopefully become part of the routine documentation obtained in psychiatric treatment settings. It will have the sensitivity to detect small increases in physical activity and exercise participation that can be achieved by targeted interventions, which can confer real clinical improvement in both mental and physical health outcomes (Vancampfort et al., 2016).

BEHAVIORAL REGULATION IN EXERCISE QUESTIONNAIRE

The Behavioral Regulation in Exercise Questionnaire-2 (BREQ-2) (Markland & Tobin, 2004) is used as an interviewer-administered questionnaire in order to ensure that patients with any literacy problems are not excluded. The BREQ-2 considers an individual's motivation towards exercise. The questionnaire comprises 19 items relating to five motivation types from the Self-Determination Theory. Each item is measured on a 5-point Likert scale, from 0 ('not true for me') to 4 ('very true for me'). The mean of the five subscales is calculated on a 5-point scale to form an idea of the extent of each motivation type separately.

THE PHYSICAL ACTIVITY AND SPORT ANXIETY SCALE

The Physical Activity and Sport Anxiety Scale (PASAS) (Norton et al., 2004) is a 16-item self-reported questionnaire measuring social anxiety in physical activities and sports. The items are scored on a 5-point Likert scale, ranging from 1 ('absolutely not true for me') to 5 ('absolutely true for me'). The range of possible total scores is 20–80, with higher total scores indicating higher experience of social anxiety in physical activities and sports. In a sample of mentally healthy individuals, this brief questionnaire demonstrated an excellent internal consistency across a number of samples with Cronbach's alpha of .91, an excellent temporal stability with a reliability coefficient of .84 and good convergent and divergent validity (De Herdt et al., 2013).

REFERENCE

De Herdt, A., Knapen, J., Vancampfort, D., et al., 2013. Social anxiety in physical activity participation in patients with mental illness: a cross-sectional multicentre study. Depress. Anxiety 30 (8), 757–762.

Faulkner, G., Cohn, T., Remington, G., 2006. Validation of a physical activity assessment tool for individuals with schizophrenia. Schizophr. Res. 82 (2), 225–231.

Markland, D., Tobin, V., 2004. A modification to the behavioural regulation in exercise questionnaire to include an assessment of amotivation. J. Sport Exerc. Psychol. 26 (2), 191–196.

Norton, P.J., Hope, D.A., Weeks, J.W., 2004. The physical activity and sport anxiety scale (PASAS): scale development and psychometric analysis. Anxiety Stress Cop. 17 (4), 363–382.

Rosenbaum, S., Ward, P.B., 2016. The Simple Physical Activity Questionnaire. Lancet Psychiat. 3 (1), e1.

van der Ploeg, H.P., Tudor-Locke, C., Marshall, A.L., et al., 2010. Reliability and validity of the international physical activity questionnaire for assessing walking. Res. Q. Exerc. Sport 81 (1), 97–101.

Vancampfort, D., Wyckaert, S., Sienaert, P., et al., 2016. Concurrent validity of the international physical activity questionnaire in outpatients with bipolar disorder: comparison with the Sensewear Armband. Psychiat. Res. 237, 122–126.

4.2.8 Motor Assessment Instruments

TINE VAN DAMME

STANDARDIZED MOTOR ASSESSMENT INSTRUMENTS FOR CHILDREN AND ADOLESCENTS

Within the field of child and adolescent development, the assessment of motor ability has become increasingly important. Several arguments can be raised in support of this idea. First, many studies indicate that the presence of motor impairment can have far-reaching implications on other developmental domains, such as psychosocial, emotional and academic functioning (Dewey et al., 2002; Cairney et al., 2010; Piek et al., 2010; Lingam et al., 2012). Second, motor ability is an important determinant of physical fitness and physical activity outcome (Wrotniak et al., 2006; Lopes et al., 2011). Lastly, there is substantial evidence indicating a heightened prevalence of impairment in motor abilities in children and adolescents with a mental health disorder (Van Damme et al., 2015).

A wide variety of standardized motor assessment instruments are available. In a review by Cools et al. (2009), it is argued that the choice of a test should depend upon several aspects, including age, context in which the assessment is planned, purpose, time available and similarity between norm and test populations. However, internationally the Bruininks-Oseretsky test of motor proficiency, second edition (BOT-2) and the movement assessment battery for children, second edition (MABC-2) are the most frequently employed instruments, in research as well as in clinical practice (Blank et al., 2012; Van Damme et al., 2015). Other frequently used instruments are the test of gross motor development, second edition (TGMD-2) (Ulrich, 2000), the körperkoordinationstest für kinder 2 (KTK-2) (Kiphard & Shilling, 2007) and the Peabody developmental motor scales, second edition (PDMS-2) (Folio & Fewell, 2000).

Bruininks-Oseretsky Test of Motor Proficiency, Second Edition (BOT-2) (Bruininks & Bruininks, 2005)

The BOT-2 is an individually administered test that uses goal-directed activities to measure a wide range of motor abilities in individuals aged 4–21 years. The BOT-2 is by far the most comprehensive standardized motor assessment instrument, which allows assessment across the full range of motor ability, measuring

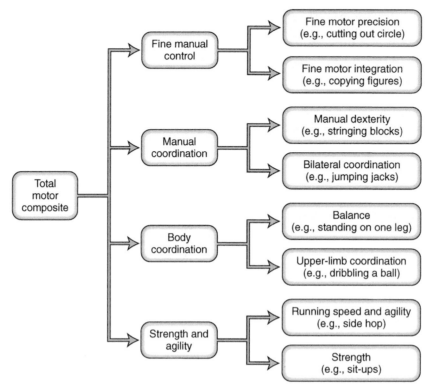

FIGURE 1 ▪ The Bruininks-Osertsky Test (2nd ed.): structure. *(Data from Bruininks & Bruininks, 2012).*

variation from well below average to well above average performance.

The BOT-2 consists of 53 items, distributed across eight subtests. Subtests that assess related aspects of a motor area are combined into a composite score. As a result, four composite scores or subscales are produced, namely fine motor control, manual coordination, body coordination, and strength and agility. Finally, a total motor composite is generated, which represents the overall motor ability of an individual. The content and structure of the BOT-2 is presented in Fig. 1.

In contrast to some other standardized motor assessment instruments, the BOT-2 provides gender-specific norms as well as gender-combined norms (based on the US population).

The authors of the BOT-2 examined the psychometric properties and report in the manual that the BOT-2 has demonstrated reliability and validity. Internal consistency data reported in the manual indicate that the reliability coefficients range from high .70 to low .80 for the eight subtests, from high .80 to low .90 for the composite subscales and in the mid .90s for the total motor composite score. Test–retest reliability coefficients ranged from .69 to low .70s for the subtests, from .77 to low .80s for the composite subscales and from mid to high .80s for the total motor composite score. Good interrater reliability has been demonstrated with Pearson correlations ranging from .92 to .99. Additionally, evidence of content validity, criterion validity and construct validity is reported in the manual.

Movement Assessment Battery for Children, Second Edition (MABC-2) (Henderson et al., 2007)

The Movement Assessment Battery for Children, Second Edition (MABC-2) is a screening instrument, designed to identify children or adolescents with motor impairment. Moreover, the European Academy for Childhood Disability recommends using this instrument as part of the diagnostic process for Developmental Coordination Disorder (Blank et al., 2012).

The MABC-2 is composed of two parts: a standardized performance test and a checklist. The checklist requires an adult (parent, teacher or caregiver) to rate the child's motor competence on a 30-item scale. The performance test is a norm-referenced and individually administered test, designed to identify motor impairment in children in different age bands (AB) from 3 to 16 years old (AB1: 3–6 years; AB2: 7–10 years; AB3: 11–16 years). The test contains eight items, which are categorized into three components: manual dexterity, aiming and catching and balance.

The test authors assume that the reliability data and validity information reported for the first edition can be generalized to the second edition. Despite reporting preliminary reliability and validity data in the MABC-2 manual, the comprehensiveness, quality and rigor of these reliability and validity studies is variable (Brown & Lalor, 2009). However, the brevity of the test enhances the utility in clinical and research settings.

REFERENCES

Blank, R., Smits-Engelsman, B., Polatajko, H., Wilson, P., 2012. European Academy for Childhood Disability (EACD): Recommendations on the definition, diagnosis and intervention of developmental coordination disorder (long version). Dev. Med. Child Neurol. 54 (1), 54–93.

Brown, T., Lalor, A., 2009. The movement assessment battery for children, second edition (MABC-2): a review and critique. Phys. Occup. Ther. Pediatr. 29 (1), 86–103.

Bruininks, R.H., Bruininks, B.D., 2005. Bruininks-Oseretsky Test of Motor Proficiency, Second ed. AGS Publishing, Circle Pines, MN.

Cairney, J., Veldhuizen, S., Szatmari, P., 2010. Motor coordination and emotional-behavioral problems in children. Curr. Opin. Psychiat. 23 (4), 324–329.

Cools, W., De Martelaer, K., Samaey, C., Andries, C., 2009. Movement skill assessment of typically developing preschool children: a review of seven movement skill assessment tools. J. Sports Sci. Med. 8 (2), 154–168.

Dewey, D., Kaplan, B.J., Crawford, S.G., Wilson, B.N., 2002. Developmental coordination disorder: associated problems in attention, learning, and psychosocial adjustment. Hum. Mov. Sci. 21 (5), 905–918.

Folio, M.R., Fewell, R.R., 2000. Peabody Developmental Motor Scales-2: Examiner's manual. Pro-Ed, Austin, TX.

Henderson, S.E., Sugden, D.A., Barnett, A.L., 2007. Movement assessment battery for children-2: Movement ABC-2: Examiner's manual. Pearson, São Paulo.

Kiphard, E.J., Shilling, F., 2007. Körperkoordinationstest für Kinder 2. Weinheim, Beltz Test GmbH.

Lingam, R., Jongmans, M.J., Ellis, M., et al., 2012. Mental health difficulties in children with developmental coordination disorder. Pediatrics 129 (4), e882–e891.

Lopes, V.P., Rodrigues, L.P., Maia, J.A., Malina, R.M., 2011. Motor coordination as predictor of physical activity in childhood. Scand. J. Med. Sci. Sports 21 (5), 663–669.

Piek, J.P., Barrett, N.C., Smith, L.M., et al., 2010. Do motor skills in infancy and early childhood predict anxious and depressive symptomatology at school age? Hum. Mov. Sci. 29 (5), 777–786.

Van Damme, T., Simons, J., Sabbe, B., van West, D., 2015. Motor abilities of children and adolescents with a psychiatric condition: a systematic literature review. World J. Psychiatry 5 (3), 315–329.

Ulrich, D., 2000. Test of Gross Motor Development-2. Pro-Ed, Austin, TX.

Wrotniak, B.H., Epstein, L.H., Dorn, J.M., et al., 2006. The relationship between motor proficiency and physical activity in children. Pediatrics 118 (6), e1758–e1765.

4.2.9 Standardized Motor Assessment Instruments for Adults and Elderly

MICHEL PROBST

BRUININKS MOTOR ABILITY TEST (BMAT)

The Bruininks motor ability test (BMAT) is an individually-administered, standardized test of gross and fine motor skills and coordination for adults of 40 years and older. The BMAT is based on the Bruininks-Oseretsky test of motor proficiency second edition (BOT-2).

The BMAT consists of 32 items across five subtests: fine motor integration, manual dexterity, coordination, balance and mobility, and strength and flexibility. Fine motor integration and manual dexterity form fine motor skills. Balance and mobility, and strength and flexibility form gross motor skills. Coordination is a subtest that stands on its own. The sum of the five subtests is the total motor composite. A short version of BMAT has also been developed, which exists of 10

TABLE 1

Bruininks Motor Ability Test: Test Content and Structure

Subtest 1: Fine Motor Integration (7 items)

These items require precise control of finger and hand movements, which must be integrated with visual stimuli. The items include three drawing tasks, a shape-recognition task, the use of scissors and folding paper.

Subtest 2: Manual Dexterity (5 items)

This subtest uses goal-directed tasks that involve reaching, grasping and bimanual coordination with small objects. These tasks include picking up and transferring plastic pennies, stringing small blocks and completing a sewing like activity.

Subtest 3: Coordination (8 items)

These items measure the ability to coordinate movements of hands, arms and feet. More concrete items involve touching the nose, simultaneous tapping of feet and fingers and catching or throwing a tennis ball.

Subtest 4: Balance and Mobility (7 items)

This subtest evaluates motor control skills that are integral for standing, walking and using stairs. The focus lies on the balance, the posture, the control and walking speed.

Subtest 5: Strength and Flexibility (7 items)

These items measure the strength and endurance of muscle groups in the legs, torso, arms and hands as well as the flexibility of the lower back. The items are important because of their relevance to gross motor performance in many daily activities.

(Data from Bruininks & Bruininks, 2012.)

items, providing an estimate of overall motor ability in 15 to 20 minutes (Bruininks & Bruininks, 2012).

The BMAT is an interesting psychomotor test battery since it will provide a lot of information about an adult's motor skills needed for primary activities of daily living in a relatively short administration time. It can be used to design treatment goals and to follow-up patients. It is very flexible and one can use it in a wide variety of circumstances. Testing can be performed in as little as 15 minutes (for a single subtest or the short form) or as long as 55 minutes (for the entire test) (Bruininks & Bruininks, 2012).

The reliability of BMAT (test–retest and interrater reliability) has been studied in the US ($N = 1000$; 32 different states). Test–retest reliability with an interval of 6 to 12 days was for fine motor integration fair ($r = .76$). The reliability coefficients of coordination ($r = .80$) and balance and mobility ($r = .83$) were good and the reliability coefficients of manual dexterity, ($r = .90$) and strength and flexibility ($r = .92$) were excellent. Mean subtest correlation for test–retest reliability was good ($r = .85$) (Bruininks & Bruininks, 2012). Interrater reliability of the different subtests was: $r = .96$ for fine motor integration, $r = .97$ for coordination and balance, and mobility, $r = .99$ for manual dexterity, and strength and flexibility. Mean subtest correlation for interrater reliability was excellent ($r = .98$) (Bruininks & Bruininks, 2012). These results indicate that the BMAT scoring guidelines seem clear and that BMAT scores are essentially unaffected by differences in how examiners score item performance in America.

The same studies also examined validity of BMAT (Bruininks & Bruininks, 2012). Validity refers to an assessment's ability to accurately measure the construct it seeks to measure. The relation between the BMAT and other motor assessment instruments (Beery-Buktenica Developmental Test of Visual-Motor Integration [Beery VMI], Nine-Hole Peg test [9-HPT] and Berg Balance Scale [BBS]) were examined. Significant correlations between scores on BMAT subtests and the other instruments were found.

According to the reliability and validity studies, BMAT in general or its subtests on their own, appear to be practical, reliable and valid standardized tests of adult motor proficiency. According to these studies you can administer all subtests or focus on one or more specific motor skill areas (Bruininks & Bruininks, 2012) (Table 1).

REFERENCES

Bruininks, B.D., Bruininks, R.H., 2012. Bruyninks Motor Ability Test. Pearson, Bloomington.

Janssens, J., Lenaerts, D., Dolferus, T., Probst, M., 2017. Bruininks Motor Ability Test in Elderly: Psychometric Properties. (Unpublished masterthesis). KU Leuven: Leuven.

PHYSIOTHERAPY WITHIN MENTAL HEALTH AND PSYCHIATRY CARE. SPECIFIC INTERVENTIONS DURING LIFE SPAN: CHILDREN, ADOLESCENTS, ADULTS AND ELDERLY

PHYSIOTHERAPY IN MENTAL HEALTH CARE

5.1.1   Musculoskeletal Pain: Evidence and Critical Factors in Rehabilitation Relevant for Physiotherapy in Mental Health

GUNVOR GARD ■ AMANDA LUNDVIK GYLLENSTEN

SUMMARY

In this chapter the area of musculoskeletal pain is outlined with a focus on evidence and critical factors for positive rehabilitation outcomes. First, psychological factors are described as they are important for a deeper understanding of the problems. Then, the use of cognitive behaviour principles in rehabilitation are presented. These principles, in combination with a treatment tailored to the individual, have been shown to reduce pain and improve social and physical function. To acknowledge and obtain a deeper understanding of the painful body has also been found to be a critical factor in pain rehabilitation. Effects of body awareness therapies, as well as other body-centred treatment methods in musculoskeletal pain rehabilitation, are described. Finally, self-management and behaviour-change strategies, as well as the use of web programmes in pain management, are briefly addressed. These techniques may improve the results of pain rehabilitation. All of these factors are relevant to consider in physiotherapy in mental health.

KEY POINTS

■ Considering psychological factors and cognitive behaviour principles is critical for the understanding and treatment of musculoskeletal pain.

■ Positive rehabilitation effects are shown after body awareness therapies; for example, reduced pain and distress and improved physical function and body image.

■ Pain rehabilitation can be improved by the use of information and communication technologies and self-management strategies; for example, web-based programmes.

LEARNING OBJECTIVES

■ Don't forget to ask a patient with musculoskeletal pain about psychological factors that may facilitate their rehabilitation.

■ Support the patient to identify and work towards activity-related goals and give feedback when goals are reached.

■ Understand the importance of asking every patient in rehabilitation about psychosocial factors.

INTRODUCTION

Musculoskeletal pain disorders are a substantial health problem and the main cause of occupational disability and sick leave in Sweden (Bergstrom et al., 2007; 2010). They are common within primary health care where the prevalence of stress-related pain disorders is high. It is important to view the problems from a systems perspective. Issues such as organizational changes, downsizing and high physical and psychosocial workloads can be seen as contributing factors to the problems. The biopsychosocial model explains persistent musculoskeletal pain as a complex process where biological, emotional, cognitive and social factors interact (Gatchel & Rollings, 2008; Gard, 2012; Laisné et al., 2012). *Persistent pain* is defined as pain with an endurance of at least 3 to 6 months (SBU, 2010). Multimodal rehabilitation is recommended for patients with persistent pain problems (SBU, 2010).

PSYCHOLOGICAL FACTORS AS CRITICAL FACTORS FOR POSITIVE RESULTS IN REHABILITATION

Today psychological factors are regarded as important for the understanding and treatment of musculoskeletal pain disorders (Linton, 2000; Gard, 2012; Laisné et al., 2012). A holistic perspective on the problem is needed for successful return to work, including not only psychological factors, but also regular physical activity and bodily treatments (SBU, 2010, Laisné et al., 2012).

To consider psychological factors in rehabilitation means to identify and consider:

1. Clients' responsibility, opportunity to influence and participate in rehabilitation.
2. Clients' opportunities for pain control.
3. Motivational factors, self-efficacy and empowerment factors in the rehabilitation process (Linton, 2000; Jensen et al, 2007; Foster et al., 2009; Gard, 2012).

High patient participation increases patient control, activity, health and well-being (SBU, 2010). Patients' pain control can be improved by physical and enjoyable activities that reduce the experience of pain. By increased control of the situation it is possible to participate in the rehabilitation to a higher extent and learn more (Dionne et al., 2007; Foster, et al. 2009).

The consideration of motivational factors in rehabilitation is important for good results (Gard, 2012). *Motivation* is often defined as everything that drives and sustains human behaviour and desire for change. It is influenced by a combination of personal and social factors, such as having individually formulated goals, future expectations and self-efficacy (Gard, 2012). Self-efficacy is also an important psychological factor in rehabilitation. Self-efficacy and coping with anxiety and fear can be focused by use of cognitive principles with positive results (Foster et al., 2009). Personal resources, such as experience of control, trust and confidence, are also important for positive results (Jensen et al., 2007), as is social support. The most critical predictors for a successful rehabilitation result have been found to be the individual's own expectations about return to work, perceived health, and participation in the treatment situation.

USE OF COGNITIVE BEHAVIOUR PRINCIPLES IN REHABILITATION AS CRITICAL FACTORS FOR POSITIVE RESULTS

The use of cognitive behaviour therapy (CBT) principles in rehabilitation, tailored to the individual, has been shown to reduce pain and improve social and physical function (Gatchel & Rollings, 2008) and work ability (Foster et al., 2009). The formulation of realistic and concrete goals together with the patient, and giving the patient regular feedback, has been shown to increase the patient's self-efficacy, motivation for change and goal attainment (Dionne et al., 2007; Foster et al., 2009). Using CBT principles in a stepwise process in the rehabilitation, with tailored progression according to clients' abilities, can increase the positive effects thanks to the clients' input and participation in the rehabilitation process. To provide social support in the coaching process may improve patients' learning and lead to a more sustainable behaviour change (Dionne et al., 2007; Foster et al., 2009). Focusing on supporting and coaching patients' goals and coping strategies are important to reduce their pain (Dionne et al., 2007; Foster et al., 2009). This also increases patients' participation in the rehabilitation process. In pain rehabilitation it is important to pay attention to cognitive and emotional aspects, such as thoughts, memories and expectations, which influence pain perception and behaviour. Fears and earlier experiences should be asked about and discussed. Combining

CBT principles and physiotherapeutic interventions from a biopsychosocial perspective may have positive effects on work ability, health behaviour and cost–effectiveness (Demmelmaier et al., 2011). Multimodal pain rehabilitation (MMR) is the recommended treatment for persistent pain, and includes both physical and psychosocial components. MMR is based on CBT principles to help the individual understand how thoughts, emotions and behaviour can affect pain.

ACKNOWLEDGING THE RELATIONSHIP TO THE PAINFUL BODY AS A CRITICAL FACTOR IN PAIN REHABILITATION

Long-lasting pain has a negative impact on an individual's general health and can also change people's self-experiences and life-world, and their relationship with their body. This has been described as a stepwise process (Gullacksen & Lidbeck, 2004). First, the opinion that health can be taken for granted has to be abandoned. Next, a reorientation to cope with future threatening situations is needed. Then a new direction towards the future with new prerequisites can be found. To live with chronic pain requires an acceptance of the fact that the pain might persist. However, not all individuals reach such an acceptance (Gullacksen & Lidbeck, 2004). An investigation looking into the relationship with the painful body (Afrell et al., 2007) with a phenomenological-hermeneutic analysis of the pain patients experience identified the following four categories:

1. the body as an aspect of identity—more or less integration,
2. body reliance—having or missing it,
3. body awareness—the quality of the perceptive flow from the body,
4. ways of understanding pain.

From these categories four typologies were inferred with regard to how the patients' self-perception and everyday actions were influenced by their painful body. In the first typology the patients did not deny that they had an aching body; they realized that the pain might not be eliminated and integrated the aching body into the self. In the second typology, 'accepting by an active

process of change', acceptance was achieved through an active change of everyday life. The integration of the aching body into the self was reached by a trusting cooperation between body and self. The patient trusts that the body will help, even in pain. The pain puts the body in the foreground when not fought against, which enhances body awareness and self-awareness. In the third typology, the aching pain puts the patient in a state of ambivalence, a balance between hope and resignation. The hopeful insight is there, that acceptance is the only way forward, but in time despair still takes over. The relationship with the body is ambiguous. The patient moves between listening to the body and shutting it off. In the fourth typology it is totally impossible to integrate the aching body. The pain is neither possible to comprehend nor accept, and it is perceived as unfair. The body is an enemy and life is felt to be a trap (Afrell et al., 2007). This study shows that patients relate in different ways to their aching body and that the process may be complex. Some patients learn to live with their pain, but cannot accept it. Critical factors in the process are if, and to what extent, the aching body can be integrated into the self and if acceptance can be reached. How the patient stands in relation to acceptance is reflected in the attitude towards the life situation and the level of integration of the body into the self. Facilitating factors in the process were body trust, confidence in coping abilities and ability to control factors in one's life situation. Body trust can, in this process, be seen as a prerequisite to reduce muscle strain and tension, and may reduce the pain. The study also indicated that body awareness and body reliance were related to the ability to integrate the aching body into the self. The patients in the second typology reached acceptance by an active process of change. Most of the patients in this study had not listened to their own bodies; they needed communication about their needs for increased body awareness and body reliance (Afrell et al., 2007).

EFFECTS OF BODY AWARENESS THERAPIES IN MUSCULOSKELETAL PAIN REHABILITATION

Enhancing body awareness has been described as important in so-called 'mind-body approaches', such as body awareness therapy, yoga, tai chi, body-orientated psychotherapy and mindfulness-based therapies (Mehling et al., 2011). The effects of these therapies have been studied to some extent (Mehling, 2005; Morone & Greco, 2007; Morone et al., 2008). Body awareness is defined in these therapies as a subjective, phenomenological aspect of proprioception and interception that enters conscious awareness, and is modifiable by mental processes, including attention, interpretation, appraisal, beliefs, memories, conditioning, attitudes and affect (Mehling et al., 2011). Body awareness is seen as an inseparable aspect of embodied self-awareness realised in action and interaction with the environment. It is an awareness of embodiment and progression towards greater unity between body and self (Mehling et al., 2011).

Basic Body Awareness Therapy (BBAT) is one of the most used bodily-centred therapies in Scandinavia. It uses movements and breathing to emphasize movement quality and unity of the self in stillness and action. The effects of BBAT have been studied within a multidisciplinary rehabilitation programme for patients with chronic musculoskeletal disorders focusing on BBAT and cognitive and relaxation therapy compared to physiotherapy treatment within primary health care. The results showed that the multidisciplinary programme that included BBAT improved health-related quality of life and was more cost-effective than the physiotherapy treatment at a 2-year follow-up (Grahn, 1999).

BBAT, Feldenkrais treatment and conventional physiotherapy were compared with regard to pain, psychological distress and self-image in patients with musculoskeletal disorders in primary healthcare. The patients received 20 sessions of treatment. The results showed that the BBAT group experienced a greater reduction in pain and psychological distress than the other groups. In all groups the body image changed to be more positive (Malmgren-Olsson et al., 2001). BBAT, Feldenkrais treatment and conventional physiotherapy have also been compared with regard to health-related quality of life for patients with musculoskeletal disorders. Improvements were shown in physical function, pain, general health, vitality, social and emotional function and psychosocial health. No significant differences were shown between the groups, but the BBAT group improved more in physical function and general

health compared with the other groups. The BBAT and Feldenkrais group improved in terms of increased self-efficacy and reduced pain at 6-month and 12-month follow-ups compared with the physiotherapy group (Malmgren-Olsson & Bränholm, 2002).

Effects of participation in physiotherapy group treatment with pool exercises including BBAT for patients with fibromyalgia has been compared with controls. The patients who participated in the physiotherapy group treatment with BBAT perceived their body more positively, were more relaxed and calm, and developed a more comfortable relationship with their bodies and selves compared to the controls (Mannerkorpi & Gard, 2003).

EFFECTS OF OTHER BODY-CENTERED TREATMENT METHODS IN MUSCULOSKELETAL PAIN CONDITIONS

A Delphi study of Pilates exercises for people with chronic lower back pain showed positive effects on functional ability, movement confidence, body awareness, posture and movement control after participation in Pilates exercises (Wells et al., 2014).

A study of yoga on body perception and psychosocial aspects of life for patients with chronic neck pain showed positive effects on body awareness (Cramer et al., 2013). Patients with chronic pain attended 90 minutes of yoga once a week for 9 weeks. Semistandardized interviews were used to explore their body perception, emotional status, everyday life and coping skills, as well as any perceived changes in these dimensions after participation. The participants reported positive physical, cognitive, emotional, behavioural and social changes. Physically, they increased their body awareness, both during their yoga practice and in their daily lives. Cognitively, they increased their perceived control over their health. Emotionally, they noted greater acceptance of their pain and life burdens. Behaviourally, they described enhanced use of active coping strategies. Socially, they increased their participation in an active life. Participants reduced their pain levels, increased their coping ability, received improved pain acceptance and increased pain control. Body awareness appeared a key mechanism in these changes (Cramer et al., 2013). An evaluation of the Body Movement and Perception (BMP) method has also shown positive effects for patients with pain due to fibromyalgia (Maddali Bongi et al., 2011). The method is based on low-impact exercises, awareness of body perception and relaxation. The effects of the BMP method were studied on 40 women with fibromyalgia syndrome in an open pilot study. The BMP sessions were performed twice a week (50 minutes each) for 8 weeks. Positive effects were shown, such as reduced pain, fatigue and irritability, and increased well-being, quality of movement, postural self-control, ability to relax mind and body and movement perception. In addition, the number of tender points and muscle contractures were reduced, which is a very relevant outcome in fibromyalgia management (Maddali Bongi et al., 2011). Experiences of body awareness in patients with chronic pain after Norwegian psychomotor physiotherapy (NPMP) have also been explored. The results showed that most participants developed their body awareness, obtained a reduction of pain and improved their coping abilities (Dragesund & Råheim, 2008).

SELF-MANAGEMENT OF PAIN AND BEHAVIOUR CHANGE

There is a link between self-management of pain and successful behaviour change. Studies focusing on self-management have shown positive results on health, well-being and work ability (Foster et al., 2009). The positive effects have often been received thanks to the focus on psychological factors in the rehabilitation process, such as motivation, coping, self-efficacy and personal resources (Linton & Shaw, 2011; Gard, 2012), and each individual's own participation in the change process through priority-making, goal formulations and feedback. To receive positive feedback when goals are reached is a critical success factor in the behaviour-change process, which also increases self-efficacy, motivation for change and goal attainment (Foster et al., 2009; Gard, 2012). Self-management of pain conditions requires individual priority-making and decision-making. To support this, self-management programmes, for example web-based programmes, can be helpful. The decision-making can also be improved with the help of a relevant monitoring and decision support system, for example the Capability,

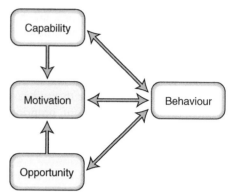

FIGURE 1 ■ The Capability, Opportunity, Motivation and Behaviour *(COM-B)* model to support behaviour change *(Michie et al., 2011).*

Opportunity, Motivation and Behaviour (COM-B) model (Michie et al., 2011) (Fig. 1).

Behaviour-change interventions are more effective when they are grounded in psychological theory and draw upon behaviour-change techniques (Webb et al., 2010). Although education that increases knowledge and understanding is essential, knowledge is not sufficient and behaviour change is often unrelated to knowledge. To be active in a behaviour-change process requires active decision-making and self-regulation. It has been recommended that interventions should include behaviour-change techniques and also clearly define these techniques. The COM-B model of behaviour change includes the necessity of three components in order for behaviour change to occur: opportunity, capability and motivation (Michie et al., 2011). In this system, capability can influence motivation and behaviour, and behaviour can also influence both of these factors. This system can be applied to a behaviour-change intervention with a target to change one or more of the components. More recent evidence recommends the inclusion of particular behaviour-change techniques, such as self-monitoring of behaviour, providing feedback on performance, promoting specific goal setting, and promoting review of behavioural goals (Waterlander et al., 2014).

USE OF WEB-BASED PROGRAMMES IN PAIN MANAGEMENT

Web-based programmes have to some extent been developed for use in pain rehabilitation (Eccleston et al., 2014). A web-based programme is based on relevant programme content developed for the specific purpose, but may also use interactive online activities, guidance and supportive feedback (Barak et al., 2009). A web programme may be guided by a therapist or not. A therapist may help with providing motivation along the process and to provide help to solve problems and give feedback. In self-guided web programmes there is no therapist support, but there may be interactive tools for symptom monitoring and online assessments (Barak et al., 2009). Web-based interventions for pain management based on CBT principles have been shown to reduce pain and improve physical and psychological functioning, but further research is needed (Eccleston et al., 2014). Recently, a randomized controlled study of the effect of comparing (1) a web-based programme added to multimodal rehabilitation and (2) multimodal rehabilitation was performed. Participants in the MMR+WEB group self-guided in the web programme, which consisted of eight modules: pain, activity, behaviour, stress and thoughts, sleep and negative thoughts, communication and self-esteem, solutions, maintenance and progress. Data was collected with a questionnaire at baseline and after 4 and 12 months. This combined treatment was shown to reduce catastrophizing and increase satisfaction with multimodal rehabilitation (Nordin, 2016). Web-based programmes need to be increasingly studied, as they may improve the effects of pain rehabilitation (Eccleston et al., 2014).

REFERENCES

Afrell, M., Biguet, G., Rudebeck, C.E., 2007. Living with a body in pain—between acceptance and denial. Scand. J. Caring Sci. 21 (3), 291–296.

Barak, A., Klein, B., Proudfoot, J.G., 2009. Defining internet-supported therapeutic interventions. Ann. Behav. Med. 38 (1), 4–17.

Bergstrom, G., Bergstrom, C., Hagberg, J., et al., 2010. A 7-year follow-up of multidisciplinary rehabilitation among chronic neck and back pain patients. Is sick leave outcome dependent on psychologically derived patient groups? Eur. J. Pain 14, 426–433.

Bergstrom, G., Bodin, L., Bertilsson, H., Jensen, I.B., 2007. Risk factors for new episodes of sick leave due to neck or back pain in a working population. A prospective study with an 18-month and a three-year follow-up. Occup. Environ. Med. 64, 279–287.

Berman, R.L., Iris, M.A., Bode, R., Drengenberg, C., 2009. The effectiveness of an online mind-body intervention for older adults with chronic pain. J. Pain 10 (1), 68–79.

Cramer, H., Lauche, R., Haller, H., et al., 2013. "I'm more in balance": a qualitative study of yoga for patients with chronic neck pain. J. Altern. Complement. Med. 19 (6), 536–542.

Demmelmaier, I., Denison, E., Lindberg, P., Åsenlöf, P., 2011. Tailored skills training of practitioners to enhance assessment of prognostic factors for persistent and disabling back pain: four quasi-experiemental single-subject studies. Physiother. Theory Pract. 28 (6), 1–14.

Denison, E., Åsenlof, P., Lindberg, P., 2004. Self-efficacy, fear avoidance, and pain intensity as predictors of disability in subacute and chronic musculoskeletal pain patients in primary health care. Pain 111, 245–252.

Dionne, C.E., Bourbonnais, R., Frémont, P., et al., 2007. Determinants of "return to work in good health" among workers with back pain who consult primary care settings: a 2-year prospective study. Eur. Spine J. 16, 641–655.

Dragesund, T., Råheim, M., 2008. Norwegian psychomotor physiotherapy and patients with chronic pain: patients' perspective on body awareness. Physiother. Theory Pract. 24 (4), 243–254.

Eccleston, C., Fisher, E., Craig, L., et al., 2014. Psychological therapies (Internet-delivered) for the management of chronic pain in adults. Cochrane Database Syst. Rev. (2), CD010152.

Foster, G., Taylor, S., Eldridge, S., et al., 2009. Self-management education programmes by lay leaders for people with chronic conditions. An interventions review. Cochrane Database Syst. Rev. (3).

Gard, G., 2012. Focus on psychological factors and body awareness in multimodal musculoskeletal pain rehabilitation. In: Bettany-Saltikov, J., Paz-Lourido (Eds.). Physical Therapy Perspectives in the 21st Century–Challenges and Possibilities. Publisher InTechOpen, DOI:10.5772/35768.

Gatchel, R.J., Rollings, K.H., 2008. Evidence-informed management of chronic low back pain with cognitive behavioral therapy. Spine 8 (1), 40–44.

Grahn, B., 1999. Quality of life, motivation and costs in multidisciplinary occupational rehabilitation. Dissertation. Lund University, Lund, Sweden.

Gullacksen, A.C., Lidbeck, J., 2004. The life adjustment process in chronic pain: psychosocial assessment and clinical implications. Pain Res. Manag. 9 (3), 145–153.

Jensen, M.P., Turner, J.A., Romano, J.M., 2007. Changes after multidisciplinary pain treatment in patient pain beliefs and coping are associated with concurrent changes in patient functioning. Pain 131, 38–47.

Laisné, F., Lecomte, C., Corbiere, M., 2012. Bio psychosocial predictors of prognosis in musculosceletal disorders: a systematic review of the literature. Disabil. Rehabil. 34 (22), 1912–1941.

Linton, S.J., 2000. A review of psychological risk factors in back and neck pain. Spine 25, 1148–1156.

Linton, S.J., Shaw, W.S., 2011. Impact of psychological factors in the experience of pain. Phys. Ther. 91 (5), 700–711.

Maddali Bongi, S., Di Felice, C., Del Rosso, A., et al., 2011. Efficacy of the "body movement and perception" method in the treatment of fibromyalgia syndrome: an open pilot study. Clin. Exp. Rheumatol. 29 (6 Suppl. 69), 12–18.

Malmgren-Olsson, E.B., Armelius, B., Armelius, K., 2001. A comparative outcome study of Body Awareness Therapy, Feldenkrais and conventional physiotherapy for patients with non-specific musculoskeletal disorders, changes in psychological symptoms, pain and self-image. Physiother. Theory Pract. 17, 77–95.

Malmgren-Olsson, E.B., Bränholm, I.B., 2002. A comparison between three physiotherapy approaches with regard to health-related factors in patients with non-specific musculoskeletal disorders. Disabil. Rehabil. 24, 308–317.

Mannerkorpi, K., Gard, G., 2003. Physiotherapy group treatment for patients with fibromyalgia—an embodied learning process. Disabil. Rehabil. 25, 1372–1380.

Mehling, W.E., 2005. Randomized, controlled trial of breath therapy for patients with chronic low-back pain. Altern. Ther. Health Med. 11 (4), 44–52.

Mehling, W.E., Wrubel, J., Daubenmier, J.J., et al., 2011. Body Awareness: a phenomenological inquiry into the common ground of mind-body therapies. Philos. Ethics Humanit. Med. 6, 6.

Michie, S., van Stralen, M.M., West, R., 2011. The behavior change wheel: a new method for characterizing and designing behavior change interventions. Implement. Sci. 6, 42. doi:10.1186/1748-5908-6-42.

Morone, N.E., Greco, C.M., 2007. Mind-body interventions for chronic pain in older adults: a structured review. Pain Med. 8 (4), 359–375.

Morone, N.E., Greco, C.M., Weiner, D.K., 2008. Mindfulness meditation for the treatment of chronic low back pain in older adults: a randomized controlled pilot study. Pain 134 (3), 310–319.

Nordin, C., 2016. Patient participation in and treatment effects of Multimodal Rehabilitation and the Web Behaviour Change Program for Activity. PhD thesis, Dept of Health Sciences, Luleå University of Technology.

SBU, 2010. Rehabilitation for long-lasting pain conditions. A systematic literature review. The Swedish Council on Technology Assessment in Health Care, SBU.

Waterlander, W., Whittaker, R., McRobbie, H., et al., 2014. Development of an evidence-based mHealth weight management program using a formative research process. JMIR Mhealth Uhealth 2 (3), e18.

Webb, T.L., Joseph, J., Yardley, L., Michie, S., 2010. Using the internet to promote health behavior change: a systematic review and meta-analysis of the impact of theoretical basis, use of behavior change techniques, and mode of delivery on efficacy. J. Med. Internet Res. 17, 12.

Wells, C., Kolt, G.S., Marshall, P.B., Bialocerkowski, A., 2014. Indications, benefits, and risks of Pilates exercise for people with chronic low back pain: a Delphi survey of pilates-trained physical therapists. Phys. Ther. 94, 806–817.

5.1.2 Touching the Lived Body: Integrating Myofascial Bodywork and Body Awareness in Mental Healthcare Practice

JOERI CALSIUS

SUMMARY

The quintessence of 'experiential bodywork' is the co-resonating use of listening touch and evocative language. Whether hands-on myofascial bodywork is combined with verbal or imagery exploration at the same time or more in a phased protocol, a concrete way into the patient's inner world of sensations and emotions is offered and serves as a tangible support for body awareness (BA). Research shows not only that BA is a bottom-up 'bodily' affair, but that it is also anchored in an interoceptive-insular pathway, which in turn is deeply connected with autonomic and emotional brain areas, as well as verbal and nonverbal memory. Because skin and myofascial tissues can be seen as interoceptive generators, if approached in the proper manual way, supportive evidence is offered to explain why a listening or haptic touch activates this interoceptive-insular pathway and eventually restores the myofascial armoured body. From a transdisciplinary angle, this article reflects on how the integration of experiential bodywork with nondirective verbal guidance can be deeply healing and resourcing for the lived body experience in psychosomatics.

KEY POINTS

■ A key aspect in personal development and well-being is the ability to contact one's own body and tune into it, i.e., *to feel it from within.*

■ Skin and myofascial tissues trigger the interoceptive-insular pathway if approached in the proper manual way, which in turn is deeply connected with autonomic and emotional brain areas, as well as verbal and nonverbal memory.

- The quintessence of experiential bodywork is the co-resonating use of listening touch and evocative language or movement, applied to the patients myofascial armouring, which can be seen as an embodied blueprint of the lived body.

- The restored embodied self-awareness puts the patient (back) at the perspectival origin of their experiences, behaviour and thoughts so they can learn once again to trust their body as a source of information and knowledge, and create the necessary counterweight to correct their often hypercognitive ways of coping with stressful situations.

REFLECTIVE QUESTIONS

- What is 'the lived body' and how or where does it appear in mental healthcare practice?

- What is the concept of 'listening touch' and why is it so central in experiential bodywork?

- Why is the interoceptive-insular pathway paramount in the process of body awareness?

INTRODUCTION

Despite its historical embedding in philosophy and psychology, *the lived body* is not as commonly implemented in mental healthcare practice (MHCP) as one would expect. Nevertheless, patients in MHCP often present themselves with a body that has become too problematic to be 'lived in' comfortably: it hurts, it weighs, it is tired, it is hyperpresent or simply absent. In fact, for a wide range of psychopathology and chronic pain in general, studies indicate that a disturbance in what is called the *'lived body'* or *'embodiment'* should be taken into account as a significant element in the process of malfunctioning (Wilde, 2003; Osborn & Smith, 2006; Fuchs & Schlimme, 2009; Stanghellini, 2009). Chronic suffering is said to disrupt the dialectic process between the individual, his body and his relation to the world: 'Persons with illness suffer not only from the physical aspects of pain and discomfort but also from a loss of identity, where one feels alienated and detached from things that used to give meaning to one's life' (Bullington, 2009).

For a comprehensive conceptualization of the lived body I draw on Stanghellini (2009), who points at its phenomenological origin where the lived body is seen as the centre of three experiential domains, i.e., the

experience of the self, the experience of other people or objects and meaning-bestowing. Thus the lived body is not only the phenomenological side of having a body (Körper) but, in particular, being one (Leib), both converging into the concept of embodiment. This 'ontological' given of being embodied has far-reaching consequences for our daily lives because one's lived body is not merely an experience of oneself and the world, it is the perspectival origin, the organizing and integrating centre of all one's experiencing. One inhabits the world, understands one's environment and gives meaning to it *through* one's bodily presence in and engagement with this world (Heidegger, 2008; Stanghellini, 2009; Merleau-Ponty, 2012). This is why patients always present and express themselves *through* their embodiment, their lived body or, as Gyllensten et al. (2010) call it, their *embodied identity*. Moreover, this 'presenting and expressing' has not only a bodily side, but also appears in language by words and metaphors because of its embodied origin (Lakoff & Johnson, 2003; Jirak et al., 2010), which means that the story a patient tells in fact is an 'embodied narrative' (Calsius et al., 2013a,b, 2015).

The ability to become aware of this being-embodied-in-the-world is generally referred to as *body awareness* (BA), which Mehling, et al. (2011) describe as 'the subjective, phenomenological aspect of proprioception and interoception that enters conscious awareness and is modifiable by mental processes including attention, interpretation, appraisal, beliefs, memories, conditioning attitude and affect'. Fogel (2009) in turn conceptualizes BA in terms of embodied self-awareness as the ability to pay attention to ourselves, to feel our sensations and movements online, along with the motivational and emotional feelings that accompany them, in the present moment, without the mediating influence of judgemental thoughts. In relation to embodiment, BA is the awareness of embodiment as an innate tendency of our organism for emergent self-organisation and wholeness (Mehling et al., 2011). A key aspect in all this is the ability to contact the body or to tune into it, i.e., *to feel it from within*, which is seen as an essential part of personal development and well-being (Fogel, 2011). Given the appearance of the lived body in clinical encounters, interventions aiming at this ability of BA are expected to be widely implemented in MHCP. Although this is the case in some psychomotor therapies or in body psychotherapy (Geuter, 2015), the main focus used in these modalities is based on movement and rarely on touch, which brings us to the main topic of this chapter on integrating myofascial bodywork and BA in MHCP.

INTEGRATING MYOFASCIAL BODYWORK AND BODY AWARENESS

Suggesting that an integration of touch-based bodywork and BA is brand new would not only be incorrect, but is not borne out by a study of the history of BA therapies. Although there is not space here to go into detail, it is necessary to mention at least that, during the heyday of body-mind therapies in the 1960s and 1970s, a dazzling variety of therapies arose, many of which are still practised today. Bioenergetics, gestalt therapy, Feldenkrais, Rolfing, postural integration, Pesso therapy and Reichian bodywork are just some examples of these attempts to implement BA in a holistic hands-on approach to the lived body.[1] Although a second, broad wave of new BA therapies originated later on from these early methods, a major drawback continued to be the lack of sufficient scientific evidence and academic support (Courtois et al., 2014). Nevertheless, a compelling body of research shows how being aware of your body is essential in normal development and health outcomes (Fuchs, 2001; Gard, 2005; Osborn & Smith, 2006; Bullington, 2009; Fuchs & Schlimme, 2009; Payne, 2009; Zeiler, 2010; Fogel, 2011; Cipolletta, 2013). Besides the presence of a rich body of knowledge (sometimes empirical, but mostly intuitive) and a common ground firmly rooted in a broad range of theoretical paradigms, working with BA from a touch-based angle, however, seems unable to get the attention it deserves.

Yet a growing interest in the concept of embodiment as a key paradigm in psychology, psychiatry, neuroscience and philosophy (Fuchs & Schlimme, 2009) on the one hand, and an exponential increase of fascia research as a transdisciplinary substrate on the other (Schleip et al., 2012), seem to offer an intriguing new momentum to explore and research the basic assumptions of BA in touch-based therapies. With

regard to these therapies and in order to avoid conceptual misunderstanding or school-dependent vocabulary, this article will use *experiential bodywork* (EBW) as an umbrella term for those body-mind therapies using an explicit hands-on approach, often in combination with movement-based strategies for emotional awareness and expression.[2]

In EBW the therapist works with BA and touch to bring patients in contact with their inner world and to facilitate interpersonal dynamics. Being a touch-based experiential approach, EBW incorporates hands-on techniques to work specifically on the patient's body, which is described in this article as the myofascial system (Box 1). On the other hand, EBW is a phenomenological approach as it focuses on the lived body experience of the patient.

Consequently one of the addressed core questions focuses on how the relationship between touch-based intervention and BA can be established more scientifically. To tackle this topic in a neurobiological as well as phenomenological way, the myofascial system is approached as an entry point to the awareness dimension in hands-on therapy. Keeping close to MHCP, the starting point is the interesting concept of 'body armouring' and its clinical manifestation in psychosomatic dysfunction.

TOUCHING THE MYOFASCIAL BODY, MOVING THE LIVED BODY

With his definition of body armouring, Wilhelm Reich (1972, 1973) introduced a psychosomatic explanation *avant la lettre* for what in MHCP is often seen in patients with stress, anxiety or persistent emotional disturbance. Namely, the body expresses its incarnated coping to a distressing reality: 'The experience-dependent development of a protective shell of muscle tension grown over time in response to a history of threat, anxiety and trauma.' To this *muscular armour* Reich (1973) attributed characteristics, for instance that it stiffens the coordination of the segments of the body, reduces the postural repertoire, inhibits

---

[1]For an extensive exploration on history, concepts and technique, see, for example, Heller (2012) and Geuter (2015).

[2]As an umbrella term, EBW tries to span existing therapies that have a firm tradition in working with BA by touch and movement from a phenomenological perspective such as the intriguing fascia method of Danis Bois (Bois, 1984; Bois & Berger, 1990).

Experiential Bodywork (EBW) offers scientific and trans-disciplinary underpinnings for an integration of hands-on bodywork, intuitive movement, phenomenology and psychodynamics in body psychotherapy.

Through deep myofascial bodywork and intuitive movement, the client in EBW learns to explore and experience his body from within. This embodied awareness helps him to understand more soundly how he participates in the world from a bodily perspective. The client learns to use his being-a-body in a more evocative and intuitive way to move, listen and express himself in relation to others and the world. In this way EBW offers a therapeutic integration of bodywork, psychotherapy and phenomenological analysis for the spectrum of psychosomatic complaints, tension-based symptoms and emotional pain.

On a scientific level EBW tries to link insights and research from different paradigms, such as body-psychotherapy, fascia-research, myofascial therapy and osteopathy, psychosomatic research, psychodynamic theories, phenomenology and integral philosophy. In this way EBW bridges ground breaking theories from the heyday of body psychotherapy and recent academic research. EBW distinguishes itself as it is not claiming to be a new or exclusive therapy, but aims to build on pre-existing concepts, paradigms and techniques while promoting an inclusive philosophy towards the strengths of all modalities in body psychotherapy.

respiration and diminishes the perception of what goes on in the body, which can easily be recognized in psychosomatic dysfunctioning. This seminal idea that the body ends up as a blueprint of the way a person has had to cope with myriad life events and as a result of the way they experienced the reactions of significant others at that time, echoes nowadays in several clinical or research domains, such as developmental psychology, neuroscience and therapy. In that way Schore (2001) states: 'The neuromuscular and autonomic nervous systems encode patterns of early object relations, so that there may be a long-term autobiographical memory of a pathological internal object relation, that becomes the unconscious working model.' Pat Ogden refers to this mutual influencing by pointing at its origins in attachment: 'All early relational dynamics with primary caregivers, traumatic or non-traumatic, serve as blueprints for the child's developing cognition and belief systems, and these belief systems influence posture, structure and movement of the body and vice

versa. [...] Chronic postural and movement tendencies serve to sustain certain beliefs and cognitive distortions, and the physical patterns, in turn, contribute to these same beliefs' (Ogden et al., 2006).

In research, these patterns and postural tendencies are studied more and more from a transdisciplinary attempt to understand the underlying pathogenic emotional influences on the myofascial system in, for example, anxiety (Schleip, 2003a,b; Younger et al., 2010; Ritz et al., 2013) and trauma (Levine, 2005; Haugstad et al., 2006; Ogden et al., 2006). On the other hand, from a therapeutic point of view this opens the question of if and how this emotionally charged and armoured myofascial body can be influenced profoundly by aiming at BA.

As mentioned previously, this is where transdisciplinary help from recent fascia research is needed to clarify a possible missing link in understanding how deep tissue work effects BA. To some extent, this link relates to the abundantly present unmyelinated polymodal C-fibre receptors in fascial tissues, called *interstitial myofascial tissue receptors* (IMTR), which follow an interoceptive pathway to awareness—if approached properly (Schleip, 2003a,b). Additionally, in (hairy) skin some other 'interoceptive' receptors, called *human tactile C-fibres*, have been identified as reacting specifically to touch that is light and sensual (McGlone et al., 2014; Ackerley et al., 2014; Björnsdotter et al., 2010; Olausson et al., 2010). Therefore, if deep bodywork[3] is applied with slow and sustained 'melting' pressure (IMTR) or 'light sensual touch' (human tactile C-fibres), the total myofascial substrate and connecting skin of the charged and armoured body can be used as an entry point to provoke interoceptive brain-body pathways and communication (Schleip & Jäger, 2012).

But why is this interoceptive involvement so important? In short, the answer lies partly in the central role of the insula. When interoceptive sensory input via parasympathetic, sympathetic, as well as enteric afferents reaches the thalamic region, it arrives at the dorsal insular cortex to form a representation of all sensory information, i.e., an 'interoceptive image' (Craig, 2010, 2011). Subsequently, this information moves on to the anterior insula and the right orbitofrontal cortex to

---

[3]For a detailed study on the integration of hands-on bodywork and body awareness, see Calsius et al. (2016).

form a re-representation of this overall sensory image (Craig, 2009; Berlucchi & Aglioti, 2010; Herbert & Pollatos, 2012). The significant role of the insula at this stage is twofold. First, there is the intertwining with several other brain structures, such as the limbic system and its relation to implicit and nonverbal memory, crucial in trauma and attachment (Levine, 1997; Ogden et al., 2006; Fogel, 2009, 2011). Second, the anterior insula is conceived by several authors, such as Cameron (2001), Craig (2002, 2011), Critchley et al. (2004), Critchley & Seth (2012) and Damasio & Carvalho (2013), as pivotal in the process of BA. At this insular stage the individual becomes *consciously* aware of their bodily status and interactions with the environment. This is why the insula is seen as a structure for the integration of hedonic, emotional, motivational and behavioural input, and as a regulator of conscious bodily experience or BA. Thus the use of the right kind of myofascial intervention—sometimes referred to as 'listening touch', 'haptic touch' or even 'limbic touch'—to the tensed and armoured body facilitates BA because of its interoceptive pathway. In short, EBW equals interoception, equals BA.

But even now a state-of-the-art neurobiological exploration has enlightened us with profound insights in how hands-on body work relates inherently to BA, the phenomenological point of departure, namely the lived body, should be kept in mind. Despite all substantial insular processing on awareness, a patient's first and foremost experience of being touched is on a phenomenological level. Not what, where or why they are touched, but the fact of *being* touched *by someone* is what moves human beings in the first place. Being moved can be seen as a focus of awareness going back and forth from what Zeiler (2010) calls bodily dis-appearance to dys-appearance.[4]

Under normal conditions, people are not aware of their body because it is not an object of their attention.

---

[4]Subsequent to this neutral (dis-appearance) and negative (dys-appearance) dialectical awareness of the lived body, it has to be mentioned that BA can also be exclusively experienced in a positive way. This is what Zeiler (2010) describes as *eu-appearance*. Here the body is experienced on the foreground of attention as pleasant and a source of enjoyment. This can be the case in sports, sexuality or sometimes even pregnancy. Now, the lived body is experienced as hyperowned and absorbed in a positive flow of consciousness, sometimes reaching extasis.

At these moments they have a prereflective relation with the body in which it seems to be absent or disappeared from their field of attention. This is why Fogel (2011) describes this type of BA as neither implicit nor explicit and not necessarily nonverbal. He looks at it as the ability to sense, in the present moment and without mediating thoughts, the sensorimotor feelings along with the motivational and emotional feelings that accompany them. For Zeiler (2010) this normal state of dis-appearance contrasts with the state she calls *bodily dys-appearance*. This happens when the implicit and harmonious relation between the body, the mind and the world gets disturbed, like in chronic suffering, pain or stress. Here the lived body feels constricted and alienated. The disrupture makes my body no longer something I *am*, but just something I *have*: my body becomes a thing that is mechanically broken and needs to be fixed or repaired. In literature this stranded BA is also referred to as *disembodiment*, where the prereflective immersion in the world is lost (Fuchs & Schlimme, 2009; de Haan, 2012).

BODY AWARENESS TRANSLATED

This bodily dys-appearance or disembodiment is often the case in the condition of body armouring where the patient does not live their body any more *from within*, but through its restrictions in movement, breathing and experiencing. Remember Reich (1973), who pointed at the stiffening of coordination of body segments, reducing its postural repertoire, inhibiting respiration and diminishing BA? Rephrased into MHCP, a phenomenological approach of the lived body reveals a dimensional spectrum where BA should be able to move from the attentional foreground to background, as well as between a negative over neutral to positive load. Using the myofascial body as an entry point to the patient's BA helps in improving their ability to contact the lived body (again) *from within* and to tune into their own bodily hermeneutics. Or, as Mooij describes it, the meaningfulness of our bodily language and (dys-)functions. So, from a therapy-orientated stance, BA can be seen as a privileged gateway to psychosomatics in general and body armouring specifically. But how can this be achieved on a concrete and therapeutic level?

In order to address this, a further differentiation of BA conceptualized by Fogel offers a possible stepping stone in fine-tuning how a specific manual approach, such as in EBW, helps patients in (re-)contacting and exploring their inner world. Fogel (2009, 2011) uses the term *embodied self-awareness* to describe the ability to be in the subjective emotional present and to explore the intricacies of senses, movements and emotions in relation to others and the world. Hereby, embodied self-awareness is labelled as spontaneous, creative and open to change, concrete and lived in the present moment, and most of all characterized by its non-verbal, translingual nature. All of these features are congruent with the prereflective and nonverbal nature of BA as a tacit but experiential primordial contact with the world. Besides the embodied outward relation to the world, there is also an inward relation that has been extensively analysed and paraphrased as the body being a source of knowledge or wisdom (Wilde, 2003; Fuchs & Schlimme, 2009; Stanghellini, 2009; Gyllensten et al., 2010). Here, the individual who listens and tunes in to their body can learn and experience an inner approval or meaning bestowing that which is sometimes labelled as a *felt sense* (Gendlin, 1969; Gendlin & Olson, 1970). From a phenomenological perspective, it has been studied why in particular this ability of BA as tuning-in and feeling the self as an embodied intelligence is often not available to people with chronic illness or pain (Price, 1993; Bullington, 2009; Calsius et al., 2015). When Fogel (2009) states that embodied self-awareness does not require language for its expression and exists prior to language, he is referring to the developmental processing of its key neurobiological correlation, namely, the amygdala. In line with Craig, Fogel sees the interoceptive-insular pathway as the backbone of BA, but although equally stressing the exclusive interest of the insular capacity to re-representation, he links the lower and limbic brain structures to embodied self-awareness.

EXPERIENTIAL BODYWORK: INTEGRATING MYOFASCIAL BODYWORK AND BODY AWARENESS

A profound therapeutic consequence of this is the use of *evocative language* (Fogel, 2009) or *imagery playing-out* (Payne & Crane-Godreau, 2015; Payne et al., 2015) to enter, explore and express embodied self-awareness in patients. In contrast to regular language, which is more under cognitive control and censorship, evocative language and imagery resonate the felt experience 'as it appears in the present moment' (Gendlin, 1969; Gendlin & Olson, 1970; Bloom, 2006; Fogel, 2009). Besides spontaneous words that capture this resonance or felt sense, metaphors, images, dreams, poetry, music, drama or meditation are also examples, and from a more psychoanalytical angle, free association, are also evocative language.

This ability to embody self-awareness is precisely what is lacking in the case of psychosomatic dysfunctioning, especially in alexithymic people, which makes them vulnerable as a wordless gap lies between the level of bodily arousal and the transfer into language or imagination. From a psychoanalytical perspective, this vulnerability is described as a representational failure of bodily arousal and tension when people do not understand what is going on in their body while experiencing, for example, stress or trivial somatic signals (Vanheule et al., 2011). Subsequently, in MHCP the importance of a progressive and patient-tailored process of finding words to describe the sensations and feelings is stressed: 'Treatment should not focus on the mental representational deficit as such, but on the underlying experiences, with which the patient fails to deal mentally' (Vanheule et al., 2011). Here, the unique feature of EBW coming in as working with embodied self-awareness from a touch-based angle is specifically aiming at closing this representational gap. Herewith, we arrive at the quintessence on how a manual, touch-based approach can be a unique entry point.

Given the use of a listening or haptic touch, EBW not only helps the patient in tuning into the aforementioned interoceptive-insular pathway and rebalancing the window of tolerance to an optimal arousal zone—mostly by silencing the sympathetic overdrive—but also specifically facilitates the ability to become body aware and to contact one's own bodily inner world. In short, EBW creates an optimal momentum for embodied self-awareness and invites, or even provokes, evocative language. In particular, the limbic load of the interoceptive-insular pathway is hypothesized to affect the experiential BA process during the hands-on approach. The combination of light and tactile manual bodywork with nondirective verbal guidance triggers the dyadic bodily resonance described by several authors as being deeply healing, restoring and resourcing (Totton, 1998; Levine, 2005; Bloom, 2006; Ogden et al., 2006; White, 2006; Heller, 2012; Cipolletta, 2013; Van der Kolk, 2014; Payne et al., 2015; Cornell, 2015). In trying to grasp the underlying mechanism of this beneficial process of EBW, research mostly points to optimizing and rebalancing a secure attachment (Ogden et al., 2006), opening up the social engagement system (Porges, 2009), engaging and integrating preverbal memories (Bloom, 2006), befriending the body, which is a metaphor for allowing and naming the physical sensations beneath the emotions (Van der Kolk, 2014) or biological completion (Payne & Crane-Goudreau, 2015; Payne et al., 2015).

Payne & Crane-Goudreau (2015) put forward a hypothesis for understanding body-mind therapies as normalizing what they call a 'preparatory set', which is essentially a unitary trauma response based on affect, posture and muscle tone, autonomic state, attention and expectation, which they call *the core response network*. Although all of these authors are, to some extent, drawing on neurophysiological frameworks, they ultimately point to the quintessence of becoming self-aware from within the body, which is convergent with the phenomenological realm in BA psychotherapies and EBW. Wilde (2003) rephrases this, more explicitly focusing on the experiential level and using BA to enter the lived body as contacting 'a silent partner of informant of embodied knowledge'. Interestingly, Payne and colleagues (2015) point at the same two principal ways on how body-mind therapies can work—by becoming aware, and by biological completion, such as trembling, crying or flushing, in which the originally obstructed energy load is enabled to complete itself.

As proposed in this present text, in EBW these two principles are intertwined, firstly because the listening touch in EBW—whether hands-on body work is combined with verbal exploration at the same time or more in a phased protocol—is offering a concrete way into the patient's inner world of sensations and emotions while serving as a tangible support for body awareness. In particular, for alexithymic patients, this guidance can be of significance regarding their representational failure of bodily arousal and tension. Secondly, given the limbic load of touch in EBW, the therapeutic frame is now expanded with an inside-out bodily experience of a safe, attentive and authentic presence, crucial for holding and containment. Although not required, this can facilitate a cathartic process, comparable with Payne's idea of biological completion and Reich's earlier thoughts on a breakthrough, where the patient is guided in expressing or acting out in a more evocative or bodily language, what is called *unmentalized material* (Grotstein, 2013; Ferro, 2013). This searching for words or symbolization puts the patient (back) at the perspectival origin of their experiences, behaviour and thoughts so they can learn once again to trust their body as a source of information and knowledge and create the necessary counterweight to correct their often hypercognitive ways of coping with stressful situations. Hereby, we not only return to the phenomenological point of departure, but moreover to the clinical reality of MHCP where our patient lost track with their body that, although crying out loud, is experienced as a tormenting bottleneck to comfort and happiness.

REFERENCES

Ackerley, R., Backlund Wasling, H., Liljencrantz, J., et al., 2014. Human C-tactile afferents are tuned to the temperature of a skin-stroking caress. J. Neurosci. 34 (8), 2879–2883.

Berlucchi, G., Aglioti, S.M., 2010. The body in the brain revisited. Exp. Brain Res. 200, 25–35.

Björnsdotter, M., Morrison, I., Olausson, H., 2010. Feeling good: on the role of C fiber mediated touch in interoception. Exp. Brain Res. 207, 149–155.

Bloom, K., 2006. The Embodied Self. Movement and psychoanalysis. Karnac, New York.

Bois, D., 1984. Concepts fondamentaux de fasciathérapie et de pulsologie profonde. Compte d'auteur, Vendôme.

Bois, D., Berger, E., 1990. Une thérapie manuelle de la profondeur. Tredaniel, Paris.

Bullington, J., 2009. Embodiment and chronic pain: implications for rehabilitation practice. Health Care Anal. 17, 100–109.

Calsius, J., Courtois, I., Feys, P., et al., 2015. How to conquer a mountain with multiple sclerosis. How a climbing expedition to Machu Picchu affects the way people with multiple sclerosis experience their body and identity: a phenomenological analysis. Disabil. Rehabil. 37, 2393–2399.

Calsius, J., Courtois, I., Stiers, J., De Bie, J., 2015. How do fibromyalgia patients with alexithymia experience their body? A qualitative approach. SAGE Open 5, 1–10.

Calsius, J., De Bie, J., Hertogen, R., Meesen, R., 2016. Touching the lived body in patients with medically unexplained symptoms. How an integration of hands-on bodywork and body awareness in psychotherapy may help people with alexithymia. Front. Psychol. 7, 253.

Calsius, J., Pott, H., Alma, H., 2013a. Going through anxiety. A phenomenological analysis of five turning points in ego development. Tijdschrift Cliëntgerichte Psychotherapie. Procesgericht Experiëntieel Interactioneel Integratief. Jg. 51, nr. 3.

Calsius, J., Pott, H., Alma, H., 2013b. The body in the process of existential awareness. Possible or not? Tijdschrift Cliëntgerichte Psychotherapie. Procesgericht Experiëntieel Interactioneel Integratief. Jg. 51, nr. 4.

Cameron, O.G., 2001. Interoception: the inside story—a model for psychosomatic processes. Psychosom. Med. 63, 697–710.

Cipolletta, S., 2013. Construing in action: experiencing embodiment. J. Constr. Psychol. 26, 293–305.

Cornell, W.F., 2015. Somatic Experience in Psychoanalysis and Psychotherapy. In the Expressive Language of The Living. Routledge, London.

Courtois, I., Cools, F., Calsius, J., 2014. Effectiveness of body awareness interventions in fibromyalgia and chronic fatigue syndrome: a systematic review and meta-analysis. J. Bodyw. Mov. Ther. 19, 35–56.

Craig, A.D., 2002. How do you feel? Interoception: the sense of the physiological condition of the body. Nat. Rev. Neurosci. 3, 655–666.

Craig, A.D., 2009. How do you feel now? The anterior insula and human awareness. Nat. Rev. Neurosci. 10, 59–70.

Craig, A.D., 2010. The sentient self. Brain Struct Funct 214, 563–577.

Craig, A.D., 2011. Significance of the insula for the evolution of human awareness of feelings from the body. Ann. N. Y. Acad. Sci. 1225, 72–82.

Critchley, H., Seth, A., 2012. Will studies of macaque insula reveal the neural mechanisms of self-awareness? Neuron 74, 423–426.

Critchley, H.D., Wiens, S., Rotshtein, P., et al., 2004. Neural systems supporting interoceptive awareness. Nat. Neurosci. 7 (2), 189–195.

Damasio, A., Carvalho, G.B., 2013. The nature of feelings: evolutionary and neurobiological origins. Nat. Rev. Neurosci. 14, 143–152.

De Haan, S., 2012. Fenomenologie van de lichaamservaring. In: Denys, D., Meynen, G. (Eds.), Handboek Psychiatrie en Filosofie. De Tijdstroom, Utrecht.

Ferro, A., 2013. Vicissitudes of the container/contained and field theory. In: Levine, H.B., Brown, L.J. (Eds.), Growth and Turbulence in the Container/Contained. Bion's Continuing Legacy. Routledge, London, pp. 79–103.

Fogel, A., 2009. The Psychophysiology of Self-Awareness. W.W. Norton, New York.

Fogel, A., 2011. Embodied awareness: neither implicit nor explicit, and not necessarily nonverbal. Child Development Perspectives 5, 183–186.

Fuchs, T., 2001. The tacit dimension. Philos Psychiatr Psychol 8, 323–326.

Fuchs, T., Schlimme, J.E., 2009. Embodiment and psychopathology: a phenomenological perspective. Curr. Opin. Psychiatry 22, 570–575.

Gard, G., 2005. Body awareness therapy for patients with fibromyalgia and chronic pain. Disabil. Rehabil. 27, 725–728.

Gendlin, E.T., 1969. Focusing. Psychotherapy: Theory, Research and Practice 6, 4–15. <http://www.focusing.org/gendlin/docs/gol _2048.html.>

Gendlin, E.T., Olsen, L., 1970. The use of imagery in experiential focusing. Psychotherapy: Theory, Research and Practice 7 (4), 221–223. <http://www.focusing.org/gendlin/docs/gol_2066 .html.>

Geuter, U., 2015. Körper-psychotherapie. Grundriss Einer Theorie für die Klinische Praxis. Springer, Berlin Heidelberg.

Grotstein, J.S., 2013. Dreaming as a curtain of illusion. Revisiting the royal road with Bion as our guide. In: Levine, H.B., Brown, L.J. (Eds.), Growth and Turbulence in the Container/Contained. Bion's continuing Legacy. Routledge, London, pp. 107–130.

Gyllensten, A.L., Skär, L., Miller, M., Gard, G., 2010. Embodied identity—a deeper understanding of body awareness. Physiother. Theory Pract. 26, 439–446.

Haugstad, G., Haugstad, T., Kirste, U., 2006. Posture, movement patterns and body awareness in women with chronic pelvic pain. J. Psychosom. Res. 61 (5), 637–644.

Heidegger, M., 2008. Being and Time. Harper and Row, New York.

Heller, M., 2012. Body Psychotherapy. History, Concepts and Methods. Norton, New York.

Herbert, B.M., Pollatos, O., 2012. The body in the mind: on the relationship between interoception and embodiment. Top. Cogn. Sci. 4, 692–704.

Jirak, D., Menz, M.M., Buccino, G., et al., 2010. Grasping language. A short story on embodiment. Conscious. Cogn. 19, 711–720.

Lakoff, G., Johnson, M., 2003. Methaphors We Live By. University Of Chicago Press, Chicago.

Levine, P., 1997. Waking the Tiger: Healing trauma. North Atlantic Books, Berkeley.

Levine, P., 2005. Panic, biology and reason. Giving the body its due. In: Totton, N. (Ed.), New Dimensions in Bodypsychotherapy. Open University Press, Maidenhead, pp. 30–39.

McGlone, F., Wessberg, J., Olausson, H., 2014. Discriminative and affective touch: sensing and feeling. Neuron 82 (4), 737–755.

Mehling, W.E., Wrubel, J., Daubenmier, J.J., et al., 2011. Body Awareness: a phenomenological inquiry into the common ground of mind-body therapies. Philos. Ethics. Humanit. Med. 6 (1), 6.

Merleau-Ponty, M., 2012. The phenomenology of Perception. Routledge, New York.

Mooij, A., 2006. The Psychological Reality. Psychiatry as Humanities. Boom, Amsterdam.

Ogden, P., Minton, K., Pain, C., 2006. Trauma and the Body. A Sensorimotor Approach to Psychotherapy. Norton, New York, London.

Olausson, H., Wessberg, J., Morisson, I., 2010. The neurophysiology of unmyelinated tactile afferents. Neurosci. Biobehav. Rev. 34, 185–191.

Osborn, M., Smith, J.A., 2006. Living with a body separate from the self. The experience of the body in chronic benign low back pain: an interpretative phenomenological analysis. Scand. J. Caring Sci. 20 (14), 216–222.

Payne, H., 2009. The BodyMind Approach TM to psychotherapeutic groupwork with patients with medically unexplained symptoms: a review of the literature, description of approach and methodology selected for a pilot study. Eur. J. Couns. Psychother. 11 (3), 287–310.

Payne, P., Crane-Goudreau, M.A., 2015. The preparatory set: a novel approach to understanding stress, trauma and the bodymind therapies. Front. Neurosci. 9, 178.

Payne, P., Levine, P.A., Crane-Goudreau, M.A., 2015. Somatic experiencing: using interoception and proprioception as core elements of trauma therapy. Front. Psychol. 6, 93.

Porges, S.W., 2009. The polyvagal theory: new insights into adaptive reactions of the autonomic nervous system. Cleve. Clin. J. Med. 76 (Suppl. 2), S86–S90.

Price, M.J., 1993. Exploration of body listening: health and physical self-awareness in chronic illness. ANS. Adv. Nurs. Sci. 15 (4), 37–52.

Reich, W., 1972. Character Analysis. Touchstone, New York.

Reich, W., 1973. The Function of the Orgasm. Sex-Economic Problems of Biological Energy. Farar, Straus & Giroux, New York.

Ritz, T.H., Meuret, A.E., Bhaskara, L., Petersen, F., 2013. Respiratory muscle tension as symptom generator in individuals with high anxiety sensitivity. Psychosom. Med. 75, 187–195.

Schleip, R., 2003a. Fascial plasticity: a new neurobiological explanation. Part 1. J. Bodyw. Mov. Ther. 11–19.

Schleip, R., 2003b. Fascial plasticity: a new neurobiological explanation. Part 2. J. Bodyw. Mov. Ther. 104–116.

Schleip, R., Jäger, H., 2012. Interoception. A new correlate for intricate connections between fascial receptors, emotion and self-recognition. In: Schleip, R., Findley, T.W., Chaitow, L., Huijing, P. (Eds.), Fascia. The Tensional Network of the Human Body. Elsevier, London, pp. 89–94.

Schore, A., 2001. Neurobiology, Developmental Psychology and Psychoanalysis: Convergent Findings on the Subject of Projective Identification. In: Edwards, J. (Ed.), Being alive: Building on the Work of Anne Alvarez. Routledge, Sussex, pp. 57–74.

Stanghellini, G., 2009. Embodiment and schizophrenia. World Psychiatry 8, 56–59.

Totton, N., 1998. The Water in the Glass. Body and Mind in Psychoanalysis. Rebus Press, London.

Van der Kolk, B.A., 2014. The Body Keeps the Score. Mind, Brain and Body in the Transformation of Trauma. Penguin Books, London.

Vanheule, S., Verhaeghe, P., Desmet, M., 2011. In search of a framework for the treatment of alexithymia. Psychol. Psychother. 84, 84–97, discussion 98–110.

White, K. (Ed.), 2006. Touch. Attachment and the Body. Karnac Books, London.

Wilde, M.H., 2003. Embodied knowledge in chronic illness and injury. Nurs. Inq. 10, 170–176.

Younger, J.W., Shen, F.Y., Goddard, G., Mackey, S.C., 2010. Chronic myofascial temporomandibular pain is associated with neural abnormalities in the trigeminal and limbic systems. Pain 149, 222–228.

Zeiler, K., 2010. A phenomenological analysis of bodily self-awareness in the experience of pain and pleasure: on dys-appearance and eu-appearance. Med. Health Care Philos. 13, 333–342.

5.1.3 Norwegian Psychomotor Physiotherapy Treatment: Change and Communication in a Long-Term Perspective—Presentation of Results From Clinical Based Research

AUD MARIE ØIEN

SUMMARY

The main aim of the three studies presented here, based on research by the Norwegian Psychomotor Physiotherapy (NPMP) treatment practice, was to increase knowledge of: (1) processes of change, and (2) communication between physiotherapist and patient during challenging episodes of processes of change. The design was a longitudinal multiple-case study of eleven cases monitored over time. Based on a purposeful sampling strategy, six physiotherapists participated, who selected altogether 11 patients from their waiting lists or early treatments. Qualitative data generated from video recordings of treatment sessions, individual and focus group interviews, patients' reflective notes and field notes were analysed looking for major patterns and details. The main results included different types of change over time and variation of communication within sessions. In the first study, patients expressed the meaning of their back pain as a long-term relationship with pain. They experienced treatment as a process of 'becoming an embodied subject', described as a narrative change from 'being detached from the body' to 'becoming in touch with the body'. The results of the second study included the emergence of change over time within and outside the space of treatment. Change included increased variety of movements and ways of breathing, and reflection on interdependence with emotional stress. Increased variation of perception emerged embedded in the different types of change. The patients experienced variations with regard to the type and degree of change. Results from the third study included variation of communication within sessions.

KEY POINTS

- In Norwegian psychomotor physiotherapy treatment, change depends on the capability of the physiotherapist and the patient to establish common ground, and deal with challenges of uncertainty and disagreement.

- Over time, patients with chronic pain experience change as variation in different areas.

- Decreasing muscle pain depends on the patient's capability to become in touch with the body.

- Move of experiences from being detached from the body to becoming in touch with the body appears as variation of self-narratives.

- Experiencing and creating variations with regard to habitual ways of moving, breathing, and reflecting within and beyond the treatment contexts open possibilities to vary ways of acting and interacting.

LEARNING OBJECTIVES

- Becoming aware of how patients develop and experience muscle tension, breathing restrictions and pain in narrative contexts of meaning, based on emotional strain over time.

- Becoming aware of how patients' experiences of change, as evidenced by improved variety of movement and ways of breathing, influence self-perception.

- Becoming aware of the physiotherapist's abilities and ways to communicate in negotiating with patients in challenging treatment session sequences.

INTRODUCTION

This chapter looks at the main results of clinical research within the field of Norwegian Psychomotor Physiotherapy (NPMP), based on studies in the thesis *Change and Communication: Long-Term Norwegian Psychomotor Physiotherapy Treatment for Patients with Chronic Muscle Pain* (Øien, 2010). Results in more detail are published in articles by Øien and colleagues (2007, 2009, 2011).

The aim of the thesis was to enhance knowledge of processes of change and communication during long-term NPMP treatments for adult patients with chronic muscle pain in the back and/or neck. Different types of change and communication were investigated in separate studies.

The specific aims and number of cases in the studies were as follows:

- Self-narratives on the foundation of patients' bodily experiences of movement and breathing prior to and during long-term NPMP treatment were investigated based on a multiple case study of two cases (Øien et al., 2007).

- Development and perception of change of movements and breathing were explored during NPMP treatment based on a multiple case study of nine cases (Øien et al., 2009).

- Communication about change in demanding NPMP physiotherapy treatment situations was explored in a multiple case study of eleven cases (Øien et al., 2011).

THEORETICAL PERSPECTIVES

Different theoretical perspectives were used in discussing the results of the different studies. The theoretical perspective of NPMP was used across the studies (Øien, 2010). Additionally, in the first study, narrative perspectives (Gergen & Kaye, 2002) were used, in the second, phenomenology of perception (Merleau-Ponty, 2012), and in the third, system theory of communication (Watzlawick et al., 1967). Comprehensive descriptions of the chosen theoretical perspectives are available in the thesis and in the particular published papers.

METHOD

The chosen design was a longitudinal multiple case study intended to catch complex social phenomena within real-life contexts. In these studies, the NPMP treatment course was defined as a single case, which included one physiotherapist and one patient. Eleven cases were monitored from early treatment and 6 to 9 months on. Applying a purposeful sample strategy, six physiotherapists and 11 patients participated. The physiotherapists were experienced clinicians with a postgraduate education in NPMP. Their clinical experience ranged from 20 to 46 years. Eleven patients with back and/or neck pain were included, based on the NPMP understanding that movements of the back and the neck are interconnected. The 11 patients were between 22 and 47 years old, with an average age of 36 years. At the end of the project, the patients' number of treatments varied from 16 to 25, with an average of 20. Qualitative data gathered from different data sources included semistructured individual interviews of patients (22) and physiotherapists (6), one focus group interview of physiotherapists with observations and video recordings of treatment sessions (44), personal notes from patients (40), and field notes (73).

RESULTS

Results from the published papers mentioned previously are given here. Discussions of specific findings are available in the particular published papers.

The results from 'the investigation of the patients' self-narratives' (narrative accounts of illness, lived life and treatment experiences) highlighted the concomitant development of self-narratives and bodily experiences on the basis of the dialogue between the patient and the physiotherapist in the treatment process (Øien et al., 2007). Two main types of narrative accounts were identified: (1) being detached from the body, and (2) being in touch with the body. During treatment, the 'being detached from the body' narrative appeared to gradually reduce and the complementary narrative, 'being in touch with the body', appeared to gradually increase in importance. This narrative change emerged as the patients' experiences of bodily change moved from 'being divided in body and mind' to 'the body is awakening'. This change appeared as a move of self-narratives built on the gradually growing variety of narratives connected to a gradually increasing variety of movement and breathing experiences. The study indicated that NPMP treatment for patients with chronic pain may productively be supplemented with a narrative approach, and consequently an increased attention to the dialogue between the patient and the physiotherapist (Øien et al., 2007).

The 'exploration of the patients' bodily changes' during NPMP treatment (Øien et al., 2009) resulted in five patterns of change connected to (1) movements, (2) breathing, (3) reflections on connections between bodily experiences of muscular tension, restricted breathing and emotional strain, and (4) transfer of use of experiences from treatment to context outside treatment. A fifth pattern, to be detached from and to be in touch with the body, emerged interwoven in each of the first four mentioned patterns. Based on the

extent of change of the different patterns over time, the patients were categorized into two groups, the group of limited change and the group of considerable change. Across the particular patterns and groups, the way patients were perceiving their body appeared as the core element of predicting change during the first body examination and the accounts of illness, as well as change underway. Long-term treatments for patients with chronic pain emerged as complex. Being aware of patients' self-perception at different levels and in different contexts at an early stage and during treatment may enhance physiotherapists' understanding of elements that may obstruct or facilitate change. Being aware of these constraints may help physiotherapists to accept the challenges and reflect on approaches to deal with them (Øien et al., 2009).

The results from the 'exploration of communication in demanding treatment situations' appeared as patterns of negotiation (Øien et al., 2011). The identified main pattern was 'seeking common ground—a demanding negotiating process'. This pattern was interrupted by short episodes of two types of challenges, the 'pattern of ambivalence and uncertainty', and the 'pattern of impatience and disagreement'. The challenging episodes involved challenging and complex negotiations of the task, emotions connected to the task or the nature of the relationship. With regard to the task, the negotiation included, for instance, how to reduce muscular tension in the lower back area when the patient was not in touch with this part of the back. With regard to emotions connected to the tasks, physiotherapists found it challenging to find an adjustable way to improve the rhythm of breathing in a situation of uncertainty. Concerning the nature of the therapeutic relationship, physiotherapists sometimes found it challenging to facilitate change when, for instance, the patients acted differently from expected with regard to passivity and activity. Negotiations emerged as processes that facilitated a change of use of the body at different levels; for instance, facilitating movements by using less muscular tension. The physiotherapists' sensitivity and capability to negotiate the different types of tasks created possibilities for change. So did the physiotherapists' and the patients' capacity to bear and come through demanding situations. Change and communication appeared as integrated. In summary, the physiotherapists' sensitivity and ability to negotiate tasks, emotions connected to tasks, and the nature of the relationships, seemed to facilitate change. The patients' and the physiotherapists' capacity to bear and come through demanding situations created new ways of interaction. Accordingly, demanding situations may generate a potential for the improvement of treatment outcomes. Understanding demanding episodes as open and dynamic, in contrast to defining the patient as demanding, was suggested as a useful perspective for treatment (Øien et al., 2011).

CONCLUSIONS

The studies demonstrated that knowledge about change and communication in patients with chronic muscle pain of the back and/or neck was built on detailed step-by-step processes of perceiving and creating meaning in a growing variety of movements and breathing. These processes emerged in close connection to how the patient and the physiotherapist negotiated details by varying their ways of communication. Based on the knowledge-producing processes, the patients explored new ways of moving and understanding. Concomitantly, learning to apply new knowledge in different contexts outside treatment took place.

REFERENCES

Gergen, K., Kaye, J., 2002. Beyond narrative in the negotiation of therapeutic meaning. In: McNamee, S., Gergen, K. (Eds.), Therapy as Social Construction. Sage Publications, London, pp. 166–185.

Merleau-Ponty, M., 2012. Phenomenology of perception. Routledge, London.

Øien, A.M., 2010. Change and Communication. Long-Term Norwegian PsychoMotor Physiotherapy Treatment for Patients with Chronic Muscle Pain. Doctoral Thesis, University of Bergen, Bergen.

Øien, A.M., Iversen, S., Stensland, P., 2007. Narratives of embodied experiences—Therapy processes in Norwegian psychomotor physiotherapy. Adv Physiother 9, 31–39.

Øien, A.M., Råheim, M., Iversen, S., Steihaug, S., 2009. Self-perception as embodied knowledge—changing processes for patients with chronic pain. Adv Physiother 11 (3), 121–129.

Øien, A.M., Steihaug, S., Iversen, S., Råheim, M., 2011. Communication as negotiation processes in long-term physiotherapy: a qualitative study. Scand. J. Caring Sci. 25 (1), 53–61.

Watzlawick, P., Bavelas, J.B., Jackson, D.D., 1967. Pragmatics of Human Communication. A Study of Interactional Patterns, Pathologies, and Paradoxes. WW Norton, New York.

5.1.4 Best Practice: Basic Body Awareness Therapy—Evidence and Experiences

AMANDA LUNDVIK GYLLENSTEN ■ GUNVOR GARD

SUMMARY

Best practice includes the best available research and the patient's experiences and wishes. Body awareness is an important aspect of rehabilitation in mental health for patients with prolonged pain and psychiatric problems. Basic Body Awareness Therapy (BBAT) is a methodology established in Scandinavia. Research studies (randomized and controlled) support the effectiveness of the method to improve health-related quality of life, self-rated depression and self-efficacy. Indications of less sick listing and reduced use of psychiatric healthcare have been found. Physiotherapists have studied movement function, movement quality and body awareness in some patient groups and certain characteristics have been found. Studies of the patients' experiences revealed feelings of being more connected to their body, stable, calmed, and more alive and vital.

KEY POINTS

Basic Body Awareness Therapy (BBAT) is a physiotherapy method used in health care. Research confirms that there is moderate evidence for the efficacy of BBAT working with patients with depression, anxiety and bodily symptoms.

Key takeaway points:

The patients express that they experience BBAT to:

■ Help them to become more aware of how they use the body.

■ Learn to listen to and trust the body.

■ Use the BBAT movements and the breathing to restore balance.

■ Increase their awareness.

■ Recognize and regulate their affects and emotions.

■ Improve social interactions.

LEARNING OBJECTIVES

■ Understand how best practice within the field of mental health physiotherapy is focused and its relation to body-awareness therapies.

■ Understand how Basic Body Awareness Therapy contributes to health and well-being for patients with prolonged pain and psychiatric diagnosis, such as depression, anxiety, posttraumatic stress disorders (PTSD) and schizophrenia.

BEST PRACTICE

Best practice is defined as the methodology that thorough research and experience has proven to reliably lead to the desired result in the best way, or a programme, activity or strategy that has the highest degree of proven effectiveness supported by objective and comprehensive research and evaluation (The National Registry of Evidence-Based Programs and Practices [NREPP], 2016). According to Haynes et al. (2002), evidence-based practice includes: research, preferably randomized controlled trials, and knowledge of the individual patient's special situation and context, as well as their experiences and wishes. It is therefore of importance to include the voice of the patient from qualitative research when trying to achieve best practice. Several research articles address the patient's perspective and experiences.

In many countries the experiences and assessments of the professional group of physiotherapists are also considered to be important to identify best practice for different patients within mental health physiotherapy and to evaluate the effects of treatment.

BACKGROUND TO BODY-AWARENESS THERAPIES

Body-awareness therapies as well as other physical activity methods and aerobic exercise are all methods used within mental health physiotherapy practice in Europe. This chapter will focus on body awareness in patients with mental health problems.

The concept of body awareness has been described as a key element, a mechanism of action for therapeutic approaches often categorized as mind-body approaches, such as yoga, tai chi, body-orientated psychotherapy, Basic Body Awareness Therapy (BBAT), mindfulness-based therapies/meditation, Feldenkrais, the Alexander method and breathing therapy (Mehling et al., 2011). Body awareness is also self-awareness, since the awareness and development of the self and one's identity is closely connected to the body. Theories of embodied cognition propose that higher order mental processes are essentially based on perceptual and motor processes. Semantic concepts have to be grounded in sensorimotor experiences in order to have meaning (Fernadino & Iacoboni, 2010).

Incidence of prolonged musculoskeletal pain (often called *chronic pain* or *prolonged pain*) is a frequent health problem in the west. In Sweden, the total amount of sick leave taken for this cause is around 25% and mostly affects women. It impacts negatively on both general health and quality of life for the individual patient (Afrell et al., 2007). Prolonged pain is costly, not only for the individual, but also for society as a whole. Costs of chronic pain include both direct costs related to treatment and provision of healthcare services, and indirect costs, such as those associated with loss of productivity, lost tax revenues and disability payments (Statistics Canada, 2001; Phillips & Schopflocher, 2008; Statistics Sweden, 2015).

Etiology of prolonged musculoskeletal pain without a clear somatic cause is considered to be multifactorial, where physical, psychological and social factors interplay. It can be viewed as a multidimensional problem (Afrell, et al., 2007; Kamper et al., 2015). Research has identified that patients with prolonged benign musculoskeletal pain also have changes in their self-experience and their experience of the world. In connection to chronic illness, the individual often experiences an identity crisis and a biographical rupture, where the known identity no longer seems to be reliable and trustworthy (Chamaz, 1995). The individual may perceive the self as chaotic and the body as no longer comprehensible (Afrell et al., 2007; Lundberg et al., 2007). In the rehabilitation of patients with chronic pain, acceptance of the pain, learning to live with it, strengthening the sense of identity, and body and self-awareness are essential aspects of physiotherapy. To help the patient to increase physical activity without more pain, fear of moving, or fear of more pain often requires the physiotherapist to work as a member of a multiprofessional/interprofessional team. Chronic pain and the biopsychosocial context is described more in depth in Chapter 5.1.1 in this book.

INCIDENCE OF MENTAL HEALTH PROBLEMS

Mental health problems, such as depression, anxiety, PTSD and chronic stress syndrome are becoming some of the leading causes of sick leave in Europe. These diagnoses are becoming more frequent, and in Sweden are now the most common cause of sick leave for women and the second most common cause for men (Social Insurance Agency, Sweden, 2015). In physiotherapy this group of patients have often been treated using a body awareness-orientated method or physical activity aiming at restoring vitality, mental health and self-efficacy, as well as relief of symptoms of pain, breathing problems and muscular tension (Mattsson et al., 1995; Gyllensten et al., 2009; Danielson et al., 2014). Deteriorating mental health alarmingly also seems to be very common in the younger healthy population; reports have shown that in particular, Swedish schoolgirls between 13 and 18 years of age have very high levels of stress-related symptoms, anxiety and depression in combination with different somatic problems, e.g., stomach ache (Hagquist 2010; Lager et al., 2012; National Board of Health and Welfare, 2013; Strömbäck et al., 2013).

BASIC BODY AWARENESS THERAPY

Evidence for Patients With Prolonged Pain

The evidence base for using BBAT for patients with prolonged pain is not so strong. Systematic high-quality research is still scarce. The frequent use of body-awareness therapies in Scandinavia is mainly based on professional expertise and small studies. The strengthening of body awareness has been found to be a way to relieve musculoskeletal pain, psychological distress and increase quality of life (Gard, 2005; Malmgren Ohlsson, et al., 2001; Mannerkorpi & Iversen, 2003). In patients with fibromyalgia, physical exercise interventions with moderate intensity reveal inconsistent results. In many research studies there seem to be difficulties with adherence to the

programme. A metaanalysis concluded that there is limited evidence that aerobic training or strength and flexibility training produces important benefits in people with fibromyalgia in global outcome measures, physical function, and possibly pain and tender points (Busch et al., 2008). Best practice for the group of patients with fibromyalgia should include low-intensity aerobic exercise, such as walking or pool exercises, and strength training at adequate load. High-intensity exercise should be undertaken with caution (Mannerkorpi & Iversen, 2003). Multidisciplinary studies show that BBAT can increase health-related quality of life and be cost effective in comparison to traditional physiotherapy, but more research is needed (Gard, 2005).

Evidence for Patients With Anxiety, Depression and Posttraumatic Stress Disorders

The use of body-awareness therapies for persons with anxiety, depression and posttraumatic or stress-related disorders is well established in physiotherapy clinical practice in most Scandinavian countries. One of the most common physiotherapy treatments is BBAT. The Swedish National Guidelines (2010) lists BBAT as an additional treatment for patients in the diagnostic group of depression and anxiety (National Guidelines for Depression and Anxiety Disorders, 2010).

The evidence base for using BBAT in mental health is moderate as an add-on to usual treatment. Research focusing on patients with anxiety, depression, personality disorders and bodily symptoms in a randomized, and controlled design study in outpatient care revealed that the BBAT group had significantly less use of social services and psychiatric healthcare 1 year after the start of a 3-month intervention with BBAT in comparison to a control group who received psychiatric treatment as usual, but no body-awareness therapy. The treatment group also showed significantly improved self-efficacy, both after treatment and at follow-up at 6 months (Gyllensten et al., 2003a, 2009).

A single-site, three-armed randomized controlled study for patients (18–65 years old) with major depression was carried out. The study had two intervention groups (aerobic exercise and BBAT) and one control group. Results revealed aerobic exercise to significantly improve depression severity. The study also indicated both aerobic exercise and BBAT to have a significant effect on self-rated depression in comparison to the control group (Danielsson et al., 2014). BBAT has also been assessed in a randomized pilot study for persons with eating disorders in addition to usual treatment. The researchers found significant improvements in the Eating Disorder Inventory in the subscales 'drive to thinness', 'body dissatisfaction' and 'ineffectiveness'. Also in the Body Attitude Test, Eating Attitude Test and the Short Form 36 significant improvements were found. The results should be viewed with caution, however, because the groups were very small (Catalan-Matamoros et al., 2011).

The evidence for BBAT as a treatment for patients with PTSD is still scarce. Presently there are several intervention studies going on, both randomized, controlled trials and submitted longitudinal studies indicating the effectiveness of BBAT on movement, experiences, PTSD symptoms and pain (Blaauweendraat, Levy-Berg & Gyllensten, 2017, submitted March 2016). BBAT has also been evaluated as a treatment for women who have been sexually abused. The researchers found that the effects of BBAT included symptom reduction, and improved self-image and self-love (Mattsson et al., 1998).

WHAT IS BBAT?

BBAT is a body and movement awareness method that has been developed in Scandinavia. BBAT aims at restoring body awareness and movement coordination, integrating physical, physiological, psychosociocultural and existential aspects (Skjaerven et al., 2008; Gyllensten et al., 2015). The aims of BBAT have previously been described as integrating the body into the total experience of the self (Roxendal, 1985; Mattsson, 1998; Gyllensten, 2001; Gyllensten et al., 2010; Skjaerven et al., 2010).

BBAT movements are inspired by everyday life situations, described in recent studies as the ability to use the body in a more stable, relaxed and coordinated way. The movement practice is carried out in different positions, such as lying, sitting, standing, walking and running. BBAT also includes practice with the voice and breathing, relational movements and massage. The movements are simple and the therapy focus is on the integration of both flexibility and stability in movements of daily life, to strengthen self-efficacy and

increase the quality of life (Skjaerven, 1999; Skjaerven et al., 2015; Gyllensten et al., 2015). The therapy is also a way to strengthen the relationship with oneself, one's own body and the ability to relate to other persons (Gyllensten et al., 2010).

The Effects of BBAT on the Autonomic Nervous System

A study focusing on the immediate effects on heart rate variability (HRV) was performed in a group of healthy youths. The youths underwent assessments of the autonomic nervous system, both sympathetic and parasympathetic activity, before and after a BBAT session. After a session of BBAT immediate significant effects on HRV activity were found. This suggests that immediately following a session of BBAT there is an improvement of the functioning of autonomic control of both the vagal and sympathetic systems (Mantovani et al., 2016)

CENTRAL CONCEPTS

Body Awareness

Mehling et al. (2011) focused on the conceptualization of body awareness in order to better understand mind-body therapies. Leading practitioners and teachers of several body-awareness approaches and their patients were invited to participate in focus groups. According to the researchers, the practice in all the different body-awareness therapies consisted of basic similarities in their approach. These included (1) the use or role of breathing, (2) training and repetition, (3) noticing body sensations, discerning and differentiating changes in the body, thoughts and/or emotions, and (4) body-mind integration as the therapeutic goal (Mehling et al., 2011).

Breathing was seen as central and connecting the body and the mind. Breathing was connected to different experiences and to the quality of movements. A central skill that patients learn through training and repetition of the movements was the ability to notice sensations, thoughts and feelings as they occur. What is noticed might or might not be verbalized. The point was that the process of noticing, as well as the learning of differentiated noticing, were viewed by the practitioners as a path to integration (Gyllensten et al., 2009; Skjaerven et al., 2010; Mehling et al., 2011).

Movement Quality

The concept of movement quality has been focused on in BBAT. Skjaerven et al. (2008, 2010) have focused on and developed the concept of movement quality after in-depth interviews and focus groups with expert physiotherapists in a couple of phenomenological studies. The results revealed four different themes of movement quality. The first theme has been described as the biomechanical aspect, relating to space. The movement aspects focused on in this theme were related to path and form, e.g., postural stability. The second theme was the physiological aspect, relating to time. The aspects focused on were breathing and centring, visible in the flow, elasticity and rhythm of the movements. In the third theme the psychosocio-cultural aspects relating to energy, awareness and intention of the movements were found. The intention could contain both aspects of emotion and/or socio-cultural phenomena. The fourth and last theme was the existential aspect of movement quality relating to the person, either as self-awareness and/or the present person and unity in movements.

Movement quality mirrors a sense of being whole and unified: Through the contact with the body— there is something in the integration between mind and body and the coordination between them. To promote movement quality has much to do with becoming conscious of a whole. To contact and sense the body as a whole is important: then you develop a sense of a unity.

(Skjaerven et al., 2008, p. 21)

How the movement quality can be promoted in a 'learning cycle' has also been studied and described by the research team (Skjaerven et al., 2010).

WHAT CAN THE PHYSIOTHERAPIST SEE WHEN THE PATIENTS MOVE?

Analysis of Movement

The physiotherapist studies how the patient moves and assesses the patient's ability to be stable/balanced, coordinated, relaxed and vital in movements. This, together with the patient's goals and wishes, is used to build the BBAT treatment. There are several ways of assessing movements, posture and body awareness described in Chapter 4.1.7. In this section, however, the focus is not on the specific tests, but on what has been documented concerning motor performance, movement coordination, balance, stability and ability to relate to the body and the physiotherapist in the movement assessments. Everybody is unique, but there are certain common characteristics on a group level that have been documented in different studies of movement assessments.

Movements in Patients With Prolonged Pain

A study of 89 patients with long-standing hip osteo-arthritis, consisting of 61 females and 28 males with an average age of 62.5 years (range 40–75 years) revealed that the patients used compensation strategies due to pain, stiffness and range of movement restrictions in daily life movements. This often led to the movements being done with too much effort and energy, and not integrating the breathing in the movements, which then became fatiguing and lacking in relaxation and ease. The stability and balance factors particularly correlated negatively with health-related quality of life measured using Short Form 36, the physical dimension (Sundén et al., 2016).

Steihaug et al. (2001) analysed the movements of women with long-standing pain. The researchers found that the women with fibromyalgia had problems moving freely, and instead carried their bodies very rigidly, especially their necks and backs. Their breathing was also found to be very controlled. The women experienced a lot of pain and also found it very difficult to move at all or to be physically active. Moving required much muscular effort. The researchers started a series of treatment with BBAT and discussions in a group setting. Training was directed at movements and experiences through the body rather than physical fitness and strength. This was very fruitful and the result revealed that the treatment led to less pain and less strenuous movements.

In summary, what does the physiotherapist see in patients with chronic pain?: In patients suffering from chronic pain there seems to be a problem of compensation and using too much energy and effort, tensing up and not integrating the breathing into movements. This can lead to movements being fatiguing, stiff and unbalanced. Physical activity is then not enjoyable and the patient often does not like to move. Research studies reveal the pattern of the group, and, of course, individual differences are found. More research is needed.

Movements in Patients With Mental Illness

A study of persons suffering from schizophrenia spectrum disorders or bipolar disorders showed that the participants' movement coordination and breathing reached the highest proportion of difficulties. A majority (77%) reached a level of obvious to severe difficulties in the ability to use the trunk, integrated into movements, turning coordination around the central axis and gait coordination especially showed the highest levels of deviation. In balance and stability, 40% of the participants showed obvious to severe difficulties and 27% showed obvious to severe difficulties in the ability to relate both to their own body and to the physiotherapist. About a quarter of the participants had severe difficulties in the ability to be mentally present and aware in the movement test (Hedlund et al., 2016).

A study of persons with different mental health problems, mostly depression, anxiety and personality disorders, enrolled in physiotherapy rehabilitation revealed problems with trunk coordination and breathing restriction, blocking flow and relaxation. There were also significantly more problems in the ability to relate to their own body and to the physiotherapist in a movement test compared with a group of patients with chronic pain and a group of healthy controls (Gyllensten et al., 1999).

In summary what does the physiotherapist see in patients in psychiatry?: In the group of patients with psychiatric problems the physiotherapist can observe significantly more difficulties in the ability to relate to their own body and the physiotherapist, compared to groups of patients with prolonged pain and to groups of healthy controls. There also seem to be great restrictions in trunk coordination and breathing, resulting in disturbances of everyday motor functions. Stiffness and difficulties in relaxing were also found in the majority of patients. The coordination problems seem to be more common than the difficulties in balance and stability, although this was a problem for about half of the group. The research studies revealed the pattern of some patient groups. Of course, individual differences within the groups were found. Research on other groups of patents is presently ongoing.

STUDIES OF PATIENT EXPERIENCES

Several studies address the patient's perspective and experiences of body-awareness therapies.

The Experience of Identity

The meaning of body awareness has also been studied in a grounded theory context by interviewing both patients with mental health problems and healthy adults. The meaning of body awareness could be expressed as becoming more in contact with the body in order to strengthen one's identity and to experience oneself through being aware of the body from within. This awareness of oneself was influenced by the relationships with important others, but also by the larger context one is living within, e.g., society. The participants explained that the experience of body awareness was connected to the experience of one's own balance, how their breathing was and their sense of stability. The experience of the body, balance and stability of the physical self, on the other hand was found to be connected to the concept of well-being and control. To understand one's emotions and needs through the awareness of the body is seen as a base for self-confidence, trust in oneself, and the ability to take care of oneself and one's needs, both physically and mentally (Fig. 1).

Living in relation to others was a seen as a need, including bodily contact with another person/other people. Improved body awareness seemed to lead to being more satisfied and at peace with oneself, and participating more actively in life. Problems with body awareness seemed to be connected to a feeling of not being alive, of missing something important in life. The authors' conclusion was that working with the body in any physiotherapy practice should include an awareness of the body as inseparable from the identity (Fig. 2; Gyllensten et al., 2010).

Patients' Experiences of BBAT With Regard to Prolonged Pain

Patients with prolonged pain often lose their sense of trust and feelings of being at home in their own bodies. Rosberg (2000) takes the starting position in the lived body. Together with the physiotherapist and working in a respectful alliance, the patients are guided to regain the understanding of themselves, the

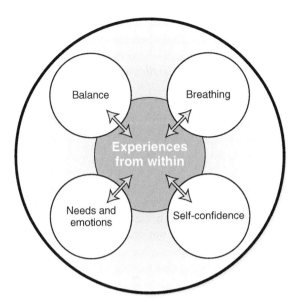

FIGURE 1 ■ Embodied Identity—Living in the Body. *(Revised from Gyllensten et al. (2010) Physiotherapy Theory and Practice 27, 439–446.)*

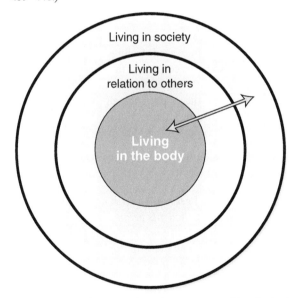

FIGURE 2 ■ Theories of Body Awareness—The Embodied Identity. *(Revised from Gyllensten et al. (2010) Physiotherapy Theory and Practice 27, 439–446.)*

connection between their symptoms and their personal history.

Gustavsson et al. (2004) described the experiences of patients with fibromyalgia and/or long-lasting widespread pain after a multiprofessional rehabilitation programme including body-awareness therapy. Analysing in-depth interviews, they identified four core categories from 'shame' to 'respect'. Three categories described a positive development and one expressed negative factors. 'Developing body awareness/knowledge', was found as a start, followed by 'Setting limits' that led to 'Changing self-image'. The fourth factor contained the negative counterbalancing factors of 'Hopelessness' and 'Frustration over one's employment situation'. The authors claim that, 'with BBAT the informants learned to be aware of how to best use their bodies, as a way to 'check' the body, to find positions and balance, to avoid unnecessary muscle tension and to prevent deterioration'. The BBAT exercises were found to be helpful in relaxing and controlling pain.

'It has been very useful to me, just to drive the car, it used to be a horror to me. Like how to stand and walk, thinking about it all the time, letting your shoulders down ...'

(Gustavsson et al., 2004, p. 99)

Patients' Experiences of BBAT in Psychiatry

The experiences of patients with different psychiatric diagnoses were studied. The following three core themes emerged after taking part in groups of BBAT for at least 6 months: increased awareness of one's own body and better knowledge of the self, threshold for taking part in time-consuming change, and relationships between oneself and others.

The process of strengthening the experience of the lived body pointed towards feelings of wholeness, and feeling more at home in themselves and in the group. The study indicated that BBAT groups contributed to better health, even though the design of the study limits the possibility to ascertain whether the changes were long-lasting (Johnsen & Råheim, 2010).

The experiences of patients suffering from major depression were studied in connection with a randomized controlled trial. The researchers concluded that the participants' experiences could be seen as a process of 'opening towards life'. The categories found were: 'vitality springing forth', 'grounding oneself', 'recognizing patterns in one's body', 'being acknowledged and allowed to be oneself', and 'grasping the vagueness', exemplified by this quotation:

> 'It was when we were trying out the standing movements, there was something, I think it was when we rocked a little from side to side and then I came to think about what I did instinctively when I felt really bad. I used to sit rocking my whole body like this [rocks back and forth in the chair with arms crossed]. But that was unconscious, I didn't think about it or analyse it until now, but it, that was really comforting, that's why I did it … and the rocking, I don't know… as a child I used to love being in the swing. So I think that when I move like that, it calms me down, I can do it now [rocks again], just a little movement makes a difference.'
>
> *(Danielsson & Rosberg, 2015, p. 8)*

The experiences of BBAT in traumatized refugees have been studied qualitatively in connection with a randomized, controlled trial (not yet published). The authors describe the evolving themes: 'symptoms', 'behavioural change', 'the role of the PT' and 'exercises'. The quote chosen is connected to 'exercises', the category 'making sounds'.

> 'It was an amazing exercise because when you inhaled you would send oxygen to certain muscle groups through the lungs and when you afterwards exhaled with sound it would bring peace to the whole body and the mind. And you would be calm.'
>
> *(Madsen et al., 2015, p. 6)*

Patients' experiences of participating in a BBAT group have been studied. In one such study involving two patient groups—one in general psychiatric out-patient care and one in-patient group consisting of patients with schizophrenia—three different themes were found: 'personal involvement and the ability to practise oneself', 'improvement of balance and posture', 'awareness and handling of body signals' and 'body movement control'. The following quotation exemplifies the theme improvements in balance and posture (Gyllensten et al., 2003b).

> 'I felt good. I was standing still and did not lose my balance or anything like that. No, completely still. I was standing still and my arms were in a good place and my legs in a good place, then I will keep my balance.'
>
> *(Gyllensten et al., 2003, p. 178)*

The experience of long-term treatment with BBAT for patients with schizophrenia has been further studied. The patients had received BBAT for 2–7 years, averaging 3.3 years. The results revealed positive treatment experiences of physiotherapy using BBAT. Four main categories were identified:

1. *Affect regulation.* This category contained the experience that the treatment resulted in a change of the emotional state towards more positive feelings.
2. *Body awareness and self-esteem.* In this category the participants reported improvements in their ability to be mentally present, be better in contact with their bodies, their movement behaviour, postural balance and experienced improved sensory awareness.
3. *Effects described in a social context.* In this category the participants reported better coping strategies, increased feelings of integrity and ability to be in contact with others.
4. *Effects on the ability to think.* This category contained the experience of increased ability to concentrate, calmer activity in the brain, or clearer thought and ability to be awake.

The following quotation exemplifies the theme 'Effects on the ability to think'.

> 'Instead, when I get more alert it affects how I feel in my head. My thoughts become maybe a little bit more alive, it feels like my level of thinking gets "more vital" or how shall I put it.'
>
> *(Hedlund & Gyllensten, 2010, p. 249)*

REFERENCES

Afrell, M., Biguet, G., Rudebeck, C.E., 2007. Living with a body in pain—between acceptance and denial. Scand. J. Caring Sci. 21 (3), 291–296.

Blaauwendraat, C., Berg, A., Gyllensten, A.L., in press 2017. One-year follow-up of Basic Body Awareness Therapy in patients with Post Traumatic Stress Disorder. A small intervention study of effects on movement quality, PTSD symptoms and movement experiences. Physiother. Theory Pract.

Busch, A., Schlater, C., Peoso, P., Bombadier, C., 2008. Exercise for fibromyalgia: a systematic review. J. Rheumatol. 35, 1130–1144.

Catalan-Matamoros, D., Skjaerven, L.H., Labajos-Manzanares, M.T., et al., 2011. A pilot study on the effect of basic body awareness therapy in patients with eating disorders: a randomized controlled trial. Clin. Rehabil. 25 (7), 617–626.

Chamaz, K., 1995. The body, identity and self: adapting to impairment. Sociol. Q. 36 (4), 857–880.

Danielsson, L., Papouilas, I., Petersson, E.L., et al., 2014. Exercise or basic body awareness therapy as add-on treatment for major depression: a controlled study. J. Affect. Disord. 168, 98–106.

Danielsson, L., Rosberg, S., 2015. Opening toward life: experiences of basic body awareness therapy in persons with major depression. Int. J. Qual. Stud. Health Well-being 10, 27069.

Fernadino, L., Iacoboni, M., 2010. Are cortical motor maps based on body parts or coordinated actions? Implications for embodied semantics. Brain Lang. 112, 44–53.

Gard, G., 2005. Body awareness therapy for patients with fibromyalgia and chronic pain. Disabil. Rehabil. 27 (12), 725–728.

Gustavsson, M., Ekholm, J., Öhman, A., 2004. From shame to respect: Musculoskeletal pain patients experience of a rehabilitation programme. A qualitative study. J. Rehabil. Med. 36, 97–103.

Gyllensten, A.L., Ekdahl, C., Hansson, L., 1999. Validity of the Body Awareness scale- Health (BAS-H). Scand. J. Caring Sci. 13, 217–226.

Gyllensten, A.L., 2001. Basic Body Awareness Therapy. (Dissertation). Department of Physical Therapy Lund University, Sweden.

Gyllensten, A.L., Ekdahl, C., Hansson, L., 2009. Long-term effectiveness of basic body awareness therapy in psychiatric out-patient care. A randomised controlled study. Adv Physiother 11, 2–12.

Gyllensten, A.L., Hansson, L., Ekdahl, C., 2003a. Outcome of basic body awareness therapy. A randomized controlled study in Psychiatric outpatient care. Adv Physiother 5, 179–190.

Gyllensten, A.L., Hansson, L., Ekdahl, C., 2003b. Patient experiences of basic body awareness therapy and the relationship with the physiotherapist. J. Bodyw. Mov. Ther. 7, 173–183.

Gyllensten, A.L., Skär, L., Miller, M., Gard, G., 2010. Embodied—A deeper understanding of body awareness. Physiother. Theory Pract. 27, 439–446.

Gyllensten, A.L., Skoglund, K., Wulf, I., 2015. Basal Kroppskännedom – Den levda kroppen. (Basic Body Awareness Therapy—The lived body). Studentlitteratur, Lund, Sweden.

Hagquist, C., 2010. Discrepant trends in mental health complaints among younger and older adolescents in Sweden: an analysis of WHO data 1985–2005. J. Adolesc. Health 46, 258–264.

Haynes, R.H., Devereau, P.J., Guyatt, G.H., 2002. Physicians' and patients choices in evidence based practice: evidence does not make decisions, people do. (editorial). Br. Med. J. 324, 1350–1351.

Hedlund, L., Gyllensten, A.L., 2010. The experiences of basic body awareness therapy in patients with schizophrenia. J. Bodyw. Mov. Ther. 14, 245–254.

Hedlund, L., Gyllensten, A.L., Waldegren, T., Hansson, L., 2016. Assessing movement quality in persons with severe mental illness—Reliability and validity of the Body Awareness Scale Movement Quality and Experience. Physiother. Theory Pract. 32, 296–306.

Johnsen, R.W., Råheim, M., 2010. Feeling more in balance and grounded in one's own body and life. Focus group interviews on experiences with basic body awareness therapy in psychiatric health care. Adv Physiother 12, 166–174.

Kamper, S.J., Apeldoorn, A.T., Chiarotto, A., et al., 2015. Multidisciplinary biopsychosocial rehabilitation for chronic low back pain: Cochrane systematic review and meta-analysis. Br. Med. J. 350, h444.

Lager, A., Berlin, M., Heimersson, I., Danielsson, M., 2012. Young people's health in Sweden: The National Public Health Report Chapter 3. Scand. J. Public Health 40 (Suppl. 9), 42–71.

Lundberg, M., Styf, J., Bullington, J., 2007. Experiences of moving with persistent pain—a qualitative study from the patients perspective. Physiother. Theory Pract. 23 (4), 199–209.

Madsen, T.S., Carlsson, J., Nordbrandt, M., Jensen, J.A., 2015. Refugee experiences of individual basic body awareness therapy and the level of transference into daily life. An interview study. J. Bodyw. Mov. Ther. 20, 243–251.

Malmgren Ohlsson, M., Armelius, K., Armelius, B.A., 2001. A comparative outcome study of body awareness therapy, feldenkrais, and conventional physiotherapy for patients with nonspecific musculoskeletal disorders: changes in psychological symptoms, pain, and self-image. Physiother. Theory Pract. 17, 77–95.

Mannerkorpi, K., Iversen, M.D., 2003. Physical exercise in fibromyalgia and related syndromes. Best Pract. Res. Clin. Rheumatol. 17 (4), 629–647.

Mantovani, A.M., Fregonesis, C.E., Lorençoni, R.M., et al., 2016. Immediate effect of basic body awareness therapy on heart rate variability. Complement. Ther. Clin. Pract. 22, 8–11.

Mattsson, M., Egberg, K., Armelius, K., Mattsson, B., 1995. Longterm effects of physiotherapeutic treatment in outpatient psychiatric care. Nord. J. Psychiatry 49 (2), 103–110.

Mattsson, M., 1998. Body Awareness – Applications in Physiotherapy. (Dissertation), Department of Psychiatry and Family Medicine, Umeå, University, Sweden.

Mattsson, M., Wikman, M., Dahlgren, L., et al., 1998. Body awareness therapy with sexually abused women. Part 2: Evaluation of body awareness in a group setting. J. Bodyw. Mov. Ther. 2, 38–45.

Mehling, W., Wrubel, J., Daubenmier, J., et al., 2011. Body Awareness: a phenomenological inquiry into the common ground of mind-body therapies. Philos. Ethics Humanit. Med. 6, 6.

National Board of Health and Welfare, 2010. National Guidelines for Depression and Anxiety- Support for Control and Management (in Swedish). Västerås, Artikelnr, pp. 3–4. ISBN: 978-91-86301-94-1.

National Board of Health and Welfare, 2013. Mental health in the young population. <https://www.socialstyrelsen.se/Lists/Artikelka talog/.../2013-5-43.pdf>

National Registry of Evidence-Based Programs and Practices (NREPP). <http://nrepp.samhsa.gov>.

Phillips, C.J., Schopflocher, D., 2008. The Economics of Chronic Pain. In: Rashiq, S., Taenzer, P., Schopflocher, D. (Eds.), Health Policy Perspectives on Chronic Pain. Wiley Press, Weinheim.

Rosberg, S., 2000. Body, being and meaning in a physiotherapeutic perspective. (Dissertation). University of Gothenborg, Sweden.

Roxendal, G., 1985. Body awareness therapy and the body awareness scale, treatment and evaluation in psychiatric physiotherapy.

(Dissertation). Department of Psychiatry, University of Gothenburg, Gothenburg, Sweden.

Skjaerven, L.H., 1999. Bevegeleskvalitet—Å vaere seg self-mer fullt og helt. En fältstudie av en bevegelsepraksis ved bevegelsepedagog og psykoterapeut Jacques Drposy, Paris. Master thesis. University of Bergen, Bergen, Norway (in Norweigan).

Skjaerven, L.H., Kristoffersen, K., Gard, G., 2008. An eye for movement quality: A phenomenological study of movement quality reflecting a group of physiotherapists' understanding of the phenomenon. Physiother. Theory Pract. 24, 13–27.

Skjaerven, L.H., Kristoffersen, K., Gard, G., 2010. How can movement quality be promoted in clinical practice? A phenomenological study of physical therapist experts. Phys. Ther. 90, 1479–1492.

Social Insurance Agency Sweden, 2015. <http://www.forsakringskassan.se/press/pressmeddelanden/sjukpenningtalet_i_juni_2015.>

Statistics Canada—A profile of disability in Canada. Statistics Canada, 89-577-XIE, 1-24. 2001 retrieved 16/06/04. http://www.statcan.gc.ca/pub/89-577-x/pdf/4228016-eng.pdf.

Statistics Sweden, 2015. <https://www.forsakringskassan.se/!ut/p/a0/LccxEkAwEAXQsyhSJxiNzi1IY3ZkhxBfJtlwfQrVm6etHrUF3X4l8RcofJ-e5ewjyabqdlBmuSAMyaxMTJzzz8nOcSA4hjJ5L0dkwGMVCizzTiiU_NyYutPxGKoXofta8Q!!/.>

Steihaug, S., Ahlsen, B., Malterud, K., 2001. From exercise and education to movement and interaction. Treatment groups in primary care for women with chronic muscular pain. Scand. J. Prim. Health Care 19, 249–254.

Strömbäck, M., Malmgren-Olsson, E.B., Wiklund, M., 2013. 'Girls need to strengthen each other as a group': experiences from a gender-sensitive stress management intervention by youth-friendly Swedish health services – a qualitative study. BMC Public Health 13, 907.

Sundén, A., Ekdahl, C., Horstman, V., Gyllensten, A.L., 2016. Analyzing movements development and evaluation of the body awareness scale movement quality (BAS MQ). Physiother. Res. Int. 21, 70–76.

5.1.5 Physiotherapy for Patients With Nonspecific Chronic Low Back Pain and Comorbid Mental Illnesses

EMANUEL BRUNNER ■ WIM DANKAERTS

SUMMARY

Mental illnesses are highly prevalent in people suffering from nonspecific chronic low back pain (NSCLBP). Complex patients with NSCLBP and comorbid somatization, depression and anxiety disorders are often seen by physiotherapists in outpatient practices. In this clinical setting the support of clinical psychologists and psychiatrists is often limited. Physiotherapists are therefore challenged to integrate psychological principles and strategies into their clinical management. This chapter provides a brief overview of biopsychosocial assessment and treatment strategies relevant for a patient-centred intervention for patients with NSCLBP and comorbid mental illnesses.

KEY POINTS

■ The prevalence of comorbid somatization disorders, anxiety and depressive disorders is high in people suffering from nonspecific chronic low back pain (NSCLBP).

■ Maladaptive cognitions, negative emotions and dysfunctional pain behaviours are important barriers for the recovery of NSCLBP.

■ Cognitive behavioural therapy (CBT)–based strategies are promising for modifying maladaptive cognitions that influence patients' emotions, behaviours and bodily experiences.

■ Physical exercise has a large antidepressant effect in patients with mental illnesses.

LEARNING OBJECTIVES

■ Review the dominant factors associated with the development and maintenance of chronic pain and disability due to NSCLBP and understand potential interactions between the contributing factors.

■ Describe and explain the importance for patients with chronic pain to remain physically active.

■ Discuss criteria to consider when integrating aerobic exercises for patients with complex NSCLBP into clinical practice.

BACKGROUND

Psychosocial factors and psychopathologies play an important role in nonspecific chronic low back pain

(NSCLBP). NSCLBP is defined as pain and discomfort in the lower back not attributed to recognizable specific pathology and lasting for longer than 12 weeks (van Tulder et al., 2006). Patients' cognitions (such as negative lower back pain [LBP] beliefs, catastrophizing and fear of movement), emotions (such as anxiety and depressed mood) and behaviour (such as fear-avoidance behaviour) play a crucial role in the development and maintenance of chronicity (Vlaeyen & Linton, 2000), and the prevalence of comorbid mental illnesses is high (Gerhardt et al., 2011; Reme et al., 2011). Patients with NSCLBP and comorbid mental illnesses are often described as complex pain patients. Physiotherapists see these patients within multidisciplinary rehabilitation settings, but also, or even more often, in outpatient practices where the support of other healthcare providers (e.g., clinical psychologist, psychiatrist) is sparse or even absent. Therefore physiotherapists involved in the management of NSCLBP are challenged to effectively deal with psychosocial factors and mental illnesses.

The vicious circle of chronicity due to musculoskeletal pain is explained by the fear-avoidance model (Vlaeyen & Linton, 2000), which describes that people who catastrophically (mis)interpret their pain experience (catastrophizing) may avoid pain-related movements, become hypervigilant to bodily sensations, and consequently are at risk of developing disability and depressive mood. Longitudinal studies have confirmed these psychosocial risk factors, based on the fear-avoidance cycle, as strong predictors of chronic pain and disability (Burton et al., 2004; Henschke et al., 2008; Campbell et al., 2013).

In addition to these psychosocial risk factors, the prevalence of psychiatric comorbidity is high in patients with NSCLBP (Gerhardt et al., 2011; Reme et al., 2011). In the USA, it was shown that 38% of patients who were sick-listed with NSCLBP had at least one clinically relevant mental illness diagnosed by applying the Mini-International Neuropsychiatric Interview (Sheehan et al., 1998), with somatoform pain disorders as the most prevalent diagnosis, followed by anxiety and major depressive disorders (Reme et al., 2011). Similar results were found in Germany, but with depression as the most prevalent diagnosis (Gerhardt et al., 2011). These epidemiological findings indicate the significance of psychiatric

comorbidity in NSCLBP. From a CBT perspective, it can be assumed that the development of pain-related disability and psychological disturbances are based on similar processes. The cognitive model proposes that dysfunctional thinking, which influences the mood and behaviour of patients, is common to all psychological disturbances (Beck, 1995). Therefore people with mental illnesses may also have a tendency to catastrophically (mis)interpret their pain experience. Although psychosocial factors and mental illnesses are highly relevant in complex NSCLBP, the clinical picture is complemented by additional physical and behavioural factors.

Alterations of the nervous system are frequently present in NSCLBP (Giesecke et al., 2004). Central sensitization is defined as an augmentation of responsiveness of central neurons in response to input from receptors (Meyer et al., 1995), resulting in an increased responsiveness to peripheral stimuli and decreased load tolerance to senses from the neuromusculoskeletal system. It is likely that the abnormal central pain processing facilitates the hypervigilance to bodily sensations in those patients who are trapped in the fear-avoidance cycle. Generally, complex pain patients often complain about symptoms that cannot be accounted for medically and are potentially related to central sensitization.

Additionally, NSCLBP is often associated with maladaptive functional behaviour. These patients perform a task in a manner that results in provocation of pain and disability (O'Sullivan et al., 2005). Experimental studies showed that patients with NSCLBP have both increased and decreased levels of abdominal wall and lumbar muscle coactivation (Dankaerts et al., 2006). Excessive (protective) muscle activation during movements may result in increased and abnormal loading forces across pain-sensitive structures (Dankaerts & O'Sullivan, 2011). Maladaptive movement behaviours resulting in self-provocation might be related to altered sensorimotor integration, decreased body awareness and maladaptive cognitions. In this context it is stated that this behaviour is reinforced by beliefs regarding core stability and training methods that tend to address the (excessive) training of trunk-stabilizing muscles (Dankaerts & O'Sullivan, 2011). Furthermore, it is often seen that psychological disturbances and maladaptive functional behaviours result in decreased levels of physical activity and physical fitness. A meta-analysis showed that patients with chronic disability are likely to have low physical activity levels (Lin et al., 2011). It can be hypothesized that physical activity and physical fitness might be even lower in patients with comorbid mental illnesses than in the general sample of NSCLBP patients. Longitudinal studies disclosed a bidirectional association between physical activity and depression. Individuals with low levels of physical activity are at a significantly higher risk of developing depression than those with high levels of activity, and depression is a significant risk factor for developing a sedentary lifestyle (Camacho et al., 1991; Roshanaei-Moghaddam et al., 2009). Additionally, sedentary lifestyle and low physical fitness are often associated with other negative lifestyle factors, such as being overweight, having an unhealthy diet, or smoking and sleep disturbances. Being physically active is important for patients with NSCLBP. Some patients with NSCLBP, however, might be overactive, meaning that their physical fitness is insufficient for their physical activity levels. Their constant physical overuse may result in fatigue as well as enhanced sensitization of the central nervous system. In summary, patients with NSCLBP and comorbid mental illness present with a complex multidimensional symptomology. Physiotherapists are challenged to understand patients' individual pain problems and furthermore, to target interventions aimed at the factors driving the patients' ongoing pain problem.

ASSESSMENT

The clinical assessment of patients with NSCLBP is highly challenging. Most patients have long histories of LBP and unsuccessful treatments. This often results in resistance towards new therapeutic interventions. Consequently, establishing a positive therapeutic relationship from the start might be quite difficult but is deemed essential. Indeed, the strength of the therapeutic alliance predicts positive treatment outcomes in NSCLBP (Hall et al., 2010; Ferreira et al., 2013). This therapeutic alliance is defined as the strength of the collaborative relationship between therapists and patients, including the agreement on goal setting and tasks, and the emotional bond (Bordin, 1979). Techniques of motivational interviewing (Miller &

Rollnick, 2012) can allow the development of this required strong therapeutic alliance. Generally, physiotherapists are challenged to develop effective communication skills in order to actively listen to the patients' stories in order to explore the multidimensional nature of the symptomology (O'Sullivan, 2012).

NSCLBP is a complex disorder associated with a complex interaction of factors. In order to address the multidimensional nature of the problem, the assessment should be based on a multidimensional clinical reasoning framework that incorporates the contemporary biopsychosocial understanding of NSCLBP (O'Sullivan, 2012), to identify modifiable and non-modifiable factors associated with a patient's individual pain problem (O'Sullivan et al., 2015a). The aim of the clinical assessment is to develop multidimensional, patient-centred interventions.

Screening for Psychosocial Factors and Mental Illnesses

Standardized screening tools should guide the physiotherapist during the patient's interview for the exploration of psychosocial factors and symptoms related to mental illnesses. Additionally, the scores from patient questionnaires can support the clinical reasoning processes. The STarT Back Tool (Hill et al., 2008) and the Orebro Musculoskeletal Pain Screening Questionnaire (Linton & Halldén, 1998) are both questionnaires developed for psychosocial screening, mainly for identifying factors associated with the fear-avoidance cycle. Alternatively, more extensive instruments can be used to identify maladaptive cognitions, such as the Fear-Avoidance Beliefs Questionnaire (Waddell et al., 1993) or the Pain Catastrophizing Scale (Sullivan et al., 1995). While these screening tools provide valuable impressions regarding psychosocial risk factors, they are often insufficient for exploring the whole psychological symptomology in patients with comorbid mental illnesses. Therefore it is recommended to use more extensive instruments for the assessment of psychological distress and symptoms of psychopathologies, such as the Four-Dimensional Symptom Questionnaire (4DSQ) (Terluin et al., 2006). The 4DSQ is a valid and reliable instrument for measuring somatization, distress, anxiety and depression in general practice patients (Terluin et al., 2006). These four subscales do sufficiently capture the psychological symptomology in complex NSCLBP.

Maladaptive Posture and Movement and Pain Behaviour

The observation of patients' functional postures and movement behaviours should include the evaluation of adaptive (protective) and maladaptive (provocative) movement behaviours (O'Sullivan et al., 2005). It has been demonstrated that patients with NSCLBP often posture and move themselves with increased levels of cocontraction of the trunk muscles during pain-provocative tasks (e.g., sitting, bending forward, standing up from sitting, walking), and they present with an inability to relax their abdominal and lumbar muscles (Dankaerts & O'Sullivan, 2011). When maladaptive posture and movement behaviours are present, it is further relevant to assess patients' body schema and body awareness.

Central Sensitization

Recognizing symptoms related to alterations of the nervous systems is highly relevant in the management of NSCLBP. Information regarding the following aspects is used for the assessment: medical diagnosis, medical history, clinical examination and the analysis of treatment responses to past interventions (Nijs et al., 2010). Hypersensitivity to touch during manual palpation should alert the physiotherapist and indicates more detailed assessments of central sensitization. The detailed procedure for assessing central sensitization is described elsewhere (Yunus, 2007).

Physical Activity and Physical Fitness

Accurate quantification of physical activity and physical fitness is essential in terms of designing a patient's specific treatment programme and in measuring treatment outcomes (Vanhees et al., 2005). In complex NSCLBP, activity diaries are useful for capturing a patient's physical activity level. While this subjective method of measurement might be of limited validity and reliability (Shephard, 2003), the instrument can build an important basis for later physical activity counselling. More objective measures of physical activity (e.g., pedometers and accelerometers) may provide more valid measurements (Vanhees et al., 2005), but are less convenient in day-to-day clinical practice. The assessment of physical fitness should, at the minimum, include a test of cardiorespiratory fitness, for example, by use of treadmill or bicycle tests. More valid and reliable assessments of physical fitness, such as the Eurofit for adults (Oja & Tuxworth, 1995), tend to be too demanding for patients with high levels of disability. Generally, the assessment of physical activity is delicate in complex NSCLBP, because of patients' strong negative affectivity towards tests targeted at their pain-related impairments, resulting in potentially low adherence to strict test protocols.

INTERVENTION

Physiotherapy should target modifiable factors related to the ongoing pain disorder, including psychosocial factors and symptoms of comorbid mental illness. However, treating complex NSCLBP solely with psychology-based approaches will often be insufficient, since these psychological factors are likely interrelated with other factors (e.g., physical factors, neurophysiological factors) as part of the multidimensional nature of NSCLBP.

Patient Education

Pain physiology education has a positive influence on maladaptive pain cognition in NSCLBP (Moseley et al., 2004), as well as in patients with chronic widespread pain (Meeus et al., 2010a). Extensive pain physiology education is indicated when the clinical picture is characterized and dominated by central sensitization and maladaptive pain cognitions are present (Nijs et al., 2011). The goal is to reconceptualize a patient's understanding of pain and knowledge about the influence of hypersensitivity of the central nervous system. Useful clinical recommendations about pain physiology education in musculoskeletal pain have recently been published (Nijs et al., 2011; Butler & Moseley, 2013) and can build the basis for this education on pain physiology. Additionally, useful material for patient education can be found on research-based webpages (e.g., *http://www.pain-ed.com* or *www.paininmotion.be*). In complex pain patients, psychoeducation regarding the influence of psychological distress and mental illness on the experience of pain needs to be integrated. Generally, education may help patients to self-reflect about the association between the different interrelated factors and their body, particularly their experience of pain.

Cognitive Behavioural Therapy–Based Treatment Strategies

CBT is promising in NSCLBP with comorbid mental illnesses, since CBT aims to alter maladaptive cognitions, emotions and dysfunctional behaviours. Clinical treatment guidelines recommend the use of CBT in NSCLBP (Koes et al., 2010). However, it is often unclear what CBT-based approaches consist of and how the treatment can be applied. McCracken & Morley (2014) classified CBT approaches into the following four models: operant behavioural, traditional cognitive behavioural, fear avoidance and psychological flexibility. This classification provides a useful overview about current concepts and theories, and allows a discussion regarding the applicability of CBT-based approaches in physiotherapy practice.

Graded activity is an individual, gradually increasing exercise programme that is based on the principles of the operant behavioural model (behaviour controlled by external situations). Although previous studies found insufficient evidence for graded activity in patients with NSCLBP (van der Giessen et al., 2012), the strategy appears to be clinical valuable for complex NSCLBP in physiotherapy. During graded activity, exercise quotas are used for increasing general activity levels, which are gradually built up towards a realistic predefined goal. Compared with other, more cognitive-orientated approaches, graded activity might be more suitable in patients without interests in psychological issues and limited language skill, as its primary focus is on a patient's functional ability.

A similar gradually increasing exercise programme is exposure in vivo, which aims to restore patients' functioning and decrease limitations. This approach aims to systematically reduce pain-related fears (fear-avoidance cycle). In comparison to graded activity, exposure in vivo is superior in diminishing pain-related fears and pain catastrophizing, but no different in improving functional disability and pain (Leeuw et al., 2008). Detailed descriptions of this exposure in vivo treatment strategy can be found elsewhere (Vlaeyen et al., 2002). In short, first fear hierarchies are established, and subsequently patients are exposed to fear-eliciting activities by use of behavioural experiments.

The application of this approach seems more challenging for physiotherapists than graded activity, and may require advanced skills of cognitive restructuring.

Traditional CBT interventions are grounded on the 'cognitive model of depression' described by Aaron Beck (Beck et al., 1979) and might be most promising in the treatment of patients with complex NSCLBP. In CBT there is always a CBT formulation that aims to develop working models of patients' individual psychological disturbances (Beck, 1995). Thereby, therapists help patients using Socratic questioning (Padesky, 1993) and strategies of motivational interviewing (Miller & Rollnick, 2012) to identify associations between their thoughts, emotions, behaviours and bodily sensations. Subsequently, as part of the CBT intervention, patients are guided to carry out behavioural experiments (e.g., exposure to fear-related situations) for testing their thoughts and beliefs related to dysfunctional behaviours, and to develop more functional behaviours. In complex NSCLBP, traditional CBT approaches have the potential to target the whole psychological symptomology of patients, and not solely the fear-avoidance cycle. However, such interventions may require a patient's ability to make sense of the use of psychological approaches, and may only be indicated when they show some interest in psychological issues.

Interventions based on the Psychology Flexibility Model with its therapies such as Acceptance and Commitment Therapy (ACT) represent the latest wave within CBT. Describing these complex new methods and discussing it is applicability in physiotherapy is beyond the scope of this chapter (see Chapter 2.5).

Traditionally, clinical psychologists and psychiatrists apply CBT-based interventions. Since associated psychological factors in NSCLBP are of importance, it was recommended that other healthcare practitioners should also be trained to deliver CBT-based treatments for pain patients (van der Windt et al., 2008). In summary, trained physiotherapists should be able to integrate CBT-based principles and strategies into their clinical practice for NSCLBP, particularly the approaches based on the operant behavioural model (Brunner et al., 2013). To apply these psychology-based strategies, it is essential that physiotherapists have knowledge of basic principles of the cognitive model, as well as effective skills in therapeutic communication and behaviour-change techniques. This might require specific extra training (Foster & Delitto, 2011).

Posture and Movement Exercises, Relaxation Techniques and Physical Exercises

Specific posture and movement exercises designed to normalize maladaptive posture and movement behaviours are indicated if this domain is a dominant factor maintaining chronic pain and disability. A promising intervention approach combining specific exercises with cognitive components has been developed by O'Sullivan (Vibe Fersum et al., 2013) and is named *cognitive functional therapy* (CFT). This approach demonstrated positive long-term effects in NSCLBP patients with mechanical behaviour to the pain (provoked and relieved with postures, movements and activities), as well as promising long-term results in patients with disabling NSCLBP (Vibe Fersum et al., 2013; O'Sullivan et al., 2015b). Combining this more functionally orientated CFT approach with specific CBT-based strategies seems highly promising in NSCLBP with comorbid mental illnesses, but it needs further investigation.

Relaxation techniques might be indicated in patients with high levels of psychological distress and dominant anxiety disorders. Owing to frequently reported difficulties in concentration during more cognitive-orientated approaches (e.g., visualization, autogenic training), bodily-orientated techniques (breathing exercises and progressive muscle relaxation) tend to be most appropriate in these patients for reducing stress levels. Patients should also be instructed to perform these exercises independently at home.

Physical activity counselling aiming to facilitate behaviour changes should always be integrated in physiotherapy interventions for patients with complex NSCLBP. Establishing adequate physical activity levels is highly relevant because of the aforementioned bidirectional association between physical activity and depression. Furthermore, recent metaanalyses on the effect of physical exercise in patients with anxiety, posttraumatic stress and depression disorders disclosed positive effects of aerobic exercises on depressive symptoms (de Souza Moura et al., 2015; Rosenbaum et al., 2015; Schuch et al., 2016). In patients with major depressive disorders, the largest effect sizes were found for supervised aerobic exercises of moderate intensity (Schuch et al., 2016). Therefore physiotherapists should support patients to reach adequate levels of physical activity and to exercise regularly with at least a moderate intensity. Delivering physical exercises for patients with NSCLBP and comorbid mental illnesses might be challenging. Firstly, those patients with central sensitization are likely to react with an exacerbation of pain-related symptoms during physical exercise (Meeus et al., 2010b). In these situations, it is important to prevent muscular ischaemia and to plan sufficient recovery breaks between exercise sessions. Secondly, patients with comorbid mental illness are likely to experience psychological barriers to being physically active. People with mental illnesses report high levels of social anxiety during physical activity situations (De Herdt et al., 2013). Social anxiety should be considered as an important barrier for physical activity participation in complex NSCLBP. Principles and techniques of motivational interviewing (Miller & Rollnick, 2012) might be useful to help patients overcome resistances to becoming physically active by enhancing patients' intrinsic motivation to change.

Measurement of Treatment Outcomes

Treatment effects should preferably be measured in the following five domains: (1) back-specific function, (2) generic health status, (3) pain, (4) work disability and (5) satisfaction with care and treatment outcome (Bombardier, 2000). In day-to-day clinical practice, pain and back-specific function might be the most relevant outcome domains for patients in complex NSCLBP. Additionally, psychological screening tools should be used to detect alterations in cognitions and symptoms of mental illness over time.

CONCLUSION

Psychosocial factors play a significant role in patients with NSCLBP, and the prevalence of comorbid mental illness is high. Generally, the clinical picture of these complex patients is multidimensional. Specific interventions are required and need to be targeted at those factors driving the ongoing pain and disability disorder. Therefore the choice of intervention strategy depends on individual patient needs.

REFERENCES

Beck, J., 1995. Cognitive therapy: basics and beyond. Guilford, New York.

Beck, A., Rush, J., Shaw, B., Emery, G., 1979. Cognitive therapy of depression. Guilford Press, New York.

Bombardier, C., 2000. Outcome assessments in the evaluation of treatment of spinal disorders: summary and general recommendations. Spine 25 (24), 3100–3103.

Bordin, E., 1979. The generalizability of the psychoanalytic concept of the working alliance. Psychother. Theor. Res. Pract. 16 (3), 252–260.

Brunner, E., De Herdt, A., Minguet, P., et al., 2013. Can cognitive behavioural therapy based strategies be integrated into physiotherapy for the prevention of chronic low back pain? A systematic review. Disabil. Rehabil. 35 (1), 1–10.

Burton, A.K., McClune, T.D., Clarke, R.D., Main, C.J., 2004. Long-term follow-up of patients with low back pain attending for manipulative care: outcomes and predictors. Man. Ther. 9 (1), 30–35.

Butler, D., Moseley, L., 2013. Explain Pain, second ed. Noigroup Publications, Adelaide.

Camacho, T.C., Roberts, R.E., Lazarus, N.B., et al., 1991. Physical activity and depression: evidence from the Alameda County Study. Am. J. Epidemiol. 134 (2), 220–231.

Campbell, P., Foster, N.E., Thomas, E., Dunn, K.M., 2013. Prognostic indicators of low back pain in primary care: five-year prospective study. J. Pain 14 (8), 873–883.

Dankaerts, W., O'Sullivan, P., 2011. The validity of O'Sullivan's classification system (CS) for a sub-group of NS-CLBP with motor control impairment (MCI): overview of a series of studies and review of the literature. Man. Ther. 16 (1), 9–14.

Dankaerts, W., O'Sullivan, P., Burnett, A., Straker, L., 2006. Altered patterns of superficial trunk muscle activation during sitting in nonspecific chronic low back pain patients: importance of subclassification. Spine 31 (17), 2017–2023.

De Herdt, A., Knapen, J., Vancampfort, D., et al., 2013. Social anxiety in physical activity participation in patients with mental illness: a cross-sectional multicentred study. Depress. Anxiety 30 (8), 757–762.

de Souza Moura, A.M., Lamego, M.K., Paes, F., et al., 2015. Effects of aerobic exercise on anxiety disorders: A systematic review. CNS Neurol. Disord. Drug Targets 14 (9), 1184–1193.

Ferreira, P., Ferreira, M., Maher, C., et al., 2013. The therapeutic alliance between clinicians and patients predicts outcome in chronic low back pain. Phys. Ther. 93 (4), 470–478.

Foster, N.E., Delitto, A., 2011. Embedding psychosocial perspectives within clinical management of low back pain: integration of psychosocially informed management principles into physical therapist practice–challenges and opportunities. Phys. Ther. 91 (5), 790–803.

Gerhardt, A., Hartmann, M., Schuller-Roma, B., et al., 2011. The prevalence and type of Axis-I and Axis-II mental disorders in subjects with non-specific chronic back pain: results from a population-based study. Pain Med. 12 (8), 1231–1240.

Giesecke, T., Gracely, R.H., Grant, M.A., et al., 2004. Evidence of augmented central pain processing in idiopathic chronic low back pain. Arthritis Rheum. 50 (2), 613–623.

Hall, A., Ferreira, P., Maher, C., et al., 2010. The influence of the therapist-patient relationship on treatment outcome in physical rehabilitation: a systematic review. Phys. Ther. 90 (8), 1099–1110.

Henschke, N., Maher, C.G., Refshauge, K.M., et al., 2008. Prognosis in patients with recent onset low back pain in Australian primary care: inception cohort study. BMJ 7 (337), a171.

Hill, J., Dunn, K., Lewis, M., et al., 2008. A primary care back pain screening tool: identifying patient subgroups for initial treatment. Arthritis Rheum. 59 (5), 632–641.

Koes, B., van Tulder, M., Lin, C., et al., 2010. An updated overview of clinical guidelines for the management of non-specific low back pain in primary care. Eur. Spine J. 19 (12), 2075–2094.

Leeuw, M., Goossens, M.E., van Breukelen, G.J., et al., 2008. Exposure in vivo versus operant graded activity in chronic low back pain patients: results of a randomized controlled trial. Pain 138 (1), 192–207.

Lin, C., McAuley, J., Macedo, L., et al., 2011. Relationship between physical activity and disability in low back pain: a systematic review and meta-analysis. Pain 152 (3), 607–613.

Linton, S., Halldén, K., 1998. Can we screen for problematic back pain? A screening questionnaire for predicting outcome in acute and subacute back pain. Clin. J. Pain 14 (3), 209–215.

McCracken, L., Morley, S., 2014. The psychological flexibility model: a basis for integration and progress in psychological approaches to chronic pain management. J. Pain 15 (3), 221–234.

Meeus, M., Nijs, J., van Oosterwijck, J., et al., 2010a. Pain physiology education improves pain beliefs in patients with chronic fatigue syndrome compared with pacing and self-management education: a double-blind randomized controlled trial. Arch. Phys. Med. Rehabil. 91 (8), 1153–1159.

Meeus, M., Roussel, N.A., Truijen, S., Nijs, J., 2010b. Reduced pressure pain thresholds in response to exercise in chronic fatigue syndrome but not in chronic low back pain: an experimental study. J. Rehabil. Med. 42 (9), 884–890.

Meyer, R., Campbell, J., Raja, S., 1995. Peripheral neural mechanisms of nociception. In: Wall, P.D., Melzack, R. (Eds.), Textbook of Pain, third ed. Churchill Livingstone, Edinburgh, pp. 13–44.

Miller, W., Rollnick, S., 2012. Motivational Interviewing: Helping People Change, third ed. The Guilford Press, New York.

Moseley, G., Nicholas, M., Hodges, P., 2004. A randomized controlled trial of intensive neurophysiology education in chronic low back pain. Clin. J. Pain 20 (5), 324–330.

Nijs, J., Van Houdenhove, B., Oostendorp, R., 2010. Recognition of central sensitization in patients with musculoskeletal pain: Application of pain neurophysiology in manual therapy practice. Man. Ther. 15 (2), 135–141.

Nijs, J., van Wilgen, P.C., van Oosterwijck, J., et al., 2011. How to explain central sensitization to patients with 'unexplained' chronic musculoskeletal pain: practice guidelines. Man. Ther. 16 (5), 413–418.

Oja, P., Tuxworth, B., 1995. Eurofit for adults. Assessment of health-related fitness. Council of Europe-UKK Institute, Tampere, Strasbourg.

O'Sullivan, P., 2012. It's time for change with the management of non-specific chronic low back pain. Br. J. Sports Med. 46 (4), 224–227.

O'Sullivan, P., Dankaerts, W., O'Sullivan, K., Fersum, K., 2015a. Multidimensional approach for the targeted management of low back pain. In: Grieve's Modern Musculoskeletal Physiotherapy, fourth ed. Elsevier, Edinburgh.

O'Sullivan, K., Dankaerts, W., O'Sullivan, L., O'Sullivan, P., 2015b. Cognitive functional therapy for disabling nonspecific chronic low back pain: multiple case-cohort study. Phys. Ther. 95 (11), 1478–1488.

O'Sullivan, P., Mitchell, T., Bulich, P., et al., 2005. The relationship between posture and back muscle endurance in industrial workers with flexion-related low back pain. Man. Ther. 11 (4), 264–271.

Padesky, C., 1993. Socratic questioning: Changing mind or guiding discovery? Invited keynote address presented at the 1993 European Congress of Behaviour and Cognitive Therapies, London.

Reme, S.E., Tangen, T., Moe, T., Eriksen, H.R., 2011. Prevalence of psychiatric disorders in sick listed chronic low back pain patients. Eur. J. Pain 15 (10), 1075–1080.

Rosenbaum, S., Vancampfort, D., Steel, Z., et al., 2015. Physical activity in the treatment of post-traumatic stress disorder: A systematic review and meta-analysis. Psychiatry Res. 230 (2), 130–136.

Roshanaei-Moghaddam, B., Katon, W.J., Russo, J., 2009. The longitudinal effects of depression on physical activity. Gen. Hosp. Psychiatry 31 (4), 306–315.

Schuch, F.B., Vancampfort, D., Richards, J., et al., 2016. Exercise as a treatment for depression: a meta-analysis adjusting for publication bias. J. Psychiatr. Res. 77, 42–51.

Sheehan, D.V., Lecrubier, Y., Sheehan, K.H., et al., 1998. The Mini-International Neuropsychiatric Interview (M.I.N.I.): the development and validation of a structured diagnostic psychiatric interview for DSM-IV and ICD-10. J. Clin. Psychiatry 59 (Suppl. 20), 22–33; quiz 34-57.

Shephard, R., 2003. Limits to the measurement of habitual physical activity by Questionnaires. Br. J. Sports Med. 37, 197–206.

Sullivan, M., Bishop, S., Pivik, J., 1995. The Pain Catastrophizing Scale: Development and validation. Psychol. Assess. 7 (4), 524–534.

Terluin, B., van Marwijk, H., Adèr, H., et al., 2006. The Four-Dimensional Symptom Questionnaire (4DSQ): a validation study of a multidimensional self-report questionnaire to assess distress, depression, anxiety and somatization. BMC Psychiatry 6, 34.

van der Giessen, R., Speksnijder, C., Helders, P., 2012. The effectiveness of graded activity in patients with non-specific low-back pain: a systematic review. Disabil. Rehabil. 34 (13), 1070–1076.

van der Windt, D., Hay, E., Jellema, P., Main, C., 2008. Psychosocial interventions for low back pain in primary care: lessons learned from recent trials. Spine 33 (1), 81–89.

van Tulder, M., Becker, A., Bekkering, T., et al., 2006. European guidelines for the management of acute nonspecific low back pain in primary care. Eur. Spine J. 15, S169–S191.

Vanhees, L., Lefevre, J., Philippaerts, R., et al., 2005. How to assess physical activity? How to assess physical fitness? Eur. J. Cardiovasc. Prev. Rehabil. 12 (2), 102–114.

Vibe Fersum, K., O'Sullivan, P., Skouen, J., et al., 2013. Efficacy of classification-based cognitive functional therapy in patients with non-specific chronic low back pain: a randomized controlled trial. Eur. J. Pain 17 (6), 916–928.

Vlaeyen, J., de Jong, J., Sieben, J., Crombez, G., 2002. Graded exposure in vivo for pain-related fear. In: Turk, D., Gatchel, R. (Eds.), Psychological Approaches to Pain Management: a Practitioner's Handbook, second ed. The Guilford Press, New York, pp. 210–233.

Vlaeyen, J., Linton, S., 2000. Fear-avoidance and its consequences in chronic musculoskeletal pain: a state of the art. Pain 85 (3), 317–332.

Waddell, G., Newton, M., Henderson, I., et al., 1993. A Fear-Avoidance Beliefs Questionnaire (FABQ) and the role of fear-avoidance beliefs in chronic low back pain and disability. Pain 52 (2), 157–168.

Yunus, M., 2007. Role of central sensitization in symptoms beyond muscle pain, and the evaluation of a patient with widespread pain. Best Pract. Res. Clin. Rheumatol. 21 (3), 481–497.

5.1.6 Physiotherapy Interventions in Individuals With Chronic Widespread Pain or Chronic Fatigue Syndrome

MERJA SALLINEN

SUMMARY

This chapter outlines the evidence-based approach of physiotherapy interventions for patients with chronic widespread pain (CWP) or chronic fatigue syndrome (CFS). To reach good physiotherapy outcomes it is necessary to understand the central sensitization as a background factor and, for example, how overly strenuous exercise may exacerbate the pain symptoms and lead to further deterioration of functioning. Physiotherapy interventions in CWP and CFS should be built on three equally important *evidence-based pillars: education, pacing the activity level and physical exercises. The reasoning behind these approaches as well as results of recent studies of outcomes among patients with CWP or CFS is introduced in this chapter.*

KEY POINTS

■ Chronic pain and fatigue combined with activity-induced muscular pain and malaise easily leads to inactivity, and may thus cause serious physical deconditioning.

■ Recent studies suggest that a combination of physical exercises and the cognitive-behavioral approach that include both patient education and activity management is the best practice in the treatment of patients with chronic pain and fatigue.

■ Physiotherapists have the skills and knowledge to tailor and implement individual exercise programmes for individuals with poor or lacking training history and various functional limitations such as individuals with chronic widespread pain (CWP) or chronic fatigue syndrome (CFS).

LEARNING OBJECTIVES

■ Understand why physiotherapy interventions of patients with CWP/CFS should include patient education and activity management in addition to exercise therapy.

■ Understand the principles of how to implement exercises according to an individual's needs and exercise tolerance in order to gain better functioning and physical condition without causing an increase in perceived postexercise pain or general fatigue.

INTRODUCTION

Chronic widespread pain (CWP) and chronic fatigue syndrome (CFS) are two overlapping conditions that may result in a substantial reduction in occupational, educational, social or personal activity level (Crooks, 2007; Arnold et al., 2008; Van Cauwenbergh et al., 2012). The most severe form of CWP is *fibromyalgia,* which is characterized by fluctuating chronic pain in all quadrants of the body, muscular tenderness, sleeping disorders and daytime tiredness (Arnold, et al., 2008; Wolfe, et al., 2010). CFS is a condition

characterized by serious mental and physical fatigue combined with at least four of the seven following minor symptoms: sore throat, new headache, tender lymph nodes, muscle pain, multiple joint pain, unrefreshing sleep and postexertional malaise that lasts more than 24 hours (Carruthers et al., 2011). Depression and anxiety are common among both individuals with CWP/fibromyalgia and CFS. Moreover, a wide range of other symptoms referring to effort and stress intolerance can be associated with these conditions (Yunus, 2008; Carruthers et al., 2011).

The etiology and pathogenesis of CWP and CFS are not fully understood, but cumulating evidence suggests that central sensitization (i.e., hyperresponsiveness of the central nervous system) dominates the clinical picture of both CWP and CFS (Yunus, 2008; Nijs et al., 2011b; Van Cauwenbergh et al., 2012). Nijs et al. (2010) points out that understanding the two-way mechanisms of central sensitivity is essential when planning and implementing physiotherapeutic interventions for individuals with CWP or CFS; on the one hand, there is the altered sensory processing in the central nervous system that leads to increased activity of pain-facilitatory pathways, temporal summation of the pain and decreased pain inhibition. It is noteworthy that this increased sensitivity may be linked to different kinds of sensory stimuli, for example, heat, cold, noise or pressure (Geisser, et al., 2007, 2008). On the other hand, repetitive musculoskeletal injuries and traumas may provide a sufficient amount of nociceptive barrage toward the central nervous system, and thus increase or perpetuate the symptoms (Nijs et al., 2010). Thus for example, overly strenuous exercise might exacerbate the pain symptoms and lead to further deterioration of functioning.

Three Pillars of Physiotherapy in Treatment of CWP and CFS

Research suggests that individuals with CWP and CFS often suffer from tendency to be overactive in their daily activities to a degree that exacerbates symptoms (Luyten et al., 2006). However, chronic pain and fatigue combined with activity-induced muscular pain and malaise easily lead to inactivity (Crooks, 2007) and fear-avoidance behavior (de Gier et al., 2003), and may thus cause serious physical deconditioning including muscle wasting and decreased cardiovascular and lung function. Therefore physiotherapy of individuals with CWP or CFS should be built on three equally important pillars, namely education, pacing and physical exercises.

Education

Patient education is recommended by various evidence-based guidelines for the management of CWP and CFS (Williams, 2003; Van Cauwenbergh et al., 2012). Patients with CWP or CFS find their symptoms emotionally distressing and difficult to understand, and they do not expect the medical treatments or therapy interventions to be effective. Moreover, inability to understand the experienced symptoms seems to increase anxiety, catastrophic thinking and desperation (van Wilgen et al., 2008; van Ittersum et al., 2009). Research indicates that catastrophizing, pain-related anxiety and fear are related to poor adjustment to pain. Patients with greater self-efficacy are more likely to respond favorably to treatment programmes and to experience better outcomes (Keefe et al., 2004; Sowden et al., 2006; Sarzi-Puttini et al., 2008) (Box 1).

Besides educating patients about the nature of their symptoms and illness, education is used to introduce and implement various other treatment options such as activity management, stress management, relaxation exercises and exercise therapy (Nijs et al., 2010). The educational approach aims at reducing anxiety, increasing treatment compliance, enhancing self-efficacy, improving coping skills and drawing attention away from the symptoms (Sarzi-Puttini et al., 2008).

Researchers point out that changes in cognitions are important to achieve because they are known to be closely linked to perceived disability and pain. Furthermore, catastrophizing appears to be related to exercise capacity in patients with CFS. In consequence, decreased catastrophizing may result in increased exercise capacity and activity levels, which may be responsible for improved physical performance, leading to increased pain thresholds and pain tolerance in the longer term (Meeus et al., 2010). They conducted a double-blinded randomized controlled trial (RCT) among 46 patients with CFS. Pain physiology education covered the physiology of the nervous system in general and of the pain system in particular. These topics were discussed with every participant and were the basis for a further individualized interactive education session, adopted on particular life situations of the patient. The researchers noticed that in addition to significant improvement in a knowledge test, catastrophic thinking reduced and changes towards more adaptive coping strategies were found in the experimental group. The difference was significant in comparison to the control group (Meeus et al., 2010). Similar results were reported in a study among patients with CWP (van Wilgen et al., 2007).

Although patient education can be used successfully as a stand-alone treatment in both CWP and CFS, it is often combined with other treatment modalities, such as exercise or medication. Patient education can be easily and effectively implemented within physiotherapy sessions both in individual therapy sessions and in group interventions. In fibromyalgia, combining cognitive-behavioral education and aerobic exercise in general is proven to be effective, resulting in significant improvements in pain, pain behavior, fatigue, general well-being, distress and physical fitness (Mannerkorpi et al., 2000; van Wilgen et al., 2007).

Group-based interventions, which combine educational issues with moderate aerobic exercise, have the additional benefit of peer support, which gives the possibility of sharing experiences and knowledge, as well as to conduct social comparisons with other people with similar illnesses (Mannerkorpi et al., 2002; Williams, 2003; Kukkurainen, 2006).

BOX 1

Tell your CWP/CFS patient about the central nervous system and hypersensitivity that is in the background of their symptoms. It helps her to understand the nature of the symptoms, which reduces the level of anxiety and worry, and increases treatment compliance and motivation to exercise.

Pacing

Patients with CWP or CFS are often tempted to be overactive on a 'good day', which may lead to deterioration of the pain and fatigue symptoms on the following days (Luyten et al., 2006). Patients need to learn to cope with their illness, which often requires permanent lifestyle modifications (Nijs et al., 2010).

Pacing is an activity-management strategy in which the patients are encouraged to achieve an appropriate balance between rest and activity. Pacing takes into account the delayed recovery from exercise and the considerable fluctuations in symptom severity that are typical of both patients with CWP and CFS (Nijs et al., 2010). The first goal of the pacing approach is to help the patient to manage the daily activities in a way so that he/she no longer experiences the fluctuation in symptoms (stabilization phase). In the second stage exercises are gradually started. The physiotherapist needs to pay attention to both the activity level in daily activities and the exercise level when planning the interventions, in order to prevent overactive patients from exceeding their own limits (Nijs et al., 2006) (Box 2).

Successful pacing requires that the patient learns to set realistic activity goals on a daily basis and to regularly monitor and manipulate their activity level in terms of intensity, duration and rest periods in order to avoid possible overexertion, which can result in worsening of the symptoms. However, it is also important to emphasize that the patients must not stay or become dependent on their symptoms like pain or fatigue. Rather than that, they should be encouraged to perform different physical and intellectual tasks, starting from a tolerable level and then gradually increasing the length and frequency of the tasks as the tolerance improves (Van Cauwenbergh et al., 2012). Body-awareness and relaxation exercises may be beneficial in learning to listen to one's body (Gard, 2005; Anderson et al., 2007; Persson et al., 2008) and continuous heart rate monitoring could be used as a biofeedback tool to control the intensity level of the exercises.

This strategy can help patients return to appropriate physical activities by reducing perceived fatigue and disability, and by encouraging them towards a more active lifestyle. However, we must bear in mind that there is still little research on pacing as a stand-alone intervention, but it can be understood as one approach within cognitive-behavioral interventions that is widely recommended for use in the treatment of patients with CWP or CFS, in particular when combined with physical exercises (Price et al., 2008; Häuser et al., 2010).

Physical Exercises

Sarzi-Puttini et al. (2008) state that healthcare workers do not hesitate to advise patients to engage in regular physical activities, but often fail to notice that advice or instructions are insufficient to motivate the patients in the absence of self-efficacy or self-confidence. Self-efficacy, in turn, is perceived to be essential when undertaking and continuing any activity. Physiotherapists have the skills and knowledge to tailor and implement individual exercise programmes for individuals with poor or lacking training history, and various functional limitations such as individuals with CWP or CFS.

According to Nijs et al. (2010), exercise therapy may have several goals depending on the patient's prominent symptoms, body functions, motivation and preferences. They point out that a realistic goal for a patient with severe pain, distress and disabilities is to increase the overall activity level and the tolerance to exercise, whereas a goal for a patient with milder symptoms might be to increase muscle strength (force-generating capacity) or cardiovascular fitness.

Häuser et al. (2010) conducted a meta-analysis of RCTs comparing different types of aerobic exercises in the treatment of fibromyalgia. Twenty-eight RCT studies totalling almost 2500 patients were analysed. Aerobic exercise in general was found to be beneficial with regard to reduced pain, fatigue, depressed mood and improved health-related quality of life and physical fitness. However, aerobic exercise had no effect on sleep problems, and continuing exercise was found to be necessary to maintain the positive effects on pain in a longer perspective. Moreover, no differences were reported between different exercise types (e.g., walking vs. cycling), and there was no evidence of superiority of water-based over land-based exercises. Very low-intensity exercise (<50% of maximal heart rate [maxHR]) was found to be ineffective, and even with moderate intensity (50–80% of maxHR) the positive effects on symptom reduction could be seen only after exercising 2–3 times a week for 4–6 weeks.

BOX 3

Regular exercise over a long period of time, even at a low-intensity level, is beneficial in these patient groups, but a gradual increase is intensity in plausible to reach good results. The most common reason for dropout is exercise-induced muscle pain and increased fatigue. This can be avoided with careful planning of the exercises.

These results confirm the earlier recommendations of the Ottawa Panel Guidelines for aerobic exercise in fibromyalgia (Brosseau et al., 2008a).

Mannerkorpi et al. (2010) studied moderate-to-high intensity Nordic walking in patients with fibromyalgia in an RCT. The Nordic walking group (NW group) exercised under supervision twice a week with moderate-to-high intensity for 15 weeks. The control group participated in low-intensity exercise sessions once a week for 15 weeks. The NW group showed significant improvement in physical capacity measured with the 6-minute walking test, and a significantly reduced heart rate in the ergometer test in comparison to baseline and controls. Limitations in daily life decreased and overall health status improved significantly in the NW group. However, with regard to pain ratings, there were no differences between the two groups. In follow-up after 6 months, a significant decrease in general and physical fatigue was seen in both groups, indicating that regular exercise over a long period of time, even when on a low-intensity level, is beneficial in reducing fatigue in fibromyalgia.

Strength training is recommended for patients with fibromyalgia in order to avoid the decline of muscle strength and physical functioning that is caused by inactivity (Mannerkorpi & Iversen, 2003). Häkkinen et al. (2002) compared fibromyalgia patients with healthy controls in an RCT where patients either participated in a 21-week strength-training programme or continued with their usual activities. The results showed improvements in muscle strength, muscle-firing patterns (EMG activity) and in mood in the exercise group compared to controls. In comparison, Kingsley et al. (2005) conducted a 12-week strength-training programme for patients with fibromyalgia and wait-listed controls. The results showed significant improvements in strength and functioning in routine household tasks in comparison to both baseline measurements and controls. Valkeinen et al. (2006) pointed out that regular strength training twice a week with progressively increasing loading (from 50% to 80% of maximum) led to significant improvements in muscle strength in postmenopausal women with fibromyalgia, and that it did not exacerbate, but slightly attenuated, perceived pain and fatigue.

In a meta-analysis by Brosseau et al. (2008b), the positive effects of strength training were indicated in terms of pain relief, increased muscle strength, improved health-related quality of life and a decrease in perceived physical disability, depression and anxiety. They recommended individualized exercise instructions to increase exercise adherence and to avoid dropout due to exercise-induced pain, which is a common problem, especially in sedentary patients with CWP or CFS.

The benefits of physical exercises concerning patients with fibromyalgia are well established in several studies, but the evidence regarding patients with CFS remains insufficient due to the lack of uniformity in outcome measures and inclusion criteria of the studies, which makes it difficult, if not impossible, to compare the findings (Nijs, et al., 2011a; Van Cauwenbergh et al., 2012).

Van Cauwenbergh et al. (2012) conducted a literature review of 12 RCTs in order to identify the appropriate exercise modalities (i.e., exercise duration, mode, number of treatment sessions, session length, duration of treatment, exercise intensity and whether or not to apply home exercise programmes) for people with CFS. According to the review, people with CFS can perform home exercises five times a week with an initial duration of 5–15 minutes per exercise session. The exercise duration can be gradually increased up to 30 minutes/session. Home exercises should be supported by guided exercise therapy for at least 10–11 sessions spread over a period of 4–5 months. Aerobic activities like walking, swimming or cycling, and strength, balance and stretching exercises were found useful in the treatment of CFS. However, particular attention needs to be paid to avoiding postexercise malaise and fatigue. Moreover, the researchers point out that most studies admitted people with CFS who could come independently to the hospital, which implies a mild or moderate disability. Those who were not able to walk or get out of bed were automatically excluded, and therefore it was not possible to examine whether exercise therapy was effective, ineffective or even harmful for a more seriously disabled group of people with CFS.

Moss-Morris et al. (2005) conducted an RCT to investigate the outcomes of graded exercise among patients with CFS. Forty-nine patients were randomized to an exercise group and a standard medical-care group. After the baseline measurements, the participants of the exercise group met with one of the researchers in order to set individual goals collaboratively between the researcher and participant. The exercise intervention took 12 weeks and the target heart rate was initially set to approximately 40% of VO_2max to be maintained for 10–15 minutes 4–5 times a week. During the first 6 weeks, increases focused on duration of the exercise rather than intensity, but after 6 weeks the intensity was increased gradually. The final goal was for each participant to be exercising for 30 minutes 5 days a week at an intensity level relating to 70% of VO_2max.

The results showed a significant reduction in perceived mental and physical fatigue and improvement in physical functioning, and these results remained at 6-month follow-up. Patients in the exercise group significantly reduced the amount they focused on their symptoms, but in the control group there was no change. A reduction in symptom focusing was strongly associated with a reduction in mental and physical fatigue, as well as with a self-rated global improvement score and increase in physical functioning. Interestingly, there were no statistically significant group effects for the physiological variables including maximum heart rate and VO_2max peak. However, the researchers remind us that this result should be treated with caution due to the high drop-out rate from the second treadmill testing; complete data were available for just over half of the sample. They concluded that the key mechanisms of improvement in functioning appear to be psychological rather than physiological. Reductions in the symptom focusing and increased ability to exert oneself were seen as significant mediators of the treatment effect.

CONCLUDING REMARKS

According to the current evidence, physical activity in daily life and exercising with mild-to-moderate intensity combined with education and activity management are useful in the physiotherapy of individuals with CWP or CFS. The physical exercises should be started with a low dose in regard to intensity and duration in order to avoid delayed onset of muscle soreness and excessive fatigue following the exercise sessions. The intensity and duration can be increased gradually, and may eventually reach the same level as exercise recommendations for healthy individuals.

In a their review, Nijs et al. (2010) pointed out that the evidence supporting spinal manipulation, massage therapy, trigger-point injections or use of transcutaneous nerve stimulation is limited, if not lacking, although these modalities are commonly used as a part of physiotherapy. Furthermore, they emphasize that treatments triggering more pain may serve as a physical stressor attacking the already deregulated stress-response system, thereby initiating a vicious cycle. They emphasize that passive treatments should never be the core feature of the treatment, and it should be acknowledged that their use might confirm maladaptive illness beliefs and strengthen passive coping strategies.

REFERENCES

Anderson, B., Strand, L.I., Råheim, M., 2007. The effect of long-term body-awareness exercise training succeeding a multimodal cognitive behavior program for patients with widespread pain. J. Musculoskelet. Pain 15 (3), 19–29.

Arnold, L., Crofford, L., Mease, P., et al., 2008. Patient perspectives on the impact of fibromyalgia. Patient Educ. Couns. 73, 114–120.

Brosseau, L., Wells, G.A., Tugwell, P., et al., 2008a. Ottawa panel evidence-based clinical practice guidelines for aerobic fitness in the management of fibromyalgia. Phys. Ther. 88, 857–871.

Brosseau, L., Wells, G.A., Tugwell, P., et al., 2008b. Ottawa panel evidence-based clinical practice guidelines for strengthening exercises in the management of fibromyalgia. Phys. Ther. 88, 873–885.

Carruthers, B.M., van de Sande, M.I., De Meirleir, K.L., et al., 2011. Myalgic encefalomielitis: International consensus criteria. J. Intern. Med. 270, 327–338.

Crooks, V.A., 2007. Exploring the altered daily geographies and life-world of women living with fibromyalgia syndrome: a mixed-method approach. Soc. Sci. Med. 64, 577–588.

de Gier, M., Peters, M.L., Vlayen, J.W., 2003. Fear of pain, physical performance, and attentional processes in patients with fibromyalgia. Pain 104, 121–130.

Gard, G., 2005. Body awareness therapy for patients with fibromyalgia and chronic pain. Disabil. Rehabil. 27 (12), 725–728.

Geisser, M.E., Glass, J., Rajcevska, L.D., et al., 2008. A psychophysical study of auditory and pressure sensitivity in patients with fibromyalgia and healthy controls. J. Pain 9, 417–422.

Geisser, M.E., Gracely, R.H., Giesecke, T., et al., 2007. The association between experimental and clinical pain measures among persons with fibromyalgia and chronic fatigue syndrome. Eur. J. Pain 11, 202–207.

Häkkinen, K., Pakarinen, A., Hannonen, P., et al., 2002. Effects of strength training on muscle strength, sross-sectional area, maximal electromyographic activity, and serum hormones in premenopausal women with fibromyalgia. J. Rheumatol. 29, 1287–1295.

Häuser, W., Klose, P., Langhorst, J., et al., 2010. Efficacy of different types of aerobic exercise in fibromyalgia syndrome: a systematic review and meta-analysis of randomised controlled trials. Arthritis Res. Ther. 12, R79.

Häuser, W., Thieme, K., Turk, D., 2010. Guideline for management of fibromyalgia suyndrome—a systematic review. Eur. J. Pain 14, 5–10.

Keefe, F.J., Rumble, M.E., Scipio, C.C., et al., 2004. Psychologiacal aspects of persistent pain: current state of the science. J. Pain 5 (4), 195–211.

Kingsley, J.D., Panton, L.B., Toole, T., et al., 2005. The effects of a 12-week strength-training program on strength and functionality in women with fibromyalgia. Arch. Phys. Med. Rehabil. 86, 1713–1721.

Kukkurainen, M.L., 2006. Fibromyalgiaa sairastavien koherenssintunne, sosiaalinen tuki ja elämänlaatu [Fibromyalgia patients' sense of coherence, social support and quality of life]. Dissertation. University of Oulu, Oulu.

Luyten, P., Van Houdenhove, B., Cosyns, N., Van den Broek, A.L., 2006. Are patients with chronic fatigue syndrome perfectionistic—or were they? A case-control study. Pers. Individ. Dif. 40, 1473–1483.

Mannerkorpi, K., Ahlmén, M., Ekdahl, C., 2002. Six and 24 month follow-up of pool exercise therapy and education for patients with fibromyalgia. Scand. J. Rheumatol. 31, 306–310.

Mannerkorpi, K., Iversen, M., 2003. Physical exercise in fibromyalgia and related syndromes. Best Pract. Res. Clin. Rheumatol. 17, 629–647.

Mannerkorpi, K., Nordeman, L., Cider, Å., Jonsson, G., 2010. Does moderate-to-high intensity Nordic walking imporve functional capacity and pain in fibromyalgia? A prospective randomized controlled trial. Arthritis Res. Ther. 12, R189.

Mannerkorpi, K., Nyberg, B., Ahlmén, M., Ekdahl, C., 2000. Pool exercise combined with an education program for patients with fibromyalgia syndrome. J. Rheumatol. 27, 2473–2481.

Meeus, M., Nijs, J., Van Oosterwijck, J., et al., 2010. Pain physiology education improves pain beliefs in patients with chronic fatigue syndrome compared with pacing and self-management education: a double-blind randomized controlled trial. Arch. Phys. Med. Rehabil. 91, 1153–1159.

Moss-Morris, R., Sharon, C., Tobin, R., Baldi, J.C., 2005. A randomized controlled graded exercise trial for chronic fatigue syndrome: outcomes and mechanisms of change. J. Health Psychol. 10 (2), 245–259.

Nijs, J., Aelbrecht, S., Meeus, M., et al., 2011a. Tired of being inactive: a systematic literature review of physical activity, physiological

exercise capacity and muscle strength in patients with chronic fatigue syndrome. Disabil. Rehabil. 33 (17-18), 1493–1500.

Nijs, J., Mannerkorpi, K., Descheemaeker, F., Van Houdenhove, B., 2010. Primary care physical therapy in people with fibromyalgia: opportunities and boundaries within a monodisciplinary setting. Phys. Ther. 90 (12), 1815–1822.

Nijs, J., Meeus, M., De Meirleir, K., 2006. Chronic musculoskeletal pain in chronic fatigue syndrome: recent develpments and therapeutic implications. Man. Ther. 11 (3), 187–191.

Nijs, J., Meeus, M., Van Oosterwijck, J., et al., 2011b. In the mind or in the brain? Scientific evidence for central sensitisation chronic fatigue syndrome. Eur. J. Clin. Invest. 42 (2), 203–212.

Persson, A.L., Veenhuizen, H., Zachrison, L., Gard, G., 2008. Relaxation as treatment for chronic musculoskeletal pain – a systematic review of randomised controlled studies. Phys. Ther. Rev. 13 (5), 355–365.

Price, J.R., Mitchell, E., Tidy, E., Hunot, V., 2008. Cognitive behavior therapy for chronic fatigue syndrome in adults. Cochrane Database Syst. Rev. (3), Art. No.: CD001027.

Sarzi-Puttini, P., Buskila, D., Carrabba, M., et al., 2008. Treatment strategy in fibromyalgia: where are we now? Semin. Arthritis Rheum. 37, 353–365.

Sowden, M., Hatch, A., Gray, S.E., Coombs, J., 2006. Can four key psychosocial ris factors for chronic pain and disability (Yellow Flags) be modified by a pain management programme? A pilot study. Physiotherapy 92, 43–49.

Valkeinen, H., Häkkinen, A., Hannonen, P., et al., 2006. Acute heavy resistance exercise-induced pain and neuromuscular fatigue in elderly women with fibromyalgia and in healthy controls. Arthritis Rheum. 54 (4), 1334–1339.

Van Cauwenbergh, D., De Kooning, M., Ickmans, K., Nijs, J., 2012. How to exercise people with chronic fatigue syndrome: evidence-based practice guidelines. Eur. J. Clin. Invest. 42, 1136–1144.

van Ittersum, M.W., van Wilgen, C.P., Hilberdink, W.K., et al., 2009. Illness perceptions in patients with fibromyalgia. Patient Educ. Couns. 74, 53–60.

van Wilgen, C.P., Bloten, H., Oeseburg, B., 2007. Results of a multidisciplinary program for patients with fibromyalgia implemented in primary care. Disabil. Rehabil. 29 (15), 1207–1213.

van Wilgen, C.P., van Ittersum, M.W., Kaptein, A.A., van Wijhe, M., 2008. Illness perception in patients with fibromyalgia and their relation to quality of life and catastrophizing. Arthritis Rheum. 59, 3618–3626.

Williams, D.A., 2003. Psychological and behavioural therpies in fibromyalgia and related syndromes. Best Pract. Res. Clin. Rheumatol. 17 (4), 640–665.

Wolfe, F., Clauw, D., Fitzcharles, M., et al., 2010. The American College of Rheumatology preliminary diagnostic criteria for fibromyalgia and measurement of symptom severity. Arthritis Care Res. 62, 600–610.

Yunus, M.B., 2008. Central sensitivity syndromes: a new paradigm and group nosology for fibromyalgia and overlapping conditions, and the related issue of disease versus illness. Semin. Arthritis Rheum. 37, 339–352.

5.1.7   The Role of Adaptive Pacing Therapy and Graded Exercise in Treatment for Chronic Fatigue Syndrome and Myalgic Encephalomyelitis

MICHEL PROBST ▪ JOLIEN DIEDENS ▪ BEELEKE BREDERO

SUMMARY

In this chapter myalgic encephalomyelitis (ME) and chronic fatigue syndrome (CFS) are explained. Secondly, current treatment options for these two syndromes are considered, and finally recommendations for further research are discussed.

KEY POINTS

▪ Several etiological factors can cause ME and CFS.

▪ Adaptive pacing therapy (APT) and graded exercise (GE) are current treatment modalities used to treat CFS and ME; however, there is no consensus about an optimal treatment approach.

▪ It is important to be patient during the treatment and explain to your patient that symptoms can fluctuate.

LEARNING OBJECTIVES

▪ Become familiar with the symptoms of ME and CFS.

▪ Understand the main treatment principles for ME and CFS.

▪ Be able to explain the differences between graded exercise therapy and APT.

INTRODUCTION

In this chapter, *myalgic encephalomyelitis* and *chronic fatigue syndrome* are used interchangeably and this illness is referred to as *ME/CFS*.

The international criteria for ME/CFS are: (1) severe chronic fatigue for at least 6 months, with other known medical conditions (whose manifestation includes fatigue) excluded by clinical diagnosis; (2) concurrently have four or more of the following symptoms: postexertional malaise (PEM), impaired memory or concentration, unrefreshing sleep, muscle pain, multijoint pain without redness or swelling, tender cervical or axillary lymph nodes, sore throat, or

headache; and (3) light-to-moderate exercise leading to extreme fatigue and a general feeling of malaise that is abnormally prolonged, sometimes lasting several weeks. The prevalence of CFS is estimated at 0.2%–2.6% worldwide (Prins et al., 2006).

The pathophysiology of CFS is still unknown. A current hypothesis is that CFS results from a disordered immune response to an infection, sometimes in combination with other forms of physical and/or psychological stress (Becker et al., 2002; Hickie et al., 2006). Several studies reported a high prevalence of psychopathology in patients with CFS—depression, anxiety, hypochondria, somatization (Garralda et al., 1999; Garralda & Rangel, 2002).

Cairns & Hotopf (2005) have found that the prognosis of ME/CFS is poor if left untreated. Complete recovery from CFS or ME is rare without any intervention. The prognosis for an improvement in symptoms is less gloomy. However, there is increasing evidence for the effectiveness of cognitive-behavioural and graded exercise therapies (GETs). Medical retirement should be postponed until a trial of such treatment has been given.

TREATMENT MODALITIES

Adaptive pacing therapy (APT) is a treatment method for CFS and/or ME. Patients often experience extreme fatigue in these illnesses, which is medically inexplicable (Prins et al., 2006; National Institute for Health and Clinical Excellence, 2007).

There are several interventions to treat patients with ME/CFS. The first intervention is cognitive behavioural therapy (CBT). Other possible interventions are: APT and GET.

Adaptive Pacing Therapy

Pacing was initially devised during the 1980s for patients with ME (UK) and epidemic neuromyasthenia (USA)

(Ramsay, 1978, 1988; Goudsmit & Howes, 2008). The basic principle of APT is that patients stay as active as possible but avoid excessive efforts (Goudsmit, 2008). APT can be defined as follows: 'pacing is an energy management strategy in which sufferers are encouraged to achieve an appropriate balance between rest and activities. This usually involves living within physical and mental limitations imposed by the illness and avoiding activities that exacerbate symptoms or interspersing activity with planned rest. The aim is to prevent sufferers entering a vicious cycle of over activity and setbacks, whilst assisting them to set realistic goals for increasing their activity when appropriate' (Burns et al., 2012).

APT consists of four core elements: (1) activity, (2) rest and relaxation, (3) forming a sustainable baseline and (4) and increasing their activities to own possibilities (White et al., 2015).

In terms of pacing, the activity includes more than just the physical aspect; it includes any activity that requires energy, from waking up to worrying or feeling angry. In addition, patients with CFS often find emotional activities the most energy intensive and therefore the hardest to control. It is important to take into account activities that urge concentration and memory; this may trigger symptoms (Rimes & Chalder, 2005; Goudsmit et al., 2009).

An adapted lifestyle is reached by dosing the patient's activities. This depends on current symptoms, the patient's situation and their preferences. In practice, it implies that patients should stop an activity if the body indicates that it is too much. Activities that require much energy should be alternated with less strenuous activities and planned breaks. One should take care that not (always) the same body parts are used during activities. Therefore the patient should pace and switch between physical and mental activities. Resting in between is possible, to recuperate from previous activity. The advice to pace and switch is based on the observation that ME tends to affect some muscles more than others (Ramsay, 1988) and the hypothesis that switching before or at the first sign of PEM may abort the mechanisms underlying activity-induced increases in symptoms (Goudsmit & Howes, 2008, Goudsmit et al., 2009, 2012; White et al., 2010). In general, it is better to avoid sleep during the day, because this may disturb the night-time sleep

cycle. The duration of the recovery period should be limited to avoid rumination and over-focusing on the symptoms (Ray et al., 1993; Goudsmit et al., 2009).

Pacing is a treatment strategy that aims to encourage patients to achieve an optimal balance between doing activities and resting. It is important to avoid any exacerbation of the patient's symptoms, therefore the patient has to make realistic goals, if necessary, in consultation with the physiotherapist.

This approach can be seen as an alternative to the CBT approach (Shepherd, 2016). Namely, it takes into account that symptoms of the patient can fluctuate in severity. Also, the patient must know that sometimes fatigue can increase after doing sports, but that must not be an excuse to be sedentary the whole day.

Phases of Adaptive Pacing Therapy

At first, the patient must manage his/her daily activities in a way he/she no longer experiences fluctuations in symptoms (stabilization phase). Next, the physiotherapist can start to grade activity and exercise levels (grading phase). During the grading phase, the same pacing techniques are applied to grade both activity level and exercise level (i.e., flexible, accounting for the fluctuating nature of the disorder). To prevent overactive patients in exceeding their own limits, heart rate monitoring can be applied for intensity control (heart rate guidelines are obtained from the exercise stress test with continuous cardiorespiratory monitoring). Results of the study by Nijs et al. (2006) have shown that GET is a better intervention than relaxation or flexibility training in CFS patients.

Practical Guidelines for APT

It is important that clinicians spend sufficient time explaining the rationale for this strategy to the patient prior to commencement of APT. Therefore it is appropriate to make a weekly schedule to distribute the work. For example, it is unadvisable to vacuum clean and iron directly after each other. These activities are more convenient if distributed over 2 days. A day filled with strenuous activities is best followed by a day of less energy-consuming activities. Patients should be advised to keep a journal in which they write down their fatigue, perceived energy level and sleep quality. By analysing the journal, an insight on the limits and triggers of the person is obtained. Furthermore, the patient and practitioner are able to monitor the effects of pacing and other coping strategies.

Purpose

APT is used to increase patients' confidence and to reduce unpredictability. Understanding, feeling and accepting personal physical limits ensures that the future is planned with more confidence. Doing activities between physical limits prevents exacerbation of the symptoms. APT increases the control over health, body and activities, and improves coping processes. For a natural recovery process of the body it is important to have a good balance between rest and activity. Because CFS is a chronic illness, the aspect of acceptance and dealing with the syndrome should not be underestimated.

Evidence

In some studies APT is recommend for patients in which symptoms fluctuate (Ramsay, 1988; Dowsett & Welsby, 1992) and/or for patients with an underlying disease process in which a time-contingent approach is recommended.

White et al. (2011) reported on the PACE trial in *The Lancet*. Three behavioural interventions (APT, CBT, and GET) and specialist medical care (SMC) have been assessed on their effectiveness and safety. PACE is the abbreviation for 'pacing, activity, and CBT: a randomized evaluation'. In 2015, Sharpe et al. had a prespecified two year follow-up after the PACE trial. Long-term outcomes (for at least 2 years after the trial) have been investigated and the patients received additional treatments after the trial and investigate long-term outcomes (at least 2 years after randomization) within and between original treatment groups in those originally included in the PACE trial.

Fig. 1 shows results from the PACE trial. Herein it is seen that CBT and GET were more effective in reducing both fatigue and physical disability than APT, if each was added to SMC, and were more effective than SMC alone. APT combined with medical treatment has no extra value. Bourke et al. (2014) concluded in a comparable study that CBT and GET are more effective in reducing the frequency of muscle and joint ache than with APT with SMC.

White et al. (2013) have concluded that it is possible to recover from CFS. According to White and colleagues,

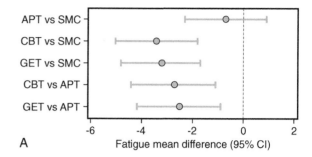

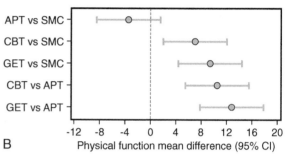

FIGURE 1 ▪ Primary outcome treatment differences for fatigue (A) and physical function (B) at 52 weeks.

CBT and GET are the most effective treatment methods. The percentages (number/total) meeting trial criteria for recovery were 22% (32/143) after CBT, 22% (32/143) after GET, 8% (12/149) after APT and 7% (11/150) after SMC. Similar proportions met criteria for clinical recovery. These results do not support pacing as a first-line treatment method for CFS.

The most fundamental difference in APT and CBT/GET is that APT encourages adaptations to the patient. The rationale in CBT and GET is to improve patient health by gradually increasing the activity level.

No targets will be planned in APT. To complete an activity is not the main goal of this treatment. APT should be offered as one component of a multidisciplinary programme that addresses the specific needs and circumstances of the individual with ME/CFS (Friedberg & Jason, 1998; Goudsmit et al., 2009; Jason et al., 2011).

Goudsmit et al. (2012) found that pacing offers practitioners an additional therapeutic option that is acceptable to the majority of patients and can reduce the severity of the exertion-related symptoms of ME/CFS; it can help to stabilize the condition and avoid

PEM. If APT is correctly applied, it prevents 'pacing' exhaustion-related relapses, deconditioning and, by definition, the 'boom-bust cycles' that are reported in the literature (Jason et al., 1999; Burgess, 2006; NICE, 2007).

APT Conclusion

APT is a frequently used therapy for CFS. An important cornerstone of this therapy is that the patient will find a balance between activity and rest, physical and mental exercise, work and free time, and needs and virtues. Pacing will not change the fundamental course of the disease; however, it can contribute to recovery (Bleijenberg & Koop, 2011).

Limited evidence is available of treatment methods for ME/CFS; furthermore, there is no uniform definition of ME/CFS. However, the results of White et al. (2011, 2015) are inspiring for further research.

For optimal treatment the therapist should explain all different treatment modalities to his patient and let him choose his favourable treatment method. It is well known that patients with ME/CFS feel unheard and not understood (Horton et al., 2010).

Graded Exercise Therapy

Another treatment modality is GET, which is a structured treatment method introduced by Lindström et al. (1992). It is based on cognitive and behavioural learning theories, in which patients learn independently of their activity level to gradually build their activities according to a time-schedule contingent (Köke et al., 2007).

Chronic pain is an indication for using GET (including chronic low-back pain, fibromyalgia, CFS-ME). GET assumes that chronic pain is perpetuated by deconditioning (lack of fitness), reduced physical strength and altered perception of exertion consequently upon reduced physical activity. Pain can be maintained, among other things, by classical and operant learning processes, even if the tissue damage is no longer present (Flor et al., 2002; Klinger et al., 2010; Goubert et al., 2011). These processes are based on associations between stimuli (classical learning) and reinforcement (operant learning) and punishment. For the operant learning processes it has been considered that the body or the mind benefits from pain and disease. Therefore it is beneficial to maintain the pain or illness. Even specific anxieties and coping styles put a serious strain on recovery and will maintain pain. Catastrophizing (Adams et al., 2007; Buitenhuis et al., 2008) and kinesiophobia (Leeuw et al., 2007) will result in chronic pain. Chronic pain should be considered in the biopsychosocial model (Engel, 1980). GET has been developed from the theory that in chronic pain the reciprocity between the patient and his environment plays an important role (Fordyce, 1976; Gatzounis et al., 2012).

What Is Graded Exercise Therapy?

GET is a behaviour-orientated treatment method that can be given by a physiotherapist. This approach is based on the idea that after a long time of sedentary behaviour the muscle system and cardiovascular system will be negatively affected, resulting in a decrease in strength and physical fitness. These factors maintain the symptoms of CFS. The aim of GET is to change the dysfunctional thoughts of the patient and to improve his physical condition. As the principles of operant conditioning will be used, healthy and sportive behaviour will be encouraged, with no attention being paid to pain and/or sedentary behaviour. Next to operant conditioning, cognitive theories will be clarified, chronic pain mechanisms will be explained and an insight is provided into the consequences of kinesiophobia. Furthermore, correcting catastrophic and irrational thoughts is a part of GET (Crul et al., 2007).

Graded exercise (GE) is a rehabilitative approach based on the principle that prolonged inactivity causes physical deconditioning of the muscles, heart and lungs, which then maintains the effects of CFS. GE programmes consist of structured, supervised activities or exercises that are progressively increased by a therapist in order to improve a patient's physical condition.

One of the main cornerstones of this therapy is a time-contingent schedule. The activity level is systematically increased regardless of the pain or symptoms. The structure of this therapy starts at a nonthreatening level for the patient. It emphasis possibilities and not restrictions. Home exercises are an important part of therapy.

The objectives of graded activity are encouraging healthy movement behaviour, increasing the level of physical activity, reducing pain behaviour and kinesio-phobia, optimizing functioning in work and leisure, promoting self-efficacy, and decreasing absenteeism. Pain reduction is not a primary goal in GA; performing more activities is central (Köke et al., 2007). Conditions for a good treatment are motivation, goodwill and cooperation.

Practical Implementations

GET principles are characterized in phases (Köke et al., 2007):

1. Problem identification
2. Problem analysis
3. Choosing activities
4. Determining baseline
5. Determining goals and their structure
6. Performing structure schedule
7. Generalization and evaluation.

The initial phase consists of a clinical examination by the physical therapist. Herein the physical fitness of the patient is determined. During problem analysis, the inhibiting and stimulating factors are identified. After that, short- and long-term objectives are worded in consultation with the patient. Next, the physiotherapist will draw up a programme with gradually increasing activities. The maxim for these activities is not to do more on good days and not less on bad days than agreed (in other words, graded exercise). During the treatment phase, the patient is working on increasing their chosen activities and the realization of their goals within the agreed time frame. The generalization phase is to apply what is learned in daily life. It is important to maintain the long-term outcome and attempt to prevent relapse; in case of relapse, the patient should be able to cope with their relapse.

Evidence

GET is an evidence-based strategy that has a positive outcome with variable effect sizes in the literature (Malouff et al., 2008; Price et al., 2008; Macedo et al., 2010; Castell et al., 2011; Knoop, 2011; White et al., 2011). CBT and GET are two treatment methods for CFS patients that provide significant improvements (Prins et al., 2006). A recent study by White et al. (2013), wherein the different methods of treatment of CFS were compared, concluded that recovering from

CFS is possible. CBT and GET are the most effective treatment methods. Bourke et al. (2014) concluded in a study that CBT and GET were more effective in reducing the frequency of muscle and joint pain than APT and SMC. An important effect of GET is that it diminishes catastrophic cognitions and vigilance (Geraets et al., 2005; Moss-Morris et al., 2005).

Gatzounis et al. (2012) suggested that increasing activities without tissue damage can be a valuable learning aspect of GA. Besides that, it will lead to an increase in activities outside and after therapy. Studies show that GA leads to quicker resumption of work (Staal et al., 2004; Hlobil et al., 2005; Lambeek et al., 2010). GA is more cost effective than usual care and no treatment.

In patients with low-back pain, GET is next applied to GE. With GE, patients are asked to create a hierarchy of feared activities. The exposure starts with the least feared activity. Once the negative associations are extinguished, activities associated with higher levels of anxiety are addressed in the same way. Both treatments have been endorsed in clinical guidelines for the management of persistent low-back pain (Airaksinen et al., 2006; Rossignol et al., 2007). Macedo et al. (2010) concluded in a review that limited evidence suggests that GE is as effective as GA for persistent low-back pain.

GET Conclusion

GET is a therapy in which the aim is toward a progressive increase in the patient's physical capacity. GET is based on the physiopathology model of deconditioning. It tries to break the vicious cycle so that the fitness of the person will increase and the symptoms that a de-conditioned chronic pain patient experiences will abate.

Pacing, on the other hand, tries to change the patient's dysfunctional thoughts about fatigue and his inactive lifestyle. Therefore, some principles from CBT are used. It is important that the patient understands the fluctuation of his symptoms. In consultation with the physiotherapist, the patient should plan daily activities. This ensures that a balanced activity programme can be made in which the patient will not overdo activity or remain sedentary all day. Over time the patient should try to improve his physical fitness by following the principles of GET. APT is often succeeded by GET.

REFERENCES

Adams, H., Ellis, T., Stanish, W.D., Sullivan, M.J., 2007. Psychosocial factors related to return to work following rehabilitation of whiplash injuries. J. Occup. Rehabil. 17 (2), 305–315.

Airaksinen, O., Brox, J.I., Cedraschi, C., et al., 2006. European guidelines for the management of chronic nonspecific low back pain. Eur. Spine J. 15 (Suppl. 2), S192–S300.

Becker, P.D., McGregor, N., Meirleirxy, K.D., 2002. Possible triggers and mode of onset of chronic fatigue syndrome. J. Chronic Fatigue Syndr. 10 (2), 3–18.

Blijenberg, G., Knoop, H., 2011. Chronic fatique syndrome: where to Pace from here? Lancet 377, 786–788.

Bourke, J.H., Johnson, A.L., Sharpe, M., et al., 2014. Pain in chronic fatigue syndrome: response to rehabilitative treatments in the PACE trial. Psychol. Med. 44 (07), 1545–1552.

Buitenhuis, J., de Jong, P.J., Jaspers, J.P., Groothoff, J.W., 2008. Catastrophizing and causal beliefs in whiplash. Spine 33 (22), 2427–2433.

Burgess, M., 2006. Physiological aspects of CFS. <https://www.kcl.ac.uk.>

Burns, D., Bennett, C., McGough, A., 2012. Chronic fatigue syndrome or myalgic encephalomyelitis. Nurs. Stand. 26 (25), 48–56.

Cairns, R., Hotopf, M., 2005. A systematic review describing the prognosis of chronic fatigue syndrome. Occup. Med. 55 (1), 20–31.

Castell, B.D., Kazantzis, N., Moss-Morris, R.E., 2011. Cognitive behavioural therapy and graded exercise for chronic fatigue syndrome: A meta-analysis. Clin. Psychol. Sci. Pr. 18 (4), 311–324.

Crul, B.J.P., Van Houdenhove, B., Perez, R.S.G.M. e.a., 2007. Pijn info: Thema Cognitieve gedragstherapie bij patiënten met chronische pijn. Bohn Stafleu van Loghum, Houten.

Dowsett, E.G., 1992. Conversation piece. Postgrad. Med. J. 68, 63–65.

Engel, G.L., 1980. The clinical application of the biopsychosocial model. Am. J. Psychiatry 137, 535–544.

Flor, H., Birbaumer, N., Schulz, R., et al., 2002. Pavlovian conditioning of opioid and nonopioid pain inhibitory mechanisms in humans. Eur. J. Pain 6 (5), 395–402.

Fordyce, W.E., 1976. Behavioural methods for chronic pain and illness. C. V Mosby, St. Louis, MO.

Friedberg, F., Jason, L.A., 1998. Understanding chronic fatigue syndrome. An empirical guide to assessment and treatment. APA, Washington DC, pp. 150–158.

Garralda, M.E., Rangel, L., 2002. Annotation: chronic fatigue syndrome in children and adolescents. J. Child Psychol. Psychiatry 43 (2), 169–176.

Garralda, M.E., Rangel, L., Levin, M., et al., 1999. Psychiatric adjustment in adolescents with a history of chronic fatigue syndrome. J. Am. Acad. Child Adolesc. Psychiatry 38 (12), 1515–1521.

Gatzounis, R., Schrooten, M.G., Crombez, G., Vlaeyen, J.W., 2012. Operant learning theory in pain and chronic pain rehabilitation. Curr. Pain Headache Rep. 16 (2), 117–126.

Geraets, J.J., Goossens, M.E., de Groot, I.J., et al., 2005. Effectiveness of a graded exercise therapy program for patients with chronic shoulder complaints. Aust. J. Physiother. 51 (2), 87–94.

Goubert, L., Vlaeyen, J.W., Crombez, G., Craig, K.D., 2011. Learning about pain from others: an observational learning account. J. Pain 12, 167–174.

Goudsmit, E.M., Howes, S., 2008. Pacing: a strategy to improve energy management in chronic fatigue syndrome. Health Psychol Update 17, 46–52.

Goudsmit, E.M., Ho-Yen, D.O., Dancey, C.P., 2009. Learning to cope with chronic illness. Efficacy of a multi-component treatment for people with chronic fatigue syndrome. Patient Educ. Couns. 77, 231–236. doi:10.1016/j.pec.05.015.

Goudsmit, E.M., Jason, L.A., Nijs, J., Wallman, K.E., 2012. Pacing as a strategy to improve energy management in myalgic encephalomyelitis/chronic fatigue syndrome: a consensus document. Disabil. Rehabil. 34 (13), 1140–1147.

Hickie, I., Davenport, T., Wakefield, D., et al., 2006. Post-infective and chronic fatigue syndromes precipitated by viral and non-viral pathogens: prospective cohort study. BMJ 333 (7568), 575. <http://dx.doi.org/10.1136/bmj.38933.585764.AE.>

Hlobil, H., Staal, J.B., Twisk, J., et al., 2005. The effects of a graded activity intervention for low back pain in occupational health on sick leave, functional status and pain: 12-month results of a randomized controlled trial. J. Occup. Rehabil. 15 (4), 569–580.

Horton, S.M., Poland, F., Kale, S., et al., 2010. Chronic fatigue syndrome/myalgic encephalomyelitis (CFS/ME) in adults: a qualitative study of perspectives from professional practice. BMC Fam. Pract. 11 (1), 1.

Jason, L.A., Sorenson, M., Porter, N., Belkairous, N., 2011. An etiological model for myalgic ncephalomyelitis/chronic fatigue syndrome. Neurosci. Med. 2, 14–27.

Jason, L.A., Tryon, W.W., Taylor, R.R., et al., 1999. Monitoring and assessing symptoms of chronic fatigue syndrome: use of time series regression. Psychol. Rep. 85, 121–130.

Klinger, R., Matter, N., Kothe, R., et al., 2010. Unconditioned and conditioned muscular responses in patients with chronic back pain and chronic tension-type headaches and in healthy controls. Pain 150 (1), 66–74.

Knoop, H., 2011. Cognitive behavior therapy for chronic fatigue syndrome: where to go from here? Clin. Psychol. Sci. Prac. 18, 325–330.

Köke, A., Wilgen, P., van Engers, A., Geilen, M., 2007. Graded activity: Een gedragsmatige behandelmethode voor paramedici. Bohn Stafleu van Loghum, Houten, Nederland.

Lambeek, L.C., Mechelen, W., van Knol, D.L., et al., 2010. Randomised controlled trial of integrated care to reduce disability from chronic low back pain in working and private life. Br. Med. J. 340, c1035.

Leeuw, M., Goossens, M.E., Linton, S.J., et al., 2007. The fear-avoidance model of musculoskeletal pain: current state of scientific evidence. J. Behav. Med. 30 (1), 77–94.

Lindström, I., Öhlund, C., Eek, C., et al., 1992. Mobility, strength, and fitness after a graded activity program for patients with subacute low back Pain: a randomized prospective clinical study with a behavioral therapy approach. Spine 17 (6), 641–652.

Macedo, L.G., Smeets, R.J., Maher, C.G., et al., 2010. Graded activity and graded exposure for persistent nonspecific low back pain: a systematic review. Phys. Ther.

Malouff, J.A., Thorsteinsson, E.B., Rooke, S.E., et al., 2008. Efficacy of cognitive behavioral therapy for chronic fatigue syndrome: a meta-analysis. Clin. Psychol. Rev. 28, 736–745.

Moss-Morris, R., Sharon, C., Tobin, R., Baldi, J.C., 2005. A randomized controlled graded exercise trial for chronic fatigue syndrome: outcomes and mechanisms of change. J. Health Psychol. 10 (2), 245–259.

National Institute for Health and Clinical Excellence. 2007. Clinical guideline CG53. Chronic fatigue syndrome/myalgic encephalomyelitis (or encephalopathy): diagnosis and management. <http://guidance.nice.org.uk/CG53.>

Price, J.R., Mitchell, E., Tidy, E., Hunot, V., 2008. Cognitive behaviour therapy for chronic fatigue syndrome in adults. Cochrane Database Syst. Rev. (3). doi:10.1002/14651858.CD001027.pub2.

Prins, J.B., Van der Meer, J.W., Bleijenberg, G., 2006. Chronic fatigue syndrome. Lancet 367, 346–355.

Ramsay, A.M., 1978. 'Epidemic neuromyasthenia' 1955–1978. Postgrad. Med. J. 54, 718–721.

Ramsay, A.M., 1988. Myalgic encephalomyelitis and postviral fatigue states: the saga of Royal Free disease. Gower Medical for the Myalgic Encephalomyelitis Association.

Ray, C., Weir, W., Stewart, D., et al., 1993. Ways of coping with chronic fatigue syndrome: development of an illness management questionnaire. Soc. Sci. Med. 37 (3), 385–391.

Rimes, K.A., Chalder, T., 2005. Treatments for chronic fatigue syndrome. Occup. Med. 55 (1), 32–39.

Rossignol, M., Arsenault, B., Dionne, C., et al., 2007. Clinic on Low-Back Pain in Interdisciplinary Practice (CLIP) Guidelines.

Montreal, Quebec, Canada: Direction de Santé Publique, Agence de la Santé et des Services Sociaux de Montréal.

Sharpe, M., Goldsmith, K.A., Johnson, A.L., et al., 2015. Rehabilitative treatments for chronic fatigue syndrome: long-term follow-up from the PACE trial. Lancet Psychiatry 2 (12), 1067–1074.

Shepherd, C., 2016. Patient reaction to the PACE trial. Lancet Psychiatry. 3 (2), e7–e8. doi:10.1016/S2215-0366(15)00546-5.

Staal, J.B., Hlobil, H., Twisk, J.W., et al., 2004. Graded activity for low back pain in occupational health care: a randomized, controlled trial. Ann. Intern. Med. 140 (2), 77–84. doi:10.7326/0003-4819-140-2-200401200-00007.

White, P.D., Chalder, T., Sharpe, M., 2015. The planning, implementation and publication of a complex intervention trial for chronic fatigue syndrome: the PACE trial. BJPsych. Bull 39 (1), 24–27.

White, P., Goldsmith, K., Johnson, A., et al., 2011. 'Comparison of adaptive pacing therapy, cognitive behaviour therapy, graded exercise therapy, and specialist medical care for chronic fatigue syndrome (PACE): a randomised trial'. Lancet 377 (9768), 823–836. doi:10.1016/S0140-6736(11)60096-2.

White, P.D., Goldsmith, K., Johnson, A.L., et al., 2013. 'Recovery from chronic fatigue syndrome after treatments given in the PACE trial'. Psychol. Med. 1–9. doi:10.1017/S0033291713000020.

White, A.T., Light, A.R., Hughen, R.W., et al., 2010. Severity of symptom flare after moderate exercise is linked to cytokine activity in chronic fatigue syndrome. Psychophysiology 47 (4), 615–624.

5.1.8   Medically Unexplained Physical Symptoms

ANNET DE JONG ■ MATTHIJS RÜMKE

SUMMARY

Patients with medically unexplained physical symptoms (MUPS) are a burden for caregivers. In this chapter we focus on what the mental health physiotherapist can contribute for patients with moderate-to-severe MUPS in primary care, in many cases in collaboration with other health professionals. Central sensitization is an etiological key mechanism in MUPS, which is a working hypothesis. Exploration of the symptoms using adequate communication is crucial, in order to respect the patient in his often-exhausting medical history. The low-threshold physical contact acts as a catalyst in the process of understanding the delayed or failed recovery. Before starting the intervention, a mental health physiotherapist should come to terms with the patient about an explanation model, of which four are presented. Interventions follow a stepped-care approach. Mental health physiotherapists should to complement the (potential) future blended care, especially in the more severe cases, because of their conducive personal and physical contact. Subsequently, 11 intervention methods are described; some of them are more explicit than others. Insight and self-regulation are the main goals in the intervention, where patients are invited to formulate their personal goals on a participation level. As an example, a case study is presented. Finally, an innovative group intervention in The Netherlands is described and evaluated.

KEY POINTS

■ Mental health physiotherapist, MUPS, sensitization, explanation model, low-threshold approach, inadequate coping, neurophysiological education.

■ The two preferred general approaches in MUPS are stepped care and blended care.

■ Elements of the beneficial Acceptance and Commitment Therapy are easily applicable.

■ Group therapy in MUPS addresses patients need of recognition and sharing.

LEARNING OBJECTIVES

■ Understand why a physiotherapist, specialized in mental health, takes a key position in coaching patients with medically unexplained physical symptoms (MUPS) in primary care.

■ Understand the importance of finding an explanation model that fits to the patient; possibly chosen from one of the described examples.

■ Become familiar with what the aims and the repertoire of a (primary care) physiotherapist in mental health in patients with MUPS are, individually as well as in a group.

INTRODUCTION

Patients with chronic pain and other physical symptoms make disproportionately high demands on healthcare workers. The search for the cause as well as for the solution of their symptoms is a burden for both patients and therapists, and costs them a lot in time, money and energy (den Boeft et al., 2016). This patient category is complicated and deserves enhanced care, usually by more than one profession (Rosendal et al., 2013).

Physiotherapists specialized in mental health are trained in coaching people with chronic pain and other symptoms that prevent them from participating in the community. In general physiotherapy the starting point in this specialism is a limitation in movement functioning. The very powerful instrument of physical contact enables the physiotherapist to deepen the patient's understanding of the origin of his chronic symptoms.

Definition

In health care, many definitions are used to characterize this group of chronic symptom sufferers. In this chapter we chose the term medically unexplained physical symptoms (MUPS; in Dutch SOLK: Somatisch Onvoldoende Verklaarde Klachten), which is defined as:

'Physical symptoms that last for longer than a few weeks and which cannot be satisfactorily explained after adequate medical examination.'
(Olde Hartman et al., 2013)

Despite the fact that proving a somatic symptom as being medically unexplained is contentious (Sykes, 2012), we will use this term because of the scientific research that has started on the topic, after the appearance of two Dutch guidelines (Fisher et al., 2010, Olde Hartman et al., 2013). These provide some opportunity to define diagnostic as well as therapeutic solutions. In addition, MUPS is broader than the DSM-5 'somatic symptom disorder' (SSD); where 92% of patients with MUPS met the diagnostic criteria of the DSM IV (defined as somatoform disorder, undifferentiated somatoform disorder and pain disorder), only 46% of the same population fulfilled the more restrictive criteria of the DSM-5 on SSD (APA, 2013; Claassen-van Dessel et al., 2016). In this way, MUPS fits better with the primary care focus of this chapter.

In accordance with the guidelines of the Dutch College of General Practitioners, we distinguish three severity levels of MUPS, as shown in Box 1 (Olde Hartman et al., 2013).

It is important to stress that MUPS is a working hypothesis, based on the justified assumption that

---

BOX 1

1. Mild MUPS
   ■ light functional impairments, and
   ■ one or more MUPS symptoms in one or two clusters of symptoms[a]
2. Moderate-to-severe MUPS
   ■ moderate-to-severe functional symptoms, and
   ■ several MUPS symptoms in at least three clusters, and/or
   ■ duration longer than expected, related to the normal course of the concerning symptom
3. Severe MUPS
   prevalence of 2.5% of all MUPS cases *(Verhaak et al., 2006)*
   ■ serious functional impairments, and
   ■ MUPS in all clusters, and/or
   ■ duration at least 3 months

[a]Cardiopulmonary; gastrointestinal; general/neurological; musculoskeletal; nonspecific.

somatic pathology has been sufficiently excluded (Sharpe et al., 2006).

Prevalence

The prevalence of medically unexplained functional somatic symptoms in primary care in The Netherlands is high. The Dutch Multidisciplinary Guideline SOLK (2010) states that 30% to 60% of the somatic symptoms reported by general practitioners and medical specialists remain medically unexplained (Fisher et al., 2010). The most frequently occurring medically unexplained somatic symptoms in general practice are joint pain, lower back pain, headache, fatigue, chest pain and pain in the arms or legs (Breivik et al., 2006; Bekkering et al., 2011).

In some cases, especially dizziness in the elderly and tiredness, the illness which primarily was classified as MUPS appears to have a somatic cause after 1 year (Koch et al., 2009; Maarsingh et al., 2010).

Etiology

The etiology of MUPS is multifactorial. Especially with regard to chronic, musculoskeletal pain, central sensitization (CS) appears to be an important key mechanism (Woolf, 2011). Psychological distress as well as depression and anxiety can increase the level of CS (Jones & O'Shaughnessy, 2014).

Parental medically unexplained symptoms, sexual and physical abuse in childhood and childhood neglect are associated with a greater risk of medically unexplained symptoms in adulthood (Khan et al., 2003). In addition, risk factors in developing MUPS are: a long existing period of the symptoms, the experience of many different symptoms and also the experience of many functional impairments (Olde Hartman et al., 2013).

Paradigm

Instead of endless medical investigations and treatments, it is essential for patients with MUPS that their worries and concerns about their health are carefully addressed. The mere 10 minutes allocated to each patient for a general practitioner in The Netherlands will hardly be enough to guarantee the supposed positive effect of a good patient-physician relationship and communication. A physiotherapist specialized in

mental health has some more time available for patients. Moreover, this specialized physiotherapist is able to act on the cutting edge of soma and psyche, and can make patients aware of the relationship between those two elements by means of a physical, practical and thence low-threshold approach.

Mental health physiotherapy is preeminently an instrument to make patients, through experience and interpretation, understand how they can influence their body.

Levels of Complexity

In The Netherlands, mental health physiotherapeutic care uses four levels of complexity, which facilitate the therapist making therapeutic choices (Box 2) (Mulders et al., 2009). This division can be especially useful in MUPS.

Each level is also defined by the feasibility of the relationship between the patient and therapist. The mental health physiotherapist determines the complexity of the therapeutic relationship and the degree

---

BOX 2

COMPLEXITY LEVEL 1: UNCOMPLICATED
- Psychologically stable with a meaningful life
- Self-regulation is adequate, with respect to health problems and problems in life

COMPLEXITY LEVEL 2: SLIGHTLY COMPLICATED
- Some dysfunctional ideas about illness and/or illness behaviour
- Slightly limited self-efficacy

COMPLEXITY LEVEL 3: MODERATELY COMPLICATED
- Ideas about illness and illness behaviour are dysfunctional to such an extent that education alone is insufficient
- Health problem affects several areas of the patient's life
- Personality characteristics that are unbeneficial for the patient's recovery process
- Self-direction is hampered by life issues

COMPLEXITY LEVEL 4: SEVERELY COMPLICATED
- Ideas about illness and illness behaviour are dysfunctional to such an extent that education alone is insufficient
- Personality characteristics that hamper the patient's recovery
- Psychopathological problems (e.g., depression)

of responsiveness relating to it. On a scale of 1–4, each larger level of complexity requires a broader arsenal of competences.

Whereas the domain of the general physiotherapist is confined to slightly complicated symptoms, the domain of the mental health physiotherapist, through far-reaching knowledge and skills, extends to moderately and severely complicated symptoms. The level of complexity dictates the intensity of the cooperation with other care providers. This classification matches the later discussed stepped-care method, which is recommended in the treatment of MUPS.

Diagnostic Phase

When, in daily practice, can a physical symptom for which a patient sees a physical therapist, like musculoskeletal pain, tiredness or dizziness, be classified as MUPS? As a matter of fact, we do not have a clear-cut answer to this question, nor any scientific proof. A suggested, practical implication of the mentioned Guideline of the Dutch College of General Practitioners for the mental health physiotherapist is the criterion that recovery, or at least the beginning of recovery, should set in within 4 weeks of the patient's first visit to the physiotherapist. This term, among other factors, is the physical recovery time for damaged collagen. When, however, there are no signs of recovery after 4 weeks, factors that hamper normal physical recovery could be involved (de Morree, 2009).

A careful physical examination and good communication are essential (Stewart, 1995). To be sure that he does not forget any aspect of the patient's experience, the mental health physiotherapist uses the SCEBS acronym, indicating the exploration of the somatic, cognitive, emotional, behavioural and social dimension of the symptoms (Olde Hartman et al., 2013). In addition, we need to investigate the patient's medical history, in the context of his life history, and the way he deals with it. Working out the various elements of this procedure could very well be the core competency of mental health physiotherapy.

Physical contact during the examination is very important and contributes to the respect for the presented complaint and, in this way, also for the individual. The physiotherapist in mental health can point directly at a detected increase in muscle tension and he can ask questions about it in order to make the patient become aware of this tension. Because he is the specialist in muscles and joints he will be able to speak with a certain authority. He can, for example, explain that the reaction of the muscles, although aberrant, still falls within the normal, physiological definitions, and therefore is no cause for concern.

Clinimetrics

The mental health physiotherapist uses various measurement instruments, as well diagnostics, to assess the factors that impede recovery, as well as to evaluate interventions. The instruments in Table 1 are not comprehensive; it would not be difficult to find other instruments on similar constructs, in an appropriate language.

Explanation Model

When physical recovery fails without any somatic reason, there are three possibilities: the involvement of an illness perception that hampers recovery, factors that negatively influence the coping style required for recovery or a combination of the two. The psychosomatic physiotherapist can make these possibilities transparent and, within certain limits, control them. As mentioned before, this requires clear communication between patient and therapist. But first of all, the general association of patients who suffer from symptoms that cannot be explained from a medical point of view should be taken into account. Within established healthcare, one tends to label MUPS as 'problems that are all in the patient's head'. From there, it is a small step to associating MUPS with affectation, fabrication and even mental illness; a widespread misunderstanding! Therefore, explicit capacities are required from the mental health physiotherapist in order to make the right translation of the patient's physical problems into an acceptable explanation model (Nijs et al., 2013). Direct acknowledgement of the symptoms opens the way to a clear look at illness perception as well as (other) factors that hamper the recovery process.

In deploying an explanation model, the therapist must take into account a number of things:

- Connect to the patient's perception.
- Acknowledge the physical component of the complaint.

	TABLE 1	
	Screening and Evaluative Questionnaires in MUPS	
Instrument (Abbreviation)	**Full Name**	**Construct**
4DSQ	Four Dimensional Symptoms Questionnaire	The presence of psychiatric diseases (distress, fear, depression, somatization)
CSI	Central Sensitization Inventory	Sensitization
PSS	Perceived Stress Scale	Stress
AAQ	Acceptance and Action Questionnaire	Acceptance of the situation and willingness to take action
IPQ-k	Illness Perception Questionnaire (short version)	Illness perceptions
G/P SES	General/Pain Self-Efficacy Scale	Self-efficacy
MVI	Multidimensionele Vermoeidheids Index	Tiredness
BSQ	Body Sensation Questionnaire	Body awareness
PCI	Pain Coping Inventory	Coping style
UCL	Utrechtse Coping List	Coping style
TSK	Tampa Scale for Kinesiophobia	Fear of movement
AEQ	Avoidance Endurance Questionnaire	Level of avoidance and endurance
RAND 36	RAND-36 item Health Survey	Quality of life
PSK	Patient Specific Complaints	Impairment in functioning in daily life
VAS	Visual Analogue Scale	Severity of difficult constructs (pain, insight, etc.)

- Begin by mentioning practical examples instead of talking about the client's situation.
- Let the client formulate the answer.
- Visualize the explanation model, filled in with the specific, patient-related examples.

Continuation of the treatment with adequate interventions will only be useful if the therapist and the patient have achieved consensus on the explanation model. Among a large amount of adequate explanation models we suggest the following four models as best applicable in MUPS:

1. The sensitization model (Woolf 2011, van Wilgen & Keizer, 2012)

   Central sensitization can be defined as an amplification of neural signalling within the central nervous system that elicits pain. It is the process of overactivity of the central nervous system that especially explains chronic pain, where there is no tissue damage. In, for example, fibromyalgia, chronic low-back pain, chronic fatigue syndrome, temporomandibular joint disorder, chronic whiplash and tension type headache, this model is very useful to explain the persistence of the symptoms.

2. The avoidance endurance model (AEM)

   The well-known fear-avoidance model has been amplified by Monica Hasenbring with the AEM (Vlaeyen & Linton, 2000; Hasenbring & Verbunt, 2010). In this, she added two more inadequate response patterns to acute pain, which makes the model more nuanced and provides a therapeutic possibility for dealing with exceedance of limitations (Fig. 1).

   The first one is the pattern of endurance of physical behaviour by neglecting the acute pain. People react with unstructured distraction and get depressed. They still carry on, exceed their limitations and muscular hyperactivity leads to chronic pain.

   The second dysfunctional response pattern is about people who succeed in adequate distraction, which leads to a positive mood. But they also forget their limitations and muscular hyperactivity also leads to chronic pain.

   The last response pattern is a functional pattern. There is a flexible, healthy balance between avoidance and endurance in physical activities, which leads to pain reduction.

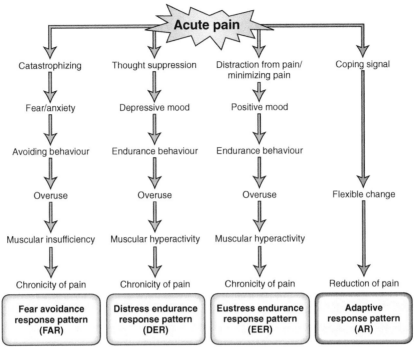

FIGURE 1 ■ The avoidance-endurance model.

3. The relational frame theory (RFT) (Hayes et al., 2006)

The RFT argues that words, pictures and observations can get a meaning or interpretation that differs from their original one. After some time, people might become caught within their inadequate thoughts and interpretations, forgetting the original perspective ('cognitive fusion'). For example, 'with my back pain I can never go to work'. In cognitive defusion this statement has to be distinguished from just 'the thought' that I can never go to work.

Acceptance and commitment therapy (ACT; mentioned later in the therapy section) is a treatment method based on the RFT and claims to increase psychological flexibility in cases of inadequate thoughts and behaviour. Besides cognitive defusion, other elements of this method are 'acceptance', strategies to accomplish personal values and goals and 'contact with the here-and-now'. Mental health physiotherapists can use these elements in a very natural way for coaching people with MUPS, possibly in collaboration with mental professionals.

4. The common-sense model

This explanatory model describes the ideas people have about the duration of a complaint and about what exactly is going on, the reasons for the complaint, how to control it, and how seriously they take their complaint. The starting point of the model is a health-threatening factor such as back pain, headache, rheumatism or arthritis. Humans react to these factors cognitively as well as emotionally, creating certain perceptions. These perceptions appear to be directive for the behaviour people show. The intention of this behaviour is to eliminate the health-threatening factor. By means of a feedback loop the patient evaluates the situation in order to determine whether the threat has decreased. In English literature, this human demeanour is known as *common sense* (Leventhal et al., 2003). The model was research tested, showing that behaviour is particularly directed by cognitive perceptions (illness perceptions). These illness perceptions are described in five domains that encompass the following questions:

- What is wrong with me?
- How long will my problem last?
- What are the consequences?
- How can I control my problem?
- What is the cause of my problem?

The answers to these questions partly (and most of the time implicitly) determine the patient's physical behaviour. This behaviour could either hamper or stimulate recovery. It could make a patient who is suffering from lower back pain think that their health problem will last for a long period of time, will have severe consequences and that there is nothing they can do about it themselves. When people think that their back pain is going to be a long-lasting problem, this will have a huge negative impact on their lives and they themselves are powerless, their level of movement dysfunction is higher than with people who do not have these ideas. These perceptions could hamper the recovery process towards normal functional movement.

Questioning the patient about his illness beliefs is both a diagnostic and a functional intervention tool. In less complicated cases, working out the illness beliefs in itself can prove to be an effective intervention, which, by drawing on the patient's medical history, gives both therapist and patient a clear understanding of the situation.

At all times, the invitation to choose a fitting explanation model should come from the patient. It is no exception that the patient needs some time to consider any possible mechanisms that slow down or, for that matter, make recovery impossible. In Box 3 the core ingredients of the diagnostic procedure are summarized.

Intervention Phase (Box 4)

The two general approaches to deal with MUPS in primary care are stepped-care approaches and blended care. The stepped-care method refers to a schedule, starting with the lightest possible effective treatment (Bower & Moseley, 2005). When this does not reach

---

BOX 3

Core ingredients of the diagnostic procedure of mental health physiotherapy in MUPS:
1. Acknowledgement of the symptoms
2. Acquiring insight into the thoughts and factors that hamper the recovery process
3. Mutual consensus on a fitting explanation model.

---

the target effect, a more severe level of treatment is used, and so on. Blended care is a promising combination of face-to-face contact and digital support, such as E-health. In patients with depression, a blended care intervention seems effective (Kooistra et al., 2016). Nevertheless, we think that the personal contact provides some extra value, especially for the more severe cases of MUPS, where the therapist is able to make a personalized link between soma and the psyche.

Before starting the therapy we advise drafting a contract with the patient, in order to increase therapy adherence. In this, the specific and time-contingent goals are formulated and signed by the patient.

Individual Intervention

An extensive collection of merely evidence-based interventions is used in moderate-severe and severe MUPS:

- Body-orientated exercises
  The patient's body is the ever-surprising gateway to understand his coping style. It is like a mirror that shows the patient how they treat their body and cope with their actual physical pain. In fact, physical behaviour is a metaphor for human behaviour. The prime objective of these interventions is to make the patient aware of his personal way of interpreting his body, when it comes to recognizing and acknowledging what his body tells him and how he copes with this information. Examples are, for instance, the body exercises with boundaries. The powerful advantage of the physical contact can be used as a catalyst in the process of understanding the origin of the symptoms.
- Neurophysiological education
  Education about the origin of the symptoms is an important task for the mental health

Frederike Blok goes to see her family doctor for the fourth time this month. She is irritated, angry and tense. For several weeks now she has suffered from severe lower back pain that is increasingly hampering her daily functioning. She is having sleeping problems as well as increasing concentration problems, and is feeling more and more miserable. It has been exactly 3 months since she misstepped while running. Since she had back problems a few years ago, that forced her to take bed rest for quite some time, she immediately went to see her family doctor, primarily to prevent a repetition of these problems at all cost. Thinking about the event alone gives her nightmares. Moreover, she is very busy at work, and the kitchen and living room are being painted; quite a daunting situation in combination with two children reaching adolescence.

At her first visit, the family doctor physically examined her. He tested her reflexes, senses, mobility, etc. Although the examination was painful, the doctor could not find anything out of the ordinary. His advice was to take it easy and, at the same time, to keep moving. Together with some painkillers, this should solve the problem. After a 10-minute consultation, Frederike left the doctor's office with a prescription for pills she could conveniently pick up at the pharmacy before going to work.

The painkillers worked—a little. But a week later, after having stopped taking them, it turned out that her back pain had worsened. Bearing in mind what had happened to her back before, Frederike once again went to see her family doctor. After having examined her, he came to the same conclusion as before: no particularities. Frederike had no intention to leave the doctor's office empty-handed. Things simply could not go on like this. With a packed waiting room in the back of his mind, the doctor eventually sent her to a physiotherapist. Although Frederike was pleased with this decision, she was not fully at ease. Was the doctor having doubts about what was wrong with her? Was something the matter after all? Perhaps the physiotherapist could help her. But after six visits to the physiotherapist she still had not made any progress. On the contrary, the physiotherapist had examined her thoroughly and, like the family doctor, had not found any peculiarities or abnormalities. As a matter of fact, he had asked a colleague of his, a manual therapist, to look into the matter. After careful examination, he too had come to the same conclusion.

physiotherapist. We suggest that this education is linked very closely to the patient-specific manifestations, from the cognitive as well as from the physical experience perspective (Butler & Moseley, 2003; Nijs et al., 2011).

■ Relaxation techniques

Progressive relaxation, applied relaxation, autogenic training and mindfulness-based stress reduction are effective methods to decrease sensitization levels in people with MUPS; besides the therapeutic session, patients are recommended to implement these exercises in their daily life (Lehrer et al., 2007; Zonneveld et al., 2012).

■ Massage

Massage has an added effect on exercises and on self-regulation, education concerning pain and function (Furlan et al., 2009). We do not particularly recommend the classic massage, but merely a massage during which the patient is invited to communicate with the physiotherapist about the various qualities of what he feels. This is part of the process of improvement of body awareness.

■ Cognitive behavioural-like interventions (for example ACT)

The mental health physiotherapist offers a suitable setting to deal with the various elements of ACT. For example, the acceptance that pain is part of life, or the capacity to focus on the here and now can be braided in a natural way into the therapy (Veehof et al., 2011 and 2016; van Ravesteijn et al., 2013).

■ Breathing exercises such as the van Dixhoorn method can be supportive to deal with breathing problems, like hyperventilation. This method focusses on the facilitation of a natural breathing pattern. The breathing does not need to be changed, but people are expected to be more aware of their breathing through very easy exercises (van Dixhoorn, 1998; Courtney et al., 2011).

■ Heart coherence training

Despite the weak evidence, heart coherence training might contribute to less pain by its propensity for self-regulation (Lehrer, 2007; McCraty & Shaffer, 2015).

■ Graded activity and graded exposure

By setting feasible goals a scheduled time-contingent programme is constructed, in order to confirm the patient's skills in performing activities. When people exhibit fear of movement a graded exposure approach is preferred (Macedo et al., 2010).

■ Aerobic exercises to increase physical condition

Physical exercises have been proven to contribute to mental health for conditions such as depression and anxiety (Danielsson et al., 2013; Wegner et al., 2014). Therefore, mental health physical therapists should incorporate these into their therapy.

■ Motivational interventions

To change persistent behavioural patterns that reinforce continuation of the MUPS symptoms, motivational interventions (such as motivational interviewing) are very well applicable for the mental health physiotherapist. They have benefits in supporting people to accomplish personal (lifestyle) goals, as well as to improve exercise adherence (McGrane et al., 2015).

■ Lifestyle interventions

It is necessary for the mental health physiotherapist to define and emphasize lifestyle prerequisites for recovery, like a healthy diet, adequate sleep pattern, regularity in activities versus rest and the amount of stress at work or in relationships. An easy way of finding out is to go through the patient's agenda from the previous week, day by day. Lifestyle coaching is a very basic and low-profile method of stress management, in which the mental health physiotherapist can fulfil an important role.

At a certain point, in higher level cases of complexity where we are faced with factors that hamper recovery such as relationship issues, problems at work or difficulties concerning the processing of traumatic experiences, we may find that we have reached the borders of our discipline. Then, explicit cooperation with other disciplines is required, such as a social worker, a psychologist, a psychiatrist or other specialists in mental healthcare. In the continuation of the case of Frederike, in Box 5, you will read a 'worse case scenario' where this cooperation is absent.

Group Intervention

Group therapy can have additional value to allow people experience that they are not alone with their complaints. Recently a group course has been developed for people with MUPS in primary care.

It contains eight sessions from 1.5 hours, led by a physiotherapist in mental health and a nurse practitioner. The general practitioner finishes the somatic procedure with the patient and screens with the 4 Dimensions Symptoms Questionnaire (4DSQ) on severe psychiatry (Terluin et al., 2006, 2014). High rates of depression and anxiety are contraindications to attend the course.

The nurse practitioner has two to three individual sessions with the patient, in which the personal goals are formulated and a commitment about the participation to the course is signed.

Each session focusses on a specific theme:

1. recognition of tension/relaxation in the body,
2. understanding the origin of the stress symptoms,
3. release/manage body tension,
4. using personal resources,
5. insight into essentials and side issues in your life,
6. awareness and communication of limitations,
7. breathing and personal space,
8. the impact of emotions on the body.

The interventions used in the course are similar to the individual sessions, except that the physical contact in the group is obviously less than in the individual sessions.

The time spent on theoretic explanation, practical exercises and group discussion is divided as 25%, 45% and 30%, respectively. The participants receive an illustrated handout, with written explanation, on what has been treated in the course. The homework and exercises are also described. There is a follow-up session 3 months after the end of the course.

The results of this group course have been evaluated in a healthcare center in The Netherlands, close to Amsterdam, in a lower socioeconomic status population. Data from 30 participants (from five groups) were collected and analysed. A small but significant increase in quality of life, on the physical as well as on the emotional part of the SF12 (i.e. Medical Outcomes Study 12-Item Short Form Health Survey), was detected after the course, which decreased somewhat after 3-months follow-up (Fig. 2). Concerning the amount at which participants reached their personal goals, a significant increase after the course was continued at 3-months follow-up (Fig. 3). This matches an important element of ACT, namely the focus on personal values and goals.

A larger trial on this group intervention is prepared, with special attention to the follow-up measures.

At the completion of the therapy, tuning with the other health professionals is necessary. In order to ratify or even celebrate the accomplished therapy goals, we suggest drafting a certificate, signed by the patient and the therapist, as a kind of final ritual.

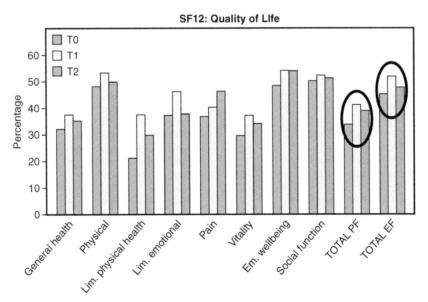

FIGURE 2 ■ Results of group intervention on quality of life (N = 30). EF, Emotional functioning; PF, physical functioning.

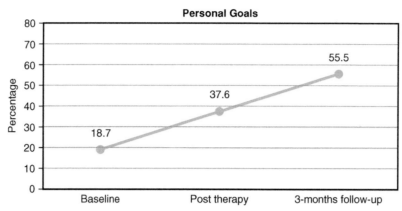

FIGURE 3 ■ Results of group intervention on the level of reaching personal goals.

REFERENCES

American Psychiatric Association, 2013. Diagnostic and Statistical Manual of Mental Disorders, fifth ed. (DSM-5). American Psychiatric Association, Arlington, VA.

Bekkering, G.E., Bala, M.M., Reid, K., et al., 2011. Epidemiology of chronic pain and its treatment in The Netherlands. Neth. J. Med. 69, 141.

Bower, P., Gilbody, S., 2005. Stepped care in psychological therapies: access, effectiveness and efficiency. Narrative literature review. Br. J. Psychiatry 186, 11–17.

Breivik, H., Collet, B., Ventafridda, V., et al., 2006. Survey of chronic pain in Europe. Eur. J. Pain 10, 287–333.

Butler, D.S., Moseley, G.L., 2003. Explain Pain. Noigroup Publications, Adelaide.

Claassen-van Dessel, N., van der Wouden, J.C., Dekker, J., van der Horst, H.E., 2016. Clinical value of DSM IV and DSM 5 criteria for diagnosing the most prevalent somatoform disorders in patients with medically unexplained physical symptoms (MUPS). J. Psychosom. Res. 82, 4–10.

Courtney, R., van Dixhoorn, J., Greenwood, K.M., Anthonissen, E.L.M., 2011. Medically unexplained dyspnea: partly moderated by dysfunctional (thoracic dominant) breathing pattern. J. Asthma Early Online, 1–7, ISSN: 0277-0903 print / 1532-4303 online.

Danielsson, L., Noras, A.M., Waern, M., Carlsson, J., 2013. Exercise in the treatment of major depression: a systematic review grading the quality of evidence. Physiother. Theory Pract. 29 (8), 573–585.

de Morree, J.J., 2009. Bindweefselbeschadiging en herstel. Bohn Stafleu van Loghum: Dynamiek van het menselijk bindweefsel; functie, beschadiging en herstel. (5ᵉ druk): 59–80.

den Boeft, M., Twisk, J.W., Terluin, B., et al., 2016. The association between medically unexplained physical symptoms and health care use over two years and the influence of depressive and anxiety disorders and personality traits: a longitudinal study. BMC Health Serv. Res. 16 (1), 100.

Fisher, E.R., Boerema, I., Franx, G., 2010. Multidisciplinaire richtlijn somatisch onvoldoende verklaarde lichamelijke klachten en somatoforme stoornissen. Trimbos-instituut in opdracht van de Landelijke Stuurgroep Multidisciplinaire Richtlijnontwikkeling, Utrecht. ISBN: 978-90-5253-699-6.

Furlan, A.D., Imamura, M., Dryden, T., Irvin, E., 2009. Massage for low back pain: an updated systematic review within the framework of the Cochrane back review Group. Spine 34 (16), 1669–1684.

Hasenbring, M.I., Verbunt, J.A., 2010. Fear-avoidance and endurance-related responses to pain: new models of behavior and their consequences for clinical practice. Clin. J. Pain 26, 747–753.

Hayes, S.C., Luoma, J., Bond, F., et al., 2006. Acceptance and commitment therapy: model, processes and outcomes. Behav. Res. Ther. 44, 1–25.

Jones, L.E., O'Shaughnessy, D.F., 2014. The pain and movement reasoning model: introduction to a simple tool for integrated pain assessment. Man. Ther. 19 (3), 2706.

Khan, A.A., Khan, A., Harezlak, J., et al., 2003. Somatic symptoms in primary care: etiology and outcome. Psychosom. 44 (6), 471–478.

Koch, H., van Bokhoven, M.A., ter Riet, G., et al., 2009. Ordering blood tests for patients with unexplained fatigue in general practice: what does it yield? Results of the VAMPIRE trial. Br. J. Gen. Pract. 59, e93–e100.

Kooistra, L.C., Ruwaard, J., Wiersma, J.E., et al., 2016. Development and initial evaluation of blended cognitive behavioural treatment for major depression in routine specialized mental health care. Elsevier Internet Interventions 4 (Pt 1), 61–71. <http://dx.doi.org/10.1016/j.invent.2016.01.003.>

Lehrer, P.M., Woolfolk, R.L., Sime, W.E. (Eds.), 2007. Principles and practice of stress management, 3rd ed. The Guilford Press, New York, pp. 227–248.

Leventhal, H., Brissette, I., Leventhal, E.A., 2003. The common sense model of self-regulation of health and illness. In: Cameron, L.D., Leventhal, H. (Eds.). behaviour. The self-regulation of health and illness behaviour. Routledge, New York, pp. 42–65.

Maarsingh, O.R., Dros, J., Schellevis, F.G., et al., 2010. Causes of persistent dizziness in elderly patients in primary care. Ann. Fam. Med. 8, 196–205.

Macedo, L.G., Smeets, R.J., Maher, C.G., et al., 2010. Graded activity and graded exposure for persistent nonspecific low back pain: a systematic review. Phys. Ther. 90 (6), 860–879.

McCraty, R., Shaffer, F., 2015. Heart rate variability: new perspectives on physiological mechanisms, assessment of self-regulatory capacity, and health risk. Glob. Adv. Health Med. 4 (1), 46–61.

McGrane, N., Galvin, R., Cusack, T., Stokes, E., 2015. Addition of motivational interventions to exercise and traditional physiotherapy: a review and meta-analysis. Physiotherapy 101 (1), 1–12.

Mulders, N., Boersma, R., Ijntema, R., Coppoolse, R., 2009. Beroepscompetentieprofiel Psychosomatische Fysiotherapie NFP. Nederlandse Vereniging voor Fysiotherapie volgens de Psychosomatiek, Amersfoort.

Nijs, J., Roussel, N., van Wilgen, P., et al., 2013. Thinking beyond muscles and joints: therapists' and patients' attitudes and beliefs regarding chronic musculoskeletal pain are key to applying effective treatment. Man. Ther. 18 (2), 96–102.

Nijs, J., van Wilgen, P., Van Oosterwijck, J., et al., 2011. How to explain central sensitization to patients with 'unexplained' chronic musculoskeletal pain: practice guidelines. Man. Ther. 16 (5), 413–418.

Olde Hartman, T., Blankenstein, A.H., Molenaar, A.O., et al., 2013. The NHG guideline medically unexplained symptoms (MUS). Huisarts Wet. 56 (5), 222–230.

Olde Hartman, T.C., Woutersen-Koch, H., Van Der Horst, H.E., 2013. Medically unexplained symptoms: evidence, guidelines, and beyond. Br. J. Gen. Pract. 63 (617), 625–626.

Rosendal, M., Blankenstein, A.H., Morriss, R., et al., 2013. Enhanced care by generalists for functional somatic symptoms and disorders in primary care. Cochrane Database Syst. Rev. (10), Art. No.: CD008142. doi:10.1002/14651858.CD008142.pub2.

Sharpe, M., Richard Mayou, R., Walker, J., 2006. Bodily symptoms: new approaches to classification. J. Psychosom. Res. 60 (4), 353–356.

Stewart, M.A., 1995. Effective physician-patient communication and health outcomes: a review. CMAJ 152, 1423–1433.

Sykes, R., 2012. Somatoform disorder and the DSM-V Workgroup's interim proposals: two central issues. Psychosomatics 53, 334.

Terluin, B., Smits, N., Miedema, B., 2014. The English version of the four-dimensional symptom questionnaire (4DSQ) measures the same as the original Dutch questionnaire: a validation study. European Journal of General Practice, 20:4, 320–326, doi:10.3109/13814788.2014.905826. [Epub 2014 Apr 29].

Terluin, B., Van Marwijk, H.W.J., Adèr, H.J., et al., 2006. The Four-Dimensional Symptom Questionnaire (4DSQ): a validation study of a multidimensional self-report questionnaire to assess distress, depression, anxiety and somatization. BMC Psychiatry 6, 34.

van Dixhoorn, J.J., 1998. Ontspanningsinstructie. Principes en oefeningen. Elsevier, Maarssen.

van Ravesteijn, H., Lucassen, P., Bor, H., et al., 2013. Mindfulness-based cognitive therapy for patients with medically unexplained symptoms: a randomized controlled trial. 82, Nijmegen. Psychother. Psychosom. 299–310.

Veehof, M.M., Oskam, M.J., Schreurs, K.M.G., Bohlmeijer, E.T., 2011. Acceptance-based interventions for the treatment of chronic pain: a systematic review and meta-analysis. Pain 152 (3), 533–542.

Veehof, M.M., Trompetter, H.R., Bohlmeijer, E.T., Schreurs, K.M.G., 2016. Acceptance- and mindfulness-based interventions for the treatment of chronic pain: a metaanalytic review. Cogn. Behav. Ther. 45 (1), 5–31. doi:10.1080/16506073.2015.1098724.

Verhaak, P.F., Meijer, S.A., Visser, A.P., Wolters, G., 2006. Persistent presentation of medically unexplained symptoms in general practice. Fam. Pract. 23, 414–420.

Vlaeyen, J.W., Linton, S.J., 2000. Fear-avoidance and its consequences in chronic musculoskeletal pain: a state of the art. Pain 85 (3), 317–332.

Wegner, M., Helmich, I., Machado, S., et al., 2014. Effects of exercise on anxiety and depression disorders: review of meta-analyses and neurobiological mechanisms. CNS Neurol. Disord. Drug Targets 13 (6), 1002–1014. Review.

van Wilgen, C.P., Keizer, D., 2012. The sensitization model to explain how chronic pain exists without tissue damage. Pain Manag. Nurs. 13 (1), 60–65.

Ware, J.E., Kosinkski, M., Keller, S.D., 1998. SF-12 How to Score the SF-12 Physical and Mental health Summary Scales. QualityMetric Incorporated, Lincoln, RI.

Woolf, C.J., 2011. Central sensitization: implications for the diagnosis and treatment of pain. Pain 152 (3 Suppl.), S2–S15.

Zonneveld, L.N.L., van Rood, Y.R., Timman, R., et al., 2012. Effective group training for patients with unexplained physical symptoms: a randomized controlled trial with a non-randomized one-year follow-up. PLoS ONE 7 (8), e42629.

5.1.9 Distress and Stress Overload

MIEKE VAN WIJK-ENGBERS ■ A. HAGEN

SUMMARY

This chapter describes distress and stress overload. Stress overload is a serious disease. Even after recovery a person remains more sensitive to (work-related) stress sources for at least 1-month. In general practice, prevalence rates vary from 2–3 to as many as 20 per 1000 patients. Stress is a large financial problem in society. In The Netherlands, physiotherapists in psychiatry and mental health specialize in recognizing and influencing the complex relationship between movement and psychological functioning. They treat physical symptoms, such as pain, fatigue and distress, in relation to psychosocial problems. This chapter describes the intervention for stress overload for the physiotherapist in psychiatry and mental health in The Netherlands.

KEY POINTS

■ Distress and stress overload.

■ Physical therapy in psychiatry and mental health in primary care.

LEARNING OBJECTIVES

■ The definition of distress and stress overload.

■ The symptoms of distress and stress overload.

■ The treatment of distress and stress overload for the physiotherapist in psychiatry and mental health in The Netherlands.

INTRODUCTION

Stress can be defined as a response to any stimulus or condition that causes tension. Stressors are conditions that are perceived as a threat. Stressors can be divided into three categories: requirements, problems and life events. When a person has difficulties in handling stressors, they may develop a condition of distress (Terluin et al., 2005), which could eventually lead to the disruption of their normal functioning. Distress has been described by Ridner (2004) as the perception of a stressor as a personal threat, an inability to handle the stressor, loss of control and a change in the person's emotional state. This is associated with feelings of discomfort, damage to health and social dysfunction. The distress symptoms can manifest themselves in both physical and psychological symptoms. As well as headaches, stomach aches, and neck and back pain, a number of specific symptoms can be defined, such as constant worrying, irritability, fatigue, general malaise, emotional lability, nervousness, sleeping disorders and impotence, as well as feelings of being overwhelmed, depression and despondency (Terluin, 1986). 'Coping' is the way a person reacts both behaviourally and cognitively in relation to their emotional adaptation abilities (Schreurs et al., 1993). Failure to cope means that a person shows an insufficiency in stress management. The person no longer knows what to do about their problem and loses their grip on the situation. These are traits of demoralization. People give up, call in sick and retreat from social interaction. In this way, a combination of psychological distress, demoralization and impairment in social and/or occupational functioning occurs (Terluin et al., 1995). In this chapter we describe this as 'stress overload' (Table 1).

TABLE 1
The Definition of Stress Overload

At least three of the following symptoms are present:

A: Fatigue, disturbed or troubled sleep, irritability, a hypersensitivity for crowds/noise, emotional lability, worrying, feeling rushed, difficulty concentrating and/or forgetfulness

B: Feelings of loss of control and/or powerlessness with regard to dealing with stressors in daily functioning. The person's stress management is inadequate: they are totally overwhelmed and feel like they are losing their grip altogether

C: Significant limitations in professional and/or social functioning

D: There could be more reasons for the patient's distress, loss of control and dysfunctional behaviour than a psychiatric disorder alone

Adapted from Verschuren et al., 2001.

The diagnosis stress overload is not mentioned in either the DSM-IV (American Psychiatric Association [APA], 1994) or in the ICD-10 (World Health Organization [WHO], 1992). However, it does have the traits of an *adjustment disorder*, a term that is used in the DSM-IV. In The Netherlands the National Primary Healthcare Collaboration Agreement (LESA) is recognized as a guide for stress overload (Verschuren et al., 2001).

RELEVANCE AND PREVALENCE

Although stress overload is an important social and economic problem, the data on incidence and prevalence are not always reliable. Estimates of relevance rates vary from 2.3 and 7.8 to as many as 20 per 1000 patients. These numbers reflect uncertain diagnoses from company doctors, general practitioners and primary care psychologists. In The Netherlands, the Second National Survey, which was carried out in 2004 among general practitioners, showed that 7.8 patients out of 1000 were diagnosed with stress overload with an average duration of 2 years. Stress overload was more often diagnosed in women than in men, with an annual incidence of 5.8 and 3.8 and a prevalence of 9.4 and 6.2, respectively (Verschuren et al., 2001; STECR, 2003)

Stress overload is a serious disease. Even after recovery, a person remains more sensitive to (work-related) stress sources for at least 1 month (Boerman et al.,

2010). Literature shows that after 1 year, 20% of people suffering from stress overload are still absent from work. Stress overload also leads to problems in other domains. The risk of acquiring a mental disorder, such as depression, increases. Surveys show that in a group of 2000 caregivers, 7% fell ill as a result of work overload (Engel, 1979). In higher education, 18% of students drop out due to stress overload. About 20,000 students are faced with study delay (Mulders et al., 2009) and some are forced to give up their studies altogether. The most important negative prognostic factor is avoidant behaviour based on unrealistic ideas; for example, the fear that problems will increase as soon as they return to work or study. Avoidance accounts for 48% of the variation influenced by factors such as illness perception, education and subjective complaints. Subjective health complaints that appear after a follow-up period of 3 months are important negative predictors with regard to returning to study or work. However, active coping significantly increases the person's chances of a successful return (Verschuren et al., 2001).

DEFINING SYMPTOMS AND TREATMENT

As yet, research shows no evidence for a fixed format for defining the severity of stress symptoms. In The Netherlands, the following sequence is applied:

stress ⇒ distress ⇒ stress overload ⇒ burnout

The specialist psychiatric and mental health physiotherapist maps the patient's (biographical) history using the SCEGS model (Van Weel-Baumgarten & Van Spaendonck, 2000). This model describes the patient's somatic symptoms, cognitions, emotions and behaviour, as well as their social environment. In Table 2 the symptoms of stress are briefly described, divided into SCEGS.

Specialist psychiatric and mental health physiotherapist in The Netherlands are trained in:

- recognizing and influencing the complex relationship between movement and psychological functioning and,
- the treatment of physical symptoms, such as pain, fatigue and distress in relation to psychosocial problems.

In The Netherlands, a protocol designed for the Dutch Association for Psychosomatic Physiotherapy (NFP) (Verschuren et al., 2001) is used for an efficient and effective approach to stress overload. Treatment is divided into three phases, defined as follows:

- crisis phase,
- problem and solution phase,
- application phase,

During the **crisis phase** (duration 1–3 weeks) the aim is to let the patient come to rest and regain control of their cognitive abilities and emotions. The patient needs to understand what has happened to them and accept their distress and stress overload. Here, an active

TABLE 2				
Frequently Occurring Symptoms With Stress Overload				
Somatic	**Cognitive**	**Emotional**	**Behavioural**	**Social**
Surfacing emotions	Forgetfulness	Emotionality	(Fear of) making mistakes	Irritability
Sleep problems	Concentration difficulties	Listlessness	Irritation	Increase in working hours
Sexual problems		Uncertainty	Changed coping abilities	Cynical attitude with respect to work and/or private life
Decreasing physical condition	Mulling	Mood swings	Increase in smoking and/or drinking behaviour	
Back, neck, muscle problems	Indecisiveness	Fatigue		
Weight change	Confused priorities	Decrease in motivation	Increase in drug abuse	Isolating
Palpitations			Inhibition	Less social interest
Gastric and/or intestinal problems		Feelings of guilt	Decreased performance	More social conflicts
Sweating				

attitude is expected from the patient. In many cases the patient finds themselves unable to carry out social or private activities and/or participate in the labour market.

Interventions at this stage provide:

1. Insight into the situation through explanation and education, for example by using the Scale Capacity and Load Capacity Models or the Burden-bearing Capacity Model (Terluin, 1996). By using the patient's personal circumstances as an example, the patient will gain insight into the possible targets regarding their individual capacity. This will stimulate the patient's motivation in following the proposed protocol.
   a. The Burden-bearing Capacity Model is a derivative of the (classic) Tax Load Model (Terluin, 1996).
   b. The Gaillard Stress Model analyses the relationship between the patient's mental-emotional load and their burden-bearing capacity. The model combines both the individual and their environment. It addresses the imbalance that may arise within, as well as outside, the individual. The individual's internal imbalance stems from the degree of nonspecific activation and selectivity on the one hand, and cognitive, emotional and behavioural functioning on the other (STECR, 2003; Van Burken, 2010).
2. Structure in the patient's immediate environment. The therapist offers the patient solid structure and uses the LESA phase model (Verschuren et al., 2001).
3. The opportunity to unwind. The therapist starts off with relaxation tools: mindfulness.
4. Activity (although in this phase one is advised to be cautious with physical activity).

During the **problem and solution phase** (duration about 3–6 weeks) the patient sorts out their problems by structuring them, asking themselves questions like: which problems are involved? how big are these problems? and what could be done about them? In general, picking up activities, such as work (whether or not on a partial basis), is useful if the patient has gained an insight into a concrete solution for at least part of their problem.

Interventions at this stage provide:

1. A cognitive behavioural approach, forming the basis of a (short) programme:
   a. The programme is aimed at improving problem-solving coping capacities
   b. Stressor identification and Problem Solving Therapy (PST)
   c. Rational Emotive Behavioural Therapy (REBT)
2. Relaxation exercises (mindfulness)
3. Physical activities
4. Homework exercises

Mindfulness, Rational Emotive Behavioural Therapy and Problem Solving Therapy

Mindfulness

Mindfulness is a form of attention and relaxation therapy. It is effective in many complaints where stress is the underlying reason. It has beneficial effects on psychological as well as physical functioning. Physical effects are, for example, pain relief and relaxation. Cognitive effects are a higher level of attention and reduced worrying. People are more aware of their emotional patterns and experience more positive emotions. In addition, people are more aware of their way of responding to situations and, as a result, respond less impulsively.

Mindfulness is a form of meditation that originates from Buddhism. It is based on the patient's focus on their physical and mental sensations at that time. It is characterized by the awareness present in the here and now, without having to judge. Jon Kabat-Zinn developed a training programme called *Mindfulness Based Stress Reduction* (MBSR). The method used in The Netherlands is based on the exercises described in the MBRS. The exercises that are used are the body scan (with attention to breathing), seated meditation and mindful movement.

Rational Emotive Behavioural Therapy

REBT is a cognitive behavioural intervention founded by Albert Ellis. The premise of this therapy is that emotional or behavioural problems are maintained by the thoughts and beliefs of the patient. Through awareness and change of these thoughts and beliefs, dysfunctional emotions and behaviour can be changed positively.

These views and thoughts are like lenses through which the patient perceives and evaluates themselves, others and the world around them. A positive turnaround is achieved by changing the dysfunctional thoughts and attitudes towards the dysfunctional behaviours and emotions. We apply the ABCD diagram:

■ A is the activating event, the reason for the occurrence of stress in the patient. In this scheme this is also called *the stressor*.
■ B stands for how situations are assessed by the patient. In other words their thoughts, opinions, ideas and beliefs about the cause of a situation.
■ C stands for the behavioural and emotional consequences of the assessment (B).
■ D stands for the review during which the dysfunctional ratings described in B are discussed and transformed into a functional view.

Problem Solving Therapy

PST is a brief psychological treatment aimed at reducing psychological symptoms associated with unresolved problems in daily life. During this treatment the therapist shows the patient the relationship between their complaints and their problems. As a result, the patient learns to accept and clearly define their issues and identify what needs to be changed. The therapist teaches the patient a systematic approach in order to deal more effectively with their obstacles.

PST has four major goals:

1. Clarifying the relationship between current complaints, symptoms and problems that one is faced with in daily life. The patient should be aware that problems are normal in everyday life, and accept that effectively solving these problems will make them feel better.
2. Teaching the patient to clearly define their current problems and to determine which problems they want to work on.
3. Offering the patient a specific procedure for dealing with structured learning problems. The patient is introduced to specific problem-solving skills, based on the issues they themselves are experiencing at that moment and which they wish to solve.

4. Providing the patient with positive experiences regarding their personal abilities in order to feel less pressurized, to improve their self-esteem and to feel more in control.

In the **application phase** (duration about 3–6 weeks) the patient applies their newly gained insights and skills in practical situations, and gradually resumes functioning in various roles. In order to be successful it is essential that the attitude of those surrounding the patient is supportive and cooperative.

The interventions applied at this stage of the treatment are similar to those used during the problem and solution phase. They are aimed at the patient's return to work and leisure activities, and the resumption of their social life.

The aforementioned protocol was specially designed for the NFP. It involves a multimodel stress programme in which a number of cognitive elements focus on problem-solving abilities:

■ Homework exercises, which are an absolute capital gain to the patient's recovery (a CD and a reader are issued),
■ The Scale Capacity and Load Capacity Models or the Burden-Bearing Capacity Model,
■ Relaxation tool (mindfulness),
■ Cognitive behavioural therapy: REBT, problem solving, positive thinking,
■ A minimum of seven sessions (up to 12) around cognitive behavioural therapy,
■ A clear therapy structure,
■ Following the phase structure,
■ Physical training combined with relaxation (a combination that has proven to be of great value).

The literature recommends that, in light of adherence, a follow-up is recommended 3 months after the final session.

CONCLUSIONS

■ Cognitive behavioural interventions show good results on several outcome measures elemental in a programme aimed at reducing psychological complaints (Van der Klink et al., 2001).
■ Research shows that relaxation interventions have a strong effect on the physiological outcome (Van der Klink et al., 2001).

■ It is plausible that physical training combined with relaxation and focus on the physical symptoms related to the work environment has a positive effect on symptoms (Van Rhenen et al., 2005).

The combination of mindfulness and cognitive therapy appears to be most effective for clients with distress (Boerman et al., 2010).

Adherence to this protocol aims to decrease complaints based on distress. When the client continues to apply the principles in their daily lives, they will experience a positive change of lifestyle as well as higher self-esteem and a positive view of their personal environment.

REFERENCES

American Psychiatric Association, 1994. Diagnostic and Statistical Manual of Mental Disorders, fourth ed. American Psychiatric Association, Washington, DC.

Boerman, H., Lelijveld, I., VanderMeer, J., et al., 2010. Dutch Association for Psychosomatic Physiotherapy (NFP). Protocol arbeidsgerelateerde stress. <http://psychosomatischefysiotherapie .nl.>

Engel, G.L., 1979. The biopsychosocial model and the education of health professionals. Gen. Hosp. Psychiatry 1 (2), 156–165.

Mulders, N., Boersma, R., Ijntema, R., Coppoolse, R., 2009. Beroepscompetentieprofiel psychosomatisch fysiotherapeut NFP. Nederlandse Vereniging voor Fysiotherapie volgens de Psychosomatiek. <http://www.psychosomatischefysiotherapie.nl/pdf/beroepscom petentieprofielnfp.pdf.>

Ridner, S.H., 2004. Psychological distress: concept analysis. J. Adv. Nurs. 45 (5), 536–545.

Schreurs, P.J.G., Van de Willige, G., Brosschot, J.F., et al., 1993. De Utrechtse Coping Lijst (UCL). Herziene handleiding. Swets & Zeitlinger, Lisse.

STECR, Platform re-integratie, 2003. Werkwijzer Werkstress: Reductie van werkstress in gezondheidszorg en onderwijs, versie 1. Hoofddorp: Platform re-integratie STECR. <http://www.stecr.nl/ uploaded_files/stecr-werkwijzer-werkstress-2004.pdf.>

Terluin, B., 1986. Surmenage in een huisartspraktijk. Een explorerend onderzoek. Huisarts Wet. 29, 261–264.

Terluin, B., 1996. De vierdimensionale klachtenlijst (4DKL). Een vragenlijst voor het meten van distress, depressie, angst en somatisatie. Huisarts Wet. 39 (12), 538–547.

Terluin, B., Van der Klink, J.J.L., Schaufeli, W.B., 2005. Stressgerelateerde klachten: Spanningsklachten, overspanning en burnout. In: Van der Klink, J.J.L., Terluin, B. (Eds.), Psychische problemen en werk. Handboek voor een activerende begeleiding door huisarts en bedrijfsarts. Bohn Stafleu Van Loghum, Houten, pp. 259–290.

Terluin, B., Winnubst, J.A.M., Gill, K., 1995. Kenmerken van patienten met de diagnose psychische surmenage in de huisartspraktijk. Ned. Tijdschr. Geneeskd 139, 1785–1789.

Van Burken, P., 2010. Gezondheidspsychologie voor de fysiotherapeut, second ed. revised. Bohn Stafleu van Loghum, Houten.

Van der Klink, J.J., Blonk, R.W., Schene, A.H., Van Dijk, F.J., 2001. The benefits of interventions for work-related stress. Am. J. Public Health 91 (2), 270–276.

Van Rhenen, W., Blonk, R.W., van der Klink, J.J., et al., 2005. The effect of a cognitive and a physical stress-reducing programme on psychological complaints. Int. Arch. Occup. Environ. Health 78 (2), 139–148.

Van Weel-Baumgarten, E.M., van Spaendonck, K.P.M., 2000. Communicatietraining in het nieuwe curriculum te Nijmegen: Van vraagverheldering naar verkenning van het referentiekader. Tijdschrift voor Medisch Onderwijs 19 (1), 16–20.

Verschuren, C.M., Nauta, A.P., Bastiaanse, M.H.H., et al., 2001. Eén Lijn in de eerste lijn bij overspanning en burnout: Multidisciplinaire richtlijn overspanning en burnout voor eerstelijns professionals. LVE, NHG, NVAB, Utrecht.

World Health Organization, 1992. The ICD-10 classification of mental and behavioural disorders: Clinical descriptions and diagnostic guidelines. World Health Organization, Geneva.

5.1.10   Physiotherapy Interventions in Individuals With a Burnout

LINDA SLOOTWEG ■ WILLEMIEN FOKKE ■ EVELIEN SWIERS

SUMMARY

This chapter describes the Dutch approach to multidisciplinary treatment for burnout syndrome. A process-contingent approach helps the patient to enhance or regain their problem-solving abilities and is divided into three phases: (1) crisis phase, (2) problem and solution phase, and (3) application phase. The physiotherapeutic approach to these phases is described. A particular emphasis is placed upon three particularly evidence-based interventions: (1) mindfulness, (2) graded activity and (3) graded exposure.

KEY POINTS

■ The recovery of burnout involves three phases.

■ Recommended therapy for burnout consists of psycho-education, mindfulness, solution focused therapy, graded activity and graded exposure.

LEARNING OBJECTIVE

■ Know the current scientific view on burnout.

■ Be able to explain the different treatment phases.

■ Understand the treatment strategy of burnout for the physiotherapist in psychiatry and mental health.

INTRODUCTION

Freudenberger first introduced *burnout* in medical and psychological literature in the early 1970s. He defined burnout as a state of fatigue or frustration that resulted from professional relationships that failed to produce the expected rewards (Freudenberger, 1974). Burnout was described by Maslach (1982) as a psychological syndrome involving emotional exhaustion, depersonalization and a diminished sense of personal accomplishment that occurred among various professionals who work with other people in challenging situations.

Currently there is no clear international definition of burnout. Burnout has been defined in the ICD-10 (10th revision of the International Statistical Classification of Diseases and Related Health Problems) as a 'state of vital exhaustion' (coded Z73.0; World Health Organization, 1992) It has many characteristics of depression. Stress plays a central role in the etiology of depression as well as in the etiology of burnout (Tennant, 2001; Sapolsky, 2004).

There is growing evidence that burnout is a stress-related illness similar to that of depression and anxiety.

The state of burnout is likely to be a form of depression.

In this chapter the following criteria are used: the person is overwrought or stressed with significant feelings of tiredness and exhaustion, which have been present for more than 6 months. Being overwrought

means that at least three of the following symptoms are present:

■ fatigue,
■ disturbed sleep,
■ irritability,
■ emotional instability,
■ concentration problems,
■ agitation,
■ fretting,
■ aversion to busy environments.

Furthermore, people with burnout syndrome suffer from loss of control as well as feelings of helplessness due to inadequate coping. This leads to demoralization, increasing loss of control, dejection and professional and social dysfunction.

Today, 13% of the working population experience burnout symptoms. A representative survey performed in Germany in 2011 showed that 1.9 million people aged 14 to 65 years were diagnosed at least once with burnout syndrome. In relation to healthcare politics, a sickness rate of 1.8 million in 2010 due to burnout resulted in a substantial economic burden (Korczak et al., 2012).

In 2011, three professional associations involved in the treatment of burnout (i.e., the National Association of Psychologists in Primary Mental Health, the Dutch Society of General Practitioners and the Dutch Association of Company Physicians) developed a multidisciplinary guideline for the treatment of burnout (Sapolsky, 2004). After extensive literature research they found that adequate management of stress or burnout, which, in fact, is a process-contingent approach that helps the patient regain their problem-solving abilities, is divided into three phases:

■ crisis phase,
■ problem and solution phase,
■ application phase.

During the crisis phase (approximately 1–3 weeks), the aim is to help the patient to unwind and regain control on both cognitive and emotional levels. In many cases the patient is unable to carry out social and private activities and participate in the labour market in this phase.

During the problem and solution phase (approximately 3–6 weeks), the patient and their environment bring structure to the problem by finding answers to questions such as: what problems are involved?; Can they be influenced?; What should be done? In general, building up their (physical) taxability and picking up activities such as work (partially or otherwise) is useful if the patient has a clear picture of concrete solutions for at least part of their problems.

In the application phase (approximately 3–6 weeks), the patient applies the newly acquired insights and skills in practical situations and gradually regains functioning in various roles (Verschuren et al., 2011).

PHYSIOTHERAPEUTIC INTERVENTIONS DURING CRISIS PHASE

The type of intervention that is selected is determined by the phase that the client is in. As mentioned previously, during the crisis phase the aim is to let the patient unwind and to regain control on cognitive and emotional levels. Through educating the client, offering perspective and by providing a rationale, the client regains control on a cognitive level. With regard to education, the etiology of the burnout syndrome can be explained. Furthermore, the importance of a normal daily rhythm and a regular sleep pattern should be explained, as well as the beneficial effects of exercising. These items should be addressed during the first intervention.

For rest and relaxation, mindfulness is recommended. Mindfulness is a safe and effective approach in reducing stress. The effect of mindfulness has been studied extensively and is proven to be successful in various occupational groups. It reduces psychological and burnout symptoms, increases psychological flexibility and participants reported a higher level of self-compassion (Flook et al., 2013). Mindfulness is a technique or skill that makes one more aware of bodily sensations, feelings and thoughts. It invites those who practise it to handle these feelings differently and to choose a response that works for them personally.

The key processes in mindfulness are:

- acceptance,
- cognitive defusing,
- self as context,
- experiencing and accepting personal boundaries,
- awareness of the present (here and now),
- personal values,
- devoted action.

PHYSIOTHERAPEUTIC INTERVENTIONS DURING PROBLEM AND SOLUTION PHASE

During the problem and solution phase, the patient and their environment bring structure to the problem. Interventions should focus on problem solving and reactivation. The technique most commonly used is called *solution focussed* (brief) *therapy* (SFT). It is a goal-directed, collaborative approach to psychotherapeutic change by means of direct observation of the client's responses to a series of precisely constructed questions (De Shazer et al., 2007).

The SFT approach assumes that clients have at least some knowledge of what could improve their lives, and minimally possess some of the skills needed to create solutions. Specialized conversation methods are used in all kinds of different therapies. In SFT, the conversation is directed towards the development of the client's ideas about possible solutions and, subsequently, the realization of these solutions (De Shazer et al., 2007). The basic SFT protocol contains the following aspects:

Role clarification: It is important to build up a cooperative relationship with the client by getting to know the *client* instead of their *complaints*. In other words, search for the client's strengths and the social support network they already have.

Problem description: Let the patient describe their problem through asking questions such as: How can I help? How is this a problem for you? What have you tried so far (What was successful)?

Goal formulation: Goal setting changes the client from problem talk to solution talk. Ask the client questions such as: what would you like to achieve with this therapy?

Compliment: Compliments are an essential part of SFT. Validating what the client is already doing well, and acknowledging how difficult their problems are encourages the client to change. At the same time, the client gets the message that the therapist has been listening, understands and cares. Compliments in therapy sessions can help punctuate the effective steps that the client is taking.

Miracle question: What would be different if the problem at hand miraculously disappears? What would you notice first? The willingness to change from problem-orientated towards solution-orientated coping, can be made by using this questions. It helps the client describe small, realistic and doable steps they can take right away.

Moving towards a solution: What was successful in the past? If nothing was successful in the past, what would be different if your situation would be a little better?

Scaling: Scaling questions can be used to help the client assess their personal situation, track their own progress or evaluate how others might rate them on a scale of 0 to 10.

Focus on the positive: Explore the progress that has been made and invite the client to keep up the good work. Focus on finding, amplifying and measuring the client's progress by opening and sustaining a dialogue about solution-orientated coping (De Jong et al., 2007).

SFT is recommended as the main intervention tool in the treatment of burnout syndrome. It is not linked to the problem and solution phase only. In fact, emphasizing the client's strengths and focusing on the positive plays an important role throughout the entire treatment process.

The cognitive behavioural intervention tool called *graded activity* (GA) is type of intervention commonly used in the problem and solution phase of burnout syndrome. The main goal of GA is to encourage physical activity and to diminish avoidance behaviour. It is a time-contingent approach in which the level of physical activity is built up gradually. It consists of three phases:

- starting phase,
- treatment phase,
- generalization phase.

With two sessions per week, the starting phase takes about 4 weeks. GA mainly focuses on educating the client about the method and theory of GA, choosing activities, determining goals and a baseline, and setting up an exercise programme. With regards to the client's motivation, it is advisable to let them choose activities that are personally significant to them, preferably activities of daily life.

The duration of the treatment is approximately 8 weeks, with approximately 10 treatment sessions.

Operant conditioning techniques predominate this phase (http://www.kennisbank.hva.nl/document/219074 Graded activity in de praktijk). Positive reinforcement of helpful behaviour, extinguishing (by ignoring) pain behaviour, shaping, as well as a time-contingent approach gradually teaches the client not to focus on negative sensations and thereby expand their activities. Shaping is the act of fractionating a difficult activity into smaller/easier pieces so that the client can fulfil the specific task and experience success. Positive reinforcement is a constant factor in GA.

In the generalization phase the client is challenged to bring their newfound level of activity into daily practice. There are no guidelines for the average duration of this phase nor for the number of sessions it requires. It all depends on the client's improvement and their degree of independence.

The last intervention often used in the problem and solution phase is called *graded exposure* (GE). GE is similar to GA, but is more focused on dealing with the emotional and psychological elements of rehabilitation. It is used to help gradually build up confidence and to establish meaningful routines that the client otherwise might avoid. Based on classic conditioning principles of GE, clients learn to create new relations between two stimuli. Once the client has described activities or situations that evoke fear and has ranked them in order of increasing severity, they are gradually exposed to those fears. The moment they develop feelings of anxiety, their associating thoughts and assumptions are explored and questioned, while the client carries out relaxation exercises to control the consequences of their fear. In burnout syndrome clients are quite often afraid to go back to work. It is found that the longer clients stay at home, the more difficult a return will be. In general guidelines for the treatment of burnout syndrome say that 'participation is usually more a condition for recovery, than recovery is a condition for participation'.

APPLICATION PHASE

In the application phase, the newfound solutions are applied in practical situations at work or in private life. The acquired insights and skills enable the client to gradually resume functioning in various roles. This phase may take 3 to 6 weeks. The essence of this phase is to support the client in their reintegration by complimenting, reinforcing the new behaviour and focusing on the positive. At the same time, reinforcement of a more phlegmatic attitude towards perfectionism and good awareness of the personal boundaries is important throughout the treatment of burnout syndrome.

When the therapist approaches the client consistently and actively, according to this model, the client will usually be able to regain grip on their performance and (partially) participate in their social roles within 3 months.

REFERENCES

De Jong, P., Berg, I.K., 2007. Interviewing for solutions, third ed. Brooks/Cole, Pacific Grove.

De Shazer, S., Dolan, Y., Korman, H., et al., 2007. More Than Miracles: the State of the Art of Solution-focused Brief Therapy. Routledge, New York, p. 101.

Flook, L., Goldberg, S.B., Pinger, L., et al., 2013. Mindfulness for teachers: a pilot study to assess effects on stress, burnout and teaching efficacy. Mind Brain Educ. 9 (7), 3.

Freudenberger, H.J., 1974. Staff burnout. J Soc Issues 30, 159–165.

Korczak, D., et al., 2012. Therapy of the burnout syndrome. GMS Health Technol. Assess. 8, 1861–8863.

Maslach, C., 1982. Burnout: the cost of caring. Prentice Hall, Englewood Cliffs, NJ.

Sapolsky, R.M. (2004). Why zebras don't get ulcers, third ed. Holt Paperbacks, New York.

Tennant, C., 2001. Work-related stress and depressive disorders. J. Psychosom. Res. 51, 697–704.

Verschuren, C.M., Terluin, B., Loo, M.A.J.M., et al., 2011. Multidisciplinaire Richtlijn Overspanning en Burn-out.

5.1.11   Working in General Practice Treating People With Comorbid Mental Health Problems

JOANNE CONNAUGHTON

SUMMARY

This chapter will review how physiotherapists working in general practice will encounter people with mental health problems from comorbid to physical health problems. We will examine the prevalence of mental health and physical health comorbidities and provide insight into modifying subjective and objective assessments and interventions to engage people of this demographic. This section is aimed at physiotherapists working in general health care.

KEY POINTS

- The prevalence of mental health issues in patients admitted to hospitals for physical illness is high.
- Mental health and physical health should not be treated in isolation.
- An holistic approach to patient care promotes successful outcomes.

LEARNING OBJECTIVES

- Define the prevalence of mental health issues amongst people with physical health problems.

- Recognize how comorbid mental health problems impact on accessing health services.
- Modify subjective, objective assessments and interventions to enhance patient engagement and participation.

INTRODUCTION

The Australian Physiotherapy Association (APA) defines the role of physiotherapy in the management of people who experience chronic pain, musculoskeletal conditions, heart disease, diabetes, neurological conditions and respiratory diseases to help them achieve the best possible physical health outcomes (Australian Physiotherapy Association, 2008, 2009, 2012). Physiotherapists working in general practice treat patients with these conditions on a daily basis. The prevalence of mental health issues in the general population is 25% and even higher amongst people with chronic physical health conditions. It stands to reason that physiotherapists working in general practice will be working with people admitted to hospital for physical health problems who have a mental health comorbidity.

HOW PHYSIOTHERAPISTS ENCOUNTER PEOPLE WITH COMORBID MENTAL ILLNESS

Physiotherapists in general practice will encounter people with comorbid mental illness. A survey undertaken in Western Australia in 2013 determined that 57% of physiotherapists working in acute care hospitals reported treating patients with mental health comorbidity on a daily basis; 85% reported treating patients with mental health problems at least once a week (Connaughton & Gibson, 2016). Of physiotherapists working in private practice, 38% reported treating patients with mental health comorbidity on a daily basis and 74% reported seeing people of this demographic at least once a week (Connaughton & Gibson, 2016).

Physiotherapists in general practice may encounter people with comorbid mental illness by seeing people:

1. who have mental health problems that lead to physical health problems requiring physiotherapeutic intervention;
2. with physical health problems that may lead to changes in mental state;
3. presenting with physical health problems completely unrelated to their mental health problems;
4. with physical health problems that may be related to behaviours associated with mental health problems.

Table 1 provides examples of each of these.

PREVALENCE OF PHYSICAL HEALTH PROBLEMS IMPACTING ON MENTAL HEALTH

Physiotherapy intervention in the management of neurological conditions such as multiple sclerosis (MS) and stroke is well documented (Australian Physiotherapy Association, 2009). Up to 44.5% of people with MS experience or develop anxiety and 18.5% experience depression (Chen et al., 2013; Wood et al., 2013). Up to 52% of people who suffer a stroke develop depression within 5 years of the event (Ayerbe

TABLE 1	
Relationship Between Physical and Mental Health Problems Encountered by Physiotherapists	
Relationship Between Physical and Mental Health Problems	**Examples of Reasons That May Present to Physiotherapists in General Practice**
Mental health problems impact on physical health	■ Fractured tibia and fibula as a result of jumping from a height in a suicide attempt ■ Diabetes as a result of weight gain from psychotropic medication and lack of motivation to exercise ■ Fall management related to dementia
Physical health impacts on mental health	■ Degenerative neurological conditions such as multiple sclerosis or motor neurone disease with subsequent development of depression
Some correlation but relationship not clearly defined	■ Heart disease and depression ■ Chronic pain and depression ■ Respiratory conditions as a result of smoking and psychotic illness
Mental health problems are independent of physical health problems	■ Cervicogenic headache in a person with schizophrenia ■ Injuries sustained as a result of a motor vehicle accident and bipolar affective disorder

et al., 2013) and 44% of people with motor neurone disease suffer from depression (Kurt et al., 2007). In the neurological rehabilitation setting it could be anticipated that almost half of the patients have comorbid mental health problems.

PREVALENCE OF MENTAL HEALTH COMORBIDITIES WHERE RELATIONSHIP IS NOT CLEARLY DEFINED

There are many more conditions than those highlighted in Table 1 where a relationship between physical and mental health problems exists but the mechanisms are not clearly defined. In Australia, one in four people with musculoskeletal health issues have a comorbid mental health problem (Australian Institute of Health and Welfare, 2010). The majority of patients attending physiotherapy private practices present with musculoskeletal problems, suggesting that a quarter of those people will have mental health comorbidities. Conditions regularly treated by physiotherapists that are associated with a significant prevalence of mental health issues include multiple pain sites, chronic pain and chronic fatigue syndrome (Korszun et al., 2002; Gureje et al., 2008; Morgan et al., 2012). The Australian study of the physical health of people experiencing psychotic illness reports that 31.8% of people experiencing psychosis also experience chronic back, neck or other pain (Morgan et al., 2012). Physiotherapists in general settings are increasingly being asked to treat musculoskeletal problems resulting from inactivity or nutritional deficits in people with eating disorders such as anorexia nervosa, binge eating or obesity.

An inactive lifestyle is linked to poor physical health and increased risk of cardiovascular disease, ischaemic heart disease, hypertension, diabetes and respiratory disease conditions (Galletly et al., 2012). An inactive lifestyle is also linked to negative symptoms of mental illness (Vancampfort et al., 2012). A strong link exists between heart disease and depression, with the exact nature of the relationships still to be explored. However, within 2 weeks of a myocardial infarction up to 27% of people develop major depression (Larsen et al., 2013).

People who smoke have frequent admissions to hospital with cardiorespiratory, vascular and oncological-related health issues. In Australia 66% of people who smoke have a comorbid lifetime mental illness (Lawrence et al., 2011). In Western Australia, 66% of people diagnosed with a psychotic illness are known to smoke an average of 21 cigarettes a day (Morgan et al., 2012), which is many more than the 25.3% of the general population (Morgan et al., 2012). These figures suggest that many people admitted to hospital with smoking-related disorders will have comorbid mental health problems. People with inactive lifestyles who also smoke are at higher risk of chronic pain, asthma, heart and circulatory problems, and diabetes.

PREVALENCE OF CONDITIONS WITHOUT CORRELATION

In Australia almost one-third of people with a psychotic illness have asthma (30.1%), over one-quarter (26.8%) of people experience heart or circulatory problems, and a further 20.5% have diabetes (Morgan et al., 2012). Some of these conditions may have a loose correlation, as described in the previous section, but many may be totally independent. Regardless of the connections, physiotherapists in mainstream health settings are involved in the long-term management of people with these conditions (Australian Physiotherapy Association, 2008, 2009).

Headache is one of the most common pains reported by people with schizophrenia (Watson et al., 1981; Kuritzky et al., 1999; Morgan et al., 2012). A recent study undertaken in Western Australia determined the 12-month prevalence of migraine headache (MH) and cervicogenic headache (CGH) in people with schizophrenia and/or schizoaffective disorder to be the same as the general population; the prevalence of tension-type headache (TTH) was lower than in the general population (Connaughton & University of Notre Dame Australia, School of Health, 2015). Forty-one percent of headache sufferers also reported associated neck pain.

Physiotherapy is the treatment of choice for CGH (Zito et al., 2006; Hall et al., 2007; Chaibi & Russell, 2012) but no-one in the study was receiving physiotherapy treatment. Management of the participants' MH did not follow best-practise guidelines as none were under the care of a neurologist nor receiving prophylactic treatment, despite experiencing MH frequently enough to meet the criteria for such intervention. Physiotherapy is not effective in the management of MH but many symptoms of MH are similar to CGH and physiotherapists are trained to differentially diagnose between the two. Physiotherapists will assist the person with MH by referring them to health professionals who can provide best-practice treatment. Physiotherapy also plays a role in the holistic management of the person with TTH (Fernández-de-Las-Peñas & Courtney, 2014), but, as mentioned earlier, no-one in the study group was receiving physiotherapy treatment.

People with comorbid mental illness who experience headache are likely being disadvantaged by not receiving best-practice, holistic management that will improve their physical health, which in turn could impact positively on their mental well-being.

CHALLENGES OF ACCESSING APPROPRIATE SERVICES IN THE GENERAL HEALTHCARE SETTING

The increased morbidity and mortality from preventable diseases amongst people with poor mental health suggests they are receiving inadequate treatment for these preventable conditions (Griswold et al., 2008; Vancampfort et al., 2011; Morgan et al., 2012; Stubbs et al., 2014). Many people with comorbid mental health problems struggle to access the general healthcare setting to receive assessment and treatment of their physical health issues, because they perceive that the challenges and barriers are too great for them to overcome (Fagiolini, 2008). Table 2 lists some of these perceived barriers. Ongoing and unmanaged poor physical health for these people could result in a further compromise to their mental health.

ENGAGING PEOPLE WITH COMORBID MENTAL ILLNESS

Physiotherapists are trained to deliver 'person-centred care' using a biopsychosocial approach, but actual practice within this paradigm becomes problematic if the body and the mind are considered in isolation rather than in unison. An holistic approach means conducting an appropriate assessment and developing realistic treatment goals to ensure successful outcomes of intervention. One generalist-physiotherapist surveyed highlighted the need to '...*treat the person first*

and not immediately dismiss other medical problem (e.g., pain) as in their head because they are a "psych case" [sic]' (Connaughton & Gibson, 2016). Table 3 lists comments from physiotherapists in relation to an holistic approach to people with both physical and mental health problems.

Communication and engagement with the person with mental health comorbidities may require a personalized approach to take into consideration symptoms and side effects of mental health problems. In addition to the side effects of the presenting physical problem, chemical neurotransmitter and neurological changes associated with mental health conditions may result in altered mood, reduced or increased energy levels, sleep disturbances, poor concentration, altered psychomotor ability and lack of motivation. Symptoms associated with depression may manifest in the assessment process with the person taking a long time to answer or formulate answers to questions, not offering any additional information and responding in a very slow, low, monosyllabic voice. Adequate time must be allowed for the person to respond without feeling pressured or inadequate. Conversely, the person with mania may speak in a very loud, fast, pressured speech pattern, making subjective and objective assessments very challenging.

Disorganized thought processes are a feature of many mental health problems and people may have difficulty forming answers to questions or following instructions. Allowing time for the individual to process the question and formulate their answer is

---

TABLE 2
Possible Barriers to Seeking Treatment for Physical Health Problems

Barriers to Seeking Treatment for Physical Conditions

Stigma

Fear of hospitalization

Health workers regarding pain as a symptom of mental illness

Waiting times

Health workers prioritizing mental health problems over physical health problems

Transport issues

Fear of unfamiliar places

Financial constraints

TABLE 3
Providing an Holistic Approach to Engage the Person With Physical and Mental Health Problems

When Working With Someone With Mental and Physical Health Problems

Do not	■ Separate mind and body
Consider	■ Communication strategies
	■ The impact mental health issues have on physical health
	■ Impact of medication and its side effects
	■ Impact of mental health issues to provide effective rehabilitation
	■ How to refer for appropriate treatment
Revise	■ Signs, symptoms and pathophysiology of mental health conditions

Tips for Physiotherapists in General Practice to Engage With the Person With Comorbid Mental Health Problems

Strategies for Physiotherapy Assessment and Intervention

Difficulty answering questions	■ Use single rather than multiple questions
	■ Consider using closed rather than open-ended questions
	■ Give plenty of time
Difficulty following instructions	■ Simplify instructions and explanations
	■ Demonstrate activity/movement
	■ Use hands to guide person through activity/movement
	■ Give plenty of time
Difficulty staying on task	■ Provide continuous guidance
	■ Reduce number of activities in task
Home programme	■ Do not overload
	■ Use SMART goals (based on patient's goals, abilities and expectations—not physiotherapists)
Avoid injury	■ Consider the type of exercise/activity
	■ Prescribe specific loads of weights, frequencies and intensities based on assessment and appropriate exercise prescription guidelines
	■ Consider precautions

SMART, Specific, measurable, achievable, realistic, timely.

essential and rushing the person to respond is not helpful. If psychomotor problems are associated with the mental health problems, then the person may have difficulty performing tasks in an objective examination or following a home programme. It is important to keep instruction clear and simple. Table 4 includes strategies for modification to assessment and intervention processes when the patient presents with any of these symptoms.

SUMMARY

Physiotherapists working in the general healthcare setting will treat patients with comorbid mental health issues. It is important to understand the nature of the mental health problem, what signs and symptoms may be present, and how to modify assessment and interventions to best engage the person to provide optimum holistic health care.

REFERENCES

Australian Institute of Health and Welfare, 2010. When musculoskeletal conditions and mental disorders occur together. <http://www.aihw.gov.au/publication-detail/?id=6442468392.>

Australian Physiotherapy Association, 2008. Primary health care and physiotherapy: position statement. <http://physiotherapy.asn.au/images/Document_Library/Position_Statements/primary%20health%20care%20and%20physiotherapy.pdf.>

Australian Physiotherapy Association, 2009. Chronic disease and physiotherapy: position statement. <http://physiotherapy.asn.au/images/Document_Library/Position_Statements/2012%20chronic%20disease.pdf.>

Australian Physiotherapy Association, 2012. Pain management: position statement. <http://physiotherapy.asn.au/images/Document_Library/Position_Statements/2016%20-%20pain%20management.pdf.>

Ayerbe, L., Ayis, S., Wolfe, C.D.A., Rudd, A.G., 2013. Natural history, predictors and outcomes of depression after stroke: systematic review and meta-analysis. Br. J. Psychiatry 202 (1), 14–21.

Chaibi, A., Russell, M.B., 2012. Manual therapies for cervicogenic headache: a systematic review. J. Headache Pain 13 (5), 351–359.

Chen, K., Fan, Y., Hu, R., et al., 2013. Impact of depression, fatigue and disability on quality of life in Chinese patients with multiple sclerosis. Stress Health 29 (2), 108–112.

Connaughton, J., University of Notre Dame Australia, School of Physiotherapy, 2015. The prevalence, characteristics, impact and management of headache in people with schizophrenia and schizoaffective disorder: A cross sectional cohort study. Doctoral Dissertation. <http://researchonline.nd.edu.au/theses/115/.>

Connaughton, J., Gibson, W., 2016. Do Physiotherapists Have the Skill to Engage in the "Psychological" in the Bio-Psychosocial Approach? Physiother. Can. 68 (4), 377–382. PubMed PMID: 27904237; PubMed Central PMCID: PMC5125500.

Fagiolini, A., 2008. Overcoming hurdles to achieving good physical health in patients treated with atypical antipsychotics. Eur. Neuropsychopharmacol. 18 (Suppl. 2), S102–S107.

Fernández-de-Las-Peñas, C., Courtney, C.A., 2014. Clinical reasoning for manual therapy management of tension type and cervicogenic headache. J. Man. Manip. Ther. 22 (1), 44–50.

Galletly, C.A., Foley, D.L., Waterreus, A., et al., 2012. Cardiometabolic risk factors in people with psychotic disorders: the second Australian national survey of psychosis. Aust. N. Z. J. Psychiatry 46 (8), 753–761.

Griswold, K.S., Zayas, L.E., Pastore, P.A., et al., 2008. Primary care after psychiatric crisis: a qualitative analysis. Ann. Fam. Med. 6 (1), 38–43.

Gureje, O., Von Korff, M., Kola, L., et al., 2008. The relation between multiple pains and mental disorders: results from the world mental health surveys. Pain 135 (1–2), 82–91.

Hall, T., Chan, H.T., Christensen, L., et al., 2007. Efficacy of a C1-C2 self-sustained natural apophyseal glide (SNAG) in the management of cervicogenic headache. J. Orthop. Sports Phys. Ther. 37 (3), 100–107.

Korszun, A., Young, E.A., Engleberg, N.C., et al., 2002. Use of actigraphy for monitoring sleep and activity levels in patients with fibromyalgia and depression. J. Psychosom. Res. 52 (6), 439–443.

Kuritzky, A., Mazeh, D., Levi, A., 1999. Headache in schizophrenic patients: a controlled study. Cephalalgia 19 (8), 725–727.

Kurt, A., Nijboer, F., Matuz, T., Kübler, A., 2007. Depression and anxiety in individuals with amyotrophic lateral sclerosis: epidemiology and management. CNS Drugs 21 (4), 279.

Larsen, K.K., Christensen, B., Søndergaard, J., Vestergaard, M., 2013. Depressive symptoms and risk of new cardiovascular events or death in patients with myocardial infarction: a population-based longitudinal study examining health behaviors and health care interventions. PLoS ONE 8 (9), e74393.

Lawrence, D., Lawn, S., Kisely, S., et al., 2011. The potential impact of smoke-free facilities on smoking cessation in people with mental illness. Aust. N. Z. J. Psychiatry 45 (12), 1053–1060.

Morgan, V., Waterreus, A., Jablensky, A., et al., 2012. People living with psychotic illness in 2010: the second Australian national survey of psychosis. Aust. N. Z. J. Psychiatry 46 (8), 735–752.

Stubbs, B., Soundy, A., Probst, M., et al., 2014. Addressing the disparity in physical health provision for people with schizophrenia: an important role for physiotherapists. Physiotherapy 100 (3), 185–186.

Vancampfort, D., Probst, M., Helvik Skjaerven, L., et al., 2012. Systematic review of the benefits of physical therapy within a multi-disciplinary care approach for people with schizophrenia. Phys. Ther. 92 (1), 11–23.

Vancampfort, D., Probst, M., Sweers, K., et al., 2011. Relationships between obesity, functional exercise capacity, physical activity participation and physical self-perception in people with schizophrenia. Acta Psychiatr. Scand. 123 (6), 423–430.

Watson, G.D., Chandarana, P.C., Merskey, H., 1981. Relationships between pain and schizophrenia. Br. J. Psychiatry 138, 33–36.

Wood, B., van der Mei, I.A.F., Ponsonby, A.L., et al., 2013. Prevalence and concurrence of anxiety, depression and fatigue over time in multiple sclerosis. Mult. Scler. 19 (2), 217–224.

Zito, G., Jull, G., Story, I., 2006. Clinical tests of musculoskeletal dysfunction in the diagnosis of cervicogenic headache. Man. Ther. 11 (2), 118–129.

5.2 PHYSIOTHERAPY IN PSYCHIATRIC CARE

5.2.1 Physiotherapy With Survivors of Torture and Trauma

MARYANN DE RUITER ■ APRIL GAMBLE ■ LAURA PIZER GUERON ■ JEPKEMOI JOANNE KIBET ■ CLAIRE O'REILLY

SUMMARY

This chapter explains some basic concepts about physiotherapy for survivors of torture and other war-related traumas. High percentages of refugees and internally displaced people (those forced to flee their homes due to violence or persecution, but still living in their country of origin) around the world have been subjected to torture and trauma. Therefore it is likely that most physiotherapists working with this population, and physiotherapists working in countries where torture is widespread, are regularly treating clients who have been tortured. There is a growing network of physiotherapists treating such clients, carrying out research studies to determine the most effective methods of treatment and willing to share information to help the physiotherapy profession continue to develop the ability to help such clients. Needs of survivors of torture are very complex, due to high rates of chronic pain and posttraumatic stress disorder that they may experience, as well other very challenging psychosocial issues. It is ideal to work in an interdisciplinary team that includes providers who can address mental health concerns. However, this is not always possible due to lack of resources in certain parts of the world.

KEY POINTS

- This chapter provides a brief overview of typical psychosocial issues experienced by survivors of torture and trauma (STT) that should influence the provision of physical therapy.

- Physiotherapists need to be aware of the common physical and psychological presentations of STT in order to be able to adjust their evaluations and treatments accordingly.

- Chronic pain, posttraumatic stress disorder, depression and anxiety often co-occur in STT and necessitate careful and specialized attention by the physiotherapist.

- The types and amounts of torture that clients experience contribute to the areas and intensities of pain even years after torture has stopped.

- While it is often not realistic to expect complete cessation of pain or complete restoration of function for many STT, physiotherapy plays a crucial role in decreasing pain and enhancing function and quality of life.

LEARNING OBJECTIVES

■ To understand four typical physical and psychological functional limitations that often result from torture and trauma.

■ To understand four typical modifications that are often made by physiotherapists when working with STT during both evaluation and treatment in order to avoid retraumatization, and to establish trust and connection.

■ To be able to describe four reasons why survivors of torture and trauma often have chronic pain years after their torture experiences have ended and to be able to describe four physiotherapy treatment strategies that can help clients to heal.

DEFINITION OF TORTURE AND SCOPE OF THE PROBLEM

According to Amnesty International's report from 2014 (Amnesty International, 2014) torture is utilized in at least 141 countries in the world. There are varying definitions of torture (Office of Public Information, United Nations, 1984; Rodley, 2002) with the most widely accepted being that contained in the UN Convention Against Torture and Other Cruel, Inhuman and Degrading Treatment or Punishment (Box 1).

PREVALENCE ESTIMATES OF TORTURE

Several studies have been conducted to estimate the prevalence of torture and trauma in the world. Some

---

BOX 1

'Torture' means any act by which severe pain or suffering, whether physical or mental, is intentionally inflicted on a person for such purpose as obtaining from him or a third person information or a confession, punishing him for an act he or a third person has committed or is suspected of having committed or intimidating or coercing him or a third person, or for any reason based on discrimination of any kind, when such pain or suffering is inflicted by, or at the instigation of, or with the consent or acquiescence of a public official or other person acting in an official capacity. It does not include pain or suffering arising from, inherent in or incidental to lawful sanctions.

---

survivors of torture and trauma (STT) are living in their country of origin as internally displaced persons (IDPs) and some as refugees or asylum seekers in Europe (Edston, 2009; Buhmann, 2014) and the United States (Jaranson et al., 2004; Willard et al., 2014; Shannon et al., 2015a,b), with an update of the estimate of survivors of torture in the United States by Higson-Smith in 2016 (Higson-Smith, 2016). Although it is difficult to obtain accurate figures, and there is wide variability based on country of origin, it is estimated that up to 1.3 million STT may live in the United States, and that between 5% and 35% of refugees in Europe are survivors of torture. With the current number of refugees and IDPs in the world at the highest levels since World War II, with an estimate of more than 60 million people displaced by war and repression (Human Rights Watch, 2016), it is clear that there are millions of STT in the world.

HISTORY OF TORTURE TREATMENT PROGRAMMES

Formal torture treatment programmes for STT began in the 1970s in Denmark and South America (Chile, Argentina and Uruguay), followed by Canada in 1983. In 1984 the United States, first torture treatment centre opened at the Center of Victims of Torture (CVT), with whom the authors of this chapter work (in programmes in Jordan, Kenya and the United States). Currently, there are at least 235 torture treatment programmes worldwide, of which 144 are members of the International Rehabilitation Council of Torture Victims (IRCT) (Goldsmith, 1986; Jaranson & Quiroga, 2011; and recent data from the IRCT). Dignity—Danish Institute Against Torture (formerly known as *RCT*) is thought to be the first torture treatment centre, as of 1983, at which physiotherapy was included as an integral part of the treatment programme.

INTERNATIONAL SURVEY OF PHYSIOTHERAPY UTILIZATION BY TORTURE TREATMENT PROGRAMMES

An unpublished survey (CVT report, 2014a,b) of approximately 200 torture treatment centres about

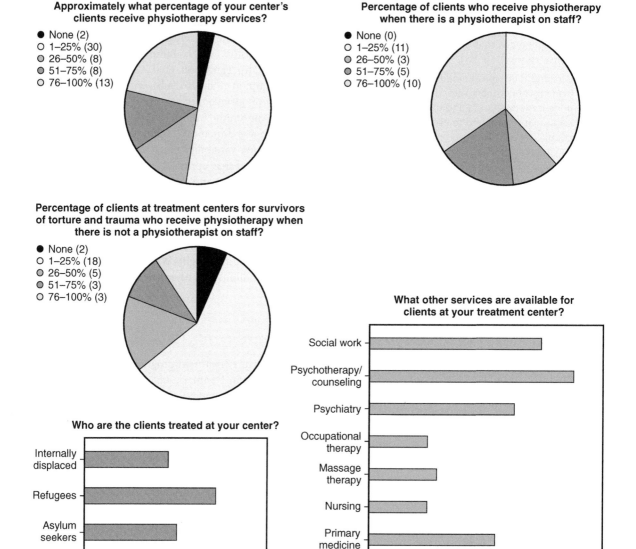

FIGURE 1 ■ Results of an international unpublished survey.

utilization of physiotherapy received 87 responses from 42 countries. Fig. 1 describes clients' access to physiotherapy and the populations served at the centres. The most common physiotherapy services received by clients, with over 60% of programmes offering them, were manual therapy, massage and individual and group exercise programmes.

TREATMENT CONSIDERATIONS

Biopsychosocial Approach

The biopsychosocial model can be applied in physiotherapy treatment of STT. This model honours the mind–body connection by acknowledging the role of mechanical and physiological processes, as well as psychological and social variables in the development of physical impairments and activity limitations (Jones et al., 2002; Turk & Ukifuji, 2002; Jette, 2006; Sanders et al., 2013; Saragiotto et al., 2016). It recognizes that physical and psychological dysfunction is a response of the entire individual, including their body structures, emotions, previous experiences, beliefs and thoughts within their unique social, cultural and environmental context (Amris, 2004; Hodas, 2006; Jette, 2006; Rundell et al., 2009; Sanders et al., 2013). Evidence indicates that due to the complexity of work with STT, interdisciplinary work with physiotherapy and counselling is most effective for achieving functional outcomes (Hough, 1992; Turk & Ukifuji, 2002; Amris, 2004; Carinci et al., 2010; Gard, 2012). If a physiotherapist is working in a setting without mental health services, a referral to an external provider should be considered. An interdisciplinary approach with STT may also warrant the involvement of additional healthcare professionals, including social services, psychiatry and medical services (Neumann et al., 2010). Additionally, when working with STT it is essential that both physiotherapists and organizations promote trauma-informed care (TIC), which serves to address the trauma-based needs of clients (Hodas, 2006). The core principles of TIC are shown in Box 5. As physiotherapy with STT has evolved to address the mind–body connection and incorporate TIC, psychological concepts have been adapted for application in physiotherapy treatment.

Trauma-Informed Care for Survivors

One model that is widely used in the psychological treatment of STT is the Judith Herman Model of Trauma Recovery (Herman, 1997; Gorman, 2001). In order to facilitate TIC, and considering the mental health context of treatment with STT, physiotherapists can use principles adapted from Judith Herman's model of trauma recovery to guide clinical decision-making (Gorman, 2001). The three main stages are (1) establishment of safety and stabilization, (2) process of reconstruction and (3) reconnection (Herman, 1997; Gorman, 2001). See Boxes 6.8 for application of these stages in clinical practice.

There are a growing number of books and articles about sensorimotor aspects of trauma healing (Levine & Frederick, 1997; Rothschild, 2000; Ogden et al.,

2006; Fabri, 2011; Gray, 2011; van der Kolk, 2014; Emerson, 2015). It is recommended that physiotherapists have a basic familiarity with this literature in order to ensure that their therapy provision is truly trauma-informed.

Moreover, culturally competent care is a key aspect of TIC. One unique application of this with STT is the recognition of cultural idioms of distress. These are defined as particular ways of expressing psychological distress within a specific culture and include somatic complaints that are common to particular cultures (Kirmayer & Young, 1998; Bentley et al., 2011; Schubert & Punamaki, 2011; Stade et al., 2015; Baird et al., 2016).

For example, the Center for Victims of Torture clinicians in Jordan report frequently observing clients with chest heaviness, while clinicians in Nairobi report that clients frequently report headache symptoms (Box 2).

IDENTIFYING CLIENTS WHO HAVE BEEN TORTURED OR TRAUMATIZED

In addition to established programmes for STT, it is important to recognize that most physiotherapists who work with clients who are refugees or IDPs are working with STTs on a regular basis, yet they may not be aware of this fact. Often, clients are fearful of disclosing their trauma history as they worry that they will not be believed, or because they are ashamed of their history. There are respectful and gentle ways to try to ascertain whether someone is an STT, which in turn can help the physiotherapist to provide optimal care, including purposefully avoiding retraumatizing the client (Miles & Garcia-Peltoniemi, 2012; Shannon, 2014; Shannon et al., 2012, 2014).

BOX 2

(Names have been changed to protect the identity of clients)

Mrs Juma was tortured 5 years ago and sustained a back injury. She had no access to treatment until recently and has had persistent back pain ever since, and is often worried that the pain will become even worse than it already is. Mrs Juma reports that she feels very worried about her pain and thinks the pain means that something bad will happen to her.

Medical Screening and Differential Diagnosis Considerations

The physiotherapist is responsible for identifying red flags or signs of an underlying medical condition or unstable medical comorbidity and making the appropriate referral (World Confederation for Physical Therapy, 2014). Survivors of trauma present with significantly higher rates of a variety of medical conditions and age-related illnesses, as well as health-risk behaviours (Hiatt, 2001; Kim et al., 2003; Killip et al., 2007; Yagihashi et al., 2007; Last & Hulbert, 2009; Bolton, 2010; Lovell & Ford, 2012) (see Table 1 for a comprehensive description). This evidence reflects the essential role of the physiotherapist in the identification and management of medical conditions in STT (Box 3).

Survivors of trauma demonstrate higher rates of chronic pain, hypertension, cardiovascular disease (McFarlane, 2010; Danese & McEwen, 2012), metabolic disorders, type 2 diabetes, dementia, fibromyalgia (Afari et al., 2013), liver disease, stroke, lung cancer, chronic obstructive pulmonary disease, autoimmune diseases (Oral et al., 2016), chronic fatigue syndrome, temporomandibular disorder, irritable bowel syndrome (Afari et al., 2013) and premature mortality (Felitti et al., 1998; Brown et al., 2009; Kelly-Irving et al., 2013). Even when controlling for other factors, survivors also present with a higher prevalence of health-risk behaviours, including higher rates of substance abuse, tobacco use and behaviours contributing to unintended pregnancies and sexually transmitted diseases (Oral et al., 2016).

Additionally, STTs consistently present with somatic complaints and physical symptoms that mimic medical conditions (Hough, 1992; Amris, 2004; Afari et al., 2014; Danneskiold-Samsøe et al., 2007). When medical conditions or tissue damage have been ruled out by the physiotherapist's assessment, a psychosomatic etiology can be considered (Amris, 2004). This can be described

TABLE 1
Differential Diagnosis Considerations

Common Symptom Presentation of STT	Differential Diagnoses
Chest heaviness, chest pain, shortness of breath, dizziness, hypertension	Hyperarousal symptoms (Kinzie, 2007); unstable cardiac pathology (Bolton, 2000); undiagnosed cardiac pathology (Bolton, 2000); respiratory pathology (Van den Bruel et al., 2010)
Stomach pain, back pain, changes in bladder and bowel function	Gastrointestinal pathology (Last & Hulbert, 2009); irritable bowel syndrome (Lovell & Ford, 2012)
Left flank pain and/or back pain, urinary incontinence, pain with urination	Kidney pathology (Last et al., 2009; Kim et al., 2003)
Dizziness, headache, fatigue, shortness of breath	Iron deficiency anaemia (Killip et al., 2007); hyperarousal symptoms (Kinzie, 2007)
Bilateral foot and calf pain, stocking pattern of paresthesia, skin changes in bilateral feet and legs	Diabetes mellitus (Yagihashi et al., 2007); intermittent vascular claudication (Hiatt, 2011)

For each symptom presentation identified, a psychosomatic etiology can be considered. In this context, a psychosomatic etiology refers to a symptom presentation or pattern that has no contributing medical condition or tissue damage (Amris, 2004). Note, this is not a comprehensive list of symptom presentations or differential diagnoses, but rather serves to demonstrate the need for the physiotherapist to engage in clinical reasoning regarding differential diagnosis and medical screening.

BOX 3

Mrs Mohamed was told by the torturers that the degenerative changes in her knee joint are progressive and she absolutely believes them. She believes that her 'joint ligaments are degenerating', and thinks that she will end up in a wheelchair someday and will never get well. During the last month, her pain has been worsening and she takes it as evidence of her inevitably degenerating condition. This perception of her pain is alarming. Because of the fear that she experiences, she responds with rest and inactivity. From her perspective, it makes all the sense in the world to rest and to remain inactive. Given her understanding that her pain is the result of a delicate orthopaedic condition that is certainly getting worse, she reasons that she must not engage in activities as a means to prevent, or at least to slow down, the degenerative process in her knee. Just as you would not walk on a broken leg, rest and diminished activity seems like the best approach for her condition. Mrs Mohamed rates her pain as intolerable and believes that she has a condition that is inevitably going to bring about severe impairments. Mrs Mohamed sees her pain as largely out of her control.

as symptoms that have no presenting medical condition or tissue damage (Amris, 2004). When working frequently with STTs, it is important to maintain a high level of vigilance to avoid a common cognitive bias of assuming a psychosomatic etiology (Bornstein & Emler, 2001). Numbness, tingling, heaviness, swelling and decreased AROM can be common symptoms, rather than, or in addition, to pain or mobility deficits. Table 1 explores the differential diagnosis considerations in the STT population. Once red flags are ruled out, it is essential that the physiotherapist explains possible reasons for the symptoms in a reassuring manner and educates about how treatment can help them reduce symptoms and improve function (Harding & Watson, 2000; Harland & Lavallee, 2003; Moseley, 2003; Turk, 2004; Louw et al., 2011; Louw & Puentedura, 2014).

The physiotherapist assessing an STT must also evaluate for possible neurological injuries. Such injuries can occur from many forms of torture, including suspension, cutting, gunshot wounds, forced stress positions and beatings. Torture of this kind can cause long-term injuries to bones, muscles, tendons, ligaments and other tissues. These types of injuries are not always simple for a healthcare provider to detect (Moreno & Grodin, 2002; Vogel et al., 2007; Nielsen, 2014).

When considering the physiotherapist's differential diagnosis it is important to recognize that symptoms of posttraumatic stress disorder (PTSD) and depression, including chronic headaches, memory and concentration impairments and fatigue, also frequently present with traumatic brain injuries (TBIs). Blows to the head during beatings are one of the most frequent causes of TBIs among STT. Prevalence rates of TBIs vary greatly across populations of STT. In one study of 337 South Vietnamese STT, 78% had sustained TBIs (Mollica et al., 2014). Moreover, TBI and PTSD, as well as depression, often co-occur, and many symptoms, such as fatigue, headaches, memory loss, irritability and decreased motivation, are common in all of these conditions, and often occur along with persistent pain (Bryant, 2011). Care needs to be taken not to confuse the symptoms of TBI with depression and PTSD, as physiotherapy and other treatments will need to be targeted differentially (Keatley et al., 2013; Mollica et al., 2014).

SPECIAL CONSIDERATIONS FOR SURVIVORS OF TORTURE AND TRAUMA

Children/Family

Children are not only casualties of war, they are often directly tortured and are witnesses to the torture of family members (Alayarian, 2009; United Nations Children's Fund, 2014; United Nations Office for the Coordination of Humanitarian Affairs, 2016). Comprehensively discussing the complex needs of children who are STT is beyond the scope of this chapter, but symptoms commonly reported in children who have been tortured include hyper/hypoarousal, sleep disorders, bed wetting, behavioural concerns and impairments of coordination and motor planning (Macksoud & Aber, 1996; van der Kolk, 2005). Additionally, based on vast research on children with adverse childhood experiences (ACE studies; Felitti et al., 1998), the more children have been exposed to adverse experiences in their youth, the greater the likelihood that they will develop psychological and physical health problems as adults. Childhood trauma and adversity has been linked to long-term changes and predisposition to both psychological and physical conditions, from depression (Heim et al., 2008) to gastrointestinal complaints (Chang et al., 2009). Considering this, it is essential to actively address and treat childhood trauma. One of the main resiliency factors for children in coping with traumatic experiences is the attachment to a parent or primary care giver (Davies, 2011; Tol et al., 2013; Center on the Developing Child at Harvard University, 2015). Therefore any rehabilitation considerations for child STT should include a child's caregiver and overall family system. An integrated approach that includes close attention to the psychological, physical and social needs of children and with the intentional inclusion of a close caregiver is essential in working with child survivors (Lobo et al., 2013).

Sexual and Gender-Based Violence

Sexual and gender-based violence (SGBV), including rape, is used as a weapon of war and torture (United Nations Office for the Coordination of Humanitarian Affairs, 2016). The term refers to 'any harmful act that is perpetrated against one person's will and that is based on socially ascribed (gender) differences between males and females. It includes acts that inflict physical, mental, or sexual harm or suffering, threats of such acts, coercion and other deprivations of liberty, whether occurring in public or in private life' (Inter-Agency Standing Committee, 2005).

Many cultures and societies have taboos with regard to talking about sexuality in general; discussing SGBV carries additional emotional difficulties and often very negative stigma that may threaten a survivor's life, family and community (Inter-Agency Standing Committee, 2015). The prevalence estimates of SGBV vary greatly by country of origin and gender. In a report on 9025 survivors of torture and trauma from 125 countries who were receiving services at any of 23 centres in the United States, 18.6% of the STT reported having been victims of SGBV, including 31% of women and 8% of men (National Consortium of Torture Treatment Programs, 2015). Effects of SGBV that should be addressed with physiotherapy can include pelvic pain, incontinence of bowel and bladder and sexual dysfunction. As with all STT, it is also essential to identify medical referral needs and to work within an interdisciplinary team to address these needs (Peel, 2004; Norredam et al., 2005; Zawati, 2007; Williams et al., 2010; Brown, 2012).

REFUGEE STATUS

STT receiving any type of physiotherapy services are most likely to be either IDPs or refugees. These individuals often face what is called the '*Triple Trauma Paradigm*':

1. The traumatic experiences that disrupted their lives and caused them to flee.
2. The uncertainties and trauma experienced during the flight for safety.
3. The adjustment and uncertainties confronted in a new country, often without an understanding of the language or culture or the ability to work (Center for Victims of Torture, 2005a,b).

While adjusting to the new country, STT may not feel safe in their current situation, may lack access to basic resources, and may have difficulty navigating in their new environments. Physiotherapy interventions for all refugees, but in particular STT, need to take into account the 'triple trauma' factors, and to adjust

treatment plans to address clients' basic, needs as well as to establish trust and safety at a pace that supports the clients' rehabilitation (Herman, 1997; Bandeira et al., 2010; Higson-Smith, 2013; Nielsen, 2014).

THE ROLE OF GROUP TREATMENT

There are several articles written about the benefits of group treatment for STT, mostly from a counselling and psychosocial group perspective, but these can be applied to the physiotherapy context. Attending group treatment sessions is beneficial for reducing isolation, providing encouragement and support, and for rebuilding trust (Kira et al., 2010; Bunn et al., 2016). In an article by Phaneth et al. (2014), the application of group treatment for STT was demonstrated by statistically significant improvements noted from a structured 10-session group 'back school' for STT in Cambodia with chronic pain.

PREVALENCE OF CHRONIC PAIN WITH A SURVIVOR OF TORTURE AND TRAUMA

There is a great deal of research describing persistent or chronic pain in survivors of torture (Amris & Prip, 2000a,b; Olsen et al., 2006a,b, 2007; Amris & Williams, 2007; Carinci et al., 2010; Williams et al., 2010; Defrin et al., 2014; Nielsen, 2014; National Consortium of Torture Treatment Programs, 2015; Teodorescu et al., 2015), as well as typical locations of pain and correlations with types of torture experienced. In one study of 61 multitraumatized outpatients, all but one had chronic pain, with a mean location of 4.6 areas of pain and comorbid pain, and PTSD was diagnosed in 57% of the clients. Head (80%), chest (74%), extremity (66%) and back (62%) were the most common locations, with 33% having pain during urination as well (Teodorescu et al., 2015). In another study of 178 male clients who had been tortured, 78% reported persistent pain in multiple areas, especially in the head and lower back. The authors stated that their findings did not support the widespread assumption that the pain in survivors is primarily a result of the clients' psychological distress (Williams et al., 2010).

STT are at this increased risk of developing persistent pain for many reasons, including that there is often no treatment provided at the acute stage of injury. One study identified that only 12% of 104 clients received medical care shortly after their torture experiences (Domovitch et al., 1984). In addition, biopsychosocial factors predispose survivors to have persistent pain (Defrin et al., 2014). The context of the initial acute injury involves the pain being delivered by other human beings at very high intensities during times of devastating emotional distress, with the survivors having no control over their suffering. STT are often living in very high-stress situations, as IDPs, refugees or asylum seekers, or living in their home community at risk of further victimization.

Pain and PTSD

Persistent pain and PTSD commonly occur together, both in survivors of torture and of other traumatic experiences (Chapman et al., 2008; Liedl & Knaevelsrud, 2008; Asmundson & Katz, 2009; Carleton et al., 2009; Moeller-Bertramm et al., 2012; Morasco et al., 2013). Extensive research has explored this co-occurrence and a variety of theories have been described to explain the relationship, including the mutual maintenance theory by Sharp and Harvey (2001). This theory recognizes the interplay and cycles between pain and anxiety where persistent pain can contribute to anxiety and PTSD, and, simultaneously, the state of hyperarousal experienced with these conditions, with typically increased muscle tension, can contribute to the persistent pain.

A study demonstrated that pain occurring after trauma among patients seen in a hospital emergency room setting was a strong risk factor for the development of PTSD (Norman et al., 2008). In addition, trauma involving physical suffering, such as rape or torture, may be more likely to result in somatization early in the development of PTSD (Deering et al., 1996). Because torture is intentionally inflicted by other human beings with the intent to cause pain and suffering, it is understandable that both the levels of chronic pain and PTSD are high among STT.

During a qualitative study about the complex interplay of persistent pain and reexperiencing of trauma by Taylor et al. (2013), four themes emerged from interviews with STT that are relevant to physiotherapy: clients felt that: (1) 'pain is the enemy', (2) their identities had changed, (3) pain and intrusive memories are connected, and the counsellors noted that clients were (4) resilient and needed more access to appropriate resources. The authors emphasize the need for interdisciplinary teams when working with survivors whenever possible, with an emphasis on counselling as well as bodily-orientated therapies, such as physiotherapy (Taylor et al., 2013).

SYMPTOMS OF HYPERAROUSAL

The stress response begins in the brain and is designed to persist for a short time, only long enough to enable the individual to survive danger (Selye, 1970; Chrousos & Gold, 1998). In situations of prolonged, acute stress this response may become maladaptive, resulting in hypo- or hyperarousal (Stratakis & Chrousos, 1995). Ongoing trauma such as prolonged captivity can create an upregulation of the nervous system, resulting in hyperarousal symptoms (Selye, 1950). In the treatment of STT, physiotherapy frequently works to identify and treat these physical signs of hyperarousal.

In order to address symptoms of hyperarousal, it is important to understand the neurochemical processes that contribute to this state. The hypothalamus–pituitary–adrenal (HPA) axis and the sympathetic nervous system make up the body's neuroendocrine stress response system. During stress or perceived danger, the amygdala sends a danger signal to the hypothalamus. This begins a chemical cascade, which communicates with the autonomic nervous system, consisting of the sympathetic and parasympathetic nervous systems. The amygdala's danger signals trigger the hypothalamus to release corticotrophin-releasing hormone (CRH), which stimulates the pituitary gland's release of adrenocorticotropic hormone (ACTH). This in turn stimulates the adrenal glands to release cortisol. This system enables the fight or flight response to prime a number of physiological systems to launch a high-power, short-term response to enable the individual to confront or flee the danger. In this situation, a number of physiological processes desirable in a precarious position occur, including dilation of the pupils, increased breathing rate and increased availability of glycogen. Less commonly, if the individual perceives neither fight nor flight as a viable option, they may 'freeze'. This is best imagined as similar to a 'deer in the headlights', or the limp immobilization of an animal caught in the jaws of a predator (Levine & Frederick, 1997). In normal functioning, this process of HPA axis activation, or fight or flight response, forms a negative feedback loop, where at a certain level, cortisol inhibits the production of CRH and ACTH, thus allowing the body to return to a state of homeostasis once the danger has been overcome or avoided. However, low cortisol levels found in individuals with PTSD (Ehlert et al., 2001) have been posited as contributing to the inhibition of this negative feedback loop, and the maintenance of a sustained state of hyperarousal. The alterations in the HPA axis have a direct influence on the brain and influence a range of symptoms that fall under the umbrella term of 'hyperarousal' (Kendall-Tackett, 2000). These symptoms may include hypervigilance, manifesting as increased responsiveness to external stimuli including touch, sound and temperature, difficulties concentrating or remembering details, and intense psychosomatic reactions to reminders of the trauma experience, such as overwhelming dread or anxiety in response to elevated heart rate (Box 3).

Hyperarousal symptoms can make an individual feel like their body is no longer within their control. They cannot predict their symptoms, as they cannot identify a connection between their psychological status and their physical symptoms. This creates a feeling of lack of safety and body trust (van der Kolk, 2014). Therefore treatment focuses on identification of triggers or predisposing psychological status, in addition to education and self-management strategies. Assessment of hyperarousal symptoms is qualitative and client specific. Physiotherapists may look at sleep patterns, reported pain and functional abilities. Assessing avoidance patterns, such as a client's reluctance to walk briskly due to the discomfort of an elevated heart rate, can help to create an understanding of the impact of symptoms on quality of life (Nielsen, 2014). Some symptoms of hyperarousal, such as poor sleep patterns, will naturally form part of the physiotherapy problem list, whereas others will require attention from the physiotherapist to facilitate focusing on other symptoms. In the authors' experience, hyperarousal symptoms rarely adhere to a standardized treatment protocol and the response may be nonlinear with regression, plateaus and sudden improvements, closely tied to psychological status (Box 4).

BOX 4

The objective assessment was as follows:
- Range of motion (ROM)
  - Limited ROM on left shoulder abduction and extension
  - Limited left ankle dorsiflexion
  - Painful right knee
- Back pain
- Headaches
- Activity limitation
  - Pain carrying small weights
  - Pain while walking for long periods
- Participation restriction
  - Playing football was a hobby for him before, now it's difficult given his physical condition

---

BODY AWARENESS

Torture and trauma results in alterations of a person's body ego, which is defined as the human being's total perception of physical identity. Body ego incorporates two dimensions, body awareness and body trust. Body awareness is the ability to recognize one's body and physical experiences or sensations, to understand ones' needs and emotions (Gyllensten et al., 2010; Mehling et al., 2011). Body trust is a psychological dimension, which when intact evokes a positive body image, satisfaction with the body, and a trust in body functions (Gard, 2007). Within the mental health context, dissociative symptoms reflect impairments of body awareness and body trust that occur as a result of trauma (van der Kolk et al., 1996; Levine & Frederick, 1997; Ogden et al., 2006; Price, 2005, 2007). An individual can experience episodic dissociative reactions, which present as discontinuities in conscious awareness. However, the focus here will be on the role of physiotherapy with more extensive dissociative symptoms (Bryant & Harvey, 1997). Dissociative symptoms occur as a result of an altered state of awareness that changes one's sense of identity. The clinical picture of dissociative symptoms includes physical and psychological dysfunction, poor concentration and memory, affect dysregulation, somatic complaints, chronic pain and an inability to differentiate relevant and irrelevant physical sensations (van der Kolk et al., 1996; Kisiel & Lyons, 2001, Price, 2005, 2007; Gard, 2007). Based on the authors' experience, dissociative symptoms can also contribute to additional impairments, including hyperarousal symptoms, increased muscle tension, altered breathing patterns, poor quality of movement, deconditioning and disuse, and impaired social functioning. See Table 1 to consider various clinical presentations associated with dissociative symptoms in STT.

Regarding STT, it is well established that the reduction of dissociative symptoms is essential for functional recovery (Price, 2005). There are several established body-awareness treatment programmes shown to be effective with survivors of trauma, including Body Awareness Program, Basic Body Awareness Therapy (BBAT) and Mindful Awareness in Body-Oriented Therapy (Roxendal, 1985, 1995; Landsman-Dijkstra et al., 2006; Price, 2007; Mehling et al., 2011; Nordbrandt et al., 2015; Stade et al., 2015). They all seek to restore the mind–body connection and share characteristics, including a focus on basic body functions and movements, an emphasis on breathing, the use of repetition, and the facilitation of increased awareness and verbalization of body sensations, thoughts and emotions (Roxendal, 1985, 1995; Price, 2007; Mehling et al., 2011; Nordbrandt et al., 2015; Stade et al., 2015). Specifically regarding STT, BBAT has been found to be an effective physiotherapy treatment (Nordbrandt et al., 2015; Stade et al., 2015).

THE UNIQUE CONTEXT OF DISSOCIATIVE SYMPTOMS WITH STT

To address dissociative symptoms with STT, consider the following precipitating factors and how both body awareness and body trust may be impaired.

Survivors of Rape and Sexual Abuse

It has been established that survivors of rape and sexual abuse frequently present with dissociative symptoms that contribute to worse mental health outcomes and higher rates of PTSD than the general population and those exposed to other forms of war trauma (Kisiel & Lyons, 2001; Kilpatrick et al., 2007; Price 2005, 2007; Johnson et al., 2008). Dissociative symptoms can contribute to clinical symptoms, including poor body image (Zarkov, 2001), urinary incontinence (Jundt et al., 2007), irritable bowel syndrome (Eriksson et al., 2007), sexual problems (Price, 2007), chronic pelvic pain (Haugstad et al., 2006) and chronic pain (Price, 2007).

Limb Amputation as a Result of Torture

It is clear that alterations of body image occur following both traumatic and nontraumatic amputations. Body image disturbances result in physical and psychological dysfunction and social impairments, including depression, social isolation, decreased sexual activity and limited functional independence (Rybarczyk et al., 1995; Wetterhahn et al., 2002). Based on the authors' experience, there are often greater impairments of body awareness and dissociation when the limb amputation is a result of torture compared with nontraumatic incidents. Additionally, based on their experience, in clinical practice with STT this presents as more significant limitations in active range of motion, sensory disturbances, pain and functional limitations than the level of tissue damage would produce in isolation.

Physical Disfigurement (e.g., Scars and Burns) as a Result of Torture or Injury During War

Research has established that burns result in alterations of body image (Stoddard, 1982) that have associated symptoms of social anxiety, maladaptive thought processes, low self-esteem, sexual disorders, social isolation, anxiety and depression (Rumsey & Harcourt, 2004; Rumsey et al., 2004). In children, body image disturbances can also contribute to nightmares, aggression and avoidance of body image and associated emotions (Stoddard, 1982).

Restraint by Binding of the Wrist

Binding of the wrist can result in specific body awareness impairments and dissociative symptoms. Symptoms are often localized to the wrist and hands, and include swelling, chronic pain, disuse and deconditioning, altered resting posture and reduced active range of motion at all joints. Additionally, it often contributes to reduced function in activities of daily living that require lifting and fine motor skills (Carinci et al., 2010).

Physical Beating (e.g., Falanga)

Falanga, or beating of the soles of the feet with a variety of instruments, is the most well-researched act of physical torture. Symptoms associated with falanga include chronic pain in feet and lower legs, skin changes, sensory disturbances in the soles and reduced elasticity of the foot pads (Amris & Prip, 2003; Amris et al., 2009a; Prip, 2014). This contributes to walking difficulties, reduced walking distance and alterations in gait pattern including reduced stride length and walking speed (Amris et al., 2009a, Prip, 2014). Considering that many survivors of falanga do not demonstrate structural changes that explain the aforementioned symptoms (Savnik et al., 2000), it can be reasoned that body-awareness impairments contribute to this complex clinical presentation (Amris et al., 2009a). Additionally, based on the authors' experience, symptoms similar to those associated with falanga can occur in any body area that has sustained physical beatings.

THE ROLE OF TRADITIONAL PHYSIOTHERAPY INTERVENTIONS IN FUNCTIONAL RECOVERY

Despite the myriad, special considerations that might seem overwhelming to the physiotherapist new to working with STT, 'traditional' physiotherapeutic interventions, such as strengthening, soft-tissue therapy and cardiovascular exercise, play a role alongside more specialized breathing, relaxation and body-awareness techniques (Hough, 1992; Nielsen, 2014; O'Sullivan, 2015).

Throughout treatment, it is important that the therapist remain sensitive to positions or equipment that may be triggering to the client. Triggers (Rothschild, 2000; Ogden et al., 2006; Nielsen, 2014; van der Kolk, 2014) can be anything that causes a visceral memory of the trauma or torture experience, and can result in dissociation, panic attacks, or a host of lesser physiological reactions, such as an increased heart and breathing rate. A trigger is specific to each client, but examples include the dominant physical position of the therapist used for some techniques, a shoulder pulley, or an ultrasound modality similar to equipment used during torture.

Education serves to help the client understand that not all triggers are avoidable, nor is avoidance a viable long-term coping strategy (Franklin, 2001; Nielsen, 2014). Recognizing physical symptoms when triggered and addressing them with physical coping strategies, such as grounding, breathing and self-massage, can be

empowering for both client and therapist, and allows faster progression in additional physiotherapeutic treatment goals.

A high level of individualization is required with this population. For example, a complaint such as lower back pain, which is common in physiotherapy, may have a broad variety of underlying mechanisms in STT. Back pain may stem from torture methods, such as suspension, forced positions, electrocution, beatings or accumulated effects of deprivation (Olsen et al., 2006a,b). Withholding appropriate medical care may be used as a form of torture (Mendez, 2013) and can result in a higher rate of secondary complications, such as fracture malunion or scar hypertrophy. Additionally, the complex underlying psychological status and fear-avoidance behaviour influencing the pain must be addressed, as discussed earlier.

Although it is a commonly expressed goal of survivors, regaining the body the STT had prior to torture may be unrealistic if irreversible harm has been caused, such as extensive scarring, limb shortening, or deformity. Difficulty accepting this can hinder physiotherapy intervention, and highlights the need to integrate physiotherapy with mental health input wherever possible (Sjolund et al., 2009). Considering this, an emphasis on functional goals is essential. Understanding what outcomes are ultimately important to clients, whether picking up their child or cooking a meal for their family, facilitates a graded and individualized treatment plan. Setting functional goals enables both parties to focus on maximizing existing capacity.

ROLE OF FEAR AVOIDANCE IN STT

Fear avoidance in the context of pain refers to the avoidance of movement on activities based on fear. Elevated levels of fear-avoidance beliefs have been shown to lead to increased disability in general populations and in clients with acute or chronic lower back pain (Buer & Linton, 2002). Pain-related fear, avoidance behaviour and hypervigilance are all concerns that affect individuals that have been tortured, and can lead to disuse and disability (Carinci et al., 2010). Fear-avoidance belief seems to be established early in the pain experience (Fritz et al., 2001). Avoidance behaviours may persist following tissue healing since they occur in anticipation of pain rather than as response to pain. Moreover, avoidance may cause a decrease in both social and physical activities (Leeuw et al., 2007). These processes directly result in disability and deconditioning, which continues to contribute to the painful experience, resulting in a perpetuating cycle (Box 4).

BRIEF EXAMPLE OF PAIN CATASTROPHIZING IN TORTURE SURVIVORS

Catastrophizing plays an important role in theoretical models of pain chronicity, including the fear-avoidance model, showing a consistent positive correlation with both pain intensity and disability (Edwards et al., 2006; Meyer et al., 2009). It has been described as a cognitive style that involves the tendency to misinterpret and exaggerate the threat value of situations (Van Damme et al., 2002) or as an exaggerated negative mental set brought to bear during an actual or anticipated painful experience (Sullivan et al., 2001a). Clients who catastrophize perceive pain as stronger than the physiological tissue damage would imply, ruminate about painful sensation and show an inability to control pain (Granot & Ferber, 2005; Fernandes et al., 2012; Raeissadat et al., 2013). Catastrophizing could be considered a coping strategy in terms of displaying distress to achieve attention or help from the social environment (Edwards et al., 2006). However, other research on the construct of catastrophizing suggests that this represents more a response to distress than a coping strategy (Sullivan et al., 2001b), and, in terms of chronicity, it seems to worsen the situation and lead to an increased perception of pain and disability (Sullivan et al., 2001). In their study Sullivan et al. (2001) described catastrophizing as a cognitive determinant of the pain experience.

Pain catastrophization has also shown associations with functional disability, pain severity, elevated disease activity and depression in chronic pain patients (Engel-Yeger & Dunn, 2011). Longitudinal research suggests that psychological factors such as catastrophizing are associated with increased risk of persistent pain (Edwards et al., 2011). It is assumed to be more pronounced in STT than in any other chronic pain population, and it often leads to development of fear-avoidance behaviours. It is well known that torture has numerous physical, psychological and pain-related sequelae that can inflict a devastating and enduring burden on its victims (Randall & Lutz, 1991).

Accordingly, in clients with chronic pain, symptoms of depression and maladaptive pain behaviors often improve when catastrophizing thoughts are addressed and diminished via treatment (Spinhoven et al., 2004).

Multiple studies have shown that physiotherapy contributes to substantial reduction of catastrophizing (Smeets et al., 2006; Sullivan & Adams, 2010). Basics of physiotherapy such as goal setting, pain education, support and graded exercise have been shown to reduce catastrophizing (Miciak et al., 2012), ranging from 12% to 14% in individuals with musculoskeletal problems taking part in physiotherapy intervention (Smeets et al., 2006). Studies have also shown that gradual exposure to movement feared by the patients has positive effects on fear-avoidance beliefs, disability and physical activity (Boersma et al., 2004).

FEAR AVOIDANCE

There appears to be little research about the role of fear avoidance or the amount of pain catastrophization in STT. One of the authors (Jepkemoi Joanne Kibet) is carrying out her dissertation research about this crucial topic (Box 5).

CONCLUSION

As physiotherapists working with the Center for Victims of Torture, we have worked with more than 4000 clients in our programmes in Jordan, Kenya and the United States (Minnesota). Work with STT is often very rewarding but can be quite complex due to the interplay of many biopsychosocial issues, and more needs to be learned about optimal physiotherapy treatment approaches to best help STT to address symptoms, increase function and to improve overall quality of life. Ideally, clients should have interdisciplinary treatment, with counselling or other mental health therapies being a crucial part of the team to help to heal the mind and body, and to be able to resume active, rewarding lives (Boxs 6, 7, 8).

There are many free online resources for physiotherapists to learn more about evaluation and treatment of STT, including Dignity—Danish Institute

BOX 5
PRINCIPLES OF TRAUMA-INFORMED CARE

1. Establish an environment where the client feels safe, connected, valued, informed, empowered and hopeful of recovery.
2. Apply the knowledge of trauma and paths to recovery to practices, policies and procedures.
3. Recognize the signs and symptoms of trauma in clients, families, staff and others involved in the system.
4. Work purposefully with individuals, family, friends and other social services agencies to promote and protect the autonomy of the clients.
5. Apply the knowledge that services can retraumatize clients to practices, policies and procedures.
6. Practise culturally competent and nondiscriminatory policies, procedures and practices.

(Muskett, 2013, Oral et al., 2016; Substance Abuse and Mental Health Services Administration, 2014)

BOX 6
ESTABLISHMENT OF SAFETY AND STABILIZATION

1. Select the most appropriate gender of therapist considering the client's cultural norms and trauma history.
2. Apply a culturally sensitive approach towards confidentiality, informed consent and use of an interpreter.
3. Provide interventions that control the body, which may include relaxation techniques, pain education and education about trauma and its effects (O'Sullivan, 2015).
4. Apply purposeful pacing of treatment based on the client's needs, with continuous discussion with the client about the treatment plan and the role of the client and physiotherapist (Carroll et al., 2016)
5. Recognize and refer to address the client's immediate situational needs including social, economic, legal or medical problems.

BOX 7
PROCESS OF RECONSTRUCTION

1. Acknowledge the loss of prior physical abilities and work together to regain or compensate for the impairments (O'Sullivan, 2015).
2. Provide individualized interventions to manage physical symptoms (Harding & Watson, 2000).

RECONNECTION

1. Facilitate functional goal achievement through shared goal-setting, pacing and an individualized home exercise programme (George & Zeppieri, 2009).
2. Facilitate independent management of symptoms through an individualized home exercise programme that facilitates the use of the body as a somatic resource (Moseley, 2010).
3. Facilitate a reconnection with the body through graded exercise and body-awareness and self-regulation exercises (Nielsen, 2014; Vargas et al., 2004).
4. Emphasize interventions, goals and discharge plans that promote reintegration into the community and social support networks.

BOX 8

High arousal level is a classic symptom of PTSD; however, fulfilling the diagnostic criteria for DSM-V diagnosis is not necessary to identify and treat symptoms of hyper-arousal.

TREATMENT STRATEGIES TO ADDRESS SYMPTOMS OF HYPERAROUSAL

1. Progressive muscle relaxation, a technique focusing on selectively contracting and relaxing muscle groups, facilitates a connection with the body that is essential for regaining a sense of control. It is often very helpful in addressing sleep issues, hypervigilance, inefficient breathing patterns and increased skeletal muscle tension.
2. Sleep hygiene facilitates stability and predictability within the individual's daily routine.
3. Interoceptive exposure involves inducing hyperarousal symptoms, such as increased heart rate, through graded cardiovascular exercise. For an STT who associates such reactions with their torture experience, gradual exposure to these symptoms in a safe environment, followed by techniques such as mindful breathing to harness the body's intrinsic ability to regain homeostasis, induces a sense of mastery and self-control should be undertaken. This facilitates functional recovery as it reduces the fear and discomfort of daily activities to allow STT to regain participation in previous functional tasks (Nielsen, 2014; O'Sullivan, 2015).

Against Torture library http://www.dignityinstitute.org/resources/library/), IRCT, which publishes the journal *Torture* with free online access (http://www.irct.org), and HealTorture PT/Physiotherapy (http://healtorture.org/content/physical-therapyphysiotherapy) where there are article reviews, physiotherapy blogs, webinars and PowerPoint presentations, as well as other resources.

BIBLIOGRAPHY

Albert, H., 1999. Psychosomatic group treatment helps women with chronic pelvic pain. J. Psychosom. Obstet. Gynaecol. 20 (4), 216–225.

Bradley, L., Tawfiq, N., 2006. The physical and psychological effects of torture in Kurds seeking asylum in the United Kingdom. Torture 16 (1), 41–47.

Busch, J., Hansen, S., Hougen, H., 2015. Geographical distribution of torture: an epidemiological study of torture reported by asylum applicants examined at the Department of Forensic Medicine, University of Copenhagen. Torture 25 (2), 12–20.

Edston, E., 2009. The epidemiology of falanga-incidence among Swedish asylum seekers. Torture 19 (1), 27–32.

Grodin, M., Piwowarczyk, L., Fulker, D., et al., 2008. Treating survivors of torture and refugee trauma: a preliminary case series using t'ai chi. J. Altern. Complement. Med. 14 (7), 801–806.

Gueron, L., 2015. HealTorture physiotherapy section; Physical therapy in Nairobi. <http://www.healtorture.org/content/physical-therapy-nairobi.>

HealTorture, 2016. Physiotherapy client outcomes at CVT-Nairobi. <http://www.healtorture.org/content/physiotherapy-outcomes-center-victims-torture-nairobi-program.>

Jaradat, R., 2016. HealTorture physiotherapy section; Building clients' trust through physiotherapy. <http://www.healtorture.org/content/building-clients%E2%80%99-trust-through-physiotherapy.>

Kaminski, K., 2016. Cadillac therapist works in Jordan to heal Syrian, Iraqi refugees. Traverse City Record Eagle. Traverse City, Michigan, USA. <http://www.record-eagle.com/news/lifestyles/cadillac-therapist-works-in-jordan-to-heal-syrian-iraqi-refugees/article_1df97674-c.>

Karoly, P., Ruehlman, L., 2007. Psychosocial aspects of pain-related life task interference: an exploratory analysis in a general population sample. Pain Med. 8 (7), 563–572.

Kim, H., Hun, S., 2015. Effects of complex manual therapy on PTSD, pain, function, and balance of male torture survivors with chronic low back pain. J. Phys. Ther. Sci. 27 (9), 2763–2766.

Kurklinsky, S., Perez, R., Lacayo, E., Sletten, C., 2016. The efficacy of interdisciplinary rehabilitation for improving function in people with chronic pain. Pain Res. Treat. 1–6.

Mattsson, M., Wilkman, M., Dahlgren, L., Mattson, B., 2000. Physiotherapy as empowerment: treating women with chronic pelvic pain. Adv. Physiother. 2 (3), 125–143.

McCracken, L., Samuel, V., 2007. The role of avoidance, pacing and other activity patterns in chronic pain. Pain 130 (1-2), 119–125.

Means-Christensen, A.J., Roy-Byrne, P.P., Sherbourne, C.D., et al., 2008. Relationships among pain, anxiety, and depression in primary care. Depress. Anxiety 25 (7), 593–600.

Morville, A.L., Erlandsson, L.K., Eklund, M., et al., 2014. Activity of Daily Living performance amongst Danish asylum seekers: a cross-sectional study. Torture 24 (1), 49–64.

Musisi, S., Kinyanda, E., Liebling, H., Mayengo-Kiziri, R., 2000. Post traumatic torture disorders in Uganda: a 3 year retrospective study of patient records at a specialized torture treatment centre in Uganda. Torture 10, 81–87.

Nijs, J., Roussell, N., Van Wilgen, P., et al., 2013. Thinking beyond muscles and joints: therapists' and patients' attitude and beliefs regarding chronic musculoskeletal pain are key to applying effective treatment. Man. Ther. 18 (2), 96–102.

Qtaishat, M., 2016. HealTorture-physiotherapy section; Physiotherapy to help survivors of torture in their darkest hours. <http://www.healtorture.org/content/physiotherapy-help-survivors-torture-their-darkest-hours.>

Quartana, P., Campbell, C., Edwards, R., 2009. Pain catastrophizing: a critical review. Expert Rev. Neurother. 9 (5), 745–758.

Salen, B.A., Spangfort, E.V., Nygren, A.L., Nordemar, R., 1994. The disability rating index: an instrument for assessment of disability in clinical setting. J. Clin. Epidemiol. 47 (12), 1423–1435.

Sledjeski, E.M., Speisman, B.A., Dierker, L.C., 2008. Does number of lifetime traumas explain a relationship between PTSD and chronic medical conditions? Answers from the National Comorbidity Survey Replication (NCS-R). J. Behav. Med. 31 (4), 341–349.

Stroud, M.W., Thorn, B.E., Jensen, M.P., Boothby, J.L., 2000. The relation between pain beliefs, negative thoughts, and psychosocial functioning in chronic pain patients. Pain 84 (2–3), 347–352.

Sullivan, M., Bishop, S., Pivik, J., 2001. The Pain Catastrophizing Scale: development and validation. J. Psychol. Assess. 7 (4), 524–532.

Woby, S.R., Watson, P.J., Roach, N.K., Urmston, M., 2004. Are changes in fear avoidance beliefs, catastrophizing and appraisals of control, predictive of changes in chronic low back pain and disability? Eur. J. Pain 8 (3), 201–210.

REFERENCES

Afari, N., Ahumada, S.M., Johnson Wright, L., et al., 2013. Psychological trauma and functional somatic syndromes: a systematic review and meta-analysis. Psychosom. Med. 76 (1), 2–11. <http://doi.org/10.1097/PSY.000000000000010.>

Afari, N., Ahumada, S.M., Wright, L.J., et al., 2014. Psychological trauma and functional somatic syndromes: a systematic review and meta-analysis. Psychosom. Med. 76 (1), 2–11.

Alayarian, A., 2009. Children, torture and psychological consequences. Torture 19 (2), 145–156.

Amnesty International, 2014. Stop Torture Media Briefing-Torture in 2014: 30 years of broken promises. ACT, 40/004/2014, 1–47.

Amris, S., 2004. Chronic pain in survivors of torture–Psyche or Soma? Psyke & Logos 25 (1), 95–124.

Amris, K., Prip, K., 2000a. Physiotherapy for torture victims (I)-Chronic pain for torture victims: possible mechanisms for the pain. Torture 10 (3), 73–76.

Amris, K., Prip, K., 2000b. Physiotherapy for torture victims (II): treatment of chronic pain. Torture 10 (4), 112–116.

Amris, K., Prip, K., 2003. Falanga Torture: Diagnostic Considerations, Assessment and Treatment. IRCT, Copenhagen.

Amris, K., Torp-Pedersen, S., Rasmussen, O., 2009a. Long-term consequences of falanga torture-what do we know and what do we need to know? Torture 19 (1), 33–40.

Amris, K., Williams, A.C., 2007. Chronic pain in survivors of torture. Pain Clinical Update 15 (7), 1–6.

Asmundson, G., Katz, J., 2009. Understanding the co-occurrence of anxiety disorders and chronic pain: state-of-the-art. Depress. Anxiety 26 (10), 888–901. <http://doi.org/10.1002/da.20600.>

Baird, E., de Williams, C., Hearn, A., & Amris, K., 2016. Interventions for treating persistent pain in survivors of torture. Cochrane Database Syst. Rev. CD012051. <http://doi.org/10.1002/14651858.>

Bandeira, M., Higson-Smith, C., Bantjes, M., Polatin, P., 2010. The land of milk and honey: a picture of refugee torture survivors presenting for treatment in a South African trauma centre. Torture 20 (2), 92–103.

Bentley, J.A., Thoburn, J.W., Stewart, D.G., Boynton, L.D., 2011. The indirect effects of somatic complaints on report of posttraumatic psychological symptomatology among Somali refugees. J. Trauma. Stress 24 (4), 479–482. <http://doi.org/10.1002/jts.20651.>

Boersma, K., Linton, S.J., Overmeer, T., et al., 2004. Lowering fear-avoidance and enhancing function through exposure in vivo. A multiple baseline study across six patients with back pain. Pain 108 (1–2), 8–16.

Bolton, P.S., Ray, C.A., 2000. Neck afferent involvement in cardiovascular control during movement. Brain Res. Bull. 53 (1), 45–49.

Bolton, M.M., 2010. Sounding the alarm about metabolic syndrome. Nursing 40 (9), 34–40. <http://doi.org/10.1097/01.NURSE .0000387152.77867.8c.>

Bornstein, B.H., Emler, A.C., 2001. Rationality in medical decision making: a review of the literature on doctors' decision-making biases. J. Eval. Clin. Pract. 7 (2), 97–107. <http://doi.org/10.104 6/j.1365-2753.2001.00284.x.>

Brown, C., 2012. Rape as a weapon of war in the Democratic Republic of the Congo. Torture 22 (1), 24–36.

Brown, D.W., Anda, R.F., Tiemeier, H., et al., 2009. Adverse childhood experiences and the risk of premature mortality. Am. J. Prev. Med. 37 (5), 389–396. <http://doi.org/10.1016/j.amepre.2009.06.021.>

Bryant, R., 2011. Post-traumatic stress disorder vs traumatic brain injury. Dialogues Clin. Neurosci. 13 (3), 251–262.

Bryant, R.A., Harvey, A.G., 1997. Acute stress disorder: a critical review of diagnostic issues. Clin. Psychol. Rev. 17 (7), 757–773. <http://doi.org/10.1016/S0272-7358(97)00052-4.>

Buer, N., Linton, S.J., 2002. Fear- avoidance beliefs and catastrophizing: occurrence and risk factor in back pain and ADL in the general population. Pain 99 (3), 485–491. <http://doi.org/10.1016/ S0304-3959(02)00265-8.>

Buhmann, C.B., 2014. Traumatized refugees: morbidity, treatment and predictors of outcome. Dan. Med. J. 61 (8), B4871.

Bunn, M., Goesel, C., Kinet, M., Ray, F., 2016. Group treatment for survivors of torture and severe violence: a literature review. Torture 26 (1), 45–67.

Carinci, A.J., Mehta, P., Christo, P.J., 2010. Chronic pain in torture victims. Curr. Pain Headache Rep. 14 (2), 73–79. <http:// doi.org/10.1007/s11916-010-0101-2.>

Carleton, R.N., Abrams, M.P., Asmundson, G.J., et al., 2009. Pain-related anxiety and anxiety sensitivity across anxiety and depressive disorders. J. Anxiety Disord. 23 (6), 791–798. <http://doi.org/ 10.1016/j.janxdis.2009.03.003.>

Carroll, L.J., Lis, A., Weiser, S., Torti, J., 2016. How well do you expect to recover, and what does recovery mean, anyway? Qualitative study of expectations after a musculoskeletal injury. Phys. Ther. 96 (6), 797–807. <http://doi.org/10.2522/ptj.20150229.>

Center for Victims of Torture, 2014a. Center for Victims of Torture PT Survey Results. Center for Victims of Torture, St. Paul, Minnesota. <http://www.healtorture.org/sites/healtorture.org/files/CVT%20 PT%20Survey%20Results%202014.pdf.>

Center for Victims of Torture, 2014a. Restoring hope and childhoods. <http://www.healtorture.org/sites/healtorture.org/files/CVT%20 PT%20Survey%20Results%202014.pdf.>

Center on the Developing Child at Harvard University, 2015. Supportive relationships and active skill-building strengthen the foundations of resilience: Working paper No. 13. <http://www .developingchild.harvard.edu.>

Chang, L., Sundaresh, S., Elliott, J., et al., 2009. Dysregulation of the hypothalamic-pituitary-adrenal (HPA) axis in irritable bowel syndrome. Neurogastroenterol. Motil. 21 (2), 149–159. <http:// doi.org/10.1111/j.1365-2982.2008.01171.x.>

Chapman, C.R., Tuckett, R.P., Song, C., 2008. Pain and stress in a systems perspective: reciprocal neural, endocrine, and immune interactions. J. Pain 9 (2), 122–145. <http://doi.org/10.1016/ j.pain.2007.09.006.>

Chrousos, G.P., Gold, P.W., 1998. A healthy body in a healthy mind-and vice versa-The damaging power of 'uncontrollable' stress. JCEM 83 (6), 1842–1845. <http://doi.org/10.1210/jcem .83.6.4908.>

Danese, A., McEwen, B.S., 2012. Adverse childhood experiences, allostasis, allostatic load, and age-related disease. Physiol. Behav. 106 (1), 26–39. <http://doi.org/10.1016/j.physbeh.2011.08/019.>

Danneskiold-Samsoe, B., Bartels, E.M., Genefke, I., 2007. Treatment of torture survivors—A longitudinal study. Torture 17 (1), 11–17.

Davies, D., 2011. Risk and protective factors: The child, family, and community contexts. In: Child Development: A Practitioner's Guide, third ed. Guilford Press, New York, pp. 60–104.

Deering, C.G., Glover, S.G., Ready, D., et al., 1996. Unique patterns of comorbidity in posttraumatic stress disorder from different sources of trauma. Compr. Psychiatry 37 (5), 336–346.

Defrin, R., Ginsburg, K., Mukulincer, M., Solomon, Z., 2014. The long -term impact of tissue injury on pain processing and modulation: a study of ex-prisoners of war who underwent torture. Eur. J. Pain 18 (4), 548–558. <http://doi.org/10.1002/j.1532-2149 .2013.00394.x.>

Domovitch, E., Berger, P.B., Wawer, M.J., et al., 1984. Human Torture: description and sequelae of 104 cases. Can. Fam. Physician 30, 827–830.

Edston, E., 2009. The epidemiology of falanga—incidence among Swedish asylum seekers. Torture 19 (1), 27–32.

Edwards, R.R., Bingham, C.O., 3rd, Bathon, J., Haythornthwaite, J., 2006. Catastrophizing and pain in arthritis, fibromyalgia, and other rheumatic diseases. Arthritis Rheum. 55 (2), 325–332. <http://doi.org/10.1002/art.21865.>

Edwards, R.R., Cahalan, C., Mensing, G., et al., 2011. Pain catastrophizing and depression in the rheumatic diseases. Nat. Rev. Rheumatol. 7 (4), 216–224. <http://doi.org/10.1038/nrrheum.2011.2.>

Ehlert, U., Gaab, J., Heinrichs, M., 2001. Psychoneuroendocrinological contributors to the etiology of depression, posttraumatic stress disorder, and stress-related bodily disorders: the role of the hypothalamus-pituitary-adrenal axis. Biol. Psychol. 57 (1), 141–152. <http://doi.org/10.1016/50301-0511(01)00029-8.>

Emerson, D., 2015. Trauma-Sensitive Yoga in Therapy: Bringing the Body Into Treatment. W.W. Norton and Company, New York.

Engel-Yeger, B., Dunn, W., 2011. Relationship between pain catastrophizing level and sensory processing patterns in typical adults. Am. J. Occup. Ther. 65 (1), e1–e10. <http://doi.org/10.5014/ajot.2011.09004.>

Eriksson, E.M., Moller, I.E., Soderberg, R.H., et al., 2007. Body awareness therapy: a new strategy for relief of symptoms in irritable bowel syndrome patients. World J. Gastroenterol. 13 (23), 3206–3214. <http://doi.org/10.3748/wjg.v13/i23.3206.>

Fabri, M.R., 2011. Best, promising and emerging practices in the treatment of trauma: What can we apply to our work with torture survivors? Torture 21 (1), 27–38.

Felitti, V.J., Anda, R.F., Nordenberg, D., et al., 1998. Relationship of childhood abuse and household dysfunction to many of the leading causes of death in adults: the Adverse Childhood Experiences (ACE) Study. Am. J. Prev. Med. 14 (4), 245–258. <http://doi.org/10.1016/S0749-3797(98)00017-8.>

Fernandes, L., Storheim, K., Lochting, I., Grothle, M., 2012. Cross-cultural adaptation and validation of the Norwegian pain catastrophizing scale in patients with low back pain. BMC Musculoskelet. Disord. 13, 111–120. <http://doi.org/10.1186/1471-2474-13-111.>

Franklin, C., 2001. Physiotherapy with torture survivors. Physiotherapy 87 (7), 374–377. <http://doi.org/10.1016/S0031-9406(05)6086903.>

Fritz, J.M., George, S.Z., Delitto, A., 2001. The role of fear avoidance beliefs in acute low back pain: relationship with current and future disability and work status. Pain 94 (1), 7–15. <http://doi.org/10.1016/S0304-3959(01)003335.>

Gard, G., 2007. Factors important for good interaction in physiotherapy treatment of persons who have undergone torture: a qualitative study. Physiother. Theory Pract. 23 (1), 47–55. <http://doi.org/10.1080/09593980701209584.>

Gard, G., 2012. Focus on psychological factors and body awareness in multimodal musculoskeletal pain rehabilitation. In: Rehabilitation in Physical Therapy Perspectives in the 21st Century–Challenges and Possibilities. InTech Open Access Publisher, pp. 1–13. <http://doi.org/10.5772/35768.>

George, S.Z., Zeppieri, G., 2009. Physical therapy utilization of graded exposure for patients with low back pain. J. Orthop. Sports Phys. Ther. 39 (7), 496–505. <http://doi.org/10.2519/jospt.2009.2983.>

Goldsmith, M.F., 1986. New center for torture victims seeks to aid the politically abused. J. Am. Med. Assoc. 255 (20), 2717–2718. <http://doi.org/10.1001/jama.1986.03370200015002.>

Gorman, W., 2001. Refugee survivors of torture: trauma and treatment. Prof. Psychol. Res. Pr. 32 (5), 443–451. <http://doi.org/10.1037/0735-7038.32.5.443.>

Granot, M., Ferber, S.G., 2005. The roles of pain catastrophizing and anxiety in the prediction of postoperative pain intensity: a prospective study. Clin. J. Pain 21 (5), 439–445. <http://doi.org/10.1097/01.ajp.0000135236.12705.2d.>

Gray, A.E.L., 2011. Expressive arts therapies: working with survivors of torture. Torture 21 (1), 39–47.

Gyllensten, A.L., Skär, L., Miller, M., Gard, G., 2010. Embodied identity–a deeper understanding of body awareness. Physiother. Theory Pract. 26 (7), 439–446.

Harding, V., Watson, P., 2000. Increasing activity and improving function in chronic pain management. Physiotherapy 86 (12), 619–630. <http://doi.org/10.1016/50031-9406(05)61298-9.>

Harland, N., Lavallee, D., 2003. Biopsychosocial management of chronic low back pain patients with psychological assessment and management tools. Physiotherapy 89 (5), 305–312. <http://doi.org/10.1016/S0031-9406(05)60043-0.>

Haugstad, G.K., Haugstad, T.S., Kirste, U.M., et al., 2006. Posture, movement patterns, and body awareness in women with chronic pelvic pain. J. Psychosom. Res. 61 (5), 637–644. <http://doi.org/10.1016/j.jpsychochores.2006.05.003.>

Heim, C., Newport, D.J., Mietzko, T., et al., 2008. The link between childhood trauma and depression: insights from HPA axis studies in humans. Psychoneuroendocrinology 33 (6), 693–710. <http://doi.org/10.1016/j.psyneuen.2008.03.008.>

Herman, J., 1997. Trauma and Recovery: The Aftermath of Violence—From Domestic Abuse to Political Terror. Basic Books, New York.

Hiatt, W.R., 2001. Medical treatment of peripheral arterial disease and claudication. NEJM 344 (21), 1608–1621. <http://doi.org/10.1056/NEJM200105243442108.>

Hiatt, W.R., 2011. Commentary. The fate of the claudicant–a prospective study of 1969 claudicants. Eur. J. Vasc. Endovasc. Surg. 42 (Suppl. 1), S7–S8.

Higson-Smith, C., 2013. Counseling torture survivors in contexts of ongoing threat: narratives from sub-Saharan Africa. Peace Confl. 19 (2), 164–179. <http://doi.org/10.1037/a0032531.>

Higson-Smith, C., 2016. Updating the Estimate of Refugees Resettled in the United States Who Have Suffered Torture (Research). The Center for Victims of Torture, St. Paul, Minnesota, USA, pp. 1–7.

Hodas, G., 2006. Responding to childhood trauma: The promise and practice of trauma informed care (p. 77). Pennsylvania Office of Mental Health and Substance Abuse Services. <http://www.childrescuebill.org/victimsOfAbuse/RespondingHodas.pdf.>

Hough, A., 1992. Physiotherapy for survivors of torture. Physiotherapy 78 (5), 323–328.

Human Rights Watch, 2016. World Report 2016: Events of 2015. Human Rights Watch, New York, United States.

Inter-Agency Standing Committee, 2005. Guidelines for gender-based violence interventions in humanitarian settings. <http://www.unhcr.org/refworld/docid/439474c74.html.>

Inter-Agency Standing Committee, 2015. Guidelines for integrating gender-based violence interventions in humanitarian action:

Reducing risk, promoting resilience and aiding recovery, p. 366. <http://www.interaction.org/document/centrality-protection-humanitarian-action-statement-iasc.>

Jaranson, J.M., Butcher, J., Halcon, I., et al., 2004. Somali and Oromo refugees: correlates of torture and trauma history. Am. J. Public Health 94 (4), 591–598. <http://doi.org/10.2105/AJPH.94.4.591.>

Jaranson, J.M., Quiroga, J., 2011. Evaluating the services of torture rehabilitation programmes: history and recommendations. Torture 21 (2), 98–140.

Jette, A.M., 2006. Toward a common language for function, disability, and health. Phys. Ther. 86 (5), 726–734.

Johnson, K., Asher, J., Rosborough, S., et al., 2008. Association of combatant status and sexual violence with health and mental health outcomes in postconflict Liberia. JAMA 300 (6), 676–690. <http://doi.org/10.1001/jama.300.6.676.>

Jones, M., Edwards, I., Gifford, L., 2002. Conceptual models for implementing biopsychosocial theory in clinical practice. Man. Ther. 7 (1), 2–9. <http://doi.org/10.1054/math.2001.0426.>

Jundt, K., Scheer, I., Schiessl, B., et al., 2007. Physical and sexual abuse in patients with overactive bladder: is there an association? Int. Urogynecol. J. Pelvic Floor Dysfunct. 18 (4), 449–453. <http://doi.org/10.1007/s00192-006-0173-z.>

Keatley, E., Ashman, T., Im, B., Rasmussen, A., 2013. Self-reported head injuries among refugee survivors of torture. J. Head Trauma Rehabil. 28 (6), 8–13. <http://doi.org/10.1097/HTR.0b013e3182776a70.>

Kelly-Irving, M., Lepage, B., Dedieu, D., et al., 2013. Adverse childhood experiences and premature all-cause mortality. Eur. J. Epidemiol. 28 (9), 721–734. <http://doi.org/10.1007/s10654-013-9832-9.>

Kendall-Tackett, K., 2000. Physiological correlates of childhood abuse: chronic hyperarousal in PTSD, depression, and irritable bowel syndrome. Child Abuse Negl. 24 (6), 799–810. <http://doi.org/10.1016/S0145-2134(00)00136-8.>

Killip, S., Bennett, J.M., Chambers, M.D., 2007. Iron deficiency anemia. Am. Fam. Physician 75 (5), 671–678.

Kilpatrick, D.G., Amstadter, A.B., Resnick, H.S., Ruggiero, K., 2007. Rape-related PTSD: Issues and interventions. Psychiatric Times, 1–8.

Kim, H.L., Belldegrun, A.S., Freitas, D.G., et al., 2003. Paraneoplastic signs and symptoms of renal cell carcinoma: implications for prognosis. J. Urol. 170 (5), 1742–1746.

Kinzie, J.D., 2007. Guidelines for psychiatric care of torture survivors. Torture 21 (1), 18–26.

Kira, I.A., Ahmed, A., Mahmoud, V., Wassim, F., 2010. Group therapy model for refugee and torture survivors. Torture 20 (2), 108–113.

Kirmayer, L.J., Young, A., 1988. Culture and somatization: clinical, epidemiological, and ethnographic perspectives. Psychosom. Med. 60 (4), 420–430.

Kisiel, C.L., Lyons, J.S., 2001. Dissociation as a mediator of psychopathology among sexually abused children and adolescents. Am. J. Psychiatry 158 (7), 1034–1039. <http://doi.org/10.1176/appi.ajp.158.7.1034.>

Landsman-Dijkstra, J.J., van Wijck, R., Groothoff, J.W., 2006. The long-term lasting effectiveness on self-efficacy, attribution style, expression of emotions and quality of life of a body awareness program for chronic a-specific psychosomatic symptoms. Patient Educ. Couns. 60 (1), 66–79. <http://doi.org/10.1016/j.pec.2004.12.003.>

Last, A.R., Hulbert, K., 2009. Chronic low back pain: evaluation and management. Am. Fam. Physician 79 (12), 1067–1074.

Leeuw, M., Goossens, M.E., Linton, S.J., et al., 2007. The fear avoidance model of musculoskeletal pain: current state of scientific evidence. J. Behav. Med. 30 (1), 77–94. <http://doi.org/10.1007/s10865-006-9085-0.>

Levine, P., Frederick, A., 1997. Waking the Tiger: Healing Trauma: The Innate Capacity to Transform Overwhelming Experiences. North Atlantic Books, Berkeley, California.

Liedl, A., Knaevelsrud, C., 2008. Chronic pain and PTSD: the Perpetual Avoidance Model and its treatment implications. Torture 18 (2), 69–76.

Lobo, M.A., Harbourne, R.T., Dusing, S.C., McCoy, S.W., 2013. Grounding early intervention: hysical therapy cannot just be about motor skills anymore. Pediatr. Phys. Ther. 93 (1), 94–103. <http://doi.org/10.2522/ptj.20120158.>

Louw, A., Diener, I., Butler, D.S., Puentedura, E.J., 2011. The effect of neuroscience education on pain, disability, anxiety and stress in chronic musculoskeletal pain. Arch. Phys. Med. Rehabil. 92 (12), 2041–2056. <http://doi.org/10.1016/j.apmr.2011.07.198.>

Louw, A., Puentedura, E.J., 2014. Therapeutic Neuroscience Education, pain, physiotherapy and the pain neuromatrix. Int. J. Health Sci. 2 (3), 33–45. <http://doi.org/10.15640/ijhs.v2n3a4.>

Lovell, R.M., Ford, A.C., 2012. Global prevalence of and risk factors for irritable bowel syndrome: a meta-analysis. Clin. Gastroenterol. Hepatol. 10 (7), 712–721. <http://doi.org/10.1016/j.cgh.2012.02.029.>

Macksoud, M.S., Aber, J.L., 1996. The war experiences and psychosocial development of children in Lebanon. Child Dev. 67 (1), 70–88.

McFarlane, A., 2010. The long-term costs of traumatic stress: intertwined physical and psychological consequences. World Psychiatry 9 (1), 3–10.

Mehling, W.E., Wrubel, J., Dubenmier, J.J., et al., 2011. Body Awareness: a phenomenological inquiry into the common ground of mind-body therapies. Philos. Ethics Humanit. Med. 6 (6), 1–12. <http://doi.org/10.1186/1747-5341-6-6.>

Mendez, J., 2013. Report of the special rapporteur on torture and other cruel, inhuman or degrading treatment or punishment (Freedom from torture, inhuman and degrading treatment No. A/HRC/22/53). United Nations Human Rights Council. <http://refworld.org/docid/51136ae62.html.>

Meyer, K., Tschopp, A., Sprott, H., Mannion, A.F., 2009. Association between catastrophizing and self-rated pain and disability in patients with chronic low back pain. J. Rehabil. Med. 41 (8), 620–625. <http://doi.org/10.2340/16501977-0395.>

Miciak, M., Gross, D.P., Joyce, A., 2012. A review of the psychotherapeutic 'common factors' model and its application in physical therapy: The need to consider general effects in physical therapy practice. Scand. J. Caring Sci. 26 (2), 394–403. <http://doi.org/10.1111/j.1471-6712.2011.00923x.>

Miles, S.H., Garcia-Peltoniemi, R.E., 2012. Torture survivors: What to ask, how to document. J. Fam. Pract. 61 (4), E1–E5.

Moeller-Bertramm, T., Keltner, J., Strigo, I.A., 2012. Pain and post-traumatic stress disorder-review of clinical and experimental evidence. Neuropharmacology 62 (2), 586–597. <http://doi.org/10.1016/j.neuropharm.2011.04.028.>

Mollica, R.F., Chernoff, M.C., Berthold, S., et al., 2014. The mental health sequelae of traumatic head injury in South Vietnamese ex-political detainees who survived torture. Compr. Psychiatry 55 (7), 1626–1638. <http://doi.org/10.1016/j.compsych.2014.04.014.>

Morasco, B.J., Lovejoy, T.I., Lu, M., et al., 2013. The relationship between PTSD and chronic pain: mediating role of coping strategies and depression. Pain 154 (4), 609–616. <http://doi.org/10.1016/j.pain.2013.01.001.>

Moreno, A., Grodin, M.A., 2002. Torture and its neurological sequelae. Spinal Cord 40 (5), 213–223. <http://doi.org/10.1038/sj/sc/3101284.>

Moseley, G., 2003. Joining forces–combining cognition-targeted motor control training with group or individual pain physiology education: a successful treatment for chronic low back pain. J. Man. Manip. Ther. 11 (2), 88–94. <http://doi.org/10.1179/106698103790826383.>

Moseley, K., Aslam, A., Speight, J., 2010. Overcoming barriers to diabetes care: Perceived communication issues of healthcare professionals attending a pilot Diabetes UK training programme. Diabetes Res. Clin. Pract. 87 (2), e11–e14.

Muskett, C., 2013. Trauma-informed care in inpatient mental health settings: a review of the literature. Int. J. Ment. Health Nurs. 23 (1), 51–59. <http://doi.org/10.1111/inm.12012.>

National Consortium of Torture Treatment Programs (NCTTP), 2015. Descriptive, inferential, functional outcome data on 9,025 torture survivors over six years in the United States. Torture 25 (2), 34–60.

Neumann, V., Gutenbrunner, C., Fialka-Moser, V., et al., 2010. Interdisciplinary team working in physical and rehabilitation medicine. J. Rehabil. Med. 42 (1), 4–8. <http://doi.org/10.2340/16501977.0483.>

Nielsen, H., 2014. Interventions for physiotherapists working with torture survivors–With special focus on chronic pain, PTSD, and sleep disturbances. Dignity Publication Series on Torture and Organised Violence–Praxis Paper.

Nordbrandt, M.S., Carlsson, J., Lindberg, L.G., et al., 2015. Treatment of traumatised refugees with Basic Body Awareness therapy versus mixed physical activity as add on treatment: study protocol of a randomized controlled trial. Trials 16, <http://doi.org/1186/s13063-015-0974-9.>

Norman, S.B., Stein, M.B., Dimsdale, J.E., Hoyt, D.B., 2008. Pain in the aftermath of trauma is a risk factor for post-traumatic stress disorder. Psychol. Med. 38 (4), 533–542. <http://doi.org/10.1016/j.acpain.2008.05.030.>

Norredam, M., Crosby, S., Munarriz, R., et al., 2005. Urologic complications of sexual trauma among male survivors of torture. Urology 65 (1), 28–32.

Office of Public Information, United Nations, 1984. Convention Against Torture and Other Cruel, Inhuman, or Degrading Treatment of Punishment. Office of Public Information, United Nations, New York, New York.

Ogden, P., Minton, K., Pain, C., 2006. Trauma and the Body: A Sensorimotor Approach to Psychotherapy. Norton and Company, New York.

Olsen, D.R., Montgomery, E., Bojholm, S., Foldspang, A., 2006a. Prevalent musculoskeletal pain as a correlate to previous exposure to torture. Scand. J. Public Health 34 (5), 496–503.

Olsen, D.R., Montgomery, E., Bojholm, S., Foldspang, A., 2007. Prevalence of pain in the head, back and feet in refugees previously exposed to torture: a ten-year follow up study. Disabil. Rehabil. 29 (2), 163–171. <http://doi.org/10.1080/09638280600474765.>

Olsen, D.R., Montgomery, E., Carlsson, J., Foldspang, A., 2006b. Prevalent pain and pain level among torture survivors. Dan. Med. J. 53, 210–214.

Oral, R., Ramirez, M., Coohey, C., et al., 2016. Adverse childhood experiences and trauma informed care: the future of health care. Pediatr. Res. 79 (1-2), 227–233. <http://doi.org/10.1038/pr.2015.197.>

O'Sullivan, V., 2015. Releasing the pain: physiotherapy with victims of torture and trauma. Refugee Transitions 30, 33–37.

Peel, M., 2004. Rape as a Method of Torture. Medical Foundation for the Care of Victims of Torture, London, UK.

Phaneth, S., Panha, P., Sopheap, T., et al., 2014. Education as a treatment for chronic pain in survivors of torture and other violent events in Cambodia: experiences of a group-based 'pain school' and evaluation of its effect in a pilot study. J. Appl. Biobehav. Res. 19 (1), 53–69. <http://doi.org/10.1111/jabr.12015.>

Price, C., 2005. Body-oriented therapy in recovery from childhood sexual abuse: an efficacy study. Altern. Ther. Health Med. 11 (5), 46–57.

Price, C., 2007. Dissociation reduction in body therapy during sexual abuse recovery. Complement. Ther. Clin. Pract. 13 (2), 116–128. <http://doi.org/10.1016/j.ctc.2006.08.004.>

Prip, K., 2014. Disability Among Tortured Refugees in Relation to Pain and Sensory Function in Their Feet (PhD dissertation). University of Southern Denmark, Osense, Denmark.

Raeissadat, S., Sadeghi, S., Montazeri, A., 2013. Validation of the pain catastrophizing scale in Iran. J. Basic Appl. Sci. Res. 3 (9), 376–380.

Randall, G., Lutz, E., 1991. Serving Survivors of Torture: A Practical Manual for Health Professionals and Other Service Providers. American Association for the Advancement of Science, Washington DC.

Rodley, N., 2002. The definition(s) of torture in international law. In: 55 Current Legal Problems. Oxford Press, Oxford, UK, pp. 467–493.

Rothschild, B., 2000. The Body Remembers: The Psychopathology of Trauma and Trauma Treatment. Norton, New York.

Roxendal, G., 1985. Body awareness therapy and the body awareness scale: Treatment and evaluation in psychiatric physiotherapy. <http://www.kineoo.nl/biblitheek/body/awareness-therapy-and.pdf.>

Roxendal, G., 1995. Psychosomatically oriented physiotherapy. In: Psychosomatic Medicine. Lund Studentlitteratur, Sweden, pp. 296–312.

Rumsey, N., Clarke, A., White, P., et al., 2004. Altered body image: appearance-related concerns of people with variable disfigurement. J. Adv. Nurs. 48 (5), 443–453. <http://doi.org/10.1111/j.1365-2648.2004.03227.x.>

Rumsey, N., Harcourt, D., 2004. Body image and disfigurement: issues and intervention. Body Image 1 (1), 83–97.

Rundell, S.D., Davenport, T.E., Wagner, T., 2009. Physical therapy management of acute and chronic low back pain using the World Health Organization's International Classification of Functioning, Disability and Health. Phys. Ther. 89 (1), 82–90. <http://doi.org/10.2522/ptj.20080113.>

Rybarczyk, B., Nyenhuis, D., Nicholas, J., et al., 1995. Body image, perceived social stigma, and the prediction of psychosocial adjustment to leg amputation. Rehabil. Psychol. 40 (2), 95–110. <http://doi.org/10.1037/0090-5550.40.2.95.>

Sanders, T., Foster, N.E., Bishop, A., Ong, B.N., 2013. Biopsychosocial care and the physiotherapy encounter: physiotherapists' accounts of low back pain consultations. BMC Musculoskelet. Disord. 14 (65), 1–10. <http://doi.org/10.1186/1471-2474-14-65.>

Saragiotto, B.T., de Almeida, M.O., Yamato, T.P., Maher, C.G., 2016. Multidisciplinary biopsychosocial rehabilitation for nonspecific chronic low back pain. Phys. Ther. 96 (6), 759–763. <http://doi.org/10.2522/ptj.20150359.>

Savnik, A., Amris, K., Rogind, H., et al., 2000. MRI of the plantar structures of the foot after falanga torture. Eur. J. Radiol. 10 (10), 1655–1659.

Schubert, C.C., Punamaki, R.L., 2011. Mental health among torture survivors; Cultural background, refugee status and gender. Nord. J. Psychiatry 65 (3), 175–182. <http://doi.org/10.3109/08039488.2010.514943.>

Selye, H., 1950. The Physiology and Pathology of Exposure to Stress. Acta Endoeringologica, Montreal, Canada.

Selye, H., 1970. The evolution of the stress concept: stress and cardiovascular disease. Am. J. Cardiol. 26 (3), 289–299. <http://doi.org/10.1016/0002-9149(70)90796-4.>

Shannon, P.J., 2014. Refugees' advice to physicians: how to ask about mental health. Fam. Pract. 31 (4), 1–5. <http://doi.org/10.1093/fampra/cmu017.>

Shannon, P.J., O'Dougherty, M., Mehta, E., 2012. Refugees' perspectives on barriers to communication about trauma history in primary care. Ment. Health Fam. Med. 9, 47–55.

Shannon, P.J., Vinson, G.A., Wieling, E., et al., 2015a. Torture, war trauma, and mental health symptoms of newly arrived Karen refugees. J. Loss Trauma 20 (6), 577–590. <http://10.1080/15325024.2014.965971.>

Shannon, P.J., Wieling, E., Simmelink-McCleary, J., Becher, E., 2014. Beyond stigma: Barriers to discussing mental health in refugee populations. Journal of Loss and Coping: International Perspectives on Stress and Aging 20 (3), 281–296. <http://doi.org/10.1080/15325024.2014.934629.>

Shannon, P.J., Wieling, L., Simmelink- McLeay, J., Becher, E., 2015b. Exploring the mental health effects of political trauma with newly arrived refugees. Qual. Health Res. 25 (4), 443–457.

Sharp, T.J., Harvey, A.G., 2001. Chronic pain and posttraumatic stress disorder: mutual maintenance? Clin. Psychol. Rev. 21 (6), 857–877. <http://doi.org/10.1016/50272-7358(00)00071-4.>

Sjolund, B.H., Kastrup, M., Montgomery, E., Persson, A.L., 2009. Rehabilitating torture survivors. J. Rehabil. Med. 41 (9), 689–696. <http://doi.org/10.2340/16501977-0426.>

Smeets, R.J., Vlaeyen, J.W., Kester, A.D., Knottnerus, J.A., 2006. Reduction of pain catastrophizing mediates the outcome of both physical and cognitive-behavioral treatment in chronic low back pain. Pain 7 (4), 261–271.

Spinhoven, P., ter Kuile, M., Kole-Snijders, A., et al., 2004. Catastrophizing and internal pain control as mediators of outcome in the multidisciplinary treatment of chronic low back pain. Eur. J. Pain 8 (3), 211–219. <http://doi.org/10.1016/j.ejpain.2003.08.003.>

Stade, K., Skammeritz, S., Hjorkjaer, C., Carlsson, J., 2015. 'After all that my body has been through, I feel good that it is still working'—Basic Body Awareness Therapy for traumatised refugees. Torture 25 (1), 33–50.

Stoddard, F.J., 1982. Body image development in the burned child. J. Am. Acad. Child Psychiatry 21 (5), 502–507. <http://doi.org/10.1016/S0002-7138(09)60802-5.>

Stratakis, C.A., Chrousos, G.P., 1995. Neuroendocrinology and pathophysiology of the stress system. Ann. N. Y. Acad. Sci. 77 (1), 1–18. <http://doi.org/10.1111/j.1749-6632.1995.tb44666.x.>

Substance Abuse and Mental Health Services Administration, 2014. SAMSHA's Concept of Trauma and Guidance for a Trauma-Informed Approach (No. HHS Publication No. (SMA) 14-4884). Substance Abuse and Mental Health Services Administration, Rockville, MD, pp. 1–27.

Sullivan, M.J.L., Adams, H., 2010. Psychological techniques to augment the impact of physiotherapy interventions for low back pain. Physiother. Can. 62 (3), 180–189. <http://doi.org/10.3138/physio.62.3.180.>

Sullivan, M.J.L., Rogers, W., Kirsch, I., 2001a. Catastrophizing, depression and expectancies for pain and emotional distress. Pain 91 (1-2), 147–154.

Sullivan, M.J.L., Thorn, B., Haythornthwaite, J., et al., 2001b. Theoretical perspectives on the relation between catastrophizing and pain. Clin. J. Pain 17 (1), 52–64.

Taylor, B., Carswell, K., Williams, A.C., 2013. The interaction of persistent pain and post-traumatic re-experiencing: a qualitative study of torture survivors. J. Pain Symptom Manage. 46 (4), 546–555. <http://doi.org/10.1016/j.jpainsymman.2012.10.281.>

Teodorescu, D.S., Heir, T., Sigveland, J., et al., 2015. Chronic pain in multi-traumatized outpatients with a refugee background resettled in Norway: a cross-sectional study. BMC Psychol. 3 (7), 1–12. <http://doi.org/10.1186/S40359-015-5064-5.>

The Center for Victims of Torture, 2005a. Core competencies in working with survivors. In: Healing the Hurt: A Guide for Developing Services for Torture Survivors. The Center for Victims of Torture, Minnesota, USA, pp. 19–38. <http://www.healtorture.org/content/chapter3-core-competencies-working-survivors.>

The Center for Victims of Torture, 2005b. Working with torture survivors. In: Healing the Hurt: A Guide for Developing Services for Torture Survivors. National Capacity Building Project, Minnesota, USA, pp. 19–38. <http://www.healtorture.org/content/chapter3-core-competencies-working-survivors.>

Tol, W.A., Song, S., Jordans, M.J., 2013. Annual Research Review: resilience and mental health in children living in areas of armed conflict-a systematic review of findings in low- and middle-income countries. J. Child Psychol. Psychiatry 54 (4), 445–460. <http://doi.org/10.1111/jcpp.12053.>

Turk, D., 2004. Understanding pain sufferers: the role of chronic processes. Spine J. 4 (1), 1–7.

Turk, D., Ukifuji, A., 2002. Psychological factors in chronic pain: evolution and revolution. J. Consult. Clin. Psychol. 70 (3), 678–690.

United Nations Children's Fund, 2014. Hidden in Plain Sight: A Statistical Analysis of Violence Against Children. UNICEF, New York, New York. <http://www.unicef.org/publications/index_74865.html.>

United Nations Office for the Coordination of Humanitarian Affairs, 2016. Sexual and Gender-Based Violence (SGBV)-SGBV Framework. United Nations Office for the Coordination of Humanitarian Affairs. <http://www.unocha.org/what-we-do/advocacy/thematic-campaigns/sgbv-framework.>

Van Damme, S., Crombez, G., Bijttebier, P., et al., 2002. A confirmatory factor analysis of the Pain Catastrophizing Scale: invariant factor structure across clinical and non-clinical populations. Pain 96 (3), 319–324. <http://doi.org/10.1016/S0304-3959(01)00463-8.>

Van den Bruel, A., Haj-Hassan, T., Thompson, M., et al., 2010. Diagnostic value of clinical features at presentation to identify serious infection in children in developed countries: a systematic review. Lancet 375 (9717), 834–845. <http://doi.org/10.1016/S0140-6736(09)62000-6.>

van der Kolk, B., 2005. Towards a rational diagnosis for chronically traumatized children. Psychiatr. Ann. 1–18.

van der Kolk, B., 2014. The Body Keeps the Score: Brain, Mind, and Body in the Healing of Trauma. Viking Press, New York.

van der Kolk, B., Pelcovitz, D., Roth, S., et al., 1996. Dissociation, somatization, and affect dysregulation: The complexity of adaptation to trauma. Am. J. Psychiatry 153 (7), 83–93. <http://doi.org/10.1176/ajp.153.7.83.>

Vargas, C., O'Rourke, D., Esfandiari, M., 2004. Complementary therapies for treating survivors of torture. Refuge: Canada's Periodical on Refugees 22 (1), 129–137.

Vogel, H., Schmitz-Engels, F., Grillo, C., 2007. Radiology of torture. Eur. J. Radiol. 63 (2), 187–204. <http://doi.org/10.106/j.ejrad.2007.03.036.>

Wetterhahn, K.A., Hanson, C., Levy, C.E., 2002. Effect of participation in physical activity on body image of amputees. Am. J. Phys. Med. Rehabil. 81 (3), 194–201. <http://doi.org/10.1097/00002060-200203000-00007.>

Williams, A.C., Pena, C.R., Rice, A.S., 2010. Persistent pain in survivors of torture: a cohort study. J. Pain Symptom Manage. 40 (5), 715–722. <http://doi.org/10.1016/j.jpainsymman.2010.02.018.>

Willard, C.L., Rabin, M., Lawless, M., 2014. The prevalence of torture and associated symptoms in United States Iraqi refugees. J. Immigr. Minor. Health 16 (6), 1069–1076. <http://doi.org/10.1007/s10903-013-9817-5.>

World Confederation for Physical Therapy, 2014. Policy: Description of Physical Therapy. World Confederation for Physical Therapy, Zambia, pp. 1–12. <http://www.wcpt.ps-descriptionPT.>

Yagihashi, S., Yamagishi, S.I., Wada, R., 2007. Pathology and pathogenic mechanisms of diabetic neuropathy: Correlation with clinical signs and symptoms. Diabetes Res. Clin. Pract. 77 (3 Suppl.), S184–S189. <http://doi.org/10.1016/j.diabres.2007.01.054.>

Zarkov, D., 2001. The body and the other man: Sexual violence and the construction of masculinity, sexuality and ethnicity in creation media. In: Victims, Perpetrators or Actors? Gender, Armed Conflict and Political Violence. Zed Books, London, pp. 69–81.

Zawati, H., 2007. Impunity or immunity: Wartime male rape and sexual torture as a crime against humanity. Torture 17 (1), 27–47.

5.2.2 Physiotherapy for Sexually Abused Women

MONICA MATTSSON

KEY POINTS

■ Global prevalence studies of child sexual abuse (CSA) estimate an occurrence of 20% for females, but most authors on the subject of prevalence remark on the great number of hidden statistics.

■ CSA has been shown to be a powerful predictor of health problems in adulthood, and indicates that sexual abuse poses a great threat to girls' and women's lives and health all over the world.

■ Physiotherapy is an established and effective way to relieve consequences of sexual abuse when working

according to principles that take care of processes related to the trauma dynamics of stigmatization in child and adolescent victims of sexual abuse.

■ Working with adjusted Basic Body Awareness is one way to bring back vitality to life and to foster a self-caring attitude through movement and reflections.

LEARNING OBJECTIVES

■ Can you see any disadvantages for a physiotherapist asking the patient about abuse history and connect such experiences to examination and treatment?

■ Do you agree that Basic Body Awareness Therapy (BBAT) is a sensible treatment for women suffering from sexual abuse? If not, why do you reject BBAT as an appropriate physiotherapy treatment in these circumstances?

■ Which principle from the nine specified would you denote as the most important for a physiotherapist to be aware of? And which is the most difficult principle to work according to?

INTRODUCTION AND PREVALENCE OF SEXUAL ABUSE

Substantial research has revealed that the prevalence of sexual abuse (SA) is 12% for females, and remained at the same level for four decades from the 1960s until the 1990s. According to Finkelhor, the lifetime experience of 17-year-olds with SA and sexual assault was 26% for girls (Finkelhor et al., 2014). However, in the psychiatric population the prevalence is around 50% (Jacobson & Herald, 1990; Craine et al., 1988).

A global prevalence study of child sexual abuse (CSA) published in 2009 estimated an occurrence of 19.7% for females, according to a study that examined 65 studies from 22 countries (Pereda et al., 2009). These findings are in line with the report by the World Health Organization (WHO) on violence against children (Newell & O'Neill, 2008).

According to the European Council's report on CSA, one of five children are exposed. The outcome from this report has resulted in suggestions and policymaking in the European Council to undertake powerful actions to protect children from SA, and prevention measures and therapeutic interventions have been suggested (Lalor & McElvaney, 2010).

Most authors on the subject of prevalence remark that there are a great number of hidden statistics and that it is impossible to know the true incidence or prevalence of CSA. One reason is that victims rarely disclose to official sources. Another difficulty in verifying prevalence is the use of different definitions and measurements in the studies, and if methodological variations are at hand. To tell the number of unrecorded cases is difficult, but consensus prevails regarding the complexity of acquiring the true figures, as reporting is connected with feelings of shame and guilt combined with fear of punishment by the perpetrator or fear of not being believed (Feiring et al., 1996; Paine & Hansen, 2002; Rädda Barnen, 2012).

However, it is estimated that almost half of all SA cases are taking place against girls younger than 16 years old (Rädda Barnen, 2012). As adults, many of these girls will never be given the opportunity to understand the cause of their suffering. They will not even be given the chance to process their conscious memories in spite of being heavy consumers of health care. One reason is the healthcare providers' lack of knowledge and lack of courage in recognizing the issue. This shortcoming could, however, be dealt with by information and education (Schachter et al., 2009; WHO, 2003).

CONSEQUENCES FOR ADULT HEALTH

The association between a reported history of child abuse and adult health problems has repeatedly been documented, including groups of patients with chronic pelvic pain, headaches, backache, fibromyalgia syndrome and gastroenterological symptoms. The case for SA adversely affecting the future health is seen in a wide variety of studies and meta-analyses (Briere & Elliot, 2003; Paras, 2009).

Many researchers have studied chronic pain in particular and its association with childhood abuse (Davis et al., 2005; Van der Kolk, 1994). Association between posttraumatic stress disorders (PTSD) and CSA is also commonly reported. Wijma et al. investigated CSA in a gynaecological population and found that 4.5% met the criteria for PTSD, and this finding was related to patients with multiple experiences of abuse (Wijma et al., 2000).

Some authors, however, are less convinced by the association between CSA and pain in later life, and question the recommended clinical routine of assessing abuse histories. A prospective study on SA did not reveal an absolute correlation, but on the other hand, when the same patients gave their retrospective self-report of SA, the association was significant (Raphael, 2005).

Clinical researchers and clinicians seem to be more inclined to suggest that SA is associated with multiple health problems and see the value in investigating patients' life history when appropriate (Davis et al., 2005; Van Houdenhove, 2006).

Politicians and medical and user organizations are advocating the need to ask the client about experiences of sexual violence in most healthcare situations. Strong justifications have been brought forward for asking the patient about abuse history and connecting such experiences to examination and treatment. A tricky question asked in a humble and professional way can at best lead to empowerment for the patient (Wijma et al., 2002; Wijma & Siwa, 2004).

RECOGNITION OF SEXUAL ABUSE IN SOCIETY AND CONSEQUENCES FOR HEALTHCARE SERVICES

The reported high rates of SA, with a preponderance of female victims, indicate that SA poses a great threat to girls' and women's lives and health all over the world (Leserman, 2005; Rädda Barnen, 2014).

While not everyone who reports a history of CSA develops great health problems, many survivors live with a variety of chronic physical, behavioural, and psychological problems that bring them into frequent contact with healthcare practitioners such as physiotherapists (PTs) (Schachter et al., 1999).

Clinicians, researchers, social workers and nongovernmental organizations have currently addressed the issues of SA and implications for consultations in healthcare services, and formulated plans of action for health staff. Ignorance of the aftermath of the abuse is common and patients seeking professionals are not always directly aware of the consequences of sexual abuse in relation to seeing healthcare professionals. Survivors' illnesses and disorders are often hidden in unclear bodily or psychological signs and symptoms.

Avoiding offering a respectful and professional encounter can do much harm and hinder further treatment interventions (Savell et al., 2005). During the last 20 years more knowledge of long-term consequences of SA has been developed and spread. Guidelines have been formulated for proper care and treatment directed at specific clinical situations; for instance, in gynaecological examination procedures and midwifery (Hilden et al., 2003; Wood & Van Esterik, 2010, Siwe, 2013).

Summing up prevalence and health: CSA has been shown to be a powerful predictor of health problems in adulthood.

CLINICAL PITFALLS

In spite of good intensions, effectively managing respectful communication in nonegalitarian relationships, as in patient–expert situations, is in practice a task laden with potential pitfalls. Staff–patient interactions can easily result in psychological stress for both patient and professional, thereby constituting a form of abuse that generally receives little attention. The likelihood of experiencing healthcare abuse is also greater for patients having a life history of abuse (Hilden et al., 2004). This phenomenon is also equally true for physiotherapy.

PHYSIOTHERAPY AND SEXUAL ABUSE

Few curricula provide adequate education to prepare PTs to be adequately equipped to provide appropriate help for the open or hidden harm that survivors may be presenting.

A physiotherapy treatment for SA may offer inbuilt multiple opportunities to heal and cure, as well as damage and harm. To protect both PT and patient from insidious pitfalls, some health authorities have provided regulations relating to sexual behaviour in therapy. For instance: patients are encouraged to react and take actions if these standards are exceeded (Understanding sexual abuse, 2014, http://collegept.org/public/protectingthepublic/understandingsexualabuse).

In physiotherapy little attention has been paid towards addressing treatments and encounters in connection with SA, and few studies have been carried out to investigate how PTs handle disclosure of SA or unexpected reactions and behaviours while touching survivors of SA.

By listening to patients' own views and stories, Mattsson and colleagues investigated the aftermaths of CSA with the objective of learning from women survivors. The aim was to develop a suitable physiotherapeutic method of treating and responding to women with CSA (Mattsson et al., 1997, 1998). The research was organized by offering a group treatment model, and during the treatment to search for an optimal design that considered both individual psychological difficulties as well as the women's needs of improved somatic functioning. Basic Body Awareness Therapy (BBAT) was used for that purpose. The treatment process is described in Mattsson et al. (1997) and the evaluation of the treatment in Mattsson et al. (1998).

BASIC BODY AWARENESS THERAPY: A SHORT DESCRIPTION

BBAT is a well-established physiotherapeutic treatment modality within psychiatric and psychosomatic physiotherapy and has been developed for patients with longstanding complex illnesses (Roxendal, 1985). It is well researched, both the methodology and the outcome, and is often recommended, not only in relation to psychosomatic problems. Balance, free breathing and mental presence can be promoted through BBAT and the treatment starts in accordance with the patient's existing recourses and focuses on health-generating elements. Within BBAT specific movements have been developed for coping with demands of daily life, and by regular practice the person will gain better health and well-being. The movements aim at normalizing balance, muscle tension, breathing and coordination, and the interaction between them, and are performed in laying, sitting, standing and walking positions. The therapist's own movement awareness and how she is communicating her own movements, is critical for the quality and effectiveness of the therapy (Skjaerven et al., 2010). The most central therapeutic components in BBAT include creating a movement dialogue as well as a verbal channel of communication between patient and therapist (Mattsson et al., 2000). BBAT is described in more detail elsewhere in this book.

PATIENT NEEDS AND PREFERENCES IN RELATION TO PHYSIOTHERAPY

In-depth qualitative interviews of female survivors have been undertaken in order to gain insight into the needs and preferences in relation to physiotherapy of persons suffering from SA (Schachter et al., 1999). The unconditional need to create a trustful relationship was a significant result from the studies and also the professional's search to produce active participation throughout the treatment. The benefits of the physiotherapy can be maximized by attending to the needs of the individual and to their sense of safety throughout the whole treatment.

The findings from this important and unique study prepared the ground for a 10-year project, which ended up with an extensive handbook for healthcare professionals of all categories (Schachter et al., 1999, 2004, 2009; Stalker et al., 2005). This handbook, distributed by the Public Health Agency of Canada, presents information that will help all practitioners practise in a manner that is sensitive to the needs of adult survivors of CSA.

The nine principles of advice given in the article *Towards a sensitive practice* (Schachter et al., 1999) can easily be transferred into most clinical physiotherapy.

PRINCIPLES OF 'SENSITIVE PRACTICE' TRANSFERRED INTO PHYSIOTHERAPY

Child abuse is a serious betrayal of trust. Many situations in the healthcare setting may trigger the feeling of being abused and out of control, not least in physiotherapy. As a result of abuse history, safety is of utmost importance for patient and practitioner. Otherwise, little progress and much misunderstanding and incorrect treatment could take place.

I will later describe how BBAT practice, principles and therapeutic components can contribute to safe and sensitive treatment, taking into account Schachter's nine principles. By adopting these principles as the standard of care, PTs convey respect, support clients' autonomy and decrease the likelihood of unintentional retraumatization.

A description of how BBAT can be modified in the treatment of survivors of CSA in a clinical PT setting, along with some examples *in italics* of how the issue was developed in my own research project by offering a group treatment model to SA survivors follows.

1. Establish and Maintain a Positive Rapport

The first encounter is crucial and cannot be repeated. There is often a conflict between the need to seek health care for a physical problem and the ambivalence or dislike of one's body, which affects the trust and disturbs the relationship. Although this distrust originates in the past, survivors constantly scrutinize healthcare providers for confirmation that they are taking active and ongoing steps to demonstrate their trustworthiness. The first minutes of the first encounter should be used to give the survivor friendly attention, and find an opening where she gets the opportunity to tell or ask whatever is on her mind.

Before the group started every woman was seen individually and BBAT was presented, the aims of the study explained and time given to examine the fears and doubts of participating in the group. We were two leaders, one female gynaecologist and one BBAT PT. At the end of the first meeting the PT tried out some practice with the client. This concrete approach was of importance to give the women an idea of the outline of the group and the possible stress. However, most of the women were interested in joining the group.

PTs are used to observe, analyse and describe the body, movement coordinations and to interpret body communication. A BBAT PT is trained in acknowledging what is going on in the body and in identifying healthy resources and reactions. She/he can offer an atmosphere that is calming and comforting on body reactions, which has consequences for the movement quality. Calm promotes a feeling of security and is a mediator for a good relationship. The PT has to attend to her own behaviour, movements, use of her voice, and be able to recognize when she is disturbing the situation and be able to admit if she has distressed the client.

2. Establish a Partnership With the Client

Survivors were, as children, often not allowed control over themselves and their own bodies. In adulthood, having control is of high importance and a great issue for feeling safe.

A first step for everybody was to find security in the treatment area. The participants were encouraged to choose a place where they could sit and 'feel secure enough', feeling rooted. Settling down on that self-selected place helped both the feeling of control and encouraged the sharing of responsibility for the treatment.

From that platform the participants could start to explore simple movements like 'close your legs together and let go', or 'let the arms come up above your head and find a place where your arms can rest'.

To be able to control one's body's movements and function gives a feeling of control and confidence. With movements performed within the limits of stability, the control grows, and self-consciousness and individual freedom is promoted.

When working with BBAT there are many opportunities for handing over the control to the client. Particularly when touch or massage is used, it is essential to collaborate around how that can be done and how the giver of massage would know that the survivor is feeling uncomfortable. Preferably there should be an expressed agreement of saying 'Stop', if the receiver wants to finish. In BBAT there are specific movements with the aim to develop the coordination of the closing around the centre of the body. When saying 'Stop', the movement and expression becomes quick and powerful, and works as a protection against being hurt.

The women gave massage to each other, one sitting on a low stool, the other standing behind. The giver's hands were placed on top of the receiver's shoulders. One aim was to stimulate the contact with the ground and the central line in the body with a targeted intermittent light pressure down-and-up. This massage is also working on balancing the rhythm of the breathing, while listening and being present. The receiver could at any time say, 'Stop' and if so, the massage ceased.

This method of giving massage is often tolerated, particularly when given by a survivor mate.

For a survivor it is very important to experience that a 'Stop' is respected and that there are different ways to build up control and contact with the body in various positions (lying, sitting or standing) that are manageable.

What is experienced and reported to be good for the client one day could be far too much provocation at the next session. In order to make progress an appropriate dosage is needed, always staying within the safety margin. If there is a discrepancy between what the client is saying and what the client's body and movements are expressing, it needs to be addressed and 'laid on the table'. 'How was this for you?' Honesty and courage in bringing up tricky things in a good way can often contribute to increased trust and improved collaboration.

3. Offer Choice of Gender of PT

In psychosomatic physiotherapy PTs are mostly female, and PTs with a specialization in BBAT are regrettably mostly women. That makes the choice of gender not so simple for the client. The topic may sometimes be brought up and if the survivor wants a therapist of another gender, the professional could offer to contact a colleague whom she trusts.

4. Share Information: a Critical Two-Way Exchange of Dialogue

Basic information is crucial for safety, and must start right away. During the whole treatment period this attitude to two-way exchange is needed. The PT explains what is going to happen, for instance, 'Now I will put my hand on your left arm'. Sometimes she demonstrates movement coordinations with her own body and asks for willingness to explore it. In BBAT with SA the PT frequently asks for feedback in relation to what has been worked with or explored, and stimulates the client to say when she is confused or uncomfortable.

We gave the group much time for reflection about experiences from the movements practice, and if something particularly had been evoked that had to be handled. The leaders suggested themes. For instance; 'How is it for you to move up and down along the vertical line in your body?' 'Do you sense when you are going to lose balance?' 'Can you find words to describe your sensations?'

The shared information is central for the patient's process of change but also for the PT's security in the treatment. PTs working with survivors know that everything with the body and its movements can be a trigger and release associations and memories from the abuse, but easily also the opposite, finding very small signs of health and relief. The shared information will be like a gauge, helping both of them to control and secure the treatment.

5. Convey Understanding and Work With Survivors' Attitudes About the Body and Pain

Understanding the body and its movements in a dialectic way, both as object and as subject, have implications for treatment and communication. The body is an anatomical matter but also the centre of thoughts, perceptions and meaning, the lived body. These aspects are important in the treatment. BBAT treatment affects the quality of movements, strengthens the self-awareness and furthers acceptance of the body and its pains. To experience and perceive are keys in the movement learning process. It is important to listen to the experiences expressed by the survivor. The PT helps the survivor to put together her understanding and knowledge so personal meaning and acceptance develop by listening to bodily sensations.

Aching feet was a common recurring problem, described by the patients. It was also common that they were disgusted over their feet, which were swollen and discoloured indicating poor circulation. To accept a standing position for a while was a great challenge. To tolerate one's sensations was a greater challenge, but also an opportunity to describe in more detail what it felt like. Slowly greater acceptance grew around the painful parts and unpleasant body. By working with gravity and the postural reflexes, health was promoted while greater stability in the body and its movements evolved.

In BBAT the client is supported by the PT to gain a more optimal balance, experience the centring process in the body and its consequence for the movement quality. Thereby bodily competence and more functional movements build up, which leads to self-control. Gaining improved access to breathing may open up more sensations and connections to the 'I am', the true self or the embodied identity.

Every session comprised moments of listening to one's breathing when being still and in movement. By resting the hands lightly on the soft area around the centre of the body, the breathing rhythm was experienced, calm or rapid. Awareness of one's breathing was not always comfortable. Gradually it became easier to just surrender to what was sensed and to tolerate different rhythms in the breathing. The breathing became a reliable partner.

Slowly the survivor receives positive experiences in relation to the body and how to move, and how to use the body in daily life, which can smooth out bodily disconnection and sensations of hate and shame about the body. A sense of being a victim and helplessness may dissolve.

6. Work With the Client on the Difficult Physical Environmental Factors

In the physical world around healthcare facilities there may be frightening or disturbing environmental factors preventing the survivors from getting to the appointment. The physiotherapy exercise room is often an open space with more or less strange training tools. Many survivors and PTs prefer to meet in a small separate room, with few obstacles around and quiet colours on the walls.

We put much effort into finding an adequate practice room for feeling safe and comfortable. The room was sparsely equipped, only tools needed for the class were visible. To start with we also gave the survivors much time to get acquainted with the room and comment on their dislikes. In spite of the absence of windows we could build up a warm environment in the room.

It is the task of the PT to determine what is preferable for the client and how different arrangements influence the relationship. Small things that the PT is unaware of in the environment can trigger the fight and flight reaction, and destroy the fragile contact. If the client suffers from PTSD this is often the case.

It is well known that survivors of SA report on discomfort and vulnerability related to undressing. In BBAT the therapy is mostly performed with clothes on. Even in massage the client is dressed comfortably for the purpose.

The participants were asked to wear trousers that were easy to move in. We wanted to highlight that the therapy was about movement practice and to take care of the body's needs and well-being.

7. Understand and Respond Sensitively to 'Triggers' and Dissociation

Many survivors hesitate to attend physiotherapy because of fears of getting flashbacks when the body and movements are the objects of the treatment. It seems to be necessary to inform and educate the survivors about the phenomenon of flashback and PTSD, and to find strategies to handle the painful body memories.

Survivors want information from professionals and release from their painful sensations and flashbacks. We could not always give answers but we gave clients time to present their own experiences and asked them to suggest alternative interpretations, which did settle their concerns. Most important was also to try moving using the principles in BBAT, which could be done whenever they needed a support from outside. Many preferred a movement called the 'Arm-wave'; bringing the arms up to the horizon line, and in a circle pushing them back again. Inviting the organic breathing into the movement enhanced the effect, and helped to improve stabilization.

Sometimes the survivor is aware of the connection between flashbacks and abuse, but many times they are totally unaware. Whatever is the case, it is most important for the PT to provide the patient with strategies for use in daily life and to promote their awareness and presence, and to use strategies to calm down the arousal. The focus is on supporting them in gaining mastery of themselves.

8. Respond Carefully to Disclosure of Abuse

Most survivors are not referred to physiotherapy *because of CSA* (but some are). Most commonly the client is referred because of pain in the musculoskeletal system or possibly because of stress and anxiety. During the course of treatment the PT might notice verbal or nonverbal signs of discomfort. At that point some sort of disclosure may occur, sometimes only as hints, other times the whole abuse history is presented. How the disclosure is taken care of is crucial for the person and for the ongoing treatment. Being present and listening empathically can often be enough. It may be the first time the survivor tells the story to somebody. There are no standard right answers to put forward. Even if the PT's verbal response may not be as important, it is essential that she is showing her acceptance and acknowledgement of the abuse and its consequences for the physical and mental health of the survivor.

The aim of the study was not to ask for survivors' disclosures in particular, but the group setting and the mutual trust encouraged them to disclose. Being among like-minded sisters the disclosures were taken with much empathy. As leaders we mostly listened and limited the amount of stuff being brought up. Although there was much despair and sorrow, the disclosure often had a liberating effect on the discloser. After an intense emotional episode we played down the emotional storm with attention to balance in a stable standing position.

9. Practise Holistic Health Care

BBAT is considered to be a holistic physiotherapy movement awareness modality, which means to see the individual at all times as a whole inseparable person with a body, where bone and flesh interacts with thoughts, feelings and experiences, and with movements.

BBAT is built up around four perspectives: the physical, physiological, psychological and purely human perspectives. While working from a PT point of view, on the whole it is possible to address one or more perspectives at a time. One particular movement can be practised from a purely physiological perspective, but the same movement can also be used for exploring all four perspectives. In BBAT the patient is learning to practise a more stable balance, more free breathing and awareness, and how these elements are integrated into movements. The three aspects are interrelated and dependent on each other. How they interact is expressed in movement quality (Skjaerven et al., 2008).

Movement quality can be seen, experienced, observed and assessed, and is the core phenomenon in BBAT. It has also been investigated in several studies, and by addressing the four perspectives, mental awareness and movement quality are furthered.

Standing upright, we moved up and down in the vertical line, by flexing the knees and coming up again. The participants were invited to look for the path of the movement (physical perspective). After a while the focus was directed at finding the flow and ease of the movement (physiological dimension). Later on the same movement was performed but the participant was now encouraged to invite related thoughts or emotions when doing the movement (psychological dimension). Some participants also found the existential dimension in the movement expressing 'now I see more clearly that I must be more protective of myself'.

As a result of the process of change, becoming more aware and having better insight, the survivor occasionally confronts the perpetrator. Such an action can be a disturbing event, but at the same time tremendously empowering for the survivor.

SUMMARY AND CONCLUSION

A psychological trauma affects the body, its movement coordination and movement habits in daily life. In CSA it is a betrayal of trust as well as a physical trauma the child has gone through. The aftermaths affect adulthood and compromise the survivors' quality of life and health. Many survivors appreciate the way bodily aspects are cared for by BBAT, giving them opportunities to resolve the consequences through movement practice.

BBAT aims to evoke the existential human perspective that influences people's unique ability to make conscious choices. That includes accepting and being responsible for the consequences of choices and the courage to engage with the world.

BBAT is one way to bring back vitality to life and to foster a self-caring attitude through movement and reflections. BBAT has been built up in a structured way, taking into account the effect on the organism. It is grounded and underpinned by theoretical suppositions, which are anchored in practice and research. Its strength has roots in the phenomenological approach helping the practitioners of the method to gain insight into the experienced world, and also to structure a movement pedagogy that increases movement quality and strengthens the self for suffering individuals.

REFERENCES

Briere, J., Elliott, D.M., 2003. Prevalence and psychological sequelae of self-reported childhood physical and sexual abuse in a general population sample of men and women. Child Abuse Negl. 27 (10), 1205–1222.

Craine, L.S., Henson, C.E., Colliver, J.A., MacLean, D.G., 1988. Prevalence of a history of sexual abuse among female psychiatric patients in a state hospital system. Hosp. Community Psychiatry 39 (3), 300–304.

Davis, D.A., Leuken, L.J., Zautra, A.J., 2005. Are reports of childhood abuse related to the experience of chronic pain in adulthood? A meta-analytic review of the literature. Clin. J. Pain 21, 398–405.

Feiring, C., Taska, L., Lewis, M., 1996. A process model for understanding adaptation to sexual abuse: the role of shame in defining stigmatization. Child Abuse Negl. 20 (8), 767–782.

Finkelhor, D., Shattuck, A., Turner, H.A., Hamby, S.L., 2014. The lifetime prevalence of child sexual abuse and sexual assault assessed in late adolescence. J. Adolesc. Health 55, 329–333.

Gyllensten, A.L., Skär, L., Miller, M., Gard, G., 2010. Understanding body awareness—a model of embodied identity. Physiother. Prac. 26 (7), 439–446.

Hedlund, L., Gyllensten, A.L., 2010. The experiences of basic body awareness therapy in patients with Schizophrenia. J. Bodyw. Mov. Ther. 14, 245–254.

Hilden, M., Schei, B., Swahnberg, K., et al., 2004. A history of sexual abuse and health: a Nordic multicentre study. Br. J. Obstet. Gynaecol. 111 (10), 1121–1127.

Hilden, M., Sidenius, K., Langhoff-Roos, J., et al., 2003. Women's experiences of the gynaecologic examination: factors associated with discomfort. Acta Obstet. Gynecol. Scand. 82 (11), 1030–1036.

Jacobson, A., Herald, C., 1990. The relevance of childhood sexual abuse to adult psychiatric inpatient care. Hosp. Comm. Psychiatry 41 (2), 154–158.

Lalor, K., McElvaney, R., 2010. Overview of the nature and extent of child sexual abuse in Europe. In: Council of Europe, Protecting Children From Sexual Violence—A Comprehensive Approach. Council of Europe, Strasbourg.

Leserman, J., 2005. Sexual abuse history: prevalence, health effects, mediators, and psychological treatment. Psychosom. Med. 67 (6), 906–915.

Mattsson, M., Wikman, M., Dahlgren, L., et al., 1997. Body awareness therapy with sexually abused women. Description of a teatment modality. J. Bodyw. Mov. Ther. 1 (5), 280–288.

Mattsson, M., Wikman, M., Dahlgren, L., et al., 1998. Body awareness therapy with sexually abused women. Evaluation of body awareness in a group setting. J. Bodyw. Mov. Ther. 2 (1), 38–45.

Mattsson, M., Wikman, M., Dahlgren, L., Mattsson, B., 2000. Physiotherapy as empowerment—treating women with chronic pelvic pain. Adv. Physiother. 2, 125–143.

Newell, P., O'Neill, K., 2008. Challenging Violence Against Children: A Handbook for NGOs Working on Follow-up to the UN Study. Save the Children, London.

Paine, M., Hansen, D., 2002. Factors influencing children to self-disclose sexual abuse. Clin. Psychol. Rev. 22 (2), 272–295.

Paras, M.L., Murad, M.H., Chen, L.P., et al., 2009. Sexual abuse and lifetime diagnosis of somatic disorders. A systematic review and meta-analysis. JAMA 302, 550–561.

Pereda, N., Guilera, G., Forns, M., Gómez-Benito, J., 2009. The international epidemiology of child sexual abuse: a continuation of Finkelhor (1994). Child Abuse Negl. 33 (6), 331–342.

Rädda Barnen (Save the Children), 2012. Garantinivå för stöd till barn i utsatta situationer, (Guaranteed level of support for children at risk) (Article in Swedish). <http://www.raddabarnen.se/Documents/medlemssidor/verksamhet/barn-drabbade-av-vald/Forandrings-arbete/rapport_garantinivae_2013.pdf.>

Rädda Barnen (Save the Children), 2014. Frågor och svar om sexuella övergrepp på barn. (Questions and answers on sexual abuse in children) (Article in Swedish). <http://www.raddabarnen.se/min-kropp-ar-min/fragor-och-svar/.

Raphael, K., 2005. Childhood abuse and pain in adulthood more than a modest relationship? Clin. J. Pain 21, 371–373.>

Roxendal, G., 1985. Body Awareness Therapy and The Body Awareness Scale, Treatment and Evaluation in Psychiatric Physiotherapy. Department of Rehabilitation Medicine. University of Göteborg and Psychiatric Department II, Lillhagen Hospital, Hisings Backa, Göteborg. (Thesis).

Savell, S., 2005. Child sexual abuse: are health care providers looking the other way? J. Forensic Nurs. 1, 78–85.

Schachter, C., Radomsky, N., Stalker, C., Teram, E., 2004. Women survivors of child sexual abuse. How can health professionals promote healing? Can. Fam. Physician 50, 405–412.

Schachter, C., Stalker, C., Teram, E., 1999. Toward sensitive practice: issues for physical therapists working with survivors of childhood sexual abuse. Phys. Ther. 79, 248–261.

Schachter, C.L., Stalker, C.A., Teram, E., et al., 2009. Handbook on Sensitive Practice for Health Care Practitioner: Lessons From Adult Survivors of Childhood Sexual Abuse. Public Health Agency of Canada, Ottawa.

Siwe, K., Wijma, B., 2013. The first pelvic examination for an adolescent: is this rite of passage used to its full potential? Curr. Opin. Obstet. Gynecol. 25, 357–363.

Skjaerven, L.H., Kristoffersen, K., Gard, G., 2008. An eye for movement quality: a phenomenological study of movement quality reflecting a group of physiotherapists' understanding of the phenomenon. Physiother. Theory Pract. 24 (1), 13–27.

Skjaerven, L.H., Kristoffersen, K., Gard, G., 2010. How can movement quality be promoted in clinical practice? a phenomenological study of physical therapy experts. Phys. Ther. 90, 1479–1492.

Stalker, C., Palmer, S., Wright, D., Gebotys, R., 2005. Specialized inpatient trauma treatment for adults abused as children: a follow-up study. Am. J. Psychiatry 162, 552–559.

Understanding Sexual Abuse, 2014. College of Physiotherapists of Ontario, Canada. <http://collegept.org/public/protectingthepublic/understandingsexualabuse.>

Van der Kolk, B., 1994. The body keeps the score: memory and the evolving psychobiology of posttraumatic stress. Harv. Rev. Psychiatry 1, 253–265.

Van Houdenhove, B., 2006. Assessing adverse childhood experiences in chronic pain: it does matter. Clin. J. Pain 22 (6), 584–585.

Wijma, B., Heimer, G., Wijma, K., 2002. Kan patienten ha utsatts för våld? Skall man ställa frågan – och i så fall hur? (Is it possible that the patient has been exposed to violence? Should we ask–and how?). (Article in Swedish). Läkartidningen (Swedish Medical Journal) 99, 2260–2264.

Wijma, B., Siwe, K., 2004. Examiner's unique possibilities to catalyze women's empowerment during a pelvic examination. Acta Obstet. Gynecol. Scand. 83, 1102–1103.

Wijma, K., Söderquist, J., Björklund, I., Wijma, B., 2000. Prevalence of post-traumatic stress disorder among gynaecological patients with a history of sexual and physical abuse. J. Interpers. Violence 15, 944–958.

Wood, K., Van Esterik, P., 2010. Infant feeding experiences of women who were sexually abused in childhood. Can. Fam. Physician 56, 136–141.

5.2.3   Physiotherapy and Substance Misuse

DANIEL CATALÁN-MATAMOROS ■ ANTONIA GÓMEZ-CONESA

SUMMARY

Substance misuse is considered an important public health problem in current society. Alcohol, smoking and the use of other drugs is a growing problem among adolescents and adults. Quitting substance misuse is not easy because dependence is a cluster of behavioural, cognitive and physiological phenomena. The limitations of pharmacotherapy and behavioural therapy, combined with knowledge from studies on nerophysiological abnormalities in substance dependence, underline the need for alternative and/or complementary therapies for these disorders, with long-lasting effects and minimal side-effects. Moreover, substance misuse can have a destructive effect on an individual's mental and physical health. Consequently, the role of the physiotherapist in the management of people suffering from substance misuse is crucial because of highly prevalent physical harm produced and the positive effect of physiotherapy in people suffering from mental health problems. Physiotherapists are involved in the multidisciplinary teams in order to alleviate the addiction, anxiety and psychological disorders, and treat musculoskeletal and neurological problems that can result from long-term abuse of alcohol, for example, osteoporosis, muscle weakness, peripheral neuropathy, impaired balance and gait, and injuries resulting from accidents. Exercise, Basic Body Awareness Therapy (BBAT), massage, transcutaneous electrical nerve stimulation (TENS), biofeedback, relaxation and acupuncture are the most common evidence-based interventions applied by physiotherapists. This chapter shows the important role of the physiotherapist in the management of substance misuse.

KEY POINTS

■ Substance misuse treatment depends on the type of the substance and length of the abuse.

■ Physiotherapists are actively involved in the multidisciplinary teams aiming to reduce the addiction, anxiety and psychological disorders, as well as improve musculoskeletal, neurological, respiratory and cardiovascular problems that can result from substance misuse.

■ The nonpharmacological approaches are potential treatments for addiction that can be applied in individuals at both acute and chronic stages.

■ Exercise, Basic Body Awareness Therapy, massage, transcutaneous electrical nerve stimulation (TENS), biofeedback, relaxation and acupuncture are the most common evidence-based interventions applied by physiotherapists.

■ Further research is needed in the use of physiotherapy interventions in substance misuse.

LEARNING OBJECTIVES

■ To understand the concept of substance misuse of drugs, alcohol and smoking as well as the morbidity, risk factors and psychological, social and health effects of substance misuse in society.

■ To recognize the effects of physiotherapy on people suffering from substance misuse.

■ To discern how the following physiotherapeutic interventions can make a positive effect on substance misuse: exercise, Basic Body Awareness Therapy, massage, TENS, biofeedback, relaxation and acupuncture.

INTRODUCTION

In the 21st century, substance misuse remains a social and psychological problem for society and is still considered as a public health problem. Addiction to various substances (i.e., alcohol, smoking and use of other drugs) is a growing global problem among adolescents, as well as adults of all ages (Kaur et al., 2013). Society has learned to coexist with drugs and alcohol, and its views of which drugs should be legal or illicit changes with time and economic and political considerations. Nevertheless, substance misuse can be dangerous for three main reasons: the user could become addicted to the substance, the substance could cause physical and psychological harm, and misuse can eventually have a negative effect on the quality of life.

The Diagnostic and Statistical Manual of Mental Disorders (DSM) adopted the term *substance misuse* as a blanket term to include drug abuse (Teresi, 2011).

However, the International Classification of Diseases (ICD) refrains from using either substance abuse or drug abuse, instead using the term *harmful use* to cover physical or psychological harm to the user from use. However, in general all agree that 'substance misuse' is a patterned use of a substance in which the user consumes the substance in amounts or with methods that are harmful to themselves or others. More harmful drugs are called *hard drugs* and less harmful drugs are called *soft drugs*.

Quitting substance abuse is not easy, as dependence is a cluster of behavioural, cognitive and physiological phenomena. Very few patients can successfully quit their habit on the first attempt. Understanding influences on substance misuse requires looking at several systems in a person's life including the individual and their family, their community and society as a whole (Fig. 1). Risk factors increase an individual's likelihood of substance misuse and abuse, and protective factors reduce the risk. It is important to note that when looking at the information presented in Fig. 1 or when assessing a patient's situation, the risk factors do not necessarily cause substance misuse, but rather they put the person more at risk for developing such a problem. Conversely, if many protective factors are present, then behaviours like substance abuse are less likely under these conditions.

Substance misuse can have a destructive effect on an individual's mind and body. Drug harmfulness is the degree to which a drug is harmful to a user and it is measured in various ways, such as by addictiveness or dependence and the potential for physical harm (Fig. 2). Substance misuse increases morbidity and mortality among their users and it is directly related to the existence of many other disorders. Depression, schizophrenia, paranoia, anxiety, panic and confusion are among the most common psychological harms. On the other hand, substance misuse also has a tremendous

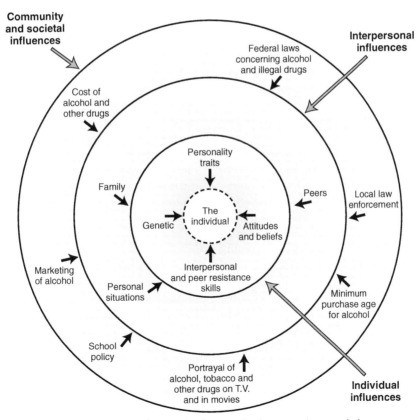

FIGURE 1 ■ Risk and protective factors of substance misuse and abuse.

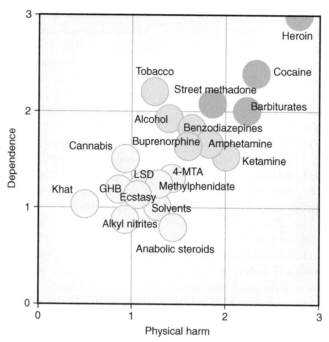

FIGURE 2 ■ Comparison of the perceived harm for various psychoactive drugs *(Nutt et al.,* The Lancet, *369, 1047–1053).*

negative effect on the physical health and the body, such as loss of coordination and muscle control, skeletal myopathy, reduced muscle strength and muscle mass, paralysis, body stiffness, respiratory problems, dizziness, insomnia, body temperature increase, heart failure, extreme weight loss, malnutrition, impotence, serious damage to the nasal passages, restlessness, and damage in the liver, kidney and brain. Moreover, substance misuse can also have a negative effect on the quality of life and relationships with others. Hobbies, interests and ambitions can be forgotten as drugs become more and more important, and eventually it can become increasingly difficult to hold down a job.

Because substance misuse produces a negative effect on mental and physical health, healthcare services need to include therapeutic approaches aiming to cover both. Consequently, the role of the physiotherapist in the management of people suffering from substance misuse is crucial because of the highly prevalent physical harm produced and the positive effect of body-orientated therapies in people with mental health problems.

Therefore this chapter aims to introduce the field of substance misuse and identify elements of good physiotherapeutic experiences in people suffering from these disorders. Alcohol consumption, smoking and drugs are the most prevalent types of substance misuse in our current society, so this chapter will examine these in greater detail. In addition, physiotherapeutic interventions will be discussed from the perspective of evidence-based practice.

ALCOHOL ADDICTION

Alcohol is a psychoactive substance with dependence-producing properties, and harmful use ranks among the top five risk factors for disease, disability and death throughout the world (Lim et al., 2012). As described in the latest status report of the World Health Organization (2014a), consumption of alcohol and problems related to alcohol vary widely around the world, but the burden of disease and death remains significant in most countries. In many parts of the world, drinking alcoholic beverages is a common feature of social gatherings. At some time in their lives, more than 30% of

Americans experienced alcohol abuse or alcohol dependence (Johnston et al., 2007). Problem drinking has a multifaceted aetiology, including environmental, cultural, genetic and social factors (Donaghy & Mutrie, 1999).

The consumption of alcohol carries a risk of adverse health and social consequences related to its inebriating, toxic and dependence-producing properties. The health risks of excess alcohol consumption include weight problems, stomach upsets, headaches, anxiety, stress, depression, poor concentration, difficulty in sleeping, raised blood pressure, liver disease, cancers, strokes, memory loss and sexual difficulties. In addition to the chronic diseases that may develop in those who drink large amounts of alcohol over a number of years, alcohol use is also associated with an increased risk of acute health conditions, such as injuries, including from traffic accidents. Thus harmful use of alcohol accounts for 5.9% of all deaths worldwide.

SMOKING

According to the World Health Organization (2014b), global consumption of cigarettes has been rising steadily since manufactured cigarettes were introduced at the beginning of the 20th century. While consumption is levelling off and even decreasing in some countries, the worldwide number of people who smoke has increased and a smoker now smokes more cigarettes. As a result, the smoking epidemic is one of the biggest public health threats the world has ever faced, killing nearly 6 million people a year. More than 5 million of those deaths are the result of direct smoking use, whereas more than 600,000 are the result of nonsmokers being exposed to second-hand smoke. Approximately one person dies every 6 seconds because of smoking, accounting for 1 in 10 adult deaths.

Smoking harms nearly every organ of the body and diminishes a person's overall health. Smoking is a leading cause of cancer and death from cancer. It causes cancers of the lung, oesophagus, larynx, mouth, throat, kidney, bladder, pancreas, stomach and cervix, as well as acute myeloid leukaemia. Smoking also causes heart disease, stroke, aortic aneurysm, chronic obstructive pulmonary disease (chronic bronchitis and emphysema), asthma, hip fractures and cataracts. Moreover, smokers are at higher risk of developing pneumonia and other airway infections (US Department of Health and Human Services, 2004, 2010).

DRUG MISUSE

Drug misuse refers to the use of a drug for purposes for which it was not intended or using a drug in excessive quantities. Drug addiction is a state of physical or psychological dependence on a drug. Physical addiction is characterized by the presence of tolerance (needing more and more of the drug to achieve the same effect) and withdrawal symptoms that disappear when further medication is taken. In fact, many different drugs can be misused, including illegal drugs (such as heroin or cannabis), prescription medicines (such as tranquilizers or painkillers) and other medicines that can be bought off the supermarket shelf (such as cough mixtures or herbal remedies). According to the United Nations Organization on Drugs and Crimes (UNODC, 2014), 3.5% to 5.7% of the world's population aged 15–64 years has used psychoactive substances, such as cannabis, amphetamines, cocaine, opioids and nonprescribed psychoactive prescription medication. Globally, cannabis is the most commonly used (129–190 million people), followed by amphetamine-type stimulants, then cocaine and opioids. The use of psychoactive substances causes significant health and social problems for the people who use them and also for others in their families and communities. WHO estimated that 0.7% of the global burden of disease in 2004 was caused by cocaine and opioid use.

According to the World Drugs Report (United Nations Office on Drugs and Crime [UNODC], 2014), drug use can alter the function and structure of the brain. The main consequences of drug use are having trouble with thinking clearly, decreased attention span and problems with memory. As a result, students who use drugs may do poorly in school or even drop out. Adults might have trouble with their work performance and maintaining employment. Some drugs, for example heroin, cocaine and certain sleeping pills or painkillers, are physically addictive. They have a specific effect on the body, which leads to tolerance and withdrawal symptoms. Other drugs may lead to a psychological addiction if people have a craving for the effect that the drug causes.

PHYSIOTHERAPEUTIC INTERVENTIONS IN SUBSTANCE MISUSE

Substance misuse is associated with tremendous costs for society and there is a need to develop effective treatment and preventive strategies. The limitations of pharmacotherapy and behavioural therapy, combined with knowledge from studies on neurophysiological abnormalities in substance dependence, underline the need for alternative and/or complementary therapies for these disorders, with long-lasting effects and minimal side-effects (Dehghani-Arani et al., 2013). The treatment depends on the type of drug used by the patient and the duration of abuse, and it should include physical, mental, social and vocational rehabilitation (Kaur et al., 2013). Thus in addition to substance abuse treatment and other multidisciplinary treatments, physiotherapy may be helpful in these individuals.

Rehabilitation programmes since the early 1990s have attempted to treat these patients, moving away from the traditional approach encompassing one model of care to a newer, more collaborative approach that offers a range of options for the patient (Bartu, 2000). The use of prescribed drugs as an adjunct to psychosocial and behavioural interventions still plays a major role in treatment, especially in maintaining postdetoxification abstinence. Other frequent options include family or group therapy, education about alcohol and general health, cognitive-behavioural therapies, cue exposure, practical life skills and relationship enhancement. Therapeutic interventions should cover both acute and chronic care needs of the patient.

Physiotherapists are involved in the multidisciplinary teams in order to alleviate the addiction, anxiety and psychological disorders, and treat musculoskeletal and neurological problems that can result from long-term abuse of alcohol, for example, osteoporosis, muscle weakness, peripheral neuropathy, impaired balance and gait, and injuries resulting from accidents. Many traditional physiotherapy approaches may be used such as exercise, massage, body awareness therapy, transcutaneous electrical nerve stimulation (TENS), acupuncture, relaxation techniques, etc. (Everett et al., 2003). Existing evidence on some

of these physiotherapeutic interventions is further discussed in this chapter.

Exercise

Exercise may provide an effective, low-cost adjunct to substance abuse treatment and has secondary health benefits, e.g., prevention of obesity and secondary diseases such as diabetes (Kaur et al., 2013). Researchers have hypothesized that exercise may be beneficial, although few studies have actually tested this relationship and the evidence is still controversial.

Kendzor et al. (2008) found that the most frequent physical activities in a sample of 620 heavy drinkers included walking, gardening/yardwork, calisthenics, biking, swimming, weight lifting, golfing and dancing. However, results revealed no significant relationships between energy expenditure from exercise and reductions in alcohol consumption. On the other hand, experimental research has shown that exercise may offer an effective clinical approach to reducing alcohol intake (Hammer et al., 2010). A recent randomized controlled trial (RCT) indicated that a moderate-intensity group aerobic exercise intervention is an efficacious adjunct to alcohol treatment (Brown et al., 2014).

Exercise may also make a positive effect in other addictions such as drugs and smoking reduction. A pilot study on using exercise to alter the behaviour and body image of drug addicts showed that physical exercise can provide important support in the treatment of drug abuse and that the main problem is maintaining change in behaviour and peer-group influence to ensure long-term change (Roessler, 2010). Another study assessed the efficacy of an 8-week endurance and resistance-training program on fitness measures in individuals undergoing residential treatment for methamphetamine dependence. These individuals showed substantial improvements in aerobic exercise performance, muscle strength and endurance and body composition, demonstrating the feasibility of exercise interventions in these participants and showing excellent responsiveness to the exercise stimulus resulting in physiological changes that might enhance recovery from drug dependency (Dolezal et al., 2013). Another RCT on the effect of isometric exercises in a smoking-cessation programme found that they were perceived as somewhat helpful by quitters (Al-Chalabi et al.,

2008). A recent study (Kurti & Dallery, 2014) found that moderate-intensity exercise is effective to reduce cravings when reducing cigarette smoking.

Exercise is therefore a potential nonpharmacological treatment for addiction that targets individuals implicated in both early and late stages of the addiction process. However, research on exercise and addictions remains limited. Larger trials should be developed to examine the influence of exercise on reducing addictions and increasing abstinence.

Basic Body Awareness Therapy

One of the most common therapeutic approaches used in mental health physiotherapy is Basic Body Awareness Therapy (BBAT). This therapy represents a health-orientated and person-centred approach, focusing on movement awareness, movement quality and function in daily life. It includes the means for reliable and valid assessment of evaluating clinical outcome. BBAT is based on the hypothesis of the human being's lack of contact with the body and how such a state can be expressed in poor balance, blocked breathing, dysfunctional movement quality and relationship with others. It offers a strategy for integrating balance, free breathing and mental awareness into human movements, function and relationships to strengthen resources and identity.

A recent project (Serranos de Andrés, 2013) studied how BBAT is experienced as a treatment of inpatients suffering from alcohol-dependence syndrome in the process of dishabituation. All informants reported positive experiences with BBAT. They gave value to the qualities of movement as facilitators for awareness, balance and well-being, considering that movements were carefully selected and meaningful for them. Informants expressed positive effects in physical and mental spheres, and improvement both in relation with themselves and with others. They reported well-being, concentration, relaxation, harmony and increased self-esteem, as well as improvement in balance, breathing and self-awareness. It was interesting to see how they reported changes in relation to their bodies, expressing that, when they were drinking, they abandoned them and that BBAT helped informants to appreciate and take care of their bodies again.

Although the aforementioned results are promising, further research studies are needed to deepen the understanding of experiences of BBAT in people suffering from substance misuse.

Massage

Despite the importance of manual therapy and massage in physiotherapy, there has been little research on the effectiveness of massage as a therapeutic intervention in substance misuse. One reason that massage can be particularly helpful in the treatment of alcohol addiction is that the body reacts to massage in a similar way to alcohol and drugs. Massage is pleasurable for most people, and triggers the release of so-called *happiness hormones* such as dopamine and endorphins. Thus massage can play a unique and important part in reawakening these reward and pleasure pathways in the nervous system and swaying them away from alcohol use.

An RCT investigated how massage could be beneficial in smoking cessation. The findings revealed that massage may be an effective adjunct treatment for adults attempting smoking cessation to alleviate smoking-related anxiety, reduce cravings and withdrawal symptoms, improve mood and reduce the number of cigarettes smoked (Hernandez-Reif et al., 1999). Black et al. (2010) studied the effectiveness of chair massage for reducing anxiety in persons participating in an inpatient withdrawal management program for psychoactive drugs. Chair massage was more effective than relaxation in reducing anxiety.

Other Interventions

Some research studies have focused in other interventions providing positive results in the field of substance misuse through biofeedback (Dehghani-Arani et al., 2013; Thurstone & Lajoie, 2013), relaxation (Dickson-Spillmann et al., 2013), TENS and acupuncture (Everett et al., 2003).

CONCLUSIONS

This chapter has shown the important role of the physiotherapist in the management of substance misuse. Exercise, BBAT, massage, TENS, biofeedback, relaxation and acupuncture seem to be the most common evidence-based interventions applied by physiotherapists. Although existing growing evidence recommends physiotherapy interventions in people suffering from substance misuse, further research is needed.

REFERENCES

Al-Chalabi, L., Prasad, N., Steed, L., et al., 2008. A pilot randomised controlled trial of the feasibility of using body scan and isometric exercise for reducing urge to smoke in a smoking cessation clinic. BMC Public Health 8, 349.

Bartu, A., 2000. Treatment and therapeutic interventions. In: Cooper, D.B. (Ed.), Alcohol Use. Radcliffe Medical Press, Abingdon, UK, pp. 185–193.

Black, S., Jacques, K., Webber, A., et al., 2010. Chair massage for treating anxiety in patients withdrawing from psychoactive drugs. J. Altern. Complement. Med. 16 (9), 979–987.

Brown, R.A., Abrantes, A.M., Minami, H., et al., 2014. A preliminary, randomized trial of aerobic exercise for alcohol dependence. J. Subst. Abuse Treat. 47 (1), 1–9.

Dehghani-Arani, F., Rostami, R., Nadali, H., 2013. Neurofeedback training for opiate addiction: improvement of mental health and craving. Appl. Psychophysiol. Biofeedback 38 (2), 133–141.

DeWit, D., McKee, C., Fjeld, J., Karioja, K., 2003. The critical role of school culture in student success. Toronto, ON, Center for addiction and mental health.

Dickson-Spillmann, M., Haug, S., Schaub, M.P., 2013. Group hypnosis vs. relaxation for smoking cessation in adults: a cluster-randomised controlled trial. BMC Public Health 23, 1227.

Dolezal, B.A., Chudzynski, J., Storer, T.W., et al., 2013. Eight weeks of exercise training improves fitness measures in methamphetamine-dependent individuals in residential treatment. J. Addict. Med. 7 (2), 122–128.

Donaghy, M.E., Mutrie, N., 1999. Is exercise beneficial in the treatment and rehabilitation of the problem drinker? A critical review. Phys. Ther. Rev. 4, 153–166.

Everett, T., Donaghy, M., Feaver, S. (Eds.), 2003. Interventions for Mental Health. An Evidence-Based Approach for Physiotherapists and Occupational Therapies. Butterworth Heinemann, London, UK.

Hammer, S.B., Ruby, C.L., Brager, A.J., et al., 2010. Environmental modulation of alcohol intake in hamsters: effects of wheel running and constant light exposure. Alcohol. Clin. Exp. Res. 34 (9), 1651–1658.

Hernandez-Reif, M., Field, T., Hart, S., 1999. Smoking cravings are reduced by self-massage. Prev. Med. 28 (1), 28–32.

Johnston, L.D., O'Malley, P.M., Bachman, J.G., Schulenberg, J.E., 2007. Monitoring the Future National Results on Adolescent Drug Use: Overview of Key Findings, 2006 (NIH Publication No. 07-6202). National Institute on Drug Abuse, Bethesda, MD.

Kaur, J., Garnawat, D., Bhatia, M.S., 2013. Rehabilitation for substance abuse disorders. Delhi Psych. J. 16 (2), 400–403.

Kendzor, D.E., Dubbert, P.M., 2008. The influence of exercise on alcohol consumption among heavy drinkers participating in an alcohol treatment intervention. Addict. Behav. 33 (10), 1337–1343.

Kurti, A.N., Dallery, J., 2014. Effects of exercise on craving and cigarette smoking in the human laboratory. Addict. Behav. 13 (39), 1131–1137.

Lim, S.S., Vos, T., Flaxman, A.D., et al., 2012. A comparative risk assessment of burden of disease and injury attributable to 67 risk factors and risk factor clusters in 21 regions, 1990–2010: a systematic analysis for the Global Burden of Disease Study 2010. Lancet 380, 2224–2260.

Nutt, D., King, L.A., Saulsbury, W., Blakemore, C., 2007. Development of a rational scale to assess the harm of drugs of potential misuse. Lancet 369, 1047–1053.

Roessler, K.K., 2010. Exercise treatment for drug abuse—A Danish pilot study. Scand. J. Public Health 38 (6), 664–669.

Serranos de Andrés, P., 2013. The experience of Basic Body Awareness Group Therapy in patients with alcohol dependence syndrome. (Master's thesis). Bergen University College, Bergen, Norway.

Teresi, L., 2011. Hijacking the Brain. How Drug and Alcohol Addiction Hijacks Our Brains. Authorhouse LLC, Bloomington, IN.

Thurstone, C., Lajoie, T., 2013. Heart rate variability biofeedback in adolescent substance abuse treatment. Global Adv. Health Med. 2 (1), 22–23.

United Nations Office on Drugs and Crime, 2014. World Drug Report, 2014. UNODC, Geneva.

US Department of Health and Human Services, 2004. The Health Consequences of Smoking: A Report of the Surgeon General. US Department of Health and Human Services, Centers for Disease Control and Prevention, National Center for Chronic Disease Prevention and Health Promotion, Office on Smoking and Health, Atlanta, Georgia.

US Department of Health and Human Services, 2010. How Smoking Smoke Causes Disease: The Biology and Behavioral Basis for Smoking-Attributable Disease: A Report of the Surgeon General. U.S. Department of Health and Human Services, Centers for Disease Control and Prevention, National Center for Chronic Disease Prevention and Health Promotion, Office on Smoking and Health, Atlanta, Georgia.

World Health Organization, 2014a. Global Status Report on Alcohol and Health, 2014. WHO, Geneva.

World Health Organization, 2014b. WHO Report on the Global Smoking Epidemic, 2013. WHO, Geneva.

5.2.4 Physiotherapy and Patients With Eating Disorders

MICHEL PROBST ▪ JOLIEN DIEDENS ▪ TINE VAN DAMME

SUMMARY

This chapter describes the role of physiotherapists who work in general practice or in a residential unit with patients with eating disorders. The inclusion of physiotherapy in the treatment of patients with eating disorders is based on the physiotherapists' experience with both the body and the body in movement, two important issues that are integral to eating disorder pathology. From our clinical experience, physiotherapeutic techniques represent a powerful clinical addition to the available treatments of eating disorders. Patients with eating disorders have an intense fear of gaining weight and have a negative body experience and disturbed body perception (weight, circumference and form). Excessive exercise and a drive for activity or hyperactivity are considered secondary symptoms in the diagnosis of patients with eating disorders, and are characterized by a voluntary increase in physical activity, a compulsive urge to move and dissociation of fatigue. These characteristics are the cornerstones of physiotherapy in children, adolescents and adults with eating disorder problems in both inpatient and outpatient treatment settings. Specifically, the objectives for physiotherapy are (1) the rebuilding of a realistic self-concept, and (2) the curbing of hyperactivity, impulses and tensions.

KEY POINTS

- Indications and objectives for physiotherapy in the treatment of patients with eating disorders.
- Specific techniques and guidelines for physical activity in the treatment of patients with eating disorders.
- Basic physiotherapy treatment principles for successful outcomes that are based on evidence-based science and clinical practice.

LEARNING OBJECTIVES

Readers should be able to complete the following:

- Define the role of physiotherapy in patients with eating disorders.
- Gain insight into and knowledge of the physiotherapy treatment for eating disorders.
- Build an elementary physiotherapy treatment programme for patients with eating disorders.

INTRODUCTION

The use of physiotherapy as an adjunctive treatment for patients with eating disorders (ED) within psychiatric health care and rehabilitation is based on the physiotherapist's expertise in both the 'body' and 'the body in movement', two important issues integral to the pathology of ED.

Based on 30 years of clinical experience and on the current body of scientific evidence, a rationale and clinical guidance for incorporating physiotherapy into treatment for patients with ED are presented.

Two main indications for physiotherapy are proposed for patients with ED: (1) a disturbed body experience with a specific focus on perception, attitudes and behaviour, and (2) the frequently observed maladaptive and excessive use of physical activity.

EATING DISORDERS

ED are considered one of the most challenging psychiatric conditions (Fairburn & Harrison, 2003). The spectrum of ED ranges from mild to severe; the severe form of this behaviour results in the clinically recognized diagnoses of anorexia nervosa (AN), bulimia nervosa (BN) and binge eating disorder (BED) (American Psychiatric Association, APA, 2013). AN is characterized by a refusal to maintain a minimally normal body weight and a distorted perception of one's body (weight, size, shape), namely a negative experience of their appearance as too fat and an intense fear of gaining weight, even when severely underweight (APA, 2013). BN is characterized by repeated episodes of binge eating followed by inappropriate compensatory behaviours, such as self-induced vomiting, misuse of laxatives (or other medications), fasting or excessive exercise (APA, 2013). BED is established as the third classical ED in addition to AN and BN, characterized by recurrent episodes of binge eating and a sense of lack of control over eating, and is associated with psychiatric comorbidity and significant medical and psychosocial impairments (Javaras et al., 2008). Physical health problems are also common and are strongly associated with obesity and physical inactivity (Vancampfort et al., 2014a, 2014b). For diagnostic criteria, see Boxes 1 and 2.

These diagnostic features can be accompanied by somatic, psychiatric, behavioural and social disturbances (APA, 2013). The most common somatic complaints (Mitchell & Crow, 2006; Mehler et al., 2010), as evaluated by medical doctors before a training programme is established, are described in Table 1.

Furthermore, psychiatric symptoms can occur, such as distorted body experience, sexual problems, attempting to prolong childhood and escape the responsibilities of adulthood, perfectionism, feelings of ineffectiveness, inflexible thinking, limited social spontaneity, overly restrained initiative and emotional expression, a strong control over one's environment, denial of illness and mood changes with

marked liability. Obsessive-compulsive features, both related and unrelated to food, are often prominent. The anorexic patient quickly develops a repertoire of behaviours in the pursuit of weight loss, including caloric restriction and caloric obsession, refusal to eat food, adoption of special diets, hyperactivity, vomiting and laxative abuse. Unusual eating rituals are frequently described. These behaviours create a vicious circle with behavioural and psychological sequelae that perpetuate the disorder. Regarding their social context, patients can become isolated, and many conflicts arise with family members. Although AN and BN differ in their behavioural features, patients with either one share an intense preoccupation with body weight and shape (Mantilla et al., 2014). Additionally, there is considerable diagnostic overlap between the two disorders, and their natural histories tend to intertwine (APA, 2013).

BOX 1

INTERNATIONAL STATISTICAL CLASSIFICATION OF DISEASES AND RELATED HEALTH PROBLEMS 10TH REVISION (ICD-10): WHO VERSION FOR 2016

EATING DISORDERS

ICD-10, Chapter 5, Mental and behavioural disorders (F00–F99).

Behavioural syndromes associated with physiological disturbances and physical factors (F50–F59).

F50.0: Anorexia Nervosa

A disorder characterized by deliberate weight loss, induced and sustained by the patient. It occurs most commonly in adolescent girls and young women, but adolescent boys and young men may also be affected, as may children approaching puberty and older women up to menopause. The disorder is associated with a specific psychopathology in which a dread of fatness and flabbiness of body contour persists as an intrusive overvalued idea, and the patients impose a low weight threshold on themselves. There is usually undernutrition of varying severity with secondary endocrine and metabolic changes and disturbances of bodily function. The symptoms include restricted dietary choice, excessive exercise, induced vomiting and purgation, and use of appetite suppressants and diuretics.

F50.1 Atypical Anorexia Nervosa

Disorders that fulfil some of the features of anorexia nervosa, but in which the overall clinical picture does not justify that diagnosis. For instance, one of the key symptoms, such as amenorrhoea or notable dread of being fat, may be absent in the presence of marked weight loss and

weight-reducing behaviour. This diagnosis should not be made in the presence of known physical disorders associated with weight loss.

F50.2: Bulimia Nervosa

A syndrome characterized by repeated bouts of overeating and an excessive preoccupation with the control of body weight, leading to a pattern of overeating followed by vomiting or use of purgatives. This disorder shares many psychological features with anorexia nervosa, including an over-concern with body shape and weight. Repeated vomiting is likely to lead to disturbances of body electrolytes and physical complications. There is often, but not always, a history of an earlier episode of anorexia nervosa, with an interval ranging from a few months to several years.

F50.3: Atypical Bulimia Nervosa

Disorders that fulfil some of the features of bulimia nervosa, but in which the overall clinical picture does not justify that diagnosis. For instance, there may be recurrent bouts of overeating and overuse of purgatives without significant weight change, or the typical over-concern about body shape and weight may be absent.

F50.4: Overeating Associated With Other Psychological Disturbances

Overeating due to stressful events, such as bereavement, accidents, childbirth, etc.

BOX 2
AMERICAN PSYCHIATRIC ASSOCIATION DIAGNOSTIC CRITERA
(American Psychiatric Association, 2013)

ANOREXIA NERVOSA

A. Restriction of energy intake relative to requirements leading to a significantly low body weight in the context of age, sex, developmental trajectory and physical health. *Significantly low weight* is defined as a weight that is less than minimally normal or, for children and adolescents, less than that minimally expected.

B. Intense fear of gaining weight or becoming fat, or persistent behavior that interferes with weight gain, even though at a significantly low weight.

C. Disturbance in the way in which one's body weight or shape is experienced, undue influence of body weight or shape on self-evaluation, or persistent lack of recognition seriousness of one's current low body weight.

Coding note: The ICD-9-CM code for anorexia nervosa is **307.1**, which is assigned regardless of the subtype. The ICD-10-CM code depends on the subtype (see below).

Specify whether:

(F50.01) Restricting type: During the last 3 months, the individual has not engaged in recurrent episodes of binge eating or purging behavior (i.e., self-induced vomiting or the misuse of laxatives, diuretics, or enemas). This subtype describes presentations in which weight loss is accomplished primarily through dieting, fasting and/or excessive exercise.

(F50.02) Binge-eating/purging type: During the last 3 months, the individual has engaged in recurrent episodes of binge eating or purging behavior (i.e., self-induced vomiting or the misuse of laxatives, diuretics, or enemas).

Specify if:

In partial remission: After full criteria for anorexia nervosa were previously met, Criterion A (low body weight) has not been met for a sustained period, but either Criterion B (intense fear of gaining weight or becoming fat or behavior that interferes with weight gain) or Criterion C (disturbances in self-perception of weight and shape) is still met.

In full remission: After full criteria for anorexia nervosa were previously met, none of the criteria have been met for a sustained period of time.

Specify current severity:

The minimum level of severity is based, for adults, on current body mass index (BMI) (see below) or, for children and adolescents, on BMI percentile. The ranges below are derived from World Health Organization categories for thinness in adults; for children and adolescents, corresponding BMI percentiles should be used. The level of severity may be increased to reflect clinical symptoms, the degree of functional disability, and the need for supervision.

Mild: BMI $\geq$ 17 kg/m^2
Moderate: BMI 16–16.99 kg/m^2
Severe: BMI 15–15.99 kg/m^2
Extreme: BMI < 15 kg/m^2

BULIMIA NERVOSA

A. Recurrent episodes of binge eating characterized by both of the following:
  - Eating in a discrete period of time (e.g. within a 2-hour period) an amount of food that is definitely larger than what most individuals would eat in a similar period of time under similar circumstances.
  - Sense of lack of control over eating during an episode e.g., a feeling that one cannot stop eating or control what or how much one is eating.

B. Recurrent inappropriate compensatory behaviours to prevent weight gain such as self-induced vomiting; misuse of laxatives, diuretics, or other medications; fasting; or excessive exercise.

C. The binge eating and inappropriate compensatory behaviours both occur, on average, at least once a week for 3 months.

D. Self-evaluation is unduly influenced by body shape and weight.

E. The disturbance does not occur exclusively during episodes of anorexia nervosa.

Specify if:

In partial remission: After full criteria for bulimia nervosa were previously met, some, but not all, of the criteria have been met for a sustained period of time.

In full remission: After full criteria for bulimia nervosa were previously met, none of the criteria have been met for a sustained period of time.

Specify current severity:

The minimum level of severity is based on the frequency of inappropriate compensatory behaviors (see below). The level of severity may be increased to reflect other symptoms and the degree of functional disability.

Mild: An average of 1–3 episodes of inappropriate compensatory behaviors per week.

Moderate: An average of 4–7 episodes of inappropriate compensatory behaviors per week.

Severe: An average of 8–13 episodes of inappropriate compensatory behaviors per week.

Extreme: An average of 14 or more episodes of inappropriate compensatory behaviors per week.

BINGE EATING DISORDERS

A. Recurrent episodes of binge eating. An episode of binge eating is characterized by both of the following:
  ■ Eating, in a discrete period of time (e.g., within any 2-hour period), an amount of food that is definitely larger than most people would eat in a similar period of time under similar circumstances
  ■ A sense of lack of control over eating during the episode (for example, a feeling that one cannot stop eating or control what or how much one is eating).
B. The binge-eating episodes are associated with three (or more) of the following:
  ■ eating much more rapidly than normal,
  ■ eating until feeling uncomfortably full,
  ■ eating large amounts of food when not feeling physically hungry,
  ■ eating alone because of feeling embarrassed by how much one is eating,
  ■ feeling disgusted with oneself, depressed, or very guilty afterwards.
C. Marked distress regarding binge eating is present.
D. Binge eating occurs, on average, at least once a week for 3 months.

E. The binge eating is not associated with the recurrent use of inappropriate compensatory behaviour (e.g., purging) and does not occur exclusively during the course of anorexia nervosa or bulimia nervosa

Specify if:

In partial remission: After full criteria for binge-eating disorder were previously met, binge eating occurs at an average frequency of less than one episode per week for a sustained period of time.

In full remission: After full criteria for binge-eating were previously met, none of the criteria have been met for a sustained period of time.

Specify current severity:

The minimum level of severity is based on the frequency of episodes of binge eating (see below). The level of severity may be increased to reflect other symptoms and the degree of functional disability.

  Mild: 1–3 binge-eating episodes per week.
  Moderate: 4–7 binge-eating episodes per week.
  Severe: 8–13 binge-eating episodes per week.
  Extreme: 14 or more binge-eating episodes per week.

INDICATIONS AND OBJECTIVES FOR PHYSIOTHERAPY IN EATING DISORDERS

Addressing the negative body experience and maladaptive physical activity are the cornerstones of a physiotherapy approach to ED. In this section, the clinical manifestations of body experience and maladaptive physical activity in ED are explained and summarized in specific physiotherapy objectives.

Body experience is a multidimensional concept that contains at least three aspects, including neurophysiological, psychological and behavioural. First, the neurophysiological aspect refers to perceptual experiences, such as visual–spatial, sensory judgements, physical sensations, body awareness, body recognition, physical appearance and body size and shape. The psychological aspect refers to cognitive (thought process and thinking styles) and subjective experiences (feelings, emotions, affect and mood). The third component, behavioural (avoidance and checking behaviour), might actually be the result of the neurophysiological

and psychological aspects (Cash, 1995; Cash & Smolak, 2011; Probst, 2006; Probst et al., 2008a). In ED pathology, body image disturbance is a central theme. The experiences of both body weight and shape are typically distorted. Persons suffering from an ED often evaluate their body structure, size or certain body parts in an unrealistic manner. Even when clearly underweight, some patients perceive their appearance as normal or even overweight (APA, 2013). The discrepancy between the way patients see themselves and the way they see others is striking: in most cases, patients can rather accurately estimate another patient's body size despite not realizing that they look the same or even thinner. Furthermore, patients often have disturbed ideas about the consequences of eating on their body structure. After a meal, patients may feel that their stomach is 'bulging', their belly is 'swelling' or that their fat is immediately deposited in their thighs, among other reactions. Although some physical complaints are directly related to fluid retention or decreased gastrointestinal motility associated with malnutrition or refeeding during treatment, other concerns are

TABLE 1	
Review of the Most Common Somatic Disturbances	
Cardiovascular disturbances	Cardiac abnormalities including bradycardia and tachycardia, ventricular arrhythmia, hypotension, cardiac failure, and a variety of electrocardiographic changes, electrolyte disturbances and acrocyanosis
Gastrointestinal disturbances	Oral or dental abnormalities, benign enlargement of the parotid salivary gland, oesophagitis
Renal disturbances	Electrolyte abnormalities, pitting and peripheral oedema, hyper- or hypophosphataemia
Haematological disturbances	Pancytopenia with mild anaemia
Skeletal disturbances	Osteoporosis
Endocrine disturbances	Amenorrhea and hormonal abnormalities
Metabolic disturbances	Sensitivity to cold, sleep abnormalities, hypothermia, hypercholesterolaemia
Dermatological complications	Atrophic dry skin, carotenodermia, lanugo hair

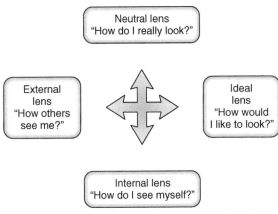

FIGURE 1 ■ The theory of lenses (Probst, 2007).

magnified or emerge due to extreme concerns about controlling body shape and weight. Most patients with ED harbour a very negative attitude towards their own bodies and their physical appearance in general (APA, 2013). Patients often engage in relentless and highly critical monitoring of their body shape and weight. Others may avoid seeing themselves (naked) and often hide in loose clothing. Generally, they are dissatisfied with certain body parts (usually their stomach, thighs or bottom), but this dissatisfaction can also apply to body parts that are entirely unrelated to weight itself (e.g., wide hips, short height, short legs and narrow shoulders). A minority of patients with AN seem to be proud of their emaciated looks (which they seem to show in an almost 'exhibitionistic' manner), although for most patients, low weight and weight loss fail to improve satisfaction with their body, and despite their low weight they continue to perceive themselves as too fat. This phenomenon is comparable to individuals suffering from 'imagined ugliness' or body dysmorphic disorder (Phillips, 2004, 2005; Rasmussen et al., 2015), who repeatedly undergo plastic surgery without resulting improvements in body image.

In addition to frequent weighing or mirror inspections, some patients develop their own rules or standards, such as 'my ribs must be visible' or 'the inner part of my thighs cannot touch when I am standing' (Probst et al., 2008a). Patients suffering from an ED lack confidence in their own body; they perceive their body as an annoyance, and they do not feel 'at home' in their body. They often dislike being touched and generally have difficulty with physical closeness. This feeling of alienation can resemble depersonalization (or a form of dissociation) similar to what occurs following physical or sexual abuse. In their mind, these patients often believe that others view them negatively, and this plays an important role in their relationships. This is comparable to seeing themselves very critically through the eyes of someone else. In this way, their opinion is constantly subject to conflicting points of view: 'how do I see myself' (the internal lens), 'how do others see me' (the external lens), 'how do I really look' (the unbiased or neutral lens) and 'how would I like to look' (the ideal lens). The internal and ideal lenses refer to their (dis-)satisfaction, and the external lens to (social) anxiety. The more the four lenses diverge, the more problematic their self-perception (Probst et al., 1995a, 2008a; Probst, 2006) (Fig. 1).

The core problem is in the discourse between being and having a body (Duesund & Skårderud, 2003; Fuchs, 2010) and in the absence of self-esteem and negative self-perception, which is expressed in a negative body image (Probst, 2006). The translation of 'discord with oneself' into 'discord with their body' is highly culturally defined (Probst, 2006).

A distorted body experience has a negative prognostic value (Vandereycken et al., 1987; Thompson, 1990; Keel et al., 2005; Danielsen & Rø, 2012). Therefore changing the way patients with AN perceive their bodies should be considered a priority in the treatment of this disorder (Bruch, 1962; Vandereycken et al., 1987; Danielsen & Rø, 2012).

Exercise plays an important role in the lives of many patients with AN (Davis & Fox, 1993; Michielli et al., 1994; Zunker et al., 2011; Ng et al., 2013). Approximately 40% to 80% of patients with AN engage in excessive physical activity (Zunker et al., 2011). Their level of exercise is substantially higher than in a clinical population. The exercises may be seemingly appropriate (e.g., riding a bicycle, walking, swimming) or meaningless (e.g., pacing a room, performing isometric exercises while sitting in class or refusing to sit back in a chair). Most of the time, the activities are practised privately and often secretly. In comparison with healthy controls, patients with AN appear to be more engaged in light physical activity (Davis et al., 1999). Some patients' lives are organized and largely dominated by an obsession with physical activity and their psychosocial functioning, including social relationships, may be severely impaired. With already severely emaciated patients in particular, this is a paradoxical behaviour that is in contrast with their physical appearance. Their drive for exercise is characterized by constant restlessness or urges to move. The voluntary increase in physical activity is not motivated by pleasure or the desire to be healthy, but out of concern for their body weight (burning calories, ignoring hunger) and appearance. Physical activity is an effective method of burning calories and losing weight, but at the same time, it is also a form of emotion regulation to diminish negative feelings, escape from feelings of emptiness, and reduce symptoms of anxiety. This could lead to behaviour that has become stereotyped, ritualized and compulsive (Van Steelandt et al., 2007).

The definition of unhealthy exercise appears to be based on two related dimensions: a quantitative dimension (excessive) and a qualitative dimension (compulsive). Exercise becomes excessive when its duration, frequency or intensity exceeds what is required for physical health and increases the risk of physical injury. Exercises become compulsive when they are characterized by the maintenance of a rigid exercise schedule, an

increasing priority over other activities to maintain the pattern of exercise, detailed recordkeeping, and feelings of guilt and anxiety when exercise sessions have been missed. In contrast with AN and BN, persons with binge eating disorders show inactive and sedentary behaviour (Adkins & Keel, 2005).

Although physical activity is a key characteristic of ED, it is not included in the diagnostic criteria of the DSM-5 (APA, 2013). The lack of an internationally accepted definition, the use of various terms with different meanings, the application of different measurements (objective versus subjective methods), and the controversial results concerning the relationship between physical activity and ED psychopathology make it difficult to draw strong conclusions.

Physiotherapy Objectives

Based on the specific conduct pattern of ED, two specific objectives for physiotherapy are suggested.

1. Rebuilding a Realistic Self-Image

A crucial precondition for recovery is the development of a more realistic and positive body image. Patients should also be prepared for changes in their body during weight restoration and the accompanying feelings and needs. The next step is to become more familiar with their body and its changes while simultaneously accepting a more physically mature body. It is essential to focus their awareness and attention on earlier negative experiences involving the body, such as trauma or abuse. Changing these negative experiences into a positive body image is extremely challenging (see also Espeset et al., 2011). In some cases, even the reconstruction of the development of body experience can be important (Kearney-Cooke, 1988). Regardless of the case, patients with AN require the development of positive and accepting attitudes towards their bodies rather than striving for sociocultural ideals of beauty. For example, they should be encouraged to identify, respect and appreciate aspects of their own physical uniqueness instead of trying to mould their bodies to fit a stereotype aggressively promoted by the fashion industry or media.

2. Limiting Hyperactivity, Impulses and Tensions

In terms of learning theory principles, it can be said that physical activity is a good reinforcing factor

TABLE 2

Review of Physiotherapeutic Interventions in Eating Disorders (Adapted From Probst et al., 2013)

Physiotherapy Intervention	Content and Explanation
Postural exercises and postural awareness	Correct posture reduces physical symptoms, but also increases self-esteem; postural abnormalities due to weakened muscles result in poor posture compensations (scoliosis, [hyper-] kyphosis, lumbar [hyper-] lordosis, scapula alata) and low back pain.
Relaxation exercises	Relaxation reduces perceived stress and anxiety and the level of salivary cortisol. Relaxation techniques: Bernstein & Berkovec's (1973) method derived from Jacobson's progressive relaxation, autogenic training, yoga (Douglas, 2011), mindfulness-orientated exercises or biofeedback.
Respiratory exercises	Respiratory exercises, especially those aimed at lowering respiration frequency, thereby amplifying abdominal respiration and lengthening expiration. The objective of breathing exercises is not simply to control respiration, but also to facilitate learning of how to sense one's own body.
Massage	The following forms of massage are used: relaxing and/or activating massage of the back and legs with or without instruments and passive mobilization of the limbs.
Exercises targeting self-perception	Exercises targeting self-perception aim to amplify the awareness of one's own body in its external appearance: mirror exercises, estimation techniques.
Sensory awareness training	Sensory awareness training aims to discover the body through the senses in a nonthreatening manner. Awareness of touch. Body boundary exploration, tactile awareness, body scanning ('trip around the body'), internal sensory exploration and a 'voyage into the body'.
Exercise, physical activity, sports and games	Supervised exercise and physical activities, such as fitness training, resistance training, exercise, aerobics and callanetics, Pilates, sports and gymnastics.

(Vandereycken et al., 1987). Appropriate physical activity connected with a certain degree of weight gain can be managed successfully and effectively in a behaviour therapy programme. It is desirable to limit hyperactivity and restlessness, which are characteristic for many anorexic patients, and transform these behaviours into a more controlled form of physical activity in which the patient is allowed to move intensively only within certain limits determined by the therapist. Learning how to limit physical activity through rest and relaxation is also an important objective. Sustaining a good physical condition can be an additional goal (Probst et al., 2013). Group and/or individual psychoeducation regarding misconceptions about exercise in general, the relationship between exercise and self-esteem and concerns about the transition from exercise during rehabilitation to exercise within the local community, can help patients accept a more realistic concept.

OBSERVATION AND EVALUATION

Different instruments to assess ED psychopathology have been developed. There are many ways to observe and evaluate body awareness and physical activity behaviour. We refer to Thompson (1990) and to Cash & Smolak (2011) for a more complete description. In the 'observation and evaluation tools' section, the reader will find the 'Musculoskeletal Strength or the Sit-up, Squat, Stand (SUSS) Test' (Robinson, 2006), the 'Body Attitude Test' (Probst et al., 1995b; Probst et al., 2008).

SPECIFIC THERAPEUTIC TECHNIQUES

There are several ways to accomplish objectives in physiotherapy. Physiotherapists have a wide array of skills that can be applied successfully to treat AN (Table 2). Each technique can be utilized in both a functional, as well as a more psychotherapeutic approach. The suggested exercises are examples of methods available to attain the desired goals and may not represent an exhaustive or exclusive list. It is important to keep in mind the overall goals of treatment and the individual treatment plan, to provide a safe and structured environment and to actively collaborate and communicate with a multidisciplinary team. The techniques can be applied in both individual and group formats. Physiotherapists should be aware that exercises can be very difficult and provoking for patients with AN, who have been in a constant struggle with their bodies for several years (Probst et al., 1995a; Wallin et al., 2000). Each person with an ED has a different story to tell, a different background and a different personality.

Guidelines for Physical Activity and Eating Disorders

In the past few decades, exercise has been contra-indicated, banned from treatment programmes and not recommended, mainly due to a lack of aware-ness of the consequences and fear of exacerbating the disorder. Ziemer & Ross (1970) were the first to introduce an integration of behavioural therapy and isometric exercises. When patients gained weight, iso-metric exercises under supervision were allowed. Since the 1980s, supervised exercise and physical activities have been increasingly incorporated into some treat-ment and physiotherapy programmes, such as fitness training (Beumont et al., 1994; Alexandridis et al., 1995; Tokumura et al., 2003), resistance training (Chantler et al., 2006; Del Valle et al., 2010), exercise (Ziemer & Ross, 1970; Sundgot-Borgen et al., 2002; Duesund & Skårderud, 2003) aerobics and callanetics (Sundgot-Borgen et al., 2002; Thiem et al., 2008), sports (swimming, volleyball, wrestling, horse riding) and gymnastics. The incorporation of supervised physical activity or exercise training into treatment for AN has largely occurred without significant negative side effects (Probst et al., 1995a; Probst, 2006; Ng et al., 2013).

The benefits of this type of training include increased strength and self-efficacy (Michielli et al., 1994), strength and cardiovascular fitness (Ng et al., 2013) and bone density (Rigotti et al., 1984).

People with AN have reduced bone mineral density, increased odds of osteoporosis and risk of fractures. Proactive monitoring and interventions are required to ameliorate bone loss in AN (Mehler & MacKenzie, 2009; Mehler et al., 2011; Solmi et al., 2016).

Physiotherapists should play a significant role in the supportive and educational management of ED through exercise prescription as well as in psycho-education programmes to explore the meaning of exercise and to clarify both the positive and nega-tive aspects of physical activity (Probst et al., 2017;

Probst, in press). Physiotherapists should avoid con-flicts and subjective discussions about the frequency, intensity, time, type and volume of exercise. They need to inform and progressively lead to a dialogue to reduce the gap and find a balance between the medical/treatment perspective and the patient's point of view, as what is obvious to the therapist is not always obvious to the patient.

Based on our clinical experience that bed rest and physical activity restrictions were not successful and led to covert exercise, we argue that it is better to allow than to forbid patients to engage in controlled activi-ties. It is essential that patients are closely involved in planning a highly individualized and tailored exercise programme based on their individual needs (Box 3).

This approach offers several therapeutic advan-tages: (1) the intensity of movement and heart rate is controlled; (2) the opportunity for the patient to engage in hidden or 'secret' physical activity is reduced; (3) the drive for physical activity is lessened; (4) the message that 'being fed' is not the sole focus of treat-ment is received; (5) the ability to cope with shape and weight changes as a result of the recovery process is

---

BOX 3

A FRAMEWORK CONSIDERING PHYSICAL ACTIVITY FOR PATIENTS WITH EATING DISORDERS

The context of the patient and the treatment modalities should always be taken into account.

BMI <15: light daily household work

BMI >15 and <17: physical activity under profes-sional supervision

BMI >17: physical activity is allowed; patient receives more responsibility. The role of the physiotherapist is to provide coaching

BMI >18: the patient receives all the responsibility. Possible guidelines following the American College of Sports Medicine are the following:

■ Moderate physical activity (cardiorespiratory): ≥30 min/day on ≥5 days/week for a total of ≥150 min/week,

■ Vigorous and intense physical activity (cardiores-piratory): ≥20 min/day on ≥3 days/week (≥75 min/week).

See Garber, C.E., et al. Medicine & Science in Sports & Exercise, *2011, 43 (7), 1334–1359.*

improved; (6) more responsibility is granted; (7) physical and psychological well-being is positively affected while maintaining good physical condition; and (8) the occurrence of social contacts is stimulated (Probst, 2006).

In rehabilitation programmes for obese people with BED, participation in physical activity, physical self-perception and perceived physical discomfort should be considered (Vancampfort, 2013). The physiotherapy care of obese individuals with BED should consist of body image treatment, physical activity and psychoeducation and might benefit from providing more attention to health-related quality of life, body image, depressive symptoms and physical fitness (Vancampfort et al., 2014b,c). Lower physical activity participation has been reported to result in a more negative body attitude (Vancampfort et al., 2014b).

Studies have revealed that significant increases in leisure-time physical activity (for instance, walking) were associated with significant improvements in physical health-related quality of life, perceived sports competence and physical fitness, and perceived body attractiveness. A significant reduction in the number of bingeing episodes was associated with significant improvements in physical health-related quality of life. Future research should focus on identifying which techniques can stimulate physical activity participation in patients with BED. Danielsen et al. (2016) found a significant reduction in thoughts and attitudes about compulsive exercise during treatment, and reported that these changes predicted outcomes, as indicated by reduced ED pathology and increased BMI in underweight participants.

GENERAL CONSIDERATIONS

When integrated into multidimensional treatment, physiotherapy has the specific purpose of influencing the patient's body experience and excessive exercise. Therefore four basic principles should be followed:

1. Physiotherapists should offer a secure and well-structured framework in which all parties understand the engagements, and in which the physiotherapist constantly provides information about the who, what, why and how.

2. Physiotherapists should bear in mind that during physiotherapy, patients are intensely confronted with their problems because they have often fought and hated their body for years. It is therefore important for patients to be well informed and aware of the objectives of the different exercises. Within a physiotherapy approach, a psychoeducation component regarding the functions of the body becomes important. For example, it is important to explain the function of the respiratory system during breathing exercises. The therapist's role will consist of thoroughly explaining that weight gain is not synonymous with feeling fat or 'puffy' but with health, attractiveness, expressiveness, and a life they may never have experienced.

3. Following a series of topics is recommended during psychoeducation sessions. These topics include the following: basic anatomy/physiology issues, osteoporosis, body and sensory awareness, stress, anxiety and coping strategies, normal healthy physical activity versus maladaptive physical activity, and the influences of the media on sociocultural ideals.

   Whenever possible, physiotherapists should design the exercises in such a way that the patients can also practise them outside of the therapy sessions, on their own, or with a partner. This can be successfully accomplished with breathing exercises, relaxation training, mirror exercises, and coping strategies. It is important that patients assume responsibility for their therapy or rehabilitation (see also Gallagher & Zahavi, 2012).

4. Within the session, physiotherapists should invite their patients to express any feelings they experience doing the exercises and encourage patients to further address their feelings during psychotherapy (Probst et al., 1995a; Probst, 2006). The continual exposure to body-orientated situations in physiotherapy enables patients to discover any changing attitudes during the exercises and to become familiar with these changes. The visual feedback intensifies the kinaesthetic sensations by providing a new perspective on the body (Probst et al., 1995a; Probst, 2006). The underlying message of all exercises and discussions

is self-respect, which will enable the patients to develop love and respect for their own body. For this purpose, it is important that patients become aware during physiotherapy sessions that in addition to outward appearance, there are other values and personal aspects that are at least equally as important in life.

DISCUSSION

Physiotherapists are uniquely well trained to help identify, prevent and treat problematic eating by teaching principles related to physical fitness, body experience, weight control, body composition and nutrition (see also Davison, 1988). The inclusion of physiotherapy in the treatment of ED does, however, depend on each country's traditions. Some countries, such as Belgium and those in Scandinavia, have a long tradition of integrating physiotherapy into psychological therapy. Other countries do not have this tradition, and their treatment approaches are more limited to the functional recovery of motor impairments and disabilities in the field of ED (Caddy & Richardson, 2012). In the USA, the focus of physiotherapy is on the female athlete triad in relation to ED (Pantano, 2009). Recently, an international cross-sectional survey was conducted with experienced physiotherapists within the field of ED. They provided information about the key role of physiotherapy in body awareness, physical activity and psychoeducation (Soundy et al., 2015). We contend that the inclusion of physiotherapeutic methods in treatment plays an important role in helping patients better understand and perceive their bodies, improve their body image and boost their confidence that they will not become 'flabby' as a result of weight gain. One important observation is that no reports exist on adverse events related to physiotherapy (Adamkova, 2010; Vancampfort et al., 2014; Ng et al., 2013). Physiotherapists are encouraged to advocate for and educate other members of the multidisciplinary team about their interventions.

In some ED units, mirror or relaxation exercises are administered by other professionals. This necessitates a close consultation and good communication between the different members of the multidisciplinary team to avoid overlap.

With regard to the effectiveness of physiotherapy, the objectives and tools of physiotherapy have substantial face validity in their application in the treatment of ED pathology. The physiotherapy approach in ED is a good illustration of the results of the combined knowledge from evidence-based sciences and professional practice. Research has revealed that body experiences do improve over time (Probst et al., 1999; Wallin et al., 2000). A recent systematic review (Vancampfort et al., 2013) demonstrated that specific physiotherapy interventions, including aerobic exercises and resistance training, massages, yoga, body awareness and body image techniques, resulted in beneficial outcomes on eating pathology, mood, quality of life, body mass index and muscular fitness. Machado and Ferreira (2014) found significant and large reductions in ED outcomes, moderate improvements in quality of life and no benefits in terms of body fat or BMI. Future quantitative and qualitative research studies should continue to investigate specific aspects of physiotherapy interventions, such as treatment indications, contraindications, side effects and posology, which may improve the existing treatment of ED. From a more clinical and qualitative point of view, patients report satisfaction with the physiotherapy approach. Although most exercises are designed for patients to experience their body in a direct and sometimes confrontational manner, patients perceive these physiotherapy interventions as very valuable and helpful as a complementary approach in their therapeutic process (Probst, 2008b). Although much remains unknown, physiotherapeutic techniques represent a powerful clinical addition to available ED treatments and similarly, may stimulate new areas of research opportunities. The absence of (empirical) evidence is not evidence of absence or ineffectiveness (Altman & Bland, 1995). This chapter is the first step in developing guidelines for the physiotherapeutic management of ED.

REFERENCES

Adamkova Ségard, M., 2010. Systematic review of researches testing movement and body techniques in the treatment of eating disorders. In: Adamkova Ségard, M., De Herdt, A., Hatlova, B., et al. (Eds.), Psychomotor Therapy in Eating Disorders. University of J.E. Purkyne, Usti nad labem, pp. 35–105.

Adkins, E.C., Keel, P.K., 2005. Does "excessive" or "compulsive" best describe exercise as a symptom of bulimia nervosa? Int. J. Eat. Disord. 38 (1), 24–29.

Alexandridis, K., Probst, M., Van Coppenolle, H., 1995. Effects of a power-training program on aspects of body experience and body composition in girls and women with anorexia nervosa. In: Van Coppenolle, H., Vanlandenwijck, Y., Simons, J., et al. (Eds.), First European Conference on Adapted Physical Activity and Sports: a white paper on research and practice. Acco, Leuven, pp. 237–240.

Altman, D.G., Bland, J.M., 1995. Absence of evidence is not evidence of absence. Br. Med. J. 311, 485.

American Psychiatric Association, 2013. Diagnostic and Statistical Manual of Mental Disorders, fifth ed. Washington, DC.

Beumont, P.J., Arthur, B., Russell, J.D., Touyz, S.W., 1994. Excessive physical activity in dieting disorder patients: proposals for a supervised exercise program. Int. J. Eat. Disord. 15, 21–36.

Bernstein, D.A., Borkovec, T., 1973. Progressive Relaxation Training. A Manual for the Helping Professions. Research Press Company, New York.

Bruch, H., 1962. Perceptual and conceptual disturbances in anorexia nervosa. Psychol. Med. 24, 187–194.

Caddy, P., Richardson, B., 2012. A pilot body image intervention programme for in-patients with eating disorders in an NHS setting. Int. J. Ther. Rehabil. 19 (4), 190–198.

Cash, J.T., 1995. What do You See When You Look in the Mirror? Helping Yourself to a Positive Body Image. Bantam Books, New York.

Cash, T., Smolak, L., 2011. Body Image. A Handbook of Science, Practice and Prevention. Guilford, New York.

Chantler, I., Szabo, C.P., Green, K., 2006. Muscular strength changes in hospitalized anorexic patients after an eight week resistance training program. Int. J. Sport Med. 27 (8), 660–665.

Danielsen, M., Rø, O., 2012. Changes in body image during inpatient treatment for eating disorders predict outcome. Eat. Disord. 20, 261–275.

Danielsen, M., Rø, O., Romild, U., Bjørnelv, S., 2016. Impact of female adult eating disorder inpatients' attitudes to compulsive exercise on outcome at discharge and follow-up. J. Eat. Disord. 4, 7.

Davis, C., Fox, J., 1993. Excessive exercise and weight preoccupations in women. Addict. Behav. 18, 201–2011.

Davis, C., Katzman, D.K., Kirsh, C., 1999. Compulsive physical activity in adolescents with anorexia nervosa: a psychobehavioral spiral of pathology. J. Nerv. Ment. Dis. 187 (6), 336–342.

Davison, K., 1988. Physiotherapy in the treatment of anorexia nervosa. Physiotherapy 74 (2), 62–64.

Del Valle, M.F., Pérez, M., Santana-Sosa, E., et al., 2010. Does resistance training improve the functional capacity and well-being of very young anorexic patients? A randomized controlled trial. J. Adolescent. Health 46 (4), 352–358.

Douglas, L., 2011. Thinking through the body: the conceptualization of yoga as therapy for individuals with eating disorders. Eat. Disord. 19 (1), 83–96.

Duesund, L., Skårderud, F., 2003. Use the body and forget the body: treating anorexia nervosa with adapted physical activity. Clin. Child Psychol. Psychiatry 8 (1), 53–72.

Espeset, E.M., Nordbø, R.H., Gulliksen, K.S., et al., 2011. The concept of body image disturbance in anorexia nervosa: an empirical inquiry utilizing patients' subjective experiences. Eat. Disord. 19 (2), 175–193.

Fairburn, C.G., Harrison, P.J., 2003. Eating disorders. Lancet 361 (9355), 407–416.

Fuchs, T., 2010. Temporality and psychopathology. Phenomenology and Cognitive Sciences. Springer, Stuttgart.

Gallagher, S., Zahavi, D., 2012. Phenomenological Mind, second ed. Routledge, London.

Javaras, K.N., Pope, H.G., Lalonde, J.K., et al., 2008. Co-occurrence of binge eating disorder with psychiatric and medical disorders. J. Clin. Psychiat. 69 (2), 266–273.

Kearney-Cooke, A., 1988. Group treatment of sexual abuse among women with eating disorders. Women Ther. 7, 5–22.

Keel, P.K., Dorer, D.J., Franko, D.L., et al., 2005. Postremission predictors of relapse in women with eating disorders. Am. J. Psychiatry 162, 2263–2268.

Machado, G.C., Ferreira, M.L., 2014. Physiotherapy improves eating disorders and quality of life in bulimia and anorexia nervosa. Br. J. Sports Med. 48 (20), 1519–1520.

Mantilla, E.F., Bergsten, K., Birgegård, A., 2014. Self-image and eating disorder symptoms in normal and clinical adolescents. Eat. Behav. 15 (1), 125–131.

Mehler, P.S., Birmingham, L.C., Crow, S., 2010. Medical complications of eating disorders. In: Grilo, L., Mitchell, J.E. (Eds.), The Treatment of Eating Disorders, a Clinical Handbook. Guilford, New York, pp. 66–82.

Mehler, P.S., Cleary, B.S., Gaudiani, J.L., 2011. Osteoporosis in anorexia nervosa. Eat. Disord. 19 (2), 194–202.

Mehler, P.S., MacKenzie, T.D., 2009. Treatment of osteopenia and osteoporosis in anorexia nervosa: a systematic review of the literature. Int. J. Eat. Disord. 42 (3), 195–201.

Mitchell, J.E., Crow, S., 2006. Medical implications of anorexia and bulimia. Curr. Opin. Psychiatry 19, 438–443.

Michielli, D.W., Dunbar, C.C., Kalinski, M.I., 1994. Is exercise indicated for the patient diagnosed as anorectic? J. Psychosoc. Nurs. 32, 33–35.

Ng, L.W.C., Ng, D.P., Wong, W.P., 2013. Is supervised exercise training safe in patients with anorexia nervosa? A meta-analysis. Physiother. 99, 1–11.

Pantano, K.J., 2009. Strategies used by physical therapists in the US for treatment and prevention of the female athlete triad. Phys. Ther. Sport 10 (1), 3–11.

Phillips, K.A., 2004. Body dysmorphic disorder: recognizing and treating imagined ugliness. World Psychiatry 3 (1), 12–17.

Phillips, K.A., 2005. The Broken Mirror. Understanding and Treating Body Dysmorphic Disorder. Revised and Expanded Version. University Press, Oxford.

Probst, M., in press. Eating disorders and exercise, a challenge. In: Stubbs, B., Rosenbaum, S. (Eds.), Exercise-based interventions for people with mental illness. Elsevier, London.

Probst, M., 2006. Body experience in eating disorders: research and therapy. Eur. B. Adapt. Phys. Act. 5, 1. <http://www.eufapa.upol.cz.> [on-line].

Probst, M., 2008b. Lichaamsbeleving (Hoofdstuk 12). In: Vandereycken, W., Noordenbos, G. (Eds.), Handboek Eetstoornissen. De Tijdstroom, Utrecht, pp. 254–267.

Probst, M., Diedens, J., Van Damme, T., 2017. The body in movement. In: Jauregui, I., Lobera, I. (Eds.), Eating Disorders. Intech (open access), Zagreb, pp. 215–236.

Probst, M., Majeweski, M.L., Albertsen, M.N., et al., 2013. Physiotherapy for patients with anorexia nervosa. Adv. Eat. Disord. 1 (3), 224–238.

Probst, M., Pieters, G., Vancampfort, G., Vanderlinden, J., 2008a. Body experience and mirror behaviour in female eating disorders patients and non-clinical subjects. Psychol. Topics 17 (2), 335–348.

Probst, M., Pieters, G., Vanderlinden, J., 2008. Evaluation of body experience questionnaire in eating disorders and non-clinical subjects. Int. J. Eat. Disord. 41, 657–665.

Probst, M., Van Coppenolle, H., Vandereycken, W., 1995a. Body experience in anorexia nervosa patients: an overview of therapeutic approaches. Eat. Disord. 3, 186–198.

Probst, M., Vandereycken, W., Van Coppenolle, H., Pieters, G., 1999. Body experience in eating disorders before and after treatment: a follow-up study. Eur. Psychiatry 14 (6), 333–340.

Probst, M., Vandereycken, W., Van Coppenolle, H., Vanderlinden, J., 1995b. The body attitude test for patients with an eating disorder: psychometric characteristics of a new questionnaire. Eat. Disord. 3, 133–144.

Rasmussen, J., Blashill, A.J., Greenberg, J.L., Wilhelm, S., 2015. Body Dysmorphic Disorder. The Wiley Handbook of Cognitive Behavioral Therapy. Wiley, London.

Rigotti, N.A., Nussbaum, S.R., Herzog, D.B., Neer, R.M., 1984. Osteoporosis in women with anorexia nervosa. New. Eng. J. Med. 311 (25), 1601–1606.

Robinson, P.H., 2006. Community Treatment of Eating Disorders. Wiley, London.

Solmi, M., Veronese, N., Correll, C.U., et al., 2016. Bone mineral density, osteoporosis, and fractures among people with eating disorders: a systematic review and meta-analysis. Acta Psychiatr. Scand. 133, 341–351.

Soundy, A., Stubbs, B., Probst, M., et al., 2015. Considering the role of physical therapists within the treatment and rehabilitation of individuals with eating disorders: an international survey of expert clinicians. Physiother. Res. Int. 21, 237–246.

Sundgot-Borgen, J., Rosenvinge, J.H., Bahr, R., Schneider, L.S., 2002. The effect of exercise, cognitive therapy, and nutritional counseling in treating bulimia nervosa. Med. Sc. Sport Exerc. 2, 190–195.

Thiem, V., Thomas, A., Markin, D., Birmingham, C.L., 2008. Pilot study of a graded exercise program 34 for the treatment of anorexia nervosa. Int. J. Eat. Disord. 28 (1), 101–106.

Thompson, J.K., 1990. Body Image Disturbance. Assessment and Treatment. Pergamon Press, New York.

Tokumura, M., Yoshiba, S., Tanaka, T., et al., 2003. Prescribed exercise training improves exercise capacity of convalescent children and adolescents with anorexia nervosa. Eur. J. Ped. 162, 430–431.

Vancampfort, D., De Herdt, A., Vanderlinden, J., et al., 2014b. Health related quality of life, physical fitness and physical activity participation in treatment-seeking obese persons with and without binge eating disorder. Psychiatry Res. 216 (1), 97–102.

Vancampfort, D., Probst, M., Adriaens, A., et al., 2014. Clinical correlates of global functioning in obese treatment seeking persons with binge eating disorder. Psychiatr. Danub. 26 (3), 256–260.

Vancampfort, D., Probst, M., Adriaens, A., et al., 2014a. Changes in physical activity, physical fitness, self-perception and quality of life following a 6-month physical activity counseling and cognitive behavioral therapy program in outpatients with binge eating disorder. Psychiatry Res. 219 (2), 361–366.

Vancampfort, D., Vanderlinden, J., De Hert, M., et al., 2013. A systematic review on physical therapy interventions for patients with binge eating disorder. Disabil. Rehabil. 35 (26), 2191–2196.

Vancampfort, D., Vanderlinden, J., De Hert, M., et al., 2014a. A systematic review of physical therapy interventions for patients with anorexia and bulimia nervosa. Disabil. Rehabil. 36 (8), 628–634.

Vancampfort, D., De Herdt, A., Vanderlinden, J., et al., 2014b. Health related quality of life, physical fitness and physical activity participation in treatment-seeking obese persons with and without binge eating disorder. Psychiatry Res. 216 (1), 97–102.

Vancampfort, D., Probst, M., Adriaens, A., et al., 2014c. Changes in physical activity, physical fitness, self-perception and quality of life following a 6-month physical activity counseling and cognitive behavioral therapy program in outpatients with binge eating disorder. Psychiatry Res. 219 (2), 361–366.

Vancampfort, D., Vanderlinden, J., De Hert, M., et al., 2014. A systematic review of physical therapy interventions for patients with anorexia and bulimia nervosa. Disabil. Rehabil. 36 (8), 628–634.

Vandereycken, W., Depreitere, L., Probst, M., 1987. Body-oriented therapy for anorexia nervosa patients. Am. J. Psychother. 41, 252–259.

Van Steelandt, K., Pieters, G., Probst, M., Vanderlinden, J., 2007. Drive for thinness, affect regulation and physical activity in eating disorders: a daily life study. Behav. Res. Ther. 45 (8), 1717–1734.

Wallin, U., Kronovall, P., Majewski, M.-L., 2000. Body Awareness Therapy in teenage Anorexia Nervosa: Outcome after 2 years. Eur. Eat. Disord. Rev. 8, 19–30.

Ziemer, R.R., Ross, J.L., 1970. Anorexia nervosa: a new approach. Am. Correct. Ther. J. 24 (2), 34–42.

Zunker, C., Mitchell, J.E., Wonderlich, S.A., 2011. Exercise interventions for women with anorexia nervosa: a review of the literature. Int. J. Eat. Disord. 44 (7), 579–584.

5.2.5   Physiotherapy for Patients with Depression

JAN KNAPEN ■ YVES MORIËN ■ YANNICK MARCHAL

SUMMARY

For more than 20 years systematic research has examined the relationship between physical activity and depression, especially aerobic exercise and resistance training. In this chapter, the characteristics of major depression and the findings of two recent meta-analyses in the area of physical exercise and depression will be presented. Depression is associated with a high incidence of comorbid somatic illnesses, especially cardiovascular diseases, diabetes mellitus type II and metabolic syndrome. The bidirectional association between major depression and metabolic syndrome, and the role of lifestyle factors in this interaction is discussed. Finally, we offer evidence-based recommendations for exercise therapy for patients with depression.

KEY POINTS

■ For mild-to-moderate depression the effect of exercise may be comparable to antidepressant medication and psychotherapy; for severe depression exercise seems to be a valuable complementary therapy to the traditional treatments.

■ Exercise therapy also improves physical health and fitness, body image, patients' coping strategies with stress, quality of life and independence in activities of daily living in older adults.

■ Motivational strategies should be incorporated in exercise therapy to enhance patients' motivation.

LEARNING OBJECTIVES

■ Discuss the evidence-based recommendations for exercise therapy in depressed patients.

■ Understand the factors that play a role in the bidirectional association between depression and metabolic syndrome.

■ Be able to discuss which motivational strategies are useful to improve exercise motivation and adherence in depressed patients.

DESCRIPTION OF MAJOR DEPRESSION

Depression refers to a wide range of mental health problems characterized by the absence of a positive affect (a loss of interest and enjoyment in ordinary things and experiences), persistent low mood, and a range of associated emotional, cognitive, physical and behavioural symptoms (National Institute for Health and Clinical Excellence, 2010). Severity of depression is classified using the Diagnostic and Statistical Manual of Mental Disorders, fifth edition (DSM-V) criteria as mild (five or more symptoms with minor functional impairment), moderate (symptoms or functional impairment are between 'mild' and 'severe') and severe (most symptoms present and interfere with functioning, with or without psychotic symptoms) (American Psychiatric Association, 2013).

Major depression consists of at least one 2-week major depressive episode. The primary symptom of a major depressive episode is either depressed mood or loss of interest or pleasure. Additionally, the symptoms must not be clearly attributable to another medical condition or to the physiological effects of a substance. The symptoms cannot be better explained by a range of psychotic, schizophrenic or delusional disorders. Symptoms that are clearly attributable to another medical condition are not counted in the required five symptoms minimum. Additionally, as with most psychiatric conditions, the symptoms must cause clinically significant distress or impairment in social, occupational or other important areas of functioning. The following is an abbreviated summary of the DSM-V symptoms of depression (at least five are needed for at least 2 weeks for a diagnosis of a major depressive episode). With the exception of suicidal ideation and weight change, symptoms must be present most of the day, nearly every day (Box 1).

MAJOR DEPRESSION, A BIG PUBLIC HEALTH PROBLEM

Recent epidemiological surveys conducted in general populations have found that the lifetime prevalence of depression is in the range of 10% to 15% (Lepine & Briley, 2011). Mood disorders, as defined by the World Mental Health and the DSM-IV, have a 12-month

BOX 1

- Depressed mood most of the day, nearly every day
- Markedly diminished interest or pleasure, in all, or almost all, activities most of the day, nearly every day
- Significant weight loss or gain when not dieting (i.e., 5% in a month), or decreased appetite nearly every day. Failure to make appropriate weight gains is considered in children
- Insomnia or hypersomnia nearly every day
- Psychomotor agitation or retardation nearly every day (observable by others)
- Fatigue or loss of energy nearly every day
- Feelings of worthlessness or excessive or inappropriate guilt (which may be delusional) nearly every day
- Diminished ability to think or concentrate, or indecisiveness nearly every day
- Recurrent thoughts of death, recurrent suicidal ideation without plan, or a suicide attempt or plan.

prevalence which varies from 3% in Japan to over 9% in the US (Demyttenaere et al., 2004). Several studies of depressive disorders have stressed the importance of the mortality and morbidity associated with depression (Osby et al., 2001; Lepine & Briley, 2011). The mortality risk for suicide in depressed patients is more than 20-fold greater than in the general population. Studies have also shown the importance of depression as a risk factor for cardiovascular death (Penninx et al., 2001; Rugulies, 2002; Lett et al., 2004; Whang et al., 2009). Greater severity of depressive symptoms has been found to be associated with a significantly higher risk of all-cause mortality including cardiovascular death and stroke. Depression increases the risk of decreased workplace productivity and absenteeism, resulting in lowered income or unemployment.

An analysis of data from the National Co-morbidity Survey Replication, a US nationally representative household survey, found that overall impairment was significantly higher for mental disorders than for chronic medical disorders (Druss et al., 2009). Severe functional impairment was reported by 42% of people with mental disorders and 24% with chronic medical disorders. Treatment, however, was provided for a significantly lower proportion of mental (21.4%) than chronic medical (58.2%) disorders.

Disability adjusted life-years (DALY) is the sum of life-years lost due to premature death and years lived with disability adjusted for severity (World Health Organization, 2004). It integrates the notions of individual mortality and disability with global disease prevalence. Using DALY, unipolar major depression was classed in 2004 as the third leading burden of disease or injury cause worldwide for both sexes, behind lower respiratory infections and diarrheal diseases. Worldwide projections by the World Health Organization for the year 2030 identify major depression as the leading cause of disease burden.

The substantial burden of major depression is due, in part, to the limited accessibility and effectiveness of treatments, with data indicating that only 55% of those with a depressive disorder seek treatment and only 32% receive an efficacious treatment (psychotherapy or antidepressant medication) (Lepine & Briley, 2011). Physical exercise has been suggested as an efficient complementary treatment to reduce symptoms of depression since it reduces cost with drugs and hospitalizations, and may also improve physical health and physiological stress responses (Cooney et al., 2013; Silveira et al., 2013). There are several hypotheses regarding the physiological and psychological mechanisms by which exercise impacts on mental health, such as enhancement of the synthesis and liberation of neurotrophic factors, as well as angiogenesis, neurogenesis and plasticity. Moreover, some studies have shown that physical exercise may improve physical and global self-esteem, quality of life, coping strategies with stress and social contact (Knapen & Vancampfort, 2014). Furthermore, it may also contribute to increased quality of life and independence in activities of daily living in older adults.

PHYSICAL EXERCISE AS INTERVENTION FOR DEPRESSION: FINDINGS OF TWO RECENT META-ANALYSES

A recent metaanalysis of the Cochrane Collaboration investigated the effectiveness of exercise in the treatment of depression in adults compared with no treatment or a comparator intervention (Cooney et al., 2013).

This metaanalysis aimed to answer the following questions:

- Is exercise more effective than no therapy for reducing symptoms of depression?

- Is exercise more effective than antidepressant medication for reducing symptoms of depression?
- Is exercise more effective than psychological therapies or other nonmedical treatments for depression?
- How acceptable to patients is exercise as a treatment for depression?

Which studies were included in the review?

The Cochrane research group used search databases to find all high-quality randomized controlled trials of how effective exercise is for treating depression in adults over 18 years of age. The authors searched for studies published up until March 2013. All studies had to include adults with a diagnosis of depression, and the physical activity carried out had to fit criteria to ensure that it met with a definition of 'exercise'. Thirty-nine studies with a total of 2326 participants were included in the systematic review.

What does the evidence from this review tell us?

The authors concluded that exercise is moderately more effective than no therapy for reducing symptoms of depression. In addition, exercise is no more or less effective than antidepressants for reducing symptoms of depression, although this conclusion is based on a small number of studies. Exercise is also no more or less effective than psychological therapies for reducing symptoms of depression, although this conclusion is based on a small number of studies. An important observation was that attendance rates for exercise treatments ranged from 50% to 100%.

Suggestions for Further Research

The authors recommend that future research should look into detail at what types of exercise could have the most benefit for people with depression. Research should also investigate the optimal dose-response relationship. Further larger trials are needed to compare the effects of exercise therapy with antidepressants or psychological treatments.

Another recent meta-analysis of 2013 by Silveira et al. (2013) evaluated the effect of aerobic and strength training as a treatment for major depression, using various aspects such as remission and response to treatment, age, severity of depression and type of exercise (aerobic training and strength training).

The following data were collected: total number of patients, age, randomized design, diagnostic criteria, assessment instruments, the percentage of remission and treatment response. The outcome variables were proportion of remission (no symptoms) and at least 50% reduction of initial depression scores (response).

The authors concluded that physical exercise moderately reduces depressive symptoms in major depression patients (SMD = 0.61). Physical exercise is an efficient alternative treatment for depression, with a 49% increase in the probability of response to treatment defined as a 50% reduction in initial depression scores. Individuals over 60 years of age showed a higher efficacy than those found in studies with populations under 60 years of age.

Patients with mild depressive symptoms showed a better treatment response than patients with mild/moderate depressive symptoms. Aerobic training was more effective than strength training.

In this meta-analysis, the efficacy of exercise in the treatment of depression was influenced by age and symptom severity. It is reasonable that physical exercise may in some cases be considered an alternative to antidepressants for the treatment of mild major-depression in older persons. This finding might contribute to decreasing the use of medication and hospitalization, and in promoting independence in activities of daily living in elderly patients. An important limitation of this meta-analysis is, however, that the samples of all studies included consisted of patients with mild or moderate depression.

MAJOR DEPRESSION AND METABOLIC SYNDROME

Depressed people have approximately a twofold increased risk of having or developing cardiovascular disease (Lett et al., 2004; Whang et al., 2009). Furthermore, after a cardiovascular event the risk of onset of depression is increased, resulting in a poorer cardiovascular outcome. The metabolic syndrome, a constellation of cardiovascular risk factors including (abdominal) obesity, hypertension, dyslipidemia and hyperglycemia, has been suggested to be one possible pathway linking depression and cardiovascular disease.

A recent metaanalysis clearly demonstrated that metabolic syndrome occurs frequently in depressed people (Vancampfort et al., 2014). The authors included 18 publications (n = 5531) with clearly defined major depression, all published between 2004 and June 2013. They reported that 30.5% of individuals with major depression suffered from metabolic syndrome. The relative risk for metabolic syndrome was 1.5-times higher for people with depression compared with general population controls.

Consistent with population studies, the research group found no significant difference between men and women, indicating that both sexes need the same attention and care. In addition, age also did not explain differences in prevalence estimates, indicating that the high risk for metabolic abnormalities should be a concern across the lifespan. However, the use of antipsychotic drugs in patients with major depression is significantly ($p < .05$) higher metabolic syndrome prevalence estimates.

Another metaanalysis on the bidirectional association between depression and metabolic syndrome concluded that metabolic syndrome is an independent risk factor major depression (Pan et al., 2012). Individuals with metabolic syndrome have a higher relative risk to develop clinical diagnosed depression (OR = 2.18) than individuals without metabolic syndrome.

The positive bidirectional longitudinal association between depression and metabolic syndrome means that depression is causing metabolic syndrome and vice versa. This association suggests a possible pathophysiological overlap (Pan et al., 2012). More specifically, elevated cortisol secretion due to hyperactivity of the hypothalamic-pituitary-adrenal axis, (pro)inflammatory processes, oxidative stress, autonomic nervous system dysregulation and insulin resistance are all interacting biological mechanisms that may mediate the association between depression and metabolic syndrome. Although biological processes might be important, socioeconomic and lifestyle factors such as lack of physical activity and poor diet are probably equally relevant (Vancampfort et al., 2014).

Conclusion: both major depression and metabolic syndrome are associated with increased mortality and morbidity, possibly through the association with various medical diseases such as cardiovascular disease and diabetes mellitus type II. Lifestyle has an impact on both physical and mental health, and desirable changes in diet and exercise can be useful in the prevention as well as treatment of depression and metabolic syndrome.

EVIDENCE-BASED RECOMMENDATIONS FOR EXERCISE THERAPY IN DEPRESSED PATIENTS

An exercise prescription includes the following key elements: (1) exercise modality; (2) frequency and duration of exercise sessions; and (3) exercise intensity. In considering exercise as a treatment option, additional key issues include (4) duration of the intervention; and (5) motivational strategies to promote adherence to the exercise program.

Rethorst & Trivedi (2013) provide the following recommendations:

Exercise Modality

Research supports the use of aerobic exercise for reducing depressive symptoms. Although findings concerning the antidepressant effects of resistance training are positive, only limited research has focused on this modality.

Frequency and Duration of Sessions

Patients should exercise at least three times per week for 45–60 minutes.

Exercise Intensity

For aerobic exercise, patients should exercise at 50%–85% of maximum heart rate. For resistance training, patients should complete a variety of upper and lower body exercises. Three sets of eight repetitions at 80% of one-repetition maximum are recommended.

Duration of Intervention

Patients may experience improvements in depressive symptoms in as little as 4 weeks; however, continued exercise for at least 10-12 weeks is necessary for the greatest antidepressant effect.

Adherence to Exercise Interventions

Depressed patients accumulate a lot of barriers for participation in exercise programs such as: a low self-concept, loss of energy, interest and motivation,

BOX 2

- Anticipate the barriers for participation by an acquaintance conversation.
- Give information about mental and physical health benefits of exercise.
- Help the person find a form of physical activity that suits them.
- Draw up an individual plan, with the patient taking into account emotional, cognitive and physiological components of depression.
- Create exercise programs based on initial physical fitness assessment and measurement of perceived exertion during exercise.
- Formulate realistic objectives improving exercise compliance and motivation.
- Adapt the moderate exercise stimulus to the individual's physical abilities, training status, expectations and goals, side effects of psychotropic medication, exercise tolerance and perceived exertion.
- Follow the programme with exercise cards and provide regular progress feedback to the patients.
- Avoid between-patient.
- Focus on perceived fitness gains, achievement of personal goals, mastery experiences and sense of control over the body and its functioning.

generalized fatigue, weak physical fitness and health condition, kinesiophobia, social fear, being overweight, a low feeling of personal control concerning own fitness and health, and psychosomatic complaints. In order to improve patient motivation and to optimize the effects of exercise therapy, the following recommendations for physical therapists are helpful (Box 2) (Knapen & Vancampfort, 2014).

REFERENCES

American Psychiatric Association, 2013. Diagnostic and Statistical Manual of Mental Disorders, fifth ed. American Psychiatric Publishing, Arlington.

Cooney, G.M., Dwan, K., Greig, C.A., et al., 2013. Exercise for depression. Cochrane Database Syst. Rev. (9), CD004366.

Demyttenaere, K., Bruffaerts, R., Posada-Villa, J., et al., 2004. Prevalence, severity, and unmet need for treatment of mental disorders in the World Health Organization World Mental Health Surveys. J. Am. Med. Assoc. 291 (21), 2581–2590.

Druss, B.G., Hwang, I., Petukhova, M., et al., 2009. Impairment in role functioning in mental and chronic medical disorders in the United States: results from the National Comorbidity Survey Replication. Mol. Psychiatry 14 (7), 728–737.

Knapen, J., Vancampfort, D., 2014. Exercise for depression and anxiety: an evidence based approach and recommendations for clinical practice. In: Probst, M., Carraro, A. (Eds.), Physical Activity and Mental Health in a Practice Oriented Perspective. Edi Ermes, Milan, pp. 91–100.

Lepine, J.P., Briley, M., 2011. The increasing burden of depression. Neuropsychiatr. Dis. Treat. 7 (Suppl. 1), 3–7.

Lett, H.S., Blumenthal, J.A., Babyak, M.A., et al., 2004. Depression as a risk factor for coronary artery disease: evidence, mechanisms, and treatment. Psychosom. Med. 66 (3), 305–315.

National Collaborating Centre for Mental Health Depression, 2010. The Treatment and Management of Depression in Adults (Update). British Psychological Society, Leicester.

Osby, U., Brandt, L., Correia, N., et al., 2001. Excess mortality in bipolar and unipolar disorder in Sweden. Arch. Gen. Psychiatry 58 (9), 844–850.

Pan, A., Keum, N., Okereke, O.I., et al., 2012. Bidirectional association between depression and metabolic syndrome: a systematic review and meta-analysis of epidemiological studies. Diabetes Care 35 (5), 1171–1180.

Penninx, B.W., Beekman, A.T., Honig, A., et al., 2001. Depression and cardiac mortality: results from a community-based longitudinal study. Arch. Gen. Psychiatry 58 (3), 221–227.

Rethorst, C., Trivedi, M., 2013. Evidence-based recommendations for the prescription of exercise for major depressive disorder. J. Psychiatr. Pract. 19 (3), 204–212.

Rugulies, R., 2002. Depression as a predictor for coronary heart disease. a review and meta-analysis. Am. J. Prev. Med. 23 (1), 51–61.

Silveira, H., Moraes, H., Oliveira, N., et al., 2013. Physical exercise and clinically depressed patients: a systematic review and meta analysis. Neuropsychobiology 67 (2), 61–68.

Vancampfort, D., Correll, C.U., Wampers, M., et al., 2014. Metabolic syndrome and metabolic abnormalities in patients with major depressive disorder: a meta-analysis of prevalences and moderating variables. Psychol. Med. 44 (10), 2017–2028.

Whang, W., Kubzansky, L.D., Kawachi, I., et al., 2009. Depression and risk of sudden cardiac death and coronary heart disease in women: results from the Nurses' Health Study. J. Am. Coll. Cardiol. 53 (11), 950–958.

World Health Organization, 2004. The Global Burden of Disease: 2004 Update. World Health Organization Press, Geneva.

5.2.6   Conversion Syndrome and Physiotherapy

JOLIEN DIEDENS ■ MICHEL PROBST ■ BEELEKE BREDERO

SUMMARY

Conversion syndrome seriously affects a person in his/her daily functioning. The loss of a physical function initially seems that it is caused by a physical or neurological disorder however, no neurological or physical disorders are found during examination. Contrary what most people think, these complaints are not feigned. In DSM-V conversion syndrome is classified under somatic symptoms and related disorders. This article shows the etiology, diagnosis and treatment for a conversion syndrome. Attention will be given to the role of a physiotherapist in the multi disciplinar treatment of this syndrome. Giving information about the syndrome and increasing daily functioning are important aspects of the treatment.

KEY POINTS

- Conversion syndrome is not feigned.
- It can really interfere with functioning in daily life.
- Multidisciplinary treatment is recommended.
- The earlier intervention starts, the better outcome patient will have.

LEARNING OBJECTIVES

- Be able to explain the etiology of conversion syndrome.
- Be able to describe several symptoms from conversion syndrome.
- Understand which factors are important in the treatment of conversion syndrome.

DEFINITION AND DESCRIPTION

The predominant feature in a conversion disorder is an alteration or a loss of physical functioning, suggesting a physical disorder. A person presents with physical symptoms such as weakness, tingling, blindness or fits which cannot be explained by a medical condition. Conversion disorder is characterized by unexplained symptoms affecting voluntary motor or sensory function in ways that suggest neurological disease and by the presence of psychological conflicts that play a significant role in initiating, aggravating and maintaining the disturbance (American Psychiatric Association, 1994, Oh et al., 2005).

The conversion patient truly believes he has the physical symptom he reports and he should be distinguished from the malingerer who attempts to convince others of his disability. With malingering, the patient has a conscious secondary gain in mind.

It is an established fact that conversion disorder develops as a reaction to emotional stress due to a series of environmental, biological and personal vulnerability factors or as a part of the current life situation (Kendell, 1974).

The common symptoms of conversion disorder include inconsistencies in repeated testing of sensation and muscle strength, manual muscle strength testing that does not correspond with the patient's functional abilities and sensory impairments that do not follow anatomical patterns (Debra, 2007).

ETIOLOGY

Freud was the pioneer on conversion disorders research (in the past this was known as *hysteria*). According to Freud, conversion is a method to cope with emotional pain. The repression of the pain would be converted into neurological symptoms (Freud, 1896). Another researcher was Janet; her hypothesis stated: 'Symptoms arise through the power of suggestion, acting on a personality vulnerable to dissociation. In this hypothetical process, the subject's experience of their leg, for example, is split-off from the rest of their consciousness, resulting in paralysis or numbness in that leg.' However, other authors have tried to do more research on these models, but none of them have succeeded in forming an empirical basis Roelofs et al., 2002; Kanaan et al., 2007).

Recent work tends to show that the onset of symptoms is related to a psychological conflict or stressful event. There are also certain populations that are vulnerable to conversion disorder, including people suffering from a medical illness or condition, people with a personality disorder and individuals with dissociative identity disorder (A.D.A.M. Medical Encyclopedia, 2012).

Nowadays, different medical imaging modalities are used to try to reveal the underlying cause of conversion disorders. Current results have shown that blood flow in patients' brains may be abnormal while they are unwell. Besides that, it is seen in people who have experienced traumatic events that their emotional processing is abnormal. Further research is required to provide a reliable neurophysiological model (Brown et al., 2007).

DIAGNOSIS

In the DSM-V, conversion disorder belongs to somatic symptoms and related disorders. The DSM-5 classification defines disorders on the basis of positive symptoms (i.e., distressing somatic symptoms plus abnormal thoughts, feelings and behaviours in response to these symptoms).

These symptoms are classified into four subtypes in the DSM-V.

1. Motor symptom/deficit; in this subtype, a patient presents with paralysis or localized weakness or with impaired balance or co-ordination. Sometimes the patient can have an impaired gait, which is defined as: astasia-basia: *"impaired balance with the falls or dramatically unbalanced gait that cannot be explained by decreased muscle strength"*.

2. Sensory symptom/deficit
Instead of motor problems, patient will now have an altered sensation: loss of touch or abnormal pain sensation. Sometimes it will occur with blindness, deafness or hallucinations.

3. Seizures/convulsions
Seizures with voluntary motor or sensory components.

4. Mixed presentation
Symptoms of more than one subtype are present. An important keynote: the presented impairments do not correspond with any anatomical and/or neurological patterns. Besides that, a neurological disease must first be excluded (Glennon, 2011).

The underlying psychological mechanism is the most difficult aspect of the diagnosis of this disorder. Further research is required to determine how a stressor or previous psychological conflict is associated with the development of the conversion disorder. It is noteworthy that for this diagnosis, deliberate feigning should be excluded. To find out whether the patient feigns or not could be distinguished by using neuroimaging. However, the results from electroencephalography (EEG) and motor-evoked potentials are usually normal. Even more, there are no laboratory results which confirm a conversion disorder.

Several features can help to diagnose a conversion disorder:

- Paralysis: the paralysis does not correspond with a corresponding neurological pattern. It just occurs 'somewhere' in the body.
- Weakness will be less intense at a distal part of the body.
- Since there are no physiologic neurological problems, all reflexes will be normal.
- Contractions of antagonist muscles are found when testing involved muscles.
- Astasia-basia (bizarre gait pattern).
- Overflow of emotion during the examination (painful expression, tooth grinding, abnormal breathing etc).
- Normal muscle tone.
- Simultaneous contraction of agonist and antagonist muscles, which can be seen while performing Hoover's test (Kaur et al., 2012).

TREATMENT

The therapist plays a central role in the treatment of conversion disorder. Dallocchio et al. (2010) has made an acronym (THERAPIST) of the essential steps to manage the treatment of patients with conversion disorder.

There are nine essential steps for an approach to management of patients with conversion disorder (Box 1).

To treat or manage conversion syndrome, a variety of treatment modalities exist. Sometimes symptoms disappear in time on their own. In some cases, a treatment is needed. Available treatment options for conversion syndrome are hypnosis, psychotherapy, physical therapy,

---

BOX 1

Terminology must engage and not alienate the patient.

Hear out the patient with interest, compassion and empathy (and patience).

Explain the diagnosis and the mechanism of symptoms.

Reassure that there is no evidence of neurological damage.

Address psychosocial and family issues.

Prognosis is likely favourable, the patient has the potential to recover fully.

Individualize the therapy and customize it.

Self-help is a crucial part of getting better.

Treat concurrent psychiatric and medical illness (if present).

---

stress management and transcranial magnetic stimulation (Mayo Foundation, 2003). If comorbid psychic disorders are present, a psychological treatment can be useful.

Duration and type of treatment depends on the presentation of symptoms. Further research is needed.

The treatment starts with an initial assessment to determine goals in consultation with the staff, patient and family. The therapy programme will be explained to the patient; this programme is based on his/her needs and what he/she would like to achieve. Furthermore, the patient will be the creator of rewards or privileges if he has achieved his/her goal. Progress of treatment will be reported on a constant basis to medical staff members.

A key feature of treatment is to incorporate behaviour modification through the Skinnerian model of learning theory. Skinner's model states that if a particular behaviour produces favourable reinforcement, there is an increased likelihood of this behaviour occurring again (Knowles et al., 2012).

Thus the therapist disregards unwanted movement patterns and only rewards desired behaviours such as smooth movement and normal gait. An important concept to integrate into the physiotherapy programme is motor learning. This is the process by which an individual acquires or modifies movement.

As the patient progresses through the programme, the therapist should provide less cueing, less physical support and more intrinsic feedback. Programmes that include strengthening, general flexibility, gait retraining in parallel bars and weight-bearing activities can influence

the patient's confidence in their ability to succeed, and thereby reintegrate into community activities.

In short, for the treatment of conversion disorders it is important to define goals in consultation with the patient and the therapy should be implemented in a multidisciplinary team. For a good prognosis, the patient should feel understood by his care workers and should work on his physical fitness.

CORNERSTONES OF PHYSICAL THERAPY INTERVENTIONS

Gelauff et al. (2014) have mentioned important steps in the treatment of conversion disorder underlining the importance of psycho-education in the treatment of conversion disorder. First of all, psychoeducation is important. Psycho-education is important for the patient as well for family members. Listen to the story of the patient and identify the expectations towards the treatment. Also explain the role of stress to the patient since many of their physical complaints are possibly caused by it. During the course of the treatment, the physiotherapist will recognize the fears, unhelpful perceptions and destructive thought patterns of the patient. For the optimal outcome, the therapist should be supportive, authentic and empathic to the patient, since most patients do not feel understood by previous caregivers (Stuart & Noyes, 2006). Avoid assumptions of the causes of the conversion disorder in communication.

Try to set goals in consultation with the patient. This will give them the feeling of having influence on their therapy. The therapy programme will be explained to the patient; this programme is based on their needs and what they would like to achieve. Furthermore, let them choose rewards or privileges if a set goal has been achieved. Progress of treatment will be reported on a constant basis to medical staff members.

Since a conversion disorder will affect several parts of the body, a multi-disciplinar treatment is recommended.

The role of the physiotherapist is treating motor dysfunction and helping the patient to maintain or improve their autonomic lifestyle (Box 2) (Hurwitz, 2003; Ness, 2007).

A physiotherapy programme is recommended from the start of the treatment. The earlier the intervention starts, the better outcome a patient will have.

By doing prescribed exercises, the patient can have a better consciousness of their body. Since inactivity is frequently observed in this population, the physiotherapist can stimulate the patient to be more active and able to complete his exercises. While doing this, the patient will be more aware of his body, which this can lead to a decrease of his complaints and, (Rosebush & Mazurek, 2006).

REFERENCES

A.D.A.M, 2012. Medical Encyclopedia, Conversion Disorder Hysterical Neurosis. November 17.

Brown, R.J., Cardena, E., Nijenhuis, E., et al., 2007. 'Should conversion disorder be reclassified as a dissociative disorder in DSM V?' Psychosomatics 48 (5), 369–378.

Dallocchio, C., Arbasino, C., Klersy, C., Marchioni, E., 2010. The effects of physical activity on psychogenic movement disorders. Mov. Disord. 25 (4), 421–425.

Debra, N., 2007. Physical therapy management for conversion disorder: case series. J. Neurol. Phys. Ther. 31, 30–39.

Eckhardt, A., 1994. Factitious disorders in the field of neurology and psychiatry. 62(1–2), pp. 56–62.

Freud, S., 1896. The aetiology of hysteria. In: Strachet, J. (Ed.), The complete works of Sigmund Freud (1893-1899): Early psychoanalytic publications, vol. 3, standard ed. Hogarth Press, London, pp. 191–221.

Gelauff, J., Stone, J., Edwards, M., et al., 2014. The prognosis of functional (psychogenic) motor symptoms: a systematic review. J. Neurol. Neurosurg. Psychiatry 85, 220–226.

Glennon, Á., 2011. A practical approach to the physiotherapy assessment and treatment of conversion disorders. R. Coll. Surg. Irel. Stud. Med. J. 4, 57–61.

Hurwitz, T., 2003. Somatisation and conversion disorder. Can. J. Psychiatry 49, 172–178.

Kanaan, R.A., Craig, T.K., Wessely, S.C., David, A.S., 2007. Imaging repressed memories in motor conversion disorder. Psychosom. Med. 69 (2), 202–205.

Kaur, J., Garnawat, D., Deepak, G., Mansi, S., 2012. Conversion Disorder and Physical Therapy. Delhi Psychiatry J. 15 (2), 394–397.

Kendell, R.E., 1974. A new look at hysteria. Medicine 30, 1780–1783.

Knowles, M.S., Holton, E.F., III, Swanson, R.A., 2012. The Adult Learner. Routledge.

Mace, C.J., 1992. Hysterical conversion. I: A history. Br. J. Psychiatry 161, 369–377.

Mayo Foundation for Medical Education and Research. Conversion disorder.

Ness, D., 2007. Physical therapy management for conversion disorder: case series. J. Neurol. Phys. Ther. 31 (1), 30–39.

Oh, D.W., Yoo, E.Y., Yi, C.H., Kwon, O.Y., 2005. Physiotherapy strategies for a patient with conversion disorder presenting abnormal gait. Physiother. Res. Int. 10 (3), 164–168.

Roelofs, K., Keijsers, G.P., Hoogduin, K.A., et al., 2002b. Childhood abuse in patients with conversion disorder. Am. J. Psychiatry 159 (11), 1908–1913.

Rosebush, P., Mazurek, M.F., 2006. Treatment of conversion disorder. In: Hallet, M., Yudofsky, S.C., Lang, A.E., et al. (Eds.), To psychogenic movement disorders. Lippincott Williams & Wilkins, Philadelphia, USA, pp. 289–301.

Stuart, S., Noyes, R., Jr., 2006. Interpersonal psychotherapy for somatizing patients. Psychother. Psychosom. 75 (4), 209–219.

5.2.7 Physiotherapy Within the Multidisciplinary Treatment of Schizophrenia

DAVY VANCAMPFORT ■ LENE NYBOE ■ BRENDON STUBBS

SUMMARY

The majority of physiotherapy interventions revolve around the promotion and support of physical activity, stress reduction and improving body awareness in people with schizophrenia. In this chapter we focus on the scientific evidence for these interventions, but also focus on the challenges that most physiotherapists working with people suffering from schizophrenia are confronted with. It is important that all physiotherapists are trained in recognizing and adequately addressing symptoms of schizophrenia, physical comorbidities and side-effects of antipsychotic medication. Policy makers should therefore offer means to physiotherapists to acquire the necessary cognitive–behavioural and motivational skills to assist physiotherapists in delivering high-quality physiotherapy. It is unequivocal that the role of physiotherapists in the multidisciplinary treatment should be further promoted.

KEY POINTS

■ Patients with schizophrenia have a drastically increased prevalence of physical morbidities and associated premature mortality compared with the general population.

■ There is rigorous evidence for aerobic exercise in improving physical, mental and social outcomes in the treatment of schizophrenia.

■ Improvements in body balance and postural control, increased self-esteem, and an improved ability to think has been reported in people with schizophrenia following physiotherapy based on basic body awareness.

LEARNING OBJECTIVES

■ Understand why physiotherapists should take a central role in the multidisciplinary treatment of schizophrenia.

■ Be able to explain the role of physiotherapists in the multidisciplinary treatment of schizophrenia.

■ Understand the most salient challenges for physiotherapists working with schizophrenia patients.

SCHIZOPHRENIA: THE FACTS

Schizophrenia spectrum disorders (including schizophrenia, schizoaffective disorder and schizophreniform disorder) are some of the most burdensome and costly illnesses (Rössler et al., 2005). According to the Global Burden of Disease Study 2010, schizophrenia spectrum disorders cause a high degree of disability, which accounts for 0.6% of the total disability-adjusted life years worldwide (Murray et al., 2012). The lifetime prevalence and incidence range from 0.30% to 0.66% and from 10.2 to 22.0 per 100,000 people-years, respectively (McGrath et al., 2008). According to the

Diagnostic Statistical Manual of Mental Disorders (DSM-V) criteria (American Psychiatric Association, 2013), schizophrenia compromises both positive and negative symptomatology severe enough to cause important social and occupational dysfunctions. Positive symptoms reflect an excess or distortion of normal functions and manifests itself in symptoms such as delusions, hallucinations, and disorganized speech and behaviour. Negative symptoms reflect a reduction or loss of normal functions consisting of symptoms such as affective flattening, apathy, avolition and social withdrawal.

Mesolimbic dopaminergic hyperactivity is believed to be part of the underlying pathology associated with positive symptoms while the pathophysiology of negative symptoms is poorly understood (Howes et al., 2012). Negative symptoms therefore remain a relatively treatment-refractory and debilitating component of schizophrenia (Abi-Dargham et al., 2000). Once the diagnosis is made, antipsychotic drugs that block dopamine receptors are the main treatment of schizophrenia (Zhang et al., 2010). Many patients continue to suffer from persistent symptoms and relapses, particularly when they discontinue the prescribed medication (Kane et al., 2013).

The Physical Health Disparity and Premature Mortality Among People With Schizophrenia

Next to severe psychiatric symptoms, patients with schizophrenia have a drastically increased prevalence of physical morbidities and associated premature mortality compared with the general population (Hoang et al., 2013; Nielsen et al., 2013). The primary cause of this premature mortality is the increased prevalence of physical comorbidities (Thornicroft, 2011; Lawrence et al., 2013). Of particular concern are metabolic and cardiovascular diseases (CVD), and patients with schizophrenia are also four times more likely to be overweight, have a twofold increased risk for diabetes and show a two to three times higher prevalence of dyslipidemia compared with the general population (Vancampfort et al., 2013a). This excess CVD morbidity results in an increased premature mortality, being two or three times as high as that in the general population. The mortality gap translates into a gap of 11 to 20 years' shortened life expectancy compared with the general population, and this mortality gap still is widening (Laursen et al., 2013; Lawrence et al., 2013). In addition, people with schizophrenia are more likely to receive suboptimal medical care and healthcare provision to address these potentially fatal physical comorbidities (Mitchell & Lawrence, 2011). People with schizophrenia are also hampered by difficulty in changing their lifestyle that can have a beneficial influence on many of the physical comorbidities seen. Much of this difficulty stems from factors related to their illness (negative symptoms, low self-esteem) and its treatment (extrapyramidal and metabolic side-effects of antipsychotic medication) (Vancampfort et al., 2012a).

Disturbed Bodily Experiences and Body-Image Aberrations in Schizophrenia

In phenomenological psychiatry as well as in the classic psychiatric literature disturbances of body experience are regarded as characteristic and frequent symptoms of schizophrenia (Priebe & Rohricht, 2001; Parnas et al., 2005). Disturbed bodily experiences in people with schizophrenia comprise a broad variety of bodily phenomena (e.g., perceptions of morphological changes of the body, perceiving the body as strange, alien or not existing, as if falling apart or going bodily into pieces, having abnormal sensory sensations, or experiencing interference, blocking or deautomation of movement) (Parnas et al., 2005). Abnormal thoughts and attitudes towards the body and disturbed bodily experiences together constitute body-image disturbances in schizophrenia (Priebe & Rohricht, 2001). In addition, psychological distress and anxiety related to the illness may place further strain on bodily function and well-being (Priebe & Rohricht, 2001; Parnas et al., 2005).

The Role of Physiotherapists in the Treatment of Schizophrenia

Because of their training and experience, physiotherapists are ideally placed to promote healthier lifestyle choices, and to improve functional outcomes and health-related quality of life of patients with schizophrenia. In particular, physiotherapists provide an important bridge between physical and mental health (Soundy et al., 2014a; Stubbs et al., 2014a,b,c,d). Whilst a significant majority of physiotherapy interventions may revolve around the promotion and

support of physical activity and improving body awareness in people with schizophrenia, physiotherapists also have a key role in other areas. For instance, a metaanalysis established that around a third of patients experience clinical pain, and physiotherapists have a key role in addressing this important and often undetected phenomenon (Stubbs et al., 2014a). Recently, a large study involving over 93,000 people with schizophrenia found that 35% and 21% are affected by arthritic pain and chronic low-back pain, respectively (Birgenheir et al., 2013). Physiotherapists are known to have an integral role in both of these areas in nonmental health settings, and clearly physiotherapists should have a leading role in addressing this type of clinical pain that can have multiple deleterious impacts upon the individual if left untreated. In addition, physiotherapists may have a key role in promoting bone health. A recent systematic review (Stubbs et al., 2014e) established that half of patients with schizophrenia have a reduced bone mass and are thus susceptible to fractures. Physiotherapists may promote physical activity and strengthening exercise, which in the general population is effective in improving bone mass.

Evidence for Physiotherapy in Patients With Schizophrenia

A systematic review investigating physiotherapy-led interventions in patients with schizophrenia (Vancampfort et al., 2012b) demonstrated that aerobic and strength training, yoga therapy and progressive muscle relaxation, offered by physiotherapists, improve the mental and physical health of patients with schizophrenia, while there are also some indications for the use of body-awareness techniques. There is emerging evidence for physiotherapy in several areas and these will briefly be explored.

Aerobic and Strength Training in the Treatment of Schizophrenia

It has been demonstrated that aerobic and strength training reduces positive and negative symptoms, and improves cardio-metabolic functioning (Vancampfort et al., 2012b). Furthermore, there is preliminary evidence that physical exercise has a beneficial influence on the brain health of people with schizophrenia (Vancampfort et al., 2014). At the moment, however, no optimal dose-response association can be defined (Vancampfort et al., 2012b). Nevertheless, there is no evidence to believe that current guidelines for physical activity for the general population are not relevant to people with schizophrenia in terms of potential cardio-metabolic benefits. The International Organization of Physical Therapy in Mental Health (IOPTMH) therefore suggests to apply the general population recommendations also to patients with schizophrenia (Vancampfort et al., 2012c). The IOPTMH states that in people with schizophrenia from the first episode on, the promotion of a healthy lifestyle, including being physically active, should be the shared responsibility of physiotherapists, general practitioners, psychiatrists, nurses, psychologists and dieticians (Vancampfort et al., 2012c).

Yoga as a Physiotherapeutic Method in the Treatment of Schizophrenia

A recent systematic review demonstrated that although the evidence still is quite limited, Hatha yoga, offered two to five times a week for 45 to 60 minutes and including postures, breathing exercises and relaxation can be a useful add-on treatment to reduce general psychopathology and positive and negative symptoms (Vancampfort et al., 2012d). In the same way, improvements in quality of life are observed following Hatha yoga in antipsychotic-stabilized patients with schizophrenia. Yoga as offered by physiotherapists should be made available, especially since patients pay for and probably experience fewer benefits with community-setting yoga classes. A reason might be that general yoga practitioners lack education on the physical and mental health barriers with which patients are confronted.

The Importance of Progressive Muscle Relation

There is compelling epidemiological evidence that psychological distress and associated anxiety are important environmental risk factors, especially in the case of cumulative exposure (van Winkel et al., 2008). People with schizophrenia experience difficulties in coping with psychological distress and anxiety, and possess a relatively limited repertoire of coping strategies. It is therefore not surprising that a better functional outcome might be achieved when psychological distress and anxiety are recognized and treated (Kern et al., 2009). The method of Bernstein and Borkovec

(1973) can be a useful add-on treatment to reduce state anxiety and psychological distress, and improve subjective well-being in people with schizophrenia (Vancampfort et al., 2013b). Nevertheless, if progressive muscle relaxation is to be used as a first-line, stepped physiotherapy care for reducing psychological stress and anxiety, we need to know the dose response and at what point other treatments should be included.

The Evidence for Basic Body Awareness Therapy

Basic Body Awareness Therapy (BBAT) was originally developed as a physiotherapeutic intervention for people with chronic schizophrenia, and the premature research findings indicated improvements in movement function, body image and anxiety (Roxendal, 1985). Recent qualitative research (Hedlund & Gyllensten, 2010; 2013) reported improvements in body balance and postural control, increased self-esteem, and an improved ability to think in people with schizophrenia following physiotherapy based on basic body awareness exercises. However, rigorous research is needed before BBAT can be considered effective in multidisciplinary treatment for people with schizophrenia.

Challenges for Physiotherapists Working With Patients With Schizophrenia

In order to motivate patients with schizophrenia to attend physiotherapy, several barriers need to be addressed. Physiotherapists should, for example, take into account the psychiatric symptoms, physical comorbidities and side-effects of antipsychotic medication (Vancampfort et al., 2012a). Disturbed bodily experiences can cause both bodily delusions and misinterpretation of normal bodily sensations, and also be a barrier for the patient's engagement in physiotherapy. It might be useful to offer safe and structured activities in a supportive environment. Although people with schizophrenia are a heterogeneous group, regardless of illness severity they do have a capacity to respond to both extrinsic and intrinsic goal properties (Vancampfort et al., 2013c). In order to increase adherence to the physiotherapy programme, physiotherapists should support patients' autonomy by offering clear choices, supporting the patients' initiatives, avoiding the use of external rewards, offering relevant information related to the goals of the physiotherapy programme and by using autonomy-supportive language (e.g., 'could' and 'choose' rather than 'should' and 'have to'). Feelings of competence are also attained when patients with schizophrenia experience success while participating. The programme needs to be tailored to the capabilities of the patient and sufficient instructions, practice and positive feedback are needed. Also, relatedness with the physiotherapist and at a later stage with other peers is important. Physiotherapists should therefore show enthusiasm and interest in their patients. When patients feel comfortable enough to participate, offering group sessions could increase the feeling of relatedness and decrease the feeling of being isolated.

How Can Physiotherapists Position Themselves to Be Leaders in the Multidisciplinary Care of People With Schizophrenia?

Physiotherapists have an integral role in the multidisciplinary care of people with schizophrenia. It is important that all physiotherapists are trained in recognizing and adequately addressing symptoms of schizophrenia, physical comorbidities and side-effects of antipsychotic medication. Policy makers should offer means for physiotherapists to acquire the necessary cognitive behavioural and motivational skills (e.g., motivational interviewing techniques) to assist them in delivering high-quality physiotherapy. It is unequivocal that the role of physiotherapists in multidisciplinary treatment should be further promoted. Policy makers should address funding for these necessary physiotherapy service improvements. They should also raise and provide adequate funding for educational campaigns, health assessment tools, and service integration. It remains unclear if mental health and indeed the role of the physiotherapists in the multidisciplinary care of schizophrenia is taught in physiotherapy-qualifying programs across the world. It is likely there are disparities, and the IOPTMH is committed to developing a minimum set standard of education to equip all physiotherapists to work with people with mental illness, including those affected by schizophrenia. The IOPTMH will take the lead in bridging the collaboration gap between physical and mental health care by promoting a policy of coordinated and integrated mental and physical health care, including physiotherapy for all people with

schizophrenia. The integration of physiotherapy in the multidisciplinary treatment of schizophrenia with the ultimate goal of providing optimal treatment of this vulnerable patient population should represent one of the most important tasks for all physiotherapy associations worldwide.

REFERENCES

Abi-Dargham, A., Rodenhiser, J., Printz, D., et al., 2000. Increased baseline occupancy of D2 receptors by dopamine in schizophrenia. Proc. Natl. Acad. Sci. U.S.A. 97 (14), 8104–8109.

American Psychiatric Association, 2013. Diagnostic and Statistical Manual of Mental Disorders, fifth ed. American Psychiatric Association, Washington DC.

Bernstein, D., Borkovec, T., 1973. Progressive Relaxation Training. Research Press, Champaign, Illinois.

Birgenheir, D.G., Ilgen, M.A., Bohnert, A.S., et al., 2013. Pain conditions among veterans with schizophrenia or bipolar disorder. Gen. Hosp. Psychiatry 35 (5), 480–484.

Hedlund, L., Gyllensten, A.L., 2010. The experiences of basic body awareness therapy in patients with schizophrenia. J. Bodyw. Mov. Ther. 14, 245–254.

Hedlund, L., Gyllensten, A.L., 2013. The physiotherapists' experience of Basic Body Awareness Therapy in patients with schizophrenia and schizophrenia spectrum disorders. J. Bodyw. Mov. Ther. 17 (2), 169–176.

Hoang, U., Goldacre, M.J., Stewart, R., 2013. Avoidable mortality in people with schizophrenia or bipolar disorder in England. Acta Psychiatr. Scand. 127 (3), 195–201.

Howes, O.D., Kambeitz, J., Kim, E., et al., 2012. The nature of dopamine dysfunction in schizophrenia and what this means for treatment. Arch. Gen. Psychiatry 69, 776–786.

Kane, J.M., Kishimoto, T., Correll, C.U., 2013. Non-adherence to medication in patients with psychotic disorders: epidemiology, contributing factors and management strategies. World Psychiatry 12 (3), 216–226.

Kern, R.S., Glynn, S.M., Horan, W.P., Marder, S.R., 2009. Psychosocial treatments to promote functional recovery in schizophrenia. Schizophr. Bull. 35, 347–361.

Laursen, T.M., Wahlbeck, K., Hällgren, J., et al., 2013. Life expectancy and death by diseases of the circulatory system in patients with bipolar disorder or schizophrenia in the Nordic countries. PLoS ONE 8 (6), e67133.

Lawrence, D., Hancock, K.J., Kisely, S., 2013. The gap in life expectancy preventable physical illness in psychiatric patients in Western Australia: retrospective analysis of population based registers. Br. Med. J. 346, 2539.

McGrath, J., Saha, S., Chant, D., Welham, J., 2008. Schizophrenia: a concise overview of incidence, prevalence, and mortality. Epidemiol. Rev. 30, 67–76.

Mitchell, A.J., Lawrence, D., 2011. Revascularisation and mortality rates following acute coronary syndromes in people with severe mental illness: comparative meta-analysis. Br. J. Psychiatry 198, 434–441.

Murray, C.J., Vos, T., Lozano, R., et al., 2012. Disability-adjusted life years (DALYs) for 291 diseases and injuries in 21 regions, 1990–2010: a systematic analysis for the Global Burden of Disease Study 2010. Lancet 380 (9859), 2197–2223.

Nielsen, R.E., Uggerby, A.S., Jensen, S.O., McGrath, J.J., 2013. Increasing mortality gap for patients diagnosed with schizophrenia over the last three decades—a Danish nationwide study from 1980 to 2010. Schizophr. Res. 146, 22–27.

Parnas, J., Moller, P., Kircher, T., et al., 2005. EASE: examination of anomalous self-experience. Psychopathology 38 (5), 236–358.

Priebe, S., Rohricht, F., 2001. Specific body image pathology in acute schizophrenia. Psychiatry Res. 101 (3), 289–301.

Rössler, W., Salize, H.J., van Os, J., Riecher-Rössler, A., 2005. Size of burden of schizophrenia and psychotic disorders. Eur. Neuropsychopharmacol. 15 (4), 399–409.

Roxendal, G., 1985. Body Awareness Therapy and the Body Awareness Scale, Treatment and Evaluation in Psychiatric Physiotherapy. Kompendietryckeriet, Kallerud.

Soundy, A., Stubbs, B., Probst, M., et al., 2014a. Barriers to and facilitators of physical activity among persons with schizophrenia: a survey of physical therapists. Psychiatr. Serv. 65 (5), 693–696.

Stubbs, B., De Hert, M., Sepehry A., et al., 2014e. A meta-analysis of prevalence estimates and moderators of low bone mass in people with schizophrenia. ACTA Psychiatr. Scand. 130 (6), 470–486.

Stubbs, B., Probst, M., Soundy, A., et al., 2014b. Physiotherapists can help implement physical activity programmes in clinical practice. Br. J. Psychiatry 204 (2), 164.

Stubbs, B., Soundy, A., Probst, M., et al., 2014a. Understanding the role of physiotherapists in schizophrenia: an international perspective from members of the International Organisation of Physical Therapists in Mental Health (IOPTMH). J. Ment. Health. 23 (3), 125–129.

Stubbs, B., Soundy, A., Probst, M., et al., 2014c. Meeting the drastic physical health disparity in people with schizophrenia: a leading role for all physiotherapists. Physiotherapy 100 (3), 185–186.

Stubbs, B., Soundy, A., Probst, M., et al., 2014d. The assessment, benefits and delivery of physical activity in people with schizophrenia: a survey of members of the International Organisation of Physical Therapists in Mental Health (IOPTMH). Physiother. Res. Int. 19 (4), 248–256.

Thornicroft, G., 2011. Physical health disparities and mental illness: the scandal of premature mortality. Br. J. Psychiatry 199, 441–442.

Vancampfort, D., Correll, C.U., Scheewe, T.W., et al., 2013b. Progressive muscle relaxation in persons with schizophrenia: a systematic review of randomized controlled trials. Clin. Rehabil. 27 (4), 291–298.

Vancampfort, D., De Hert, M., Skjaerven, L., et al., 2012c. International Organization of Physical Therapy in Mental Health consensus on physical activity within multidisciplinary rehabilitation programmes for minimising cardio-metabolic risk in patients with schizophrenia. Disabil. Rehabil. 34 (1), 1–12.

Vancampfort, D., De Hert, M., Vansteenkiste, M., et al., 2013c. The importance of self-determined motivation towards physical activity in patients with schizophrenia. Psychiatry Res. 210 (3), 812–818.

Vancampfort, D., Knapen, J., Probst, M., et al., 2012a. A systematic review of correlates of physical activity in patients with schizophrenia. Acta Psychiatr. Scand. 125 (5), 352–362.

Vancampfort, D., Probst, M., De Hert, M., et al., 2014. Neurobiological effects of physical exercise in schizophrenia: a systematic review. Disabil. Rehabil. 36 (21), 1749–1754.

Vancampfort, D., Probst, M., Skjaerven, L., et al., 2012b. Systematic review of the benefits of physical therapy within a multidisciplinary care approach for people with schizophrenia. Phys. Ther. 92 (1), 11–23.

Vancampfort, D., Vansteelandt, K., Scheewe, T.W., et al., 2012d. Yoga in schizophrenia: a systematic review of randomised controlled trials. Acta Psychiatr. Scand. 126 (1), 12–20.

Vancampfort, D., Wampers, M., Mitchell, A.J., et al., 2013a. A meta-analysis of cardio-metabolic abnormalities in drug naïve, first-episode and multi-episode patients with schizophrenia versus general population controls. World Psychiatry 12 (3), 240–250.

van Winkel, R., Stefanis, N.C., Myin-Germeys, I., 2008. Psychosocial stress and psychosis. A review of the neurobiological mechanisms and the evidence for gene-stress interaction. Schizophr. Bull. 34 (6), 1095–1105.

Zhang, J.P., Lencz, T., Malhotra, A.K., 2010. D2 receptor genetic variation and clinical response to antipsychotic drug treatment: a meta-analysis. Am. J. Psychiatry 167 (7), 763–772.

5.2.8 The Need of Embodiment in Patients With Schizophrenia Spectrum Disorders: a Physiotherapeutic Perspective

LENA HEDLUND

SUMMARY

Patients with schizophrenia are suggested to have disturbed self-recognition and show a high incidence of movement disorders. Self-recognition is based on the experience of agency and body ownership, and built on top-down and bottom-up dynamics, linking together body and cognition. To achieve a good and functional movement quality, the patient needs to be in charge of their own body, and to have a good sense of agency and body ownership. An individualized physiotherapeutic treatment with

Basic Body Awareness Therapy, based on the assessment of movement quality, may enhance the patient's embodiment, increase their movement quality, and decrease symptoms such as anxiety, pain and self-disturbances. In the long run, this is also important in enabling a higher level of physical activity and achieving a healthier lifestyle.

KEY POINTS

▪ Patients with schizophrenia have a disturbed self-recognition, a weak, inflexible and vulnerable sense of self.

▪ A disturbed self-recognition leads to symptoms of psychosis and motor disturbances.

▪ Lack of vitality is a common feature which negatively affects the treatment and rehabilitation of schizophrenia.

LEARNING OBJECTIVES

▪ Physiotherapy can be used to increase embodiment and self-recognition in patients with schizophrenia.

▪ Self-recognition is based on the experience of agency, the perception of willed action as one's own, and body ownership, the perception of the body as one's own among other higher cognitive functions, such as intentional binding and the narrative perspective of life.

▪ Multisensory integration and body image are important neurological mechanisms in establishing a good basic level of self-recognition.

EMBODIMENT

Within mental health, physiotherapists contribute to knowledge about body and mind interaction, body movement, physical activity and its contribution to health, well-being and quality of life. One basic mission is to enhance embodiment. The process of embodiment makes the body and soul inseparable; the body becomes mine and the 'me' is anchored in the body. The embodied identity includes experience of living in the body and living in society. Body awareness is a central aspect and is inseparable from identity and self-awareness (or self-recognition); it is expressed in movement quality (Skjaerven et al., 2008, 2010; Bullington, 2009; Gyllensten et al., 2010; Hedlund & Gyllensten, 2013). Patients with different kinds of mental disturbance often have difficulties with embodiment.

Schizophrenia spectrum disorders include diagnoses that share some similarities, such as symptoms of delusion and hallucinations. The main symptom of delusion often includes a disturbed self-recognition and body image. It also affects sensory motor function and body language. Recently, research has focused on the normal self-experience and the self-disturbances connected to psychosis and schizophrenia, also known as *first-rank symptoms* or *basic symptoms*. The research is expanding fast, owing to newer phenomenological research, better brain imaging techniques and innovative experimental designs (Botvinick & Cohen, 1998; Ehrsson, 2007; Lenggenhager et al., 2007; Petkova & Ehrsson, 2008; Waters & Badcock, 2010; Chiong, 2011; Hirjak et al., 2013).

SELF-RECOGNITION, BODY OWNERSHIP AND AGENCY

Patients with schizophrenia are stipulated to have a minimal self, or *ipseity*, that is weak, inflexible and vulnerable, and leads to a diminished or, in opposite, an exaggerated sense of self (Sass & Parnas, 2003; Thakkar et al., 2011; Ferrari et al., 2012; Nelson et al., 2012; Postmes et al., 2014). Human self-recognition is proposed to be reliant on several mechanisms, basically on body ownership and on agency, and on more social and psychological dimensions including the narrative perspective (Lysaker et al., 2007; Waters & Badcock, 2010). Body ownership, the perception of the body as one's own, includes both body image (our mental representation of our body, its shape, size and unique physiognomy) and body scheme (the sensory motor-generated three-dimensional experiences of the body and its position and localization in the room). Agency is the perception of willed action (such as volitional body movement) as one's own. These dimensions emanate from cognition related to afferent and efferent loops, through a dynamic bottom-up or embodied model (perception affects cognition) and top-down or disembodied model (cognition affects perception) dynamics, and the ability of the nervous system to achieve multisensory integration and intentional binding (Mahon & Caramazza, 2008; Taylor et al., 2010; Waters & Badcock, 2010). Intentional binding is the ability to link together intention with sensory feedback more quickly than it occurs in reality (Waters

& Badcock, 2010). Multisensory integration links together impressions across our senses and is central to adaptive behaviour. It enables us to have a coherent perception of the world and the body. The body scheme and multisensory integration seem to be of great importance; they overlap perceptual incoherence and centre the perception of the body towards the trunk and make our body feel like a unit in relationship to the environment (Serino et al., 2013; Postmes et al., 2014). However, we also must be able to separate ourselves from impressions from the surroundings, and body image appears to be a top-down reference for the self, excluding information that does not fit the image (Longo et al., 2009).

SELF-DISTURBANCE AND MOVEMENT DISORDER

The self-disturbances in patients with schizophrenia lead to difficulties in the basic experience of agency. Patients may compensate for or underestimate the connection between intention and activity owing to a weak ability to adequately anticipate a reaction (Voss et al., 2010). The disturbed experience of agency and vague body ownership lead to difficulties in the basic experience of the body as a unit, and also in self-compassion and vitality (de Haan & Fuchs, 2010; Ferrari et al., 2012). Studies suggest that patients with schizophrenia might have difficulties in making an inner vision of their own body movements, which leads to difficulties in sustaining the feeling of agency (Ferrari et al., 2012). This means that patients with schizophrenia may not experience their body movements with a predicted movement pattern as other people do. To assess the self-disturbance, Parnas et al. (2005) have developed an instrument, EASE (examination of anomalous self-experience), which is used in some psychiatric clinics in Europe.

A disturbed agency may result in different movement disorders through the top-down mechanism. Conversely, different movement disorders may also affect the experience of agency. Movement disorders are a common feature in patients with schizophrenia spectrum disorders. The interest in these phenomena has increased recently because of newer research within neurophysiology and neurobiology, and the fact that it appears in nonmedicated patients and persons at ultrahigh risk (Koning et al., 2011; Mittal et al., 2011; Docx et al., 2012; Walther & Strik, 2012). The movement disorders are regarded as both a sign of difficulties within the neurological function and as an indicator of developmental disturbance and predictor of later psychosocial function, or as a parallel phenomenon, not primarily linked to the disease (Mittal et al., 2011; Docx et al., 2012; Walther & Strik, 2012; Bodén et al., 2013; Hedlund et al., 2016). However, between 66% (unmedicated patients) and 80% (long-term ill and medicated patients) of all patients with schizophrenia spectrum disorders have at least one kind of motor disturbance. In a study by Docx et al. (2012), 35% of 124 patients had catatonia, 43% had problems with coordination, 51% had difficulties with complex motor sequences, 18% had motor speed difficulties and 24% had parkinsonism. Among all the patients, 91% had more than one motor disturbance, 57% had more than two kinds of disturbance, 25% more than three kinds and 7% had all kinds of motor disturbances (Docx et al., 2012). A major problem in research is the lack of clear conceptual boundaries and the overlap between different psychomotor phenomena and motor disturbance. Docx et al. (2012) identified four categories of motor disturbance: catatonia, extrapyramidal signs, psychomotor slowing connected to negative symptoms in schizophrenia, and motoric neurological soft signs, more related to cognitive function in patients with schizophrenia. Walther & Strik (2012) highlight six groups of motor disturbance: involuntary movements, neurological signs, catatonic symptoms, parkinsonism, psychomotor slowing and negative syndrome (including loss of affective experience and expression, as well as disturbances of volition). Regardless of the difficulties with conceptual boundaries and the connection to the schizophrenia etiology, movement disorders lead to difficulties in patient self-recognition, daily life and social activities (Hedlund et al., 2016).

EMBODIMENT, PHYSIOTHERAPY AND PHYSICAL ACTIVITY

Body movement is a complex activity that includes an agent with intention and motivation, multisensory integration, spatial orientation, adjusted force and vitality, among others. To stimulate the process of embodiment is a fundamental goal of physiotherapy in patients with schizophrenia spectrum disorders. Working with embodiment, either through Basic Body Awareness, tai chi chuan or yoga, may increase movement quality and care of the self, and motivate the patient towards a healthier lifestyle by increasing the level of physical activity (Hedlund & Gyllensten, 2010; Visceglia & Lewis, 2011; Ho et al., 2012). These interventions share some similarities: the body movements are performed in a slow and calm way, with a focus on balance, coordination, breathing and mindfulness (Hedlund & Gyllensten, 2010, 2013; Visceglia & Lewis, 2011; Ho et al., 2012).

In the long run, increasing a patient's level of physical activity is important in decreasing the consequences of inactivity and an unhealthy lifestyle (McNamee et al., 2013; Vassilios et al., 2014). Patients with schizophrenia are physically inactive probably for several reasons. In a qualitative study, 49 patients explained why they did not exercise or did not intend to do so in future. The main reasons included various physical health problems (overweight, back problems, unfit, unwell), disinterest and the mental illness itself (amotivation, low mood, anergia, agoraphobias, mind elsewhere) (Vassilios et al., 2014). The high prevalence of movement disorders and difficulties with movement quality hamper physical activity (Docx et al., 2012; Vancampfort et al., 2013; Hedlund et al., 2016). Clinically, many patients report pain, tension, stiffness, exhaustion and lack of well-being after physical activity. The fitness of the body is poor and patients easily become stressed and fatigued, and suffer increased anxiety due to their bad physical condition and malfunction in the hypothalamic–pituitary–adrenal axis (Vancampfort et al., 2013; Cullen et al., 2014; Green et al., 2014; Manzanares et al., 2014; Hedlund et al., 2016). This indicates the need for an individual treatment plan and close follow-up initially, to observe and respond to increased anxiety and other physical reactions, and to adjust the activity level alongside the treatment development. The level of intensity and frequency needed to profit from physical activity is still unknown. However, physical activity may not only increase physical health, studies indicate that it can also affect psychiatric symptomatology, cognition (short-term memory), state anxiety, self-esteem and quality of life. Researchers have reported increased hippocampal volume that correlates with better short-term memory (Vancampfort et al., 2011, 2014; Oertel-Knöchel et al., 2013; Pearsall et al., 2014; Firth et al., 2015). Decreased psychiatric symptomatology has also been reported in studies of yoga and tai chi chuan, along with better interpersonal function and daily living functioning (Bangalore & Varambally, 2012; Ho et al., 2012; Paikkat et al., 2012). Focusing on physical activity and brain health, one study found a correlation between the level of physical inactivity in youth at ultrahigh risk for psychosis and their medial temporal lobe health. The authors suggested that this may be a secondary outcome of prodromal negative symptoms that hinder normal physical activity in youth and thereby affect the normal development of the brain (Mittal et al., 2011). If confirmed in further studies, physical activity may have an even more prominent role in preventing negative brain changes due to schizophrenia.

Assessing Movement Quality and Lack of Vitality

Before introducing the individual treatment plan, the physiotherapist needs to assess movement quality, body image and other important aspects, for example, the patient's experience of the body and the treatment goals (Hedlund & Gyllensten, 2013). Movement quality and capacity offer a starting point for treatment, where both the difficulties (as in movement disorders) and resources are noted (Skjaerven et al., 2008, 2010, Vancampfort et al., 2013; Hedlund et al., 2016). The assessment gives the physiotherapist relevant information to communicate with the patient and other professionals concerning needs and the treatment goal (Hedlund & Gyllensten, 2013). One important aspect of movement quality is the experienced alertness, strength or vitality. When it comes to body movement and treatments, patients with schizophrenia often lack vitality, which is described as negative symptoms or fatigue (Harrington, 2012; Targum et al., 2012; Hedlund et al., 2014). To assess fatigue, the Multidimensional Fatigue Inventory (MFI-20) can be used (Hedlund et al., 2014). This self-questionnaire discriminates five dimensions of fatigue: general, mental and physical fatigue, as well as reduced motivation and activity. There are several causes for a lack of vitality: depression, anxiety, insomnia, negative symptoms and an unhealthy lifestyle. Increased levels of fatigue need to be clinically highlighted and followed up (Targum et al., 2012; Hedlund et al., 2014).

Body Awareness Movement Quality and Experience (BAS MQ-E) is a scientific and clinically developed assessment. The assessment consists of three parts: a movement test where the physiotherapist moves together with the patient, giving both verbal and non-verbal instructions; a questionnaire about body experiences, symptoms and coping strategies; and finally, a qualitative interview focusing on the experiences of the body and movement in the here and now. For patients with schizophrenia spectrum disorder, the movement scale has shown satisfactory interrater reliability. A study of the concurrent validity of both the movement scale and the questionnaire showed a correlation with neurological soft sign (NES-13), fatigue (MFI-20), anxiety (STAI), the experience of control (mastery) and alexithymia (TAS-20) (Hedlund et al., 2016). Difficulties in movement quality, as in movement disorders, have been shown to be in general much greater in persons with schizophrenia when compared with persons with other diagnoses within the schizophrenia spectrum disorders and bipolar disorder. In particular, the BAS MQ-E scale for coordination and breathing showed considerable severity in patients with schizophrenia (Hedlund et al., 2016).

Strengthening Embodiment in Patients With Schizophrenia

To achieve better embodiment in patients with schizophrenia spectrum, physical therapy in general can be used, as long as it stimulates multisensory integration, body ownership and agency. BBAT was developed to enhance body awareness and embodied identity. Physiotherapists often offer BBAT for addressing different kinds of movement disorder, pain, anxiety, lack of vitality and self-disturbances in persons with severe mental illness (Hedlund & Gyllensten, 2013). In BBAT, the physiotherapist encourages the patient to move in ways that are optimal for postural control, balance, free breathing, coordination and awareness. The experience of BBAT has been studied in patients with schizophrenia spectrum disorders. Roxendal (1985) showed in a small controlled study that after 6 months of treatment with BBAT, patients had increased movability, less anxiety, better eye contact, and increased interest in sexuality and social interaction. The patients

($n = 20$) had fewer pharmacological side effects and were less worried about target problems. In two qualitative studies, patients and physiotherapists reported a similarity in results (Hedlund & Gyllensten, 2010, 2013). The patients and physiotherapists described experiencing improvements in balance, posture, movability, alertness and conscious awareness. Better balance was linked to better self-esteem, and the improved awareness made it possible to reflect on one's own behaviour. The physiotherapists described a change in posture, as the patients became more proud and had better self-integrity. Both patients and physiotherapists described better coping strategies, a better ability to think, with clearer and calmer thoughts, and an increased level of activity, both socially and physically, among the patients. The physiotherapists give rich descriptions of the treatment process and of how they clinically guide patients to improve embodiment and movement. They used curiosity as a motivational force, and there was an important balance to achieve between more difficult and uncomfortable moments and pleasurable moments in the exercise. Both the patients and the physiotherapists believed it was important to overcome the difficulties. The physiotherapists focused on the patients' resources and their belief in the patients' inherent ability to develop (Hedlund & Gyllensten, 2010, 2013).

In summary, physiotherapists can contribute to the multidisciplinary care of patients with schizophrenia spectrum disorders by offering interventions to increase embodiment and improve physical health. It is important to highlight and assess the self-disturbances, movement quality and lack of vitality, and to offer an individualized treatment. BBAT, yoga, tai chi and different forms of more intense physical activity are complementary treatments that can be used to support the unique recovery of patients suffering from schizophrenia spectrum disorders.

REFERENCES

Bangalore, N.G., Varambally, S., 2012. Yoga therapy for schizophrenia. Int. J. Yoga 5 (2), 85–89.

Bodén, R., Abrahamsson, T., Holm, G., Borg, J., 2013. Psychomotor and cognitive deficits as predictors of 5-year outcome in first-episode schizophrenia. Nord. J. Psychiatry 68 (4), 282–288.

Botvinick, M., Cohen, J., 1998. Rubber hands "feel" touch that eyes see. Nature 391, 756.

Bullington, J., 2009. Embodiment and chronic pain: implications for rehabilitation practice. Health Care Anal. 17, 100–109.

Chiong, W., 2011. The self: from philosophy to cognitive neuroscience. Neurocase 17 (3), 190–200.

Cullen, A.E., Zunszain, P.A., Dickson, H., et al., 2014. Cortisol awakening response and diurnal cortisol among children at elevated risk for schizophrenia: relationship to psychosocial stress and cognition. Psychoneuroendocrinology 46, 1–13.

de Haan, S., Fuchs, T., 2010. The ghost in the machine: disembodiment in schizophrenia – two case studies. Psychopathology 43, 327–333.

Docx, L., Morrens, M., Bervoets, C., et al., 2012. Parsing the components of the psychomotor syndrome in schizophrenia. Acta Psychiatr. Scand. 12, 1–10.

Ehrsson, H.H., 2007. The experimental induction of out-of-body experiences. Science 317, 1048.

Ferrari, F., Frassinetti, F., Mastrangelo, F., et al., 2012. Bodily self and schizophrenia: the loss of implicit self-body knowledge. Conscious. Cogn. 21, 1365–1374.

Firth, J., Cotter, J., Elliot, R., et al., 2015. A systematic review and meta-analysis of exercise interventions in schizophrenia patients. Psychol. Med. 45, 1343–1346.

Green, M.J., Girshkin, L., Teroganova, N., Quidé, Y., 2014. Stress, schizophrenia and bipolar disorder. Current Topic Behav. Neurosci. 18, 217–235.

Gyllensten, A.L., Skär, L., Miller, M., Gard, G., 2010. Embodied identity – A deeper understanding of body awareness. Physiother. Theory Pract. 26 (7), 439–446.

Harrington, M., 2012. Neurobiological studies of fatigue. Prog. Neurobiol. 2, 93–105.

Hedlund, L., Gyllensten, A.L., 2010. The experience of basic body awareness therapy in patients with schizophrenia. J. Bodyw. Mov. Ther. 14, 245–254.

Hedlund, L., Gyllensten, A.L., 2013. The physiotherapist's experience of basic body awareness therapy in patients with schizophrenia and schizophrenia spectrum disorders. J. Bodyw. Mov. Ther. 17, 169–176.

Hedlund, L., Gyllensten, A.L., Hansson, L., 2014. A psychometric study of the multidimensional fatigue inventory to assess fatigue in patients with schizophrenia and schizophrenia disorders. Comm. Ment. Health J. 51 (3), 377–382.

Hedlund, L., Gyllensten, A.L., Waldegren, T., Hansson, L., 2016. Assessing movement quality in persons with severe mental illness – Reliability and validity of the Body Awareness Scale Movement Quality and Experience. Physiother. Theory Pract. 32 (4), 296–306.

Hirjak, D., Breyer, T., Thomann, T.B., Fuchs, T., 2013. Disturbance of intentionality: a phenomenological study of body-affecting first-rank symptoms in schizophrenia. PLoS ONE 8 (9), e73662.

Ho, R.T.H., Yeung, F.S.W.A., Lo, K.Y., et al., 2012. Tai-chi for residential patients with schizophrenia on movement coordination, negative symptoms, and functioning: a randomized controlled trial. Evid. Based Complement. Alternat. Med. 2012, 1–10.

Koning, J.P., Kahn, R.S., Tenback, D.E., et al., 2011. Movement disorders in nonpsychotic siblings of patients with nonaffective psychosis. Psychiatry Res. 188 (1), 133–137.

Lenggenhager, B., Tadi, T., Metzinger, T., Blanke, O., 2007. Video ergo sum: manipulating bodily self-consciousness. Science 317 (5841), 1096–1099.

Longo, M., Schüür, F., Krammers, M.P.M., et al., 2009. Self-awareness and the body image. Acta Psychol. (Amst.) 132, 166–172.

Lysaker, P.H., Buck, K.D., Roe, D., 2007. Psychotherapy and recovery in schizophrenia: a proposal of key elements for an integrative psychotherapy attuned to narrative in schizophrenia. Psychol. Serv. 4, 28–37.

Mahon, B.Z., Caramazza, A., 2008. A critical look at the embodied cognition hypothesis and a new proposal for grounding conceptual content. J. Physiol. Paris 102, 59–70.

Manzanares, N., Montseny, R., Montalvo, I., et al., 2014. Unhealthy lifestyle in early psychoses: the role of life stress and the hypothalamic-pituitary-adrenal axis. Psychoneuroendocrinology 39, 1–10.

McNamee, L., Mead, G., MacGillivray, S., Lawrie, S., 2013. Schizophrenia, poor physical health and physical activity: evidence-based interventions are required to reduce major health inequalities. Br. J. Psychiatry 203, 239–241.

Mittal, V., Jalbrzikowski, M., Daley, M., et al., 2011. Abnormal movements are associated with poor psychosocial function in adolescents at high risk for psychosis. Schizophr. Res. 130, 164–169.

Nelson, B., Thompson, A., Yung, A.R., 2012. Basic self-disturbance predicts psychosis onset in the ultra-high risk for psychosis "prodromal" population. Schizophr. Bull. 38 (6), 1277–1287.

Oertel-Knöchel, V., Mehler, P., Thiel, C., et al., 2013. Effects of aerobic exercise on cognitive performance and individual psychopathology in depressive and schizophrenia patients. Eur. Arch. Psychiatry Clin. Neurosci. 264 (7), 589–604.

Paikkat, B., Singh, A.R., Singh, P.K., Jahan, M., 2012. Efficacy of yoga therapy on subject well-being and basic living skills of patients having chronic schizophrenia. Ind. Psychiatry J. 21 (2), 109–114.

Parnas, J., Møller, P., Kircher, T., et al., 2005. EASE: examination of anomalous self-experience. Psychopathology 38, 236–258. doi:10.1159/000088441.

Pearsall, R., Smith, D.J., Pelosi, A., Geddes, J., 2014. Exercise therapy in adults with serious mental illness: a systematic review and meta-analysis. BMC Psychiatry 14, 117. doi:10.1186/1471-244X-14-117.

Petkova, V.I., Ehrsson, H.H., 2008. If I were you: perceptual illusion of body swapping. PLoS ONE 3 (12), e3832.

Postmes, L., Sno, H.N., Goedhart, S., et al., 2014. Schizophrenia as a self-disorder due to perceptual incoherence. Schizophr. Res. 152, 41–50.

Roxendal, G., 1985. Body awareness therapy and the body awareness scale, treatment and evaluation in psychiatric physiotherapy. Thesis, Gothenburg.

Sass, A., Parnas, J., 2003. Schizophrenia, consciousness, and the self. Schizophr. Bull. 29 (3), 427–444.

Serino, A., Al Smith, A., Costantini, M., et al., 2013. Bodily ownership and self-location: components of bodily self-consciousness. Conscious. Cogn. 22, 1239–1252.

Skjaerven, L., Kristoffersen, K., Gard, G., 2008. An eye for movement quality: a phenomenological study of movement quality reflecting a group of physiotherapists' understanding of the phenomenon. Physiother. Theory Pract. 24 (1), 13–27.

Skjaerven, L., Kristoffersen, K., Gard, G., 2010. How can movement quality be promoted in clinical practice? A phenomenological study of physical therapist experts. Phys. Ther. 90 (10), 1479–1492.

Targum, S., Hassman, H., Pinho, M., Fava, M., 2012. Development of a clinical impression scale for fatigue. J. Psychiatr. Res. 46, 370–374.

Taylor, A.G., Goehler, L.E., Galper, D.I., et al., 2010. Top-down and bottom-up mechanisms in mind-body medicine: development of an integrative framework for psychophysiological research. Explorer (Hayward) 6, 29–41.

Thakkar, K., Nichols, H., McIntosh, L., Park, S., 2011. Disturbances in body ownership in schizophrenia: evidence from the rubber hand illusion and case study of a spontaneous out-of-body experience. PLoS ONE 6 (10), e27089.

Vancampfort, D., Probst, M., De Hert, M., et al., 2014. Neurobiological effects of physical exercise in schizophrenia: a systematic review. Disabil. Rehabil. 36 (21), 1749–1754.

Vancampfort, D., Probst, M., Scheewe, T., et al., 2013. Relationship between physical fitness, physical activity, smoking and metabolic and mental health parameters in people with schizophrenia. Psychiatry Res. 207, 25–32.

Vancampfort, D., Probst, M., Skjaerven, L.H., et al., 2011. Systematic review of the benefits of physical therapy within a multidisciplinary care approach for people with schizophrenia. Phys. Ther. 92, 11–23.

Vassilios, B., Judd, F., Pattison, P., 2014. Why don't people diagnosed with schizophrenia spectrum disorders (SSDs) get enough exercise? Australas. Psychiatry 22 (1), 71–77.

Visceglia, E., Lewis, S., 2011. Yoga therapy as an adjunctive treatment for schizophrenia: a randomized, controlled pilot study. J. Altern. Complement. Med. 17, 601–607.

Voss, M., Moore, J., Hauser, M., et al., 2010. Altered awareness of action in schizophrenia: a specific deficit in predicting action consequences. Brain 133, 3104–3112.

Walther, S., Strik, W., 2012. Motor symptoms and schizophrenia. Neuropsychobiology 66, 77–92.

Waters, F., Badcock, J., 2010. First-rank symptoms in schizophrenia: reexamining mechanisms of self-recognition. Schizophr. Bull. 36, 510–517.

5.2.9   Physiotherapy for People With Bipolar Disorder: a Systematic Review

DAVY VANCAMPFORT ■ JAN KNAPEN ■ BRENDON STUBBS

SUMMARY

To date, there exists no systematic review of physical therapy in people with bipolar disorders. The question of whether physical therapy interventions are effective in the multidisciplinary management of bipolar disorder therefore remains unclear. The purpose of this chapter is to systematically evaluate the type and effectiveness of physical therapy in the treatment of people with bipolar disorder. Our comprehensive search only identified two studies. The absence of basic or applied physical therapy studies for bipolar disorder is surprising given that physical therapy is recommended as an essential treatment for improving physical and mental health outcomes of other psychiatric populations. The current review indicates that there is preliminary evidence for physical activity in reducing stress, anxiety and depression. Additionally, yoga demonstrates promise, although this study had limitations. In order to avoid adverse events and meet the individual needs, yoga and other physical activities should be provided by specialized healthcare professionals such as physical therapists. Physical therapists should provide persons with bipolar disorder with choices and options about both the type and content of their physical therapy programme.

KEY POINTS

■ The role of physical therapy is still in its infancy in the multidisciplinary treatment of bipolar disorder.

■ There is preliminary evidence for physical activity in reducing stress, anxiety and depression.

LEARNING OBJECTIVES

■ Be able to discuss the evidence for physical therapy in people with bipolar disorder.

■ Understand why physical activity should be prescribed by physical therapists.

INTRODUCTION

Bipolar disorder refers to a group of affective disorders in which an individual experiences episodes of depression, characterized by low mood and related symptoms (e.g., loss of pleasure and reduced energy), and episodes of mania, characterized by either elated or irritable mood, or both. In addition, individuals often experience related symptoms such as increased energy and a reduced need for sleep (American Psychiatric Association, 2013). Bipolar disorder is associated with high physical morbidity, mortality and risk of suicide (Carney & Jones, 2006; Novick et al., 2010). People with bipolar disorder on average die 10–20 years earlier than the general population (Laursen et al., 2013).

There is strong evidence that the excess mortality in bipolar disorder is directly related to the increased rates of cardiovascular disease observed in this population (Goldstein et al., 2009; Prieto et al., 2014). Underlying reasons for the development of cardiovascular diseases in patients with bipolar disorder are complex and multifactorial, but include genetic factors (Ellingrod et al., 2012), cardiometabolic side effects of antipsychotic treatment (Vancampfort et al., 2013a) and an unhealthy lifestyle (Cerimele & Katon, 2013). Potentially modifiable unhealthy lifestyle factors include a sedentary lifestyle (Janney et al., 2014), higher prevalence of smoking and high rates of substance abuse (Waxmonsky et al., 2005). To compound this, patients with bipolar disorder have limited access to general somatic health care (Mitchell et al., 2009; De Hert et al., 2011).

In the general population (Naci & Ioannadis, 2013) and also in other serious mental illnesses (e.g., schizophrenia; Rosenbaum et al., 2014), physical activity interventions have been demonstrated to reduce the burden of cardiovascular disease. Physical therapists are well equipped to lead the delivery of physical activity interventions in people with mental illness (Stubbs et al., 2014a) and are effective in improving cardiometabolic health and outcomes in people with schizophrenia (Vancampfort et al., 2012). Despite the additive burden of cardiovascular disease in people with bipolar disorder and other physical comorbidities (e.g., pain; Stubbs et al., 2014b), little is known about physical therapy interventions for this population. With the increasing recognition that pharmacological interventions for bipolar disorder, at best, have modest effects (Geddes & Miklowitz, 2013), there is increasing recognition for the need to deliver alternatives/adjuncts to improve the physical health and well-being of this group.

To the best of the authors' knowledge, no systematic review on physical therapy in people with bipolar disorders is currently available. The question whether physical therapy interventions are effective in the multidisciplinary management of bipolar disorder is unclear. Thus, the purpose of this systematic review is to evaluate the type and effectiveness of physical therapy in the treatment of people with bipolar disorder.

METHODS

Data Searches and Sources

A literature search was conducted according to the search strategy of Dickersin et al. (1994). No restrictions were made regarding the language of publication. PubMed, CINAHL and PEDro were searched for relevant studies from their inception until October 1, 2014. Medical subject headings included 'bipolar disorder' AND 'physical therapy' OR 'physiotherapy' OR 'exercise' OR 'physical activity' OR 'relaxation' OR 'body awareness therapy' in the title, abstract or index term fields. Titles of the publications found in the databases were screened for appropriateness, and, if available, the abstract of the publication as well. If the investigator felt that any published article potentially met the inclusion criteria, or if there was inadequate information to make a decision, a copy of the article was obtained or authors were contacted to obtain from them the necessary data. The next phase of the search strategy involved searching for unpublished intervention studies potentially overlooked or absent from the databases. This involved hand searching the references of all retrieved articles and the available systematic reviews for potential studies in order to locate (un)published research. Reviews were excluded as search results.

Participants

Inclusion in this review was restricted to intervention studies in patients with a diagnosis of bipolar disorder using any criteria, with any length of illness and in any treatment setting. We did not exclude trials due to age, nationality or gender of participants.

Types of Physical Therapy Interventions

Studies were considered eligible for inclusion if they were studies investigating physical therapy interventions. The physical therapy interventions could comprise either aerobic and strength exercises, relaxation training and/or basic body awareness exercises, which are in accordance with the World Confederation for Physical Therapy Position Statement (WCPT, 2007). A physical therapy intervention could be used alone or in conjunction with others, where physical therapy was considered to be the main or active element. Interventions which included physical therapy in a multiple-component weight-management programme were excluded because the specific effects of the physical therapy intervention could not be addressed. Other cointerventions could include any other of the following treatments: pharmacotherapy or psychoeducation and/or cognitive–behavioural and/or motivational techniques related to exercise behaviour.

Types of Outcomes

Outcomes were grouped according to assessments of mental health and physical health outcomes.

RESULTS

Study Selection

The initial electronic database search resulted in a total of 329 articles. Through an additional hand search of reference lists and after consulting websites and experts in the field, no potentially eligible articles were identified. After removal of duplicates and screening of titles/abstracts and full texts, two studies were included (Fig. 1) (Ng et al., 2007; Uebelacker et al., 2014). Reasons for exclusion are shown in Fig. 1.

Details of Intervention Studies

Ng et al. (2007) used a controlled clinical trial investigating a walking intervention over 24 weeks and compared this to standard care. Uebelacker et al. (2014) conducted an online evaluation study on the

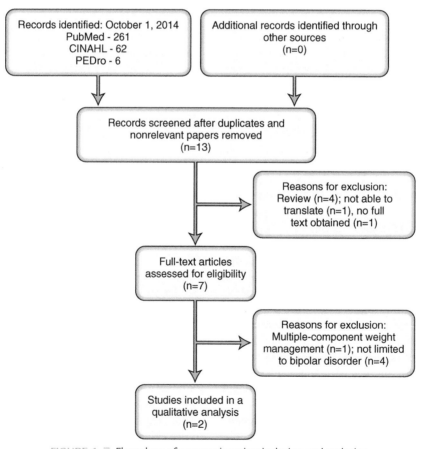

FIGURE 1 ■ Flow chart of systematic review inclusion and exclusion

self-reported health outcomes from engaging in yoga among practitioners with bipolar disorder. Further details of the studies are presented in Table 1.

Participants

In total, 135 people with bipolar disorder were included in the analyses. Ng et al. (2007) recruited only in inpatients, while Uebelacker et al. (2014) recruited outpatients only. In both studies, the majority of the included participants were female (See Table 1 for further demographical information).

Mental Health Outcomes

As reported in Table 1, adding a 24-week walking programme (40 min on weekdays) to standard care results in less anxiety, depression and stress. Also, those practising yoga report reductions in anxiety. Next to this, yoga has beneficial cognitive effects (e.g., distraction).

Physical Health Outcomes

Practicing yoga may result in a small amount of weight loss (Table 1).

Adverse Outcomes

While no adverse outcomes were reported for physical activity, some who practised yoga reported injuries, pain, agitation or lethargy (Table 1).

DISCUSSION

General Findings

Despite the increased recognition over the past decade that bipolar disorder imposes a tremendous health burden due in part to the substantial risk for cardiovascular diseases (Goldstein et al., 2009; Prieto et al., 2014), physical therapy interventions designed to address these physical health disparities are distinctly lacking. Our comprehensive search only identified two studies (Ng et al., 2007; Uebelacker et al., 2014). The absence of basic or applied physical therapy studies for bipolar disorder is surprising given that physical therapy is recommended as an essential treatment for improving physical and mental health outcomes of other psychiatric populations (Knapen et al., 2015; Stubbs et al., 2014).

Clinical Considerations

Bipolar disorder engenders unique characteristics that make adapted physical therapy interventions important for this group. For example, a recent review on physical activity correlates in people with bipolar disorder (Vancampfort et al., 2013b) established that lower self-efficacy, presence of medical comorbidity, lower educational status and social isolation were all important variables that need to be considered when developing physical activity interventions. Less consistent variables associated with lower physical activity participation included higher BMI older age, financial strains, not being connected to a healthcare service and minority ethnicity. Although medical health status is not always amenable to improvement, it could be argued that improved treatment of the increased risk for comorbid medical conditions in patients with bipolar disorder (Vancampfort et al., 2013b) may result in improvements in physical activity patterns. From a personalized care perspective, physical activity interventions need to take into account the limitations these medical comorbidities may place on the intensity of physical activity that patients with bipolar disorder can engage in without physical symptoms.

As indicated in our review, also some yoga exercises might result in pain. Physical therapists should therefore consider in particular the high risk for somatic pain. A recent meta-analysis (Stubbs et al., 2015) demonstrated that the prevalence of pain in people with bipolar disorder was 28.9%, which is over double compared with members of the general population. In terms of specific types of pain, the pooled prevalence of chronic pain was high, with almost one in four (23.7%) being affected. It is therefore imperative that this population receives adequate pain assessment and management, especially because untreated pain can reduce compliance with medication and physical activity, and may consequently have a deleterious impact on the individuals' mental health (Stubbs et al., 2015). We advocate that systematic assessment of pain should be undertaken as part of the management of bipolar disorder by physical therapists. Pain should also be monitored during the course of treatment. Physical therapists are established specialists in the nonpharmacological management of pain in

TABLE 1
Details of the Included Studies

First Author	Participants	Design	Intervention	Duration	Frequency	Intensity	Relevant Instruments	Relevant Outcomes
Ng, 2007	14 (8♀) participants (43.6±15 years) and 35 (26♀) nonparticipants (43.9±18.5 years), all inpatients, ICD-10 bipolar disorder	Clinical controlled trial	Walking additional to standard care	24 weeks	5× week, 40 min	On even terrain	CGI-S CGI-S DASS	Significant lower post-DASS depression (7.2±7.3 vs. 13.7±12.8, p=.048), DASS anxiety (6.6±4.5 vs. 13.8±8.9, p=.002) and DASS stress (9.2±7.2 vs. 17.1±11.6, p=.01) scores
Uebelacker, 2014	86 (75♀) with nonstandardized bipolar disorder (33±12 years), community-based patients	Qualitative study	Yoga	Not mentioned	In class: 1.9±1.9× week; At home 3.3±2.6× week	Not mentioned	/	Participants responded most commonly with positive emotional effects, particularly reduced anxiety, positive cognitive effects (e.g., acceptance, focus, or 'a break from my thoughts') or positive physical effects (e.g., weight loss, increased energy). Some respondents considered yoga to be significantly life changing. The most common negative effect of yoga was physical injury or pain. Five respondents gave examples of specific instances or a yoga practice that they believed increased agitation or manic symptoms; five respondents gave examples of times that yoga increased depression or lethargy.

DASS, Depression Anxiety Stress Scales; *CGI-S*, Clinical Global Impression Severity and; *CGI-I*, Improvement scales; *ICD*, International Classification of Diseases.

nonmental health settings, and can effectively use tailored exercise and other interventions to manage pain. With the increasing recognition of the importance of identifying and managing pain, physical therapists can take a clinical lead.

Our review data also demonstrate that yoga should be considered as a potential option. Physical therapists should therefore provide persons with bipolar disorder with choices and options about both type and content of their physical therapy programme. For example, the physical therapist should assess what type of exercise (e.g., yoga or aerobic exercise) would best fit a person's preference. Insurance coverage should be made available, especially because people with severe mental illness pay for and probably experience fewer benefits or, as mentioned in the current review, might have negative experiences with community-setting yoga classes. A reason might be that general yoga practitioners lack education on physical and mental health barriers with which patients are confronted. In 2005, more than 20% of psychiatric patients in the USA were reported to follow complementary therapies such as yoga, although this was not discussed with their psychiatrist (Elkins et al., 2005).

CONCLUSIONS

Despite increased recognition that bipolar disorder imposes a tremendous health burden, evidence for physical therapy interventions still is limited. The current review indicates that there is preliminary evidence for physical activity in reducing stress, anxiety and depression. In addition, yoga demonstrates promise, although this study had limitations. In order to avoid adverse events and meet the individual needs, yoga and other physical activities should be provided by specialized healthcare professionals such as physical therapists. Physical therapists should provide people with bipolar disorder with choices and options about both the type and content of their physical therapy programme.

REFERENCES

American Psychiatric Association, 2013. Diagnostic and Statistical Manual of Mental Disorders, fifth ed. American Psychiatric Association, Washington DC.

Carney, C.P., Jones, L.E., 2006. Medical comorbidity in women and men with bipolar disorders: a population-based controlled study. Psychosom. Med. 68, 684–691. doi:10.1111/j.1525-1497.2006.00563.x.

Cerimele, J.M., Katon, W.J., 2013. Associations between health risk behaviors and symptoms of schizophrenia and bipolar disorder: a systematic review. Gen. Hosp. Psychiatry 35 (1), 16–22. doi:10.1016/j.genhosppsych.2012.08.001.

De Hert, M., Correll, C.U., Bobes, J., et al., 2011. Physical illness in patients with severe mental disorders, I: prevalence, impact of medications and disparities in health care. World Psychiatry 10, 52–77.

Dickersin, K., Scherer, R., Lefebvre, C., 1994. Identifying relevant studies for systematic reviews. Br. Med. J. 309, 1286–1291. doi: <http://dx.doi.org/10.1136/bmj.309.6964.1286.>

Elkins, G., Rajab, M.H., Marcus, J., 2005. Complementary and alternative medicine use by psychiatric inpatients. Psychol. Rep. 96 (1), 163–166.

Ellingrod, V.L., Taylor, S.F., Dalack, G., et al., 2012. Risk factors associated with metabolic syndrome in bipolar and schizophrenia subjects treated with antipsychotics: the role of folate pharmacogenetics. J. Clin. Psychopharmacol. 32 (2), 261–265. doi:10.1097/JCP.0b013e3182485888.

Geddes, J.R., Miklowitz, D.J., 2013. Treatment of bipolar disorder. Lancet 381 (9878), 1672–1682. doi:10.1016/S0140-6736(13)60857-0.

Goldstein, B.I., Fagiolini, A., Houck, P., Kupfer, D.J., 2009. Cardiovascular disease and hypertension among adults with bipolar I disorder in the United States. Bipolar Disord. 11, 657–662. doi:10.1111/j.1399-5618.2009.00735.x.

Janney, C.A., Fagiolini, A., Swartz, H.A., et al., 2014. Are adults with bipolar disorder active? Objectively measured physical activity and sedentary behavior using accelerometry. J. Affect. Disord. 152-154, 498–504. doi:10.1016/j.jad.2013.09.009.

Knapen, J., Vancampfort, D., Moriën, Y., Marchal, Y., 2015. Exercise therapy improves both mental and physical health in patients with major depression. Disabil. Rehabil. 37 (16), 1490–1495.

Laursen, T.M., Wahlbeck, K., Hallgren, J., et al., 2013. Life expectancy and death by diseases of the circulatory system in patients with bipolar disorder or schizophrenia in the Nordic countries. PLoS. One 8, e67133. doi:10.1371/journal.pone.0067133.

Mitchell, A.J., Malone, D., Doebbeling, C.C., 2009. Quality of medical care for people with and without comorbid mental illness and substance misuse: systematic review of comparative studies. Br. J. Psychiatry 194, 491–499. doi:10.1192/bjp.bp.107.045732.

Naci, H., Ioannidis, J.P., 2013. Comparative effectiveness of exercise and drug interventions on mortality outcomes: meta-epidemiological study. Br. Med. J. 347, f5577. doi:10.1136/bmj.f5577.

Ng, F., Dodd, S., Berk, M., 2007. The effects of physical activity in the acute treatment of bipolar disorder: a pilot study. J. Affect. Disord. 101 (1–3), 259–262.

Novick, D.M., Swartz, H.A., Frank, E., 2010. Suicide attempts in bipolar I and bipolar II disorder: a review and meta-analysis of the evidence. Bipolar Disord. 12 (1), 1–9. doi:10.1111/j.1399-5618.2009.00786.x.

Prieto, M.L., Cuéllar-Barboza, A.B., Bobo, W.V., et al., 2014. Risk of myocardial infarction and stroke in bipolar disorder: a systematic review and exploratory meta-analysis. Acta Psychiatr. Scand. doi:10.1111/acps.12293.

Rosenbaum, S., Tiedemann, A., Sherrington, C., et al., 2014. Physical activity interventions for people with mental illness: a systematic review and meta-analysis. J. Clin. Psychiatry. 75 (9), 964–974. doi:10.4088/JCP.13r08765.

Stubbs, B., Eggermont, L., Mitchell, A.J., et al., 2015. The prevalence of pain in bipolar disorder: a systematic review and large-scale meta-analysis. Acta Psychiatr. Scand. 131 (2), 75–88. doi:10.1111/acps.12325.

Stubbs, B., Soundy, A., Probst, M., et al., 2014. Addressing the disparity in physical health provision for people with schizophrenia: an important role for physiotherapists. Physiotherapy 100 (3), 185–186. doi:10.1016/j.physio.2013.11.003.

Uebelacker, L.A., Weinstock, L.M., Kraines, M.A., 2014. Self-reported benefits and risks of yoga in individuals with bipolar disorder. J. Psychiatr. Pract. 20 (5), 345–352. doi:10.1097/01.pra.0000454779.59859.f8.

Vancampfort, D., Correll, C.U., Probst, M., et al., 2013b. A review of physical activity correlates in patients with bipolar disorder. J. Affect. Disord. 145 (3), 285–289. doi:10.1016/j.jad.2012.07.020.

Vancampfort, D., Probst, M., Skjaerven, L., et al., 2012. Systematic review of the benefits of physical therapy within a multidisciplinary care approach for people with schizophrenia. Phys. Ther. 92 (1), 11–23. doi:10.2522/ptj.20110218.

Vancampfort, D., Vansteelandt, K., Correll, C.U., et al., 2013a. Metabolic syndrome and metabolic abnormalities in bipolar disorder: a meta-analysis of prevalence rates and moderators. Am. J. Psychiatry 170 (3), 265–274. doi:10.1176/appi.ajp.2012.12050620.

Waxmonsky, J.A., Thomas, M.R., Miklowitz, D.J., et al., 2005. Prevalence and correlates of tobacco use in bipolar disorder: data from the first 2000 participants in the Systematic Treatment Enhancement Program. Gen. Hosp. Psychiatry 27, 321–328. doi:10.1016/j.comppsych.2005.08.001.

World Confederation for Physical Therapy (WCPT), 2007. WCPT Description of Physical Therapy. WCPT, London, UK.

5.3 PHYSIOTHERAPY FOR CHILDREN AND ADOLESCENTS

5.3.1 Physiotherapy in Mental Health With Children and Adolescents in Belgium

JOHAN SIMONS

SUMMARY

Physiotherapy in mental health with children and adolescents in Belgium is an extensive domain and has evolved over time. After situating the domain, the different diagnostic approaches and the most frequently used instruments in Belgium will be presented. Two major forms of physiotherapy in mental health therapy will be distinguished and evidence-based results of the effects of therapy in mental health will be presented.

KEY POINTS

■ Physiotherapy in mental health for children and adolescents tries to influence the whole personality of the child.

LEARNING OBJECTIVES

■ To gain insight and knowledge of the field of physiotherapy in mental health in children and adolescents.

■ To gain insight and knowledge of different concepts and strategies within assessments and therapies used with children and adolescents.

INTRODUCTION

For this already well-established approach with children and adolescents there are many terms, namely *psychomotricity* (Lefevere, 1976; Vallaey, 1978; Van Dun, 1981; European Forum Psychomotricity, 1996), *movement therapy* (Schipperijn, 1971; Koolen, 1974), *sensorimotor therapy* (Ayres, 1972a; Van Empelen, 1981; Van de Riet, 1985; Netelenbos, 2001), *perceptuomotor training* (Netelenbos, 2001), *psychomotor education* (Picq & Vayer, 1960; Soubiran & Mazo, 1965; Le Boulch, 1971, 1973; Decker, 1972; Defontaine, 1976; Irmischer, 1980; Mertens, 1982; Zimmer, 1982), *psychomotor therapy* (Gantenbein, 1975; Kiphard, 1979; Van Coppenolle & Simons, 1985) and *physiotherapy in mental health* (Probst & Simons, 2014).

Based on all these terms, which may not cover nor address the same content, the meaning of the approach can be confusing (Hendrickx, 1998; Vandroemme, 1998; Van Waelvelde, 1998, 1999; Netelenbos, 2001). The names indicate either a global approach of the field, or a selective approach; either a theoretically founded approach, or a pragmatic one. Besides these differences, this therapy is practised by a large mixture of disciplines, which also makes it more diffuse and difficult to define. In the research of Simons, Dufait and Pyck (1980), it appears that the professionals are located in several settings: the paramedical sector, the educational sector and in both regular and special education. In addition, all levels of educational background are found among these professionals and their training.

The multiplicity in terminology and the mixture of disciplines result in many definitions for this field. An overall definition for the approach is: *physiotherapy in mental health*. This is based on a holistic human view, a vision that starts from the unity between mind and body. It incorporates the cognitive, emotional and motor aspects, as well as the capacity to be and act in a psychosocial context (European Forum Psychomotricity, 1996; Probst & Simons, 2014). To bring some clarity in this labyrinth of terms, we will first discuss the starting points of this approach.

SITUATING THE DOMAIN

First, in the approach of physiotherapy in mental health, the dualistic thinking of Descartes whereby 'the mind and the body' are separated and the mind is superior to the body is gone. In physiotherapy in mental health, the body and mind are in unison and are the basis of being human. The somatic functioning constantly influences mental functioning, and vice versa. Personal functioning is in the centre of physiotherapy in mental health; this means that the treatment is not situated in the purely somatic area, nor is the basic aim to improve the body's shape and/or movement apparatus. In personal functioning, the motor, cognitive and social–affective aspects are always considered to be connected during motor activity (Simons, 2014a). In other words, this approach influences our understanding of the total personality. 'Personality' can be represented graphically as a triangle, thus the mutual relations between the three elements become clear (Fig. 1).

Second, for a child to function in a healthy way while growing up, it is important that this can take place in a stimulating context. It should be mentioned that a balance of all stimuli in the context is necessary for optimal growth. A shortage can be situated in the motor area by a lack of movement space, or movement experience. A lack of structure can influence the cognitive area for positive development. The social–affective

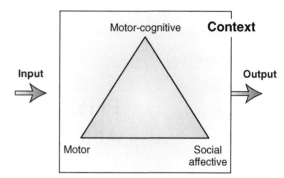

FIGURE 1 ■ Graphic representation of the different elements of the personality in the context.

area can lack the normative expectation for the child of affection and social contacts. For example, motor developmental delays often lead to low self-esteem (Rose et al., 1997), being bullied (Piek et al., 2005), being socially less accepted (Livesey et al., 2011), low self-efficacy (Engel-Yeger & Kasis, 2010), or anxiety disorders and depression (Skinner & Piek, 2001). This may lead to reduced physical activity, resulting in a negative spiral with a further decrease in motor skills, an increased risk of becoming overweight and deterioration of physical and psychosocial health.

Motor behaviour (the output) will always be the result of the information (input) processed by the child. This individual will function within a certain context, which could be their family, school and peers, and this will influence their development. The context is represented by the square in Fig. 1.

Third, identifying problems in the field of motor development is not simple because there is a strong coherence among the different developmental domains.

Adolescents, young adults, adults and the elderly have distinct developmental stages. In order to recognize pathology, a therapist must have knowledge of normal motor development in relationship with the different developmental stages (Fig. 2). They must be aware of what is typical for preschool children, school-age children or adolescents, as well as motor, motor–cognitive and social–affective development.

DIAGNOSTIC APPROACH

Between normal motor development and movement, developmental impairment is a third field: the motor

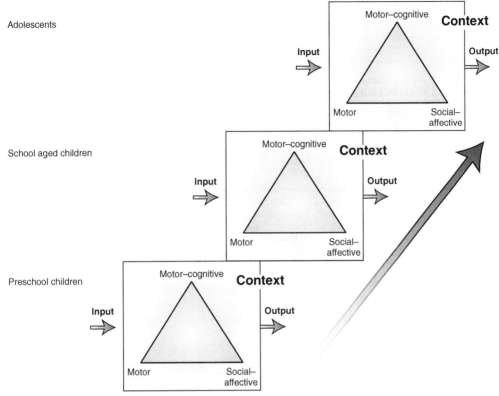

FIGURE 2 ▪ Development related to the development of the individual.

diagnostic field. Within this aspect we continue to focus on the four components: the motor, motor–cognitive and social–affective components and the context.

The mutual linkages among the different aspects mean that the physiotherapist in mental health must have knowledge of normal motor development, the forms of pathological motor expression and the normal pedagogical measures and, of course, knowledge of and skills in diagnostic and therapeutic methods (Simons, 2014a). An extensive list of mostly quantitative diagnostic tools is available to evaluate the motor, motor–cognitive and social–affective aspects and the context. On the other hand, qualitative information is gathered about functioning in groups and in the family (Verscheure & Van Roie, 2014).

Motor

To get an idea of the motor possibilities of the child or adolescent, a distinction can be made among five types

of instrument, in particular: developmental tests, basic motor skills, psychomotor developmental tests and fitness and skills tests.

Developmental Tests

The developmental tests include, among other instruments, the Bayley scales of infant and toddler development (BSITD-III; Bayley, 2005) and Peabody Developmental Motor Scales (PDMS-2; Folio & Fewell, 2000). These tools focus on very young children and are mainly interested in the early movement milestones (Fig. 3).

Basic Motor Skills

In the second group of tests is the Test of Gross Motor Development (TGMD-2; Ulrich & Sanford, 2000) and Clinical Observations of Motor and Postural Skills (COMPS-2; Wilson et al., 2000), situated where the basic motor skills of children over 5 years of age are examined.

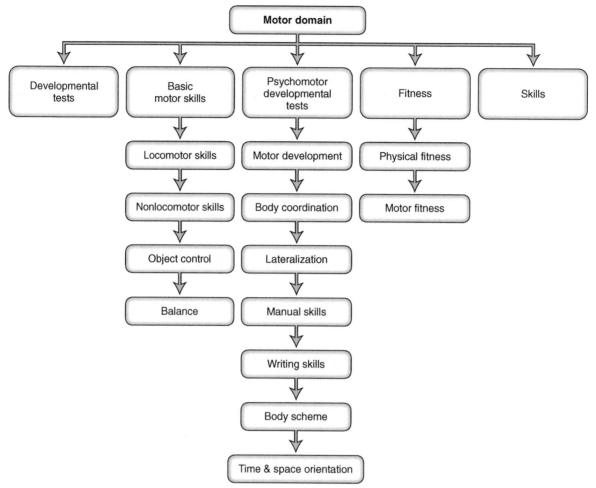

FIGURE 3 ■ Different diagnostic aspects of the motor diagnostic domains.

Perceptual-Motor Development

The third group includes motor tests for the evaluation of perceptual-motor development, such as the Oseretsky test of Motor Proficiency (BOT-2; Bruininks & Bruininks, 2005), the Movement Assessment battery for children (Movement ABC-II-NL; Smits-Engelsman et al., 2010), the Lincoln Oseretsky Test Kurzform 18 (Eggert, 1971), the Motoriktest für Vier – Bis Sechsjährige Kinder (MOT 4–6) (Zimmer & Volkamer, 1984), the Maastricht Motoriek Test (MMT) designed in 2004 by Vles, Kroes and Feron and different checklists including the Checklist Motorischer Verhaltensweisen (CMV) (Schilling, 1976), the DCDDaily Questionnaire (van der Linde et al., 2014), a parental questionnaire to evaluate the activities of daily living of children with developmental coordination disorder and the Motor Observation Questionnaire for Teachers (MOQ-T) (Schoemaker et al., 2008).

Other aspects that could be evaluated are body coordination, on the basis of the Body Coordination Test (KTK-NL; Lenoir et al., 2014), lateralization by means of the Test of Vallaey (Vallaey, 1973) or the Hand Dominanz Test HDT-3 (Steingrüber, 2011), manual skills by means of the Gibson Spiral Maze Test (Gibson, 1965) or the Purdue Pegboard (Tiffin, 1968) and/or the Beery–Buktenica Developmental Test of Visual Motor Integration (Beery & Beery, 2010). A possibility for evaluation of writing skills is the Systematische Opsporing Schrijfproblemen (SOS-2-VL) ([Systematic Detection of Writing Problems]; Van Waelvelde et al., 2014) or the Detailed Assessment of Speed of Handwriting (DASH) (Barnett et al., 2007). To assess the body scheme, the Test Eupreuve de Schema Corporel-Révisée (Meljac et al., 2010), or the Test of Pointing and Naming Body Parts (Simons, 2014b) may be used, and time and space orientation assessed using the test of Piaget–Head (Zazzo et al., 1958).

Fitness and Skills Tests

A fourth group refers to measuring instruments that make it possible to check the physical fitness of young people. Finally, the last group in Fig. 3 refers to the evaluation of certain sports skills, such as the ability to play basketball, football, etc.

Motor-Cognitive

Motor performance not only depends on motor capabilities but is also determined by the extent to which the input is undisturbed, especially when incorporating visual and auditory information. To check this many instruments are available; for example, the Test of Visual Perceptual Skills (TVPS-3; Martin, 2006) and the Developmental Test of Visual Perception (DTVP-2; Hammil et al., 1993). In addition, each individual has a typical motor learning style, which leads to faster or slower acquirement of a certain motor skill. The combination of these two elements will determine the motor learning process.

Social-Affective

This is a very extensive domain, in which various aspects occur, such as self-esteem, body esteem and kinesiophobia, or the fear of motion situations. Many instruments are available to assess these aspects, for example Self-Description Questionnaires I, II and III (SDQ; Marsh, 1990a,b,c), the Physical Self-Description Questionnaire (PSDQ-S; Marsh et al., 2010), and the Bilder Angst test (BAT; Bös & Mechling, 1983).

Additional information on existing measurement instruments in different countries can be found in: *Introductie tot de Psychomotoriek* (Simons, 2014a), the *Manuel Pour l'examen Psychologique de l'enfant* (Zazzo et al., 1958), *Motorische Testverfahren* (Rapp & Schoder, 1977), *Handbuch Motorische Tests* (Bös, 2001),

Movement Skill Assessment (Burton & Miller, 1998), the *Directory of Psychological Tests in Sport and Exercise Sciences* (Ostrow, 1996) and *Adapted Physical Activity, Recreation and Sport: Crossdisciplinary and lifespan* (Sherrill, 2003).

Finally, all instruments used by the professional provide a certain outcome. It requires expertise to analyse the data and subsequently to interpret them. We can obtain as outcome a raw score, a standard score, a quotient, a percentile and an age equivalent. A raw score is the sum of the items and gives little information. Therefore the raw score is usually converted into a standard score. This is a score that reflects the variation of the average of the group, usually equipped with a standard deviation. Examples are the motor quotient (MQ), which has an average of 100 (M = 100) and a standard deviation of 15 (SD = 15). Another example of a standard score is a T-score, having an average of 50 (M = 50) and a standard deviation of 10 (SD = 10). Even simpler and more universal is the use of percentiles (PC). This reflects the number of persons of the same age or class who score lower than the person tested. Therefore a percentile is easy to understand, even by lay people. For example PC = 16 indicates that 16% of the norm group achieves lower than the subject and 84% higher. Percentiles can easily be interpreted with five classes, namely PC 0–2: very weak; PC 3–16: weak; PC 17–84: intermediate; PC 85–97: good; PC 98–100: very good.

However, assessment clearly involves more than doing a test. An important step is the interpretation of the test data. Four parts can be distinguished:

1. The detection of the strengths and weaknesses of an individual. This is done through the checking of the trends between the results of the various tests.
2. The detection of major points of disagreement. This means listing the items and subtests of major differences with respect to children of the same age. Here it is much easier to work with quantitative tests than with process-orientated tests.
3. The detection of clusters. This means the grouping of tests to detect trends and patterns. It is the detection of the factors common to a deficit. The therapist must have knowledge of

the contents of the various tests and the various subtests, and be able to check whether the characteristics found correspond to a particular syndrome or not.

4. The identification of the degree of therapy needed.

Last but not least, abundant evidence has demonstrated an increased risk for various negative outcomes in children who demonstrate poor motor competence, such as social, emotional, physical and academic difficulties (Schoemaker & Kalverboer, 1994; Skinner & Piek, 2001; Dewey et al., 2002; Piek et al., 2008; Rivilis et al., 2011; Missiuna et al., 2014), meaning that a good psychomotor therapist has to keep in mind the holistic starting point of the therapy.

GOALS FOR PSYCHOMOTOR THERAPY

In 2008 psychomotor therapists were interviewed by means of a questionnaire to check the importance of the objectives for psychomotor therapy (Simons, 2014a). Participants were asked to judge 62 objectives on a scale of 1 to 5 points. Score 1 stood for 'the objective is not at all important' and score 5 'this is a very important objective in psychomotor therapy'. The questionnaire was carried out at the Mental Health Care facility in Flanders and had a response rate of 78% (Table 1).

The same procedure was used in a study on psychomotor therapists working in medical pedagogical institutions (Table 2). The response was 79% (Simons, 2014a).

Remarkably, only four objectives appear in both rankings within the first 10 objectives. Psychomotor therapists working in mental health care mentioned more objectives in the socio-affective field. Psychomotor therapists working in medical pedagogical institutions mentioned objectives from the three domains.

THERAPEUTIC APPROACH

As mentioned earlier, physiotherapy in mental health tries to influence the personality in a positive way, starting from movement and bodily experiences.

Two major forms of physiotherapy in mental health can be distinguished: functional training or

TABLE 1

Objectives of Physiotherapy in Services for Children in Mental Health Care

	Objective	Average Score	Standard Deviation
1	Stimulate the Self	4.67	0.55
2	Exercise self-control	4.54	0.64
3	Exercise relaxation (to prevent tension)	4.42	0.64
	Increase self-perception	4.42	0.70
	Increase self-esteem	4.42	0.70
	Stimulate to express themselves adequately emotionally	4.42	0.70
4	Stimulate perseverance	4.33	0.69
5	Stimulate the experience of fun	4.29	0.68
6	Stimulate the feeling of safety	4.25	0.83
	Increase the acceptance of one's own body	4.25	0.92
7	Teach self-responsibility	4.21	0.76
8	Increase trust in others	4.13	0.83
	Increase body contact	4.13	0.88
	Increase insight into own problems	4.13	0.88
	Teach entering relationships	4.13	0.97
9	Advance empathizing with others	4.04	0.79
10	Learning to be open to personal criticism	4.00	0.87

function-training and psychotherapeutic-orientated psychomotor therapy. If an attempt is made to improve the motor aspect of personality (such as coordination, laterality, etc.) or to work on cognitive development through locomotion (for example reading, language and solving mathematic problems) this approach is called *functional training* or *function-training*. If an attempt is made to influence the socio-affective aspect of the personality or the context by movement, it is called *psychotherapeutic-orientated psychomotor therapy* (Fig. 4). The motor domain is employed as a gateway to improve the socio-affective functioning of an individual.

Functional Training

In the past many functional training programmes were developed. They can be broadly categorized into either bottom-up or top-down approaches.

TABLE 2		
Objectives of Physiotherapy for Children in Medical Pedagogical Institutions		
Objective	Average Score	Standard Deviation
1 Improve the body scheme	4.42	0.86
2 Develop eye–hand coordination	4.39	0.76
3 Stimulating the use of sensory stimulation	4.38	0.85
4 Improve orientation in space	4.35	0.74
5 Stimulate self-confidence	4.30	0.88
6 Advance relaxation	4.23	0.88
7 Stimulate active participation in activities	4.20	0.93
8 Alter movement aversion to liking to move	4.12	0.98
9 Increase motivation	4.08	1.04
Increase the experience of fun	4.08	1.07
10 Advance body contact	4.06	0.91
Increase fine motor skills	4.06	0.97

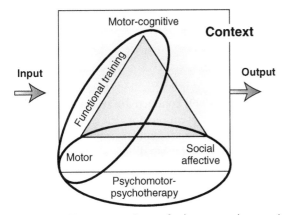

FIGURE 4 ▪ Representation of the two therapeutic approaches.

In the bottom-up approaches, a distinction can be made among different theoretical principles. Some theorists use the neurological basis and others use a basic functional model. Doman and Delacato (Doman et al., 1964) can be situated in the first group. They argue that the phylogeny is repeated in ontogenesis. This means that the development of the human species as an animal species is repeated in the development of the human spinal cord towards the cortex. When there is a deficit in the development of a human, the therapy will have to descend to the level which is not yet fully developed. To remediate, some specific exercises must be performed for each neurological level of development. For example, with damage at the midbrain level, crossed crawl must be taught: head left, lift left arm and right leg; head right, lift right arm and left leg. These authors also have the idea that a defect in brain function can be corrected or that the intact brain cells can take over the function of damaged cells. Doman (1974) suggests stimulating the transport of oxygen to the brain; for example, by hanging the child upside down.

A second group of theorists are those who emphasize basic functions. The perceptual-motor approach (Getman, 1962; Barsch, 1968; Kephart et al., 1971; Frostig, 1974) is situated within this group, as is the approach that focuses on sensory integration (Ayres, 1972b). Common to all these approaches is that they place great importance on motor development as a basis for perceptual development. They tend to explain remediation through activation of higher levels of neurological functioning of the child.

Top-down approaches were developed more recently and they use a problem-solving approach. Task-specific interventions and cognitive strategies are the two most commonly used techniques in this approach. In the task-specific interventions the motor task is broken down into different steps. Each step is trained separately and then reorganized to form the entire task.

Cognitive approaches are based on active problem solving. Most of these strategies involve the Goal, Plan, Do it and Check framework (GPDC; Goal: What am I going to do? Plan: How am I going to accomplish the skill? Do it: Perform the skill; Check: How well did my plan work?). Typical examples here are the self-instruction method of Meichenbaum (1981), the Instrumental Enrichment Program of Feuerstein (1980) (Feuerstein & Rand, 1979) and Cognitive Orientation to Daily Occupational Performance (CO-OP: Polatajka & Mandich, 2004).

Psychotherapeutic-Orientated Psychomotor Therapy

Under the pressure of the increased incidence of psychiatric symptoms, rising healthcare costs and the risk associated with psychotropic drugs and some forms of psychotherapy, a search for holistic, inexpensive and safe treatment methods has started (Dishman, 1986). In the holistic view of exercise and health behaviour, argumentation comes from the psychosomatic point of view. Given this, the potential value of exercise as a cheap and safe treatment for various mental disorders has been proposed. Emphasis is placed on the value of exercise as a prophylactic against physical disorders and to improve social well-being. Most researchers agree that, in both clinical and nonclinical populations, exercise has a positive psychological effect. To achieve this, one can rely on techniques that are inspired by psychotherapeutic methods such as behavioural therapy, systems thinking, psychoanalysis, phenomenology, etc. (Hölter, 1993). How and why exercise improves psychological well-being is still a very lively debate.

Gradually, a number of treatment protocols were developed for children and adolescents. Examples are: Stress management for young people with psychotic disorders (Emck, 1998), a workbook for children who have experienced sexual abuse (Lamers-Winkelman & Bicanic, 2000), Empowerment of Young People (Cautaert et al., 2001), a programme for behaviourally disturbed children (Simons, 2002), a protocol for relaxation training, and aggression training (Sherborne, 1990; Simons, 2000; Simons et al., 2011).

EVIDENCE-BASED RESULTS

There is an amalgam of hypotheses, theories and speculations concerning the impact of physical activity on mental health. Some studies of the therapeutic effects on mental health are presented here.

Functional Training

Research on children with Developmental Coordination Disorder (DCD) gave an effectiveness score (ES) = 1.46 for specific skills training, an ES = 0.71 for general training and an ES = 0.21 for sensory integration training (Pless & Carlsson, 2000), suggesting that specific skills training is highly efficient. Specific skill interventions work on teaching essential activities of daily living, and thereby stimulate participation of the child in school, leisure and sports.

Evidence that cognitive skills can be improved by motor training is, however, very scarce. The most cited study is that of Kavale and Mattson (1983). In this study the results of 180 studies were compared in the ES. Perceptual-motor programmes have an ES = 0.082, reduction of the class size an ES = 0.15, 9 months' reading instruction an ES = 0.67 and medication an ES = 0.85. This shows that functional training had the least favourable result.

Children with learning disabilities commonly show impaired motor proficiency. It has been hypothesized that poor motor performance and/or poor social skills lead to exclusion from games, creating a vicious cycle of decreasing participation, decreasing competence, deterioration of self-worth and increasing social maladjustment. Attempts to break the vicious cycle with programmes designed to enhance motor proficiency have been uniformly unsuccessful. There is limited experimental evidence to support the view that structured physical activity programmes with an embedded social skills training component can be an effective method of enhancing both actual motor ability and self-perception of physical and academic competence (Bluechardt et al., 1995).

Psychotherapeutic-Orientated Psychomotor Therapy

Larun et al. (2009) conducted a systematic review of five exercise interventions for depression in children and adolescents, and found a significant moderate effect (standardized mean difference [SMD] = −0.66), indicating that exercise was reducing the depression.

In their study of depressed children ($n = 9374$), Goodman and Whitaker (2002) concluded that depression is often associated with obesity. They emphasize the importance of movement as preventative treatment for obesity in depressed children. The same trend is found in the research of Rosenblum and Forman (2002) but in children with eating disorders. Physical activity in these children had the advantage of promoting a healthy lifestyle, giving the courage to continue the fight against the disease and was associated with a higher peak bone mass than in children who did not participate in sport.

Ekeland et al. (2009) conducted a systematic review to check the effectiveness of gross motor interventions on improving self-esteem in 1821 children and young people. They found an overall effect of SMD = 0.51, indicating a moderate difference in self-esteem in favour of the intervention. They concluded that, since there are no known negative effects of exercise and many positive effects on physical health, exercise may be an important measure for improving children's self-esteem.

Positive effects of physical activity were also found by Larun et al. (2009) on anxiety (SMD = −048) and depression (SMD = −0.66). Good results were found for the use of relaxation on anxiety (SMD = −0.25) and depression (SMD = −0.31 to −0.58). Less convincing results were found for running and walking as a treatment for anxiety (SMD = −0.13) and in depressed individuals (SMD = −0.10 to −0.31).

Although a number of studies have yielded positive results on the effectiveness of exercise as an adjunct treatment, evidence is limited for most psychiatric disorders. Generally, studies using equal contact control groups revealed smaller effects than studies comparing physical activity with no intervention. This leads to the assumption that nonspecific effects such as therapeutic contact, social support and distraction may drive some of the effects of lower intensity exercise in particular, which is in line with epidemiological findings (Harvey et al., 2010).

However, from the few available longitudinal studies, there is some evidence suggesting that when motor abilities are delayed in early childhood, these children fall further behind when they grow up (Cairney et al., 2010; Lloyd et al., 2013). This could be explained by the idea that poor motor ability may have an impact on early learning opportunities and activities of daily life. Furthermore, individuals with motor problems are less likely to engage in active play. Once again, this puts weight on the importance of psychomotor therapy, where in personal functioning, motor, cognitive and social–affective aspects are always considered to be connected during a motor activity (Simons, 2014a).

CONCLUSION

The authors consider that physiotherapists in mental health have many tools that contribute to the multidisciplinary diagnostics of children and young people from a holistic view of the personality. Nevertheless, more quantitative and qualitative research is needed in order to develop this field.

The significant treatment effects suggest that exercise and physical activity may play a role in the prevention and treatment of mental health problems in children and adolescents. However, high-quality outcome-focused studies are needed to confirm those findings. Future research needs to determine the most appropriate level of intervention intensity and which interventions provide long-term improvement.

REFERENCES

Ayres, A.J., 1972a. Sensory Integration and Learning Disorders. Western Psychological Services, Los Angeles.

Ayres, A.J., 1972b. Sensory Integration Functions and Learning Disabilities. Maternal and Child Health Service, Washington DC.

Barnett, A., Henderson, S.E., Scheib, B., Schulz, J., 2007. Detailed Assessment of Speed of Handwriting (DASH) Manuel. Pearson Education, Inc, London.

Barsch, R.H., 1968. Achieving Perceptual Motor Efficiency: A Space-Oriented Approach. Special Child Publications, Seattle.

Bayley, N., 2005. Bayley Scales of Infant and Toddler Development. The psychological corporation, San Antonio TX.

Beery, K.E., Beery, N.A., 2010. The Beery-Buktenica Developmental Test of Visual-Motor Integration, sixth ed. NCS Pearson, Inc, Minneapolis, MN.

Bluechardt, M.H., Wiener, J., Shephard, R.J., 1995. Exercise programmes in the treatment of children with learning disabilities. Sports Med. 19 (1), 55–72.

Bös, K., 2001. Handbuch Motorische Tests [Handbook of Motor Tests]. Hogrefe-Verlag, Göttingen.

Bös, K., Mechling, E.H., 1983. Bilder-Angst-Test fur Bewegungssituationen (BAT): Handanweisung [Pictures-Anxiety Test for Movement Situations: Manual]. Verlag für Psychology, Hogrefe, Gottingen.

Bruininks, R.H., Bruininks, B.D., 2005. Bruininks-Oseretsky Test of Motor Proficiency, second ed. Manual. Pearson Assessment, Minneapolis, MN.

Burton, A.W., Miller, D.E., 1998. Movement Skill Assessment. Human Kinetics, Champaign, Illinois.

Cairney, J., Hay, J., Veldhuizen, S., et al., 2010. Trajectories of relative weight and waist circumference among children with and without developmental coordination disorder. Can. Med. Assoc. J. 182 (11), 1167–1172.

Cautaert, S., Dupont, V., Ideler, I., 2001. Weerbaarheid van jongeren: een denk-en doeboek. [Resilience of Young People: A Think- and Action Book]. Garant, Leuven/Apeldoorn.

Decker, R., 1972. Praxis und Theorie der psychomotorischen Erziehung bei behinderten und normalen Kindern in Frankreich. In: Eggert, D., Kiphard, E.J. (Eds.), Die Bedeutung der Motorik für die Entwicklung normaler und behinderter Kinder [The meaning of Motor Skills for the Development of Normal and Disabled Children]. Verlag Karl Hofmann, Schorndorf, pp. 68–97.

Defontaine, J., 1976. Manuel de rééducation psychomotrice [Manual of Psychomotor Rehabilitation]. Maloine, Paris, pp. 68–97.

Dewey, D., Kaplan, B.J., Crawford, S.G., Wilson, B.N., 2002. Developmental coordination disorder: associated problems in attention, learning, and psychosocial adjustment. Hum. Mov. Sci. 21 (5), 905–918.

Dishman, R.K., 1986. Mental health. In: Seefelt, V. (Ed.), Physical activity and well-being. American Alliance for Health, Physical Education, Recreation & Dance, Virginia, pp. 306–338.

Doman, G., 1974. What to Do about Your Brain Injured Child. Doubleday & Co, New York.

Doman, G.J., Delacato, C.H., Doman, R.J., 1964. The Doman–Delacato developmental profile. The Institute for Achievement of Human Potential, Philadelphia.

Eggert, D., 1971. LOS KF 18. Lincoln Oseretsky Scale shortform measuring motor development of typical and disavantaged children from 5 to 13 years old. Beltz-test, Weinheim.

Ekeland, E., Heian, F., Hagen, K.B., et al., 2009. Exercise to Improve Self-Esteem in Children and Young People (Review). John Wiley & Sons, Ltd, The Cochrane Collaboration.

Emck, C., 1998. Stress management training voor jongeren met psychotische stoornissen. Een handleiding voor trainers en therapeuten [Stress Management Training for Young People with Psychotic Disorders. A Manual for Trainers and Therapists]. Acco, Leuven Amersfoort.

Engel-Yeger, B., Kasis, A.H., 2010. The relationship between Developmental Coordination Disorders, child's perceived self-efficacy and preference to participate in daily activities. Child Care Health Dev. 36 (5), 670–677.

European Forum Psychomotricity, 1996. Statuten [Statutes]. Marburg. <http://www.psychomot.org/.>

Feuerstein, R., 1980. Instrumental Enrichment. University Park Press, Baltimore.

Feuerstein, R., Rand, Y., 1979. Instrumental Enrichment. An Intervention Program for Performers. The Learning Potential Assessment Device, Theory, Instruments and Techniques. Scott-Foresman and Company, Glenview, IL.

Folio, M.R., Fewell, R.R., 2000. Peabody Developmental Motor Scales. Examiner's Manual. Pro-Ed Inc, Austin, TX.

Frostig, M., 1974. Het Frostigprogramma voor de ontwikkeling van de visuele waarneming [The Frostig Programme for the Development of the Visual Perception]. Swets & Zeitlinger, Amsterdam.

Gantenbein, H., 1975. Was ist psychomotorische Therapie? In: Heese, G. (Ed.), Rehabilitation Behinderter durch Förderung der Motorik [Rehabilitation of People with Disabilities Through Motor Training]. Carl Marhold Verlagbuchhandlung, Berlin, pp. 79–90.

Getman, G.N., 1962. How to Develop your Child's Intelligence. Luverne, Minnesota.

Gibson, J.J., 1965. Spiral Maze Test. Appleton, New York.

Goodman, E., Whitaker, R.C., 2002. A prospective study of the role of depression in the development and persistence of adolescent obesity. Pediatrics 110 (3), 497–504.

Hammill, D.D., Pearson, N.A., Voress, J.K., 1993. Developmental Test of Visual Perception, second ed. Examiners Manual. Pro-Ed, Austin, TX.

Harvey, S.B., Hotopf, M., Overland, S., Mykletun, A., 2010. Physical activity and common mental disorders. Br. J. Psychiatry 197 (5), 357–364.

Hendrickx, F.J.P., 1998. Reactie op artikel Psychomotoriek [Reaction to an article in Psychomotricity]. What's in a name? SIGnaal 7 (24), 47–52.

Hölter, G., 1993. Ansätze zu einer Methodik der Mototherapie. In: Hölter, G. (Ed.), Mototherapie mit Erwachenen. Sport, Spiel und Bewegung in Psychiatrie, psychosomatik und Suchtbehandlung [Motor Therapy with Adults. Sports, Play and Movement in Psychiatry, Psychosomatic Medicine and Addiction Treatment]. Verlag Karl Hofmann, Schorndorf, pp. 52–80.

Irmischer, T., 1980. Motopädagogik bei geistig Behinderten. [Motor Education in Persons With a Mental Disability]. Hofmann, Schorndorf.

Kavale, K., Mattson, P.D., 1983. One jumped off the balance beam: meta-analysis of perceptual–motor training. J Learn. Disabil. 16 (3), 165–173.

Kephart, N.C., Chasey, C.M., Ebersole, M., Zaad, C.P.M., 1971. Hekkesluiters [The Slow Learner in the Classroom]. Lemniscaat, Rotterdam.

Kiphard, E.J., 1979. Motopädagogik [Motor Education]. Modernes Lernen, Dortmund.

Koolen, H.J., 1974. Basis Bewegingstherapie [Basics of Movement Therapy]. Agon Elsevier, Amsterdam.

Lamers-Winkelman, F., Bicanic, I., 2000. Horizon. Een werkboek voor kinderen die seksueel misbruik hebben meegemaakt [Horizon. A Work Book for Children Who Have Experienced Sexual Abuse]. SWP, Amsterdam.

Larun, L., Nordheim, L.V., Ekeland, E., et al., 2009. Exercise in Prevention and Treatment of Anxiety and Depression Among Children and Young People (Review). John Wiley & Sons, Ltd, The Cochrane Collaboration.

Le Boulch, J., 1971. Vers une science du movement humain [Towards a Human Movement Science]. ESF, Paris.

Le Boulch, J., 1973. L'Education par le mouvement [Education Through Movement]. Les Editions ESF, Paris.

Lefevere, D., 1976. Psychomotorische training [Psychomotor Training]. De Sikkel, Kapellen.

Lenoir, M., Vandorpe, B., D'Hondt, E., et al., 2014. KTK-NL. Herwerkte, gehernormeerde en vertaalde uitgave van de KTK voor het Nederlandstalige gebied [Reworked, Normed and Translated Edition of the KTK for the Dutch-speaking area]. Sig, Destelbergen.

Livesey, D., Lum Mow, M., Toshack, T., Zheng, Y., 2011. The relationship between motor performance and peer relations in 9- to 12-year-old children. Child Care Health Dev. 37 (4), 581–588.

Lloyd, M., MacDonald, M., Lord, C., 2013. Motor skills of toddlers with autism spectrum disorders. Autism 17 (2), 133–146.

Marsh, H.W., 1990a. Self-Description Questionnaire-I. University of Western Sydney, Macarthur, Campelltown.

Marsh, H.W., 1990b. Self-Description Questionnaire-II. University of Western Sydney, Macarthur, Campelltown.

Marsh, H.W., 1990c. Self-Description Questionnaire-III. University of Western Sydney, Macarthur, Campelltown.

Marsh, H.W., Martin, A.J., Jackson, S., 2010. Introducing a short version of the physical self-description questionnaire: new strategies, short-form evaluative criteria, and applications of factor analyses. J Sport Exerc. Psychol. 32 (4), 438–482.

Martin, N.A., 2006. Test of Visual Perceptual Skills, third ed. Academic Therapy Publications, Novato, CA.

Meichenbaum, D., 1981. Cognitieve gedragsmodificatie. Een integrale benadering [Cognitive behavior modification. An Integral Approach]. Van Loghem Slaterus, Deventer.

Meljac, C., Fauconnier, E., Camilli, F., 2010. Manuel Epreuve de Schema Corporel [Test of Body Schema. Manual]. Pearson France-ECPA, Montrieul.

Mertens, K., 1982. Methodik der bewegungserziehung mit Lernbehinderten. In: Irmischer, T., Fischer, K. (Eds.), Bewegungserziehung und Sport an Schulen für Lernbehinderte [Movement Education and Sport in Schools for Students with Learning Disabilities]. Hoffmann, Schorndorf, pp. 149–158.

Missiuna, C., Cairney, J., Pollock, N., et al., 2014. Psychological distress in children with developmental coordination disorder and attention-deficit hyperactivity disorder. Res. Dev. Disabil. 35 (5), 1198–1207.

Netelenbos, J.B., 2001. Motorische ontwikkeling van kinderen. Handboek 1: Introductie [Motor Development of Children. Handbook 1: Introduction]. Boom, Amsterdam.

Ostrow, A.C., 1996. Directory of Psychological Tests in Sport and Exercise Sciences. Fitness information Technology, Inc, Morgantown, WV.

Picq, L., Vayer, P., 1960. L'Education psychomotrice et arriération mentale [Psychomotor Education and Mental Retardation]. Doin et Cie, Paris.

Piek, J.P., Barrett, N.C., Allen, L.S.R., et al., 2005. The relationship between bullying and self-worth in children with movement coordination problems. Br. J. Educ. Psychol. 75 (3), 453–463.

Piek, J.P., Bradbury, G.S., Elsley, S.C., Tate, L., 2008. Motor coordination and social–emotional behaviour in preschool-aged children. Int. J. Disabil. Dev. Educ. 55 (2), 143–151.

Pless, M., Carlsson, M., 2000. Effects of motor skill intervention on developmental coordination disorder: a meta-analysis. Adapt. Phys. Activ. Q. 17 (4), 381–401.

Polatajko, H.J., Mandich, A.D., 2004. Enabling Occupation in Children: The Cognitive Orientation to Daily Occupational Performance (CO-OP) approach. CAOT Publication ACE, Ottawa, Ontario.

Probst, M., Simons, J. (2014). De rol van de kinesitherapie in de geestelijke gezondheid [The role of physiotherapy in mental health]. Werkgroep 2. "Adequaat gebruik van psychofarmaca" Mededeling FOD Depressie en stemmingsstoornissen, 20 May 2014, Brussels.

Rapp, G., Schoder, G., 1977. Motorische Testverfahren [Motor Tests]. CD-Verlaggesellschaft, Stuttgart.

Rivilis, I., Hay, J., Cairney, J., et al., 2011. Physical activity and fitness in children with developmental coordination disorder: A systematic review. Res. Dev. Disabil. 32 (3), 894–910.

Rose, B., Larkin, D., Berger, B.G., 1997. Coordination and gender influences on the perceived competence of children. Adapt. Phys. Activ. Q. 14, 210–221.

Rosenblum, J., Forman, S., 2002. Evidence-based treatment of eating disorders. Curr. Opin. Pediatr. 14 (4), 379–383.

Schilling, F., 1976. Checklist motorischer Verhaltensweisen. Westerman Verlag, Braunschweig.

Schipperijn, L., 1971. Bewegingstherapie, zin of onzin [Movement therapy, sense or nonsense]. Tijdschrift voor Bewegingstherapie (1), 1, 4–21.

Schoemaker, M.M., Kalverboer, A.F., 1994. Social and affective problems of children who are clumsy: How early do they begin? Adapt. Phys. Activ. Q. 11, 130–140.

Schoemaker, M.M., Flapper, B.C.T., Reinders-Messelink, H.A., de Kloet, A., 2008. Validity of the motor observation questionnaire for teachers as a screening instrument for children at risk for developmental coordination disorder. Hum. Mov. Sci. 27, 190–199.

Sherborne, V., 1990. Developmental Movement for Children. Mainstream, Special Needs and Pre-School. Cambridge University Press, Cambridge.

Sherrill, C., 2003. Adapted Physical Activity, Recreation, and Sport: Crossdisciplinary and Lifespan. McGraw Hill companies, Boston.

Simons, J., 2000. Kortdurende therapeutische interventies in psychomotorische therapie [Short-term therapeutic interventions in psychomotor therapy]. Tijdschrift NVPMT 6 (3), 10–16.

Simons, J., 2002. Psychomotorische therapie bij kinderen met gedragsproblemen [Psychomotor therapy in children with behavior problems]. Informatieblad Studiegroep Vroegdiagnose, Vroegbehandeling en Ontwikkelingsstoornissen 14, 15–30.

Simons, J., 2014a. Introductie tot de psychomotoriek [Introduction to Psychomotricity]. Garant, Antwerpen/Apeldoorn.

Simons, J., 2014b. Nieuwe Vlaamse normering van de test voor lichaamsbesef: tonen en benoemen van lichaamsdelen. Psychomotorische therapie met gezinnen. In: Simons, J. (Ed.), Themata uit de psychomotorische therapie [Themes From Psychomotor Therapy]. Garant, Antwerpen/Apeldoorn, pp. 29–40.

Simons, J., Dufait, H., Pyck, K., 1980. Situering van de psychomotorische therapie in Vlaanderen [Situating the Psychomotor Therapy in Flanders]. Hermes (Wiesb) 14 (2), 107–113.

Simons, J., Simons, J., Leitschuh, C., Popa, M., 2011. The effect of body-awareness training of pre-school children based on the Sherborne developmental movement method versus regular physical education class. E. P. J. 4 (1), 38–50.

Skinner, R.A., Piek, J.P., 2001. Psychosocial implications of poor motor coordination in children and adolescents. Hum. Mov. Sci. 20 (1), 73–94.

Smits-Engelsman, B.C., Henderson, S.E., Sugden, D.A., Barnett, A.L., 2010. Movement Assessment Battery for Children, second ed. Manual, Nederlandstalige bewerking. Pearson Assessment and Information B.V, Amsterdam.

Soubiran, G.B., Mazo, P., 1965. La réadaptation scolaire des enfants intelligents par la rééducation psychomotrice [School Rehabilitation of Intelligent Children by Psychomotor Rehabilitation]. Doin et Cie, Paris.

Steingrüber, H.J., 2011. Hand-Dominanz-Test [Test of Manual Preference]. Hogrefe Verlag GmbH & Co.KG, Göttingen.

Tiffin, J., 1968. Purdue Pegboard, examiner manual. Science Research Associates Inc., Chicago, Illinois. http:// www.lafayetteinstrument .com.

Ulrich, D.A., Sanford, C.B., 2000. Test of Gross Motor Development, second ed. Examiner's manual. Pro-Ed, Austin, TX.

Vallaey, M., 1973. Lateralisatieonderzoek bij kinderen van 4 tot 10 jaar [Research on Lateralization in Children From 4 to 10 Years]. CSBO, Brussels.

Vallaey, M., 1978. Psychomotoriek bij kinderen, theoretische benadering [Psychomotricity in Children, Theoretical Approach]. Acco, Leuven.

Van Coppenolle, H., Simons, J., 1985. Algemene technieken van psychomotorische therapi. [General Techniques of Psychomotor Therapy]. Acco, Leuven.

Van de Riet, G., 1985. Sensorische integratie [Sensory Integration]. De Tijdstroom, Lochem.

van der Linde, B.W., van Netten, J.J., Otten, B.E., et al., 2014. Psychometric properties of the DCDDaily-Q: A new parental questionnaire on children's performance in activities of daily living. Res. Dev. Disabil. 35 (7), 1711–1719.

Van Dun, W., 1981. Psychomotoriek [Psychomotricity]. Van In, Lier.

Van Empelen, R., 1981. Effectiviteit van sensomotorische training [Effectiveness of Sensomotor Therapy]. De Tijdstroom, Lochem.

Van Waelvelde, H., 1998. Psychomotoriek. What's in a name? [Psychomotricity. What's in a name?]. SIGnaal 7 (22), 16–23.

Van Waelvelde, H., 1999. Psychomotoriek. De polemiek afgesloten [Psychomotricity. The polemic closed]. SIGnaal 8 (26), 21–22.

Van Waelvelde, H., De Mey, B., Smits-Engelsman, B., 2014. Systematische OpsporingSchrijfproblemen (SOS-2-VL) [Systematic Detection of Writing Problems]. Sig, Destelbergen.

Vandroemme, G., 1998. Reactie op artikel Psychomotoriek. What's in a name? [Reaction on the article Psychomotricity. What's in a name?]. SIGnaal 7 (23), 34–38.

Verscheure, B., Van Roie, E., 2014. Psychomotorische therapie met gezinnen. In: Simons, J. (Ed.), Themata uit de psychomotorische therapie [Themes from Psychomotor Therapy]. Garant, Antwerpen/Apeldoorn, pp. 41–46.

Vles, J.S.H., Kroes, M., Feron, F.J.M., 2004. Maastrichter Motoriek Test [Maastrichter Motor Test]. Handleiding. Leiden, PITS BV.

Wilson, B., Pollock, N., Kaplan, B., Law, M., 2000. Clinical Observations of Motor and Postural Skills. Therapro, Inc, Framingham, MA.

Zazzo, R., Galifret-Granjon, N., Hurtig, M.C., et al., 1958. Manuel pour l'examen psychologique de l'enfant [Manual for the Psychological Examination of the Child]. Delachaux et Niestlé, Neuchâtel.

Zimmer, R., 1982. Methodik der Bewegungserziehung mit Lernbehinderten. In: Irmischer, T., Fischer, K. (Eds.), Bewegungserziehung und Sport an Schulen für Lernbehinderte [Movement education and sport in schools for students with learning disabilities]. Hofmann, Schorndorf, pp. 140–148.

Zimmer, R., Volkamer, M., 1984. Motoriktest für vier-bis sechsjährige Kinder [Motor test in children from 4 to 6 years]. Beltz test, Weinheim.

5.3.2   Creating Space for Youth in Physiotherapy: Aspects Related to Gender and Embodied Empowerment

MARIA STRÖMBÄCK ■ MARIA WIKLUND

SUMMARY

This chapter aims to give one example of how physiotherapists can work with young people experiencing stress-related and mental health problems, by adapting a youth-friendly and gender-sensitive approach. The chapter is based on a qualitative study that illuminates young women's experiences of participating in a body-based, gender-sensitive stress management group intervention by youth-friendly health services in northern Sweden. The stress-management courses consisted of eight sessions, each lasting about 2 hours. The content of the intervention combined reflective discussions, for example on stress and pressures related to femininity and body ideals, and physiotherapeutic methods, including Basic Body Awareness Therapy and relaxation. Follow-up interviews were carried out with 32 young women (17–25 years of age) after they had completed the intervention. The overall results suggest that the stress-management course facilitated 'a space for gendered and embodied empowerment in a hectic life', implying that it both contributed to a sense of individual growth and allowed participants to unburden themselves of stress problems within a trustful and supportive context. Participants narrated experiences of 'finding a social oasis to challenge gendered expectations', 'being bodily empowered', and 'altering gendered positions and stance on life' point to empowering processes of change that allowed them to cope with distress, despite sometimes continuously stressful life situations. The participants' experiences of the intervention as a safe and exploratory space for gendered collective understanding and embodied empowerment further indicates the need to develop *gender-sensitive interventions to reduce individualization of health problems and instead encourage spaces for collective support, action, and change.*

KEY POINTS

■ Mental health, stress-related and psychosomatic problems are common among children and youth—and there are gendered patterns.

■ The complex interaction between internal bodily stress reactions and gendered external stressors is important to address in youth mental health interventions.

■ Youth-friendly and gender-sensitive intervention models need to be developed within physiotherapy.

LEARNING OBJECTIVES

■ To gain an insight into gendered patterns of youth mental health.

■ To explore if gender-sensitive interventions tailored to young women's own experiences can be used in health promotion.

■ To discern how physiotherapy with a focus on body awareness can empower young women to handle stress and societal demands.

INTRODUCTION

In Sweden, it is unusual for physiotherapists to work at youth health centres and, in addition, physiotherapy is regarded as relatively 'gender blind'. In Scandinavian and Swedish physiotherapy there are established intervention methods suitable for adults with psychiatric disorders, as well as stress and pain management for adults, yet there are few studies on young people with stress-related and mental health problems. In this chapter, we give one example of how physiotherapists can work with young people experiencing mental health problems, by adapting a youth-friendly and gender-sensitive approach. We base the chapter on our own research, a qualitative study that illuminates young women's experiences of participating in a body-based, gender-sensitive stress-management group intervention by youth-friendly health services in northern Sweden (Strömbäck et al., 2013). The chapter is a shortened version of our article: '"Girls

need to strengthen each other as a group": experiences from a gender-sensitive stress management intervention by youth-friendly Swedish health services', published in the open access journal BMC Public Health (Strömbäck et al., 2013).

GENDERED PATTERNS OF YOUTH MENTAL HEALTH AND BODY PRESSURES

Mental health and psychosomatic problems are common during adolescence and emerging adulthood (Patel et al., 2007; Patton et al., 2012). The prevalence of mental disorders is at least 20% in the general population of 18–24-year-olds (Patel et al., 2007). Mild or moderate mental health or psychosocial problems among young people have also been defined as stress-related problems, which are often interlinked with complaints such as stomach ache and headache, neck and shoulder pain, muscle tension, anxiety, depressive mood, sleeping problems and fatigue (Hagquist, 2009; Wiklund et al., 2012).

Gendered stress and mental health patterns are observed in several countries, indicating that girls and young women aged 16–24 years old report more problems than boys and young men (Moksnes et al., 2011). In the search for explanatory factors, external stressors such as youth unemployment, educational pressures, normative body and health ideals, and sexual harassment are found (Gillander Gådin & Hammarström, 2005; Lager et al., 2012). Studies also indicate that interpersonal stressors such as worries about family or peer relations are significant (Sweeting et al., 2010). Other stressors affecting young women include changing living conditions in contemporary Western societies, including increased individualization, and the focus on consumption, fitness and appearance (Wiklund et al., 2010; Wright et al., 2006).

In comparison with boys, adolescent girls have poorer body esteem (Frisén et al., 2013; Wängqvist & Frisén, 2013). This is thought to be the result of gendered objectification of girls' bodies and adverse media exposure (McLean et al., 2013; Einberg et al., 2015). Such pressures are tied to perceptions and social constructions of the body as a 'problem' and a 'burden' (Wiklund et al., 2010, 2014). Hence, gendered and sociocultural messages position the young feminine body as a venue for different societal and psychosocial pressures (Aapola et al., 2005; Liimakka, 2011a). This complex interaction between gendered external stressors and internal bodily stress reactions is an important consideration in health interventions geared towards young women experiencing distress (Wiklund, 2010; Wiklund et al., 2010, 2014; Strömbäck, 2014; Strömbäck et al., 2016).

THE NEED FOR YOUTH-FRIENDLY AND GENDER-SENSITIVE MENTAL HEALTH INTERVENTIONS

Worldwide, so-called *youth-friendly health services* are being developed to respond to young people's complex health needs. According to the World Health Organization (WHO), youth-friendly services are characterized by accessibility, acceptability and appropriateness (World Health Organization, 2010). Social support, validation and encouragement from others are aspects that are found to attract young people and facilitate their help-seeking behaviour (Tylee et al., 2007; Muir et al., 2012). In Sweden, youth clinics addressing sexual and reproductive health care are well-established, youth-friendly services. For many years, youth clinics have been offering services to young people in the range of 13–25 years of age nationwide. Still, there are few Swedish youth health services specifically geared towards late adolescents and young adults with mental health problems.

Moreover, because young people's mental health problems and help-seeking behaviour are found to be interlinked with social aspects of gender (Maclean et al., 2010; Sweeting et al., 2010), it is important to take various aspects of gender and gendered living conditions into account when developing intervention models (Danielsson et al., 2011; Wiklund et al., 2010). Nevertheless, there are, to our knowledge, few Swedish youth health services and interventions that adapt a gender-sensitive approach to late adolescents and young adults with stress and mental health problems.

In Sweden, it is unusual for physiotherapists to work at youth health centres, as described in the present study, and, in addition, physiotherapy is regarded as relatively 'gender blind' (Öhman, 2001; Strömbäck & Wiklund, 2015; Strömbäck et al., 2016). To the best

of our knowledge, no gender-sensitive interventions have yet been evaluated within physiotherapy. In Scandinavian and Swedish physiotherapy there are established and evaluated intervention methods suitable for adults with psychiatric disorders, as well as stress and pain management for adults (Malmgren-Olsson & Bränholm, 2002, Gyllensten et al., 2009), yet there are few studies on youth with stress-related and mental health problems. Such mental health studies with adults demonstrate that psychosomatically oriented and psychiatric methods, such as Basic Body Awareness Therapy (BBAT), have positive and long-term effects on pain, tension relief and self-efficacy in individuals with nonspecific musculoskeletal pain and psychiatric disorders (Malmgren-Olsson & Bränholm, 2002; Gyllensten et al., 2009), and inspire more positive experiences of the body and self in women with fibromyalgia or chronic musculoskeletal pain (Gustafsson et al., 2004). Qualitative evaluations of group interventions with BBAT in psychiatric outpatient care and chronic pain rehabilitation for adults indicate that feelings of being included in a supportive group environment encouraged empowering processes that led towards improved bodily functions and finding strategies for better health (Gustafsson et al., 2004; Johnsen & Råheim, 2010). In comparison, short-term psychological counselling was found to improve mental and general health among young adults (Winzer & Bergsten Brucefors, 2007).

In this chapter, our aim is to give one example of how physiotherapists can work with young women experiencing mental health problems by adapting a youth-friendly and gender-sensitive approach, and to present participants' experiences of such an intervention.

THE RESEARCH PROJECT: STRESS AND HEALTH IN YOUTH (UMEÅ SHY)

The results and ideas presented in this chapter refer to our research project, Stress and Health in Youth (Umeå SHY). Umeå SHY aims to develop knowledge and understanding about stress and health among young people and to develop gender-sensitive intervention models. An additional aim is to integrate sociocultural and gender-theoretical perspectives as applied within medicine and health research. The project is being conducted in close collaboration with school health and youth health services, and uses a mixed-method design (Wiklund, 2010; Strömbäck, 2014).

The qualitative study referred to in this chapter was conducted at a youth health centre in Umeå, a university city in northern Sweden (Strömbäck et al., 2013). The youth health centre specifically addressed young people 16–25 years of age with psychosocial problems and mental ill health. Between 2005 and 2009, stress-management courses for young women were initiated and implemented at the centre as part of Umeå SHY.

The intervention model has been evaluated with both qualitative and quantitative methods (Strömbäck, 2014). Before the intervention period, participants were interviewed and answered a questionnaire consisting of questions about their stress, health and bodily experiences. The findings from these substudies suggest that the symptomatology was complex and multifaceted (Wiklund et al., 2014; Strömbäck et al., 2015). Also, the external stressors and demands in young women's lives were found to be multiple, and influenced by their social context as well as by social constructions of gender (Wiklund et al., 2010; Strömbäck et al., 2014). The quantitative evaluation of the intervention model showed positive significant changes in aspects of body perception, self-image, and mental health and somatic symptoms. The changes were most significant in lowering internalization of anxiety and depression symptoms. Symptoms such as headaches and sleeping problems decreased and the participants were more satisfied with their bodies (Strömbäck, 2014; Strömbäck et al., 2016).

The Intervention Model: Gender-Sensitive Stress Management

The intervention model was announced as a stress-management course and led by the physiotherapist at the youth health centre. The physiotherapist (MS), who has specific competence in psychiatry, cognitive–behavioural therapy, psychosomatics, trauma and stress, was part of the regular staff at the youth health centre. The stress-management course had an eight-session group treatment design and each group session lasted about 2 hours. The inclusion criteria for participation in the project comprised young women 16–25 years of age with self-defined stress-related problems and interest in participating in the course concept. The

exclusion criteria were severe mental health disorders or other reasons that made group participation not relevant. In total, 55 participants joined one of the intervention groups (6–8 participants/group). The qualitative evaluation comprises 32 interviews drawn from the 46 participants who completed the course (see Strömbäck et al., 2013).

The concept was a combination of well-established and evidence-based methods used in Scandinavian physiotherapy, primarily BBAT and progressive muscular relaxation. The pedagogy was informed by group counselling and a problem-based physiotherapeutic pedagogy, combining reflective discussions and BBAT.

The gender-sensitive approach integrated into the course concept is based on our understanding of gender as a social construction, where gender is produced and reproduced in ongoing social, cultural and hierarchal relations and processes (West & Zimmerman, 1987; Annandale & Kuhlmann, 2010). Gender is viewed as reflected in the body through the process of social and gendered embodiment, for example, expressed as low body esteem and stress arousal (Connell, 2012; Wiklund et al., 2014).

Gender-sensitive interventions address and formulate constraining and demanding gender relations, perceptions and norms that may be barriers to recognizing stress and mental health symptoms. Central issues to address in stress management are the need to question and relinquish gendered responsibilities and high levels of responsibility taking in multiple areas, as well as stereotyped body ideals and harassments (Landstedt et al., 2009; Wiklund et al., 2010; Strömbäck et al., 2013, 2014).

The group pedagogy and the gender-sensitive intentions implied being sensitive to the young women's expressed needs, both in the choice of themes for discussion and during the body-orientated parts of the sessions (Strömbäck et al., 2013, 2016). Themes elaborated on during the course were identified during the initial group sessions, or originated from the research team's knowledge about young women, gender and stress, but had also emerged from the young women's own narratives told to the group leader (MS) and researcher (MW) before the course started. Themes were, for example, based on questions such as 'How do I react to stress?' 'What is stress for me?' 'How do I cope with stress?' 'What is it like to be a contemporary young woman?' and 'How can I set limits?' Themes might also address pressures in life such as sociocultural and gendered norms, body ideals, dieting, high achievement, and expectations for girls to assume responsibility in social relationships and in caring for others' needs. Rest, sleep and recovery were other central themes (see Strömbäck et al., 2016 for a more detailed description of the intervention model).

A SPACE FOR GENDERED AND EMBODIED EMPOWERMENT

Our analysis of participants' experiences of taking part in the stress-management course resulted in one main theme of 'a space for gendered and embodied empowerment in a hectic life', which together with related themes and subthemes illuminates how the young women in the study experienced participation in the stress-management course as encouraging processes of change (Table 1). The contents of the group intervention, requiring active participation, support, reflection and bodily presence, strengthened the participants' own resources to meet and handle problems of stress.

The theme 'finding a social oasis to challenge gendered expectations' represents the participants' narrated experiences of social togetherness through a process of sharing life stories in discussions with

other young women in similar situations. Sharing experiences about stress as a complex and multifaceted phenomenon gave them valuable insights into how various stressors and individual stress reactions could be related to social creations of gender and external demands from society in general, as well as in relation to their own everyday lives.

I think we have had really good discussions within the group and talked about things that individually we might not have dared to talk about, perception of our bodies or whatever.

Many of them felt it troublesome to seek help for stress-related problems, as they had associated this with personal weakness and failure. The participants brought to the surface their ideas about 'girl stress' and, to some extent, were able to challenge these from social and relational points of view. These reflections and discussions led to perceptions that young women's stress was not only a problem for them as individuals, but also was dependent upon gendered social relations, norms and structures in the society in which they were immersed.

The theme of 'being bodily empowered' represents experiences from which the participants began to approach their problematic bodies. By engaging in body-based awareness and reflections, they achieved consciousness of how bodily sensations and reactions were strongly connected to stress experiences.

"I've actually been able to sleep, that's to say I've been able to drop off quite quickly recently and I've not had so many headaches."

The young women were engrossed in bodily deficiencies and difficulties in fully controlling their bodies through training loads and food intake. In contrast to this, the body-awareness sessions created a bodily space where participants could explore their bodies as potential resources. The young womens' discovery of their flexibility and reconfigurability strengthened their feelings of hope for change. Participants also explored balance and stability in different positions, which further strengthened their sense of confidence. Close interaction and physical contact with themselves and other young women helped them to a greater acceptance of themselves and their own bodies.

TABLE 1

Main Theme, Themes and Subthemes in the Results of the Study

A Space for Gendered and Embodied Empowerment in a Hectic Life

Finding a Social Oasis to Challenge Gendered Expectations	*Being Bodily Empowered*	*Altering Gendered Positions and Stance to Life*
Being confirmed in a nonjudging and supportive atmosphere	Approaching the problematic body	Upgrading oneself and one's abilities
Making space for reflection on gender and stress	Finding breathing space	Switching pace in life
		Setting limits and resisting outer pressure

"Previously I had a lot more heart palpitations, and I had very, very tense, shallow breathing. Now it's gone down a bit, at least to my stomach, and I'm beginning to breathe a bit better. I'm not as tense and stiff as I was previously, more relaxed now…"

Moreover, the young women experienced the course as a 'breathing space' in their demanding lives. Paying attention to their own breathing involved awareness of bodily rhythm and tempo. They discovered that calmer and more open breathing reduced their stress and created space for well-being. Their stories express a process of moving towards body-anchored confidence in oneself and bodily freedom—which is our interpretation of bodily empowerment.

The theme 'altering gendered positions and stance to life' represents experiences of progression in the young women's ability to handle difficult stress situations. The course was used as a forum to challenge oneself, to try out new positions and skills, and to develop strategies and competence. By a process of confirming one another, they were able to create space for thoughts such as 'You're good enough as you are'. This more relaxed stance towards oneself included less focus on a perfect body, weight and appearance— although such pressures were still problematic to handle. 'Switching pace in life' was a central theme in the process towards altered strategies to handle time pressures and demands.

"Yes, well it feels like I have cut down on the pace of life. Earlier, I felt that I had to fill my day with many activities […] I think a lot about what I have to do today, what is the absolute most needed to do today. So I, like, prioritize between what I need and what I want."

Overall, trying out a new—often slower—pace and loosening up tight schedules resulted in an increased sense of freedom to move and act differently, which unburdened the participants from pressures and positively affected their well-being. The processes of negotiated and altered gendered positions reflect bodily and personal empowerment, embracing the possibility of 'taking a step forward', 'claiming space', 'leaning back', or withdrawing from negative or demanding attention in both a physical and metaphorical sense.

CONCLUDING REFLECTIONS

Based on our analysis of participating young womens' experiences, the group intervention worked to facilitate coping, action and change in a hectic and demanding life. Experiences of social support from similar others led to insights and new explanatory models where collective understanding and a shared gendered identity helped them to reduce the individual responsibility for, and feelings of failure and stigma associated with, distress and help seeking. Sociologists such as Thoits (2011) emphasize the value of social support from similar others. Such specific support is defined as an effective buffer against stress and mental ill health in terms of empathic understanding, validation of feelings, encouragement and inspiring hope. The results of widened explanatory models point to the development of collective understandings and a shared identity that the young women gained from the supportive group setting (Kelly et al., 2004). The concept of 'collective wisdom' captures the advantages of problem solving and reflecting together with similar others in a group (Davison et al., 2000). Processes of collective understanding are reported from interventions guided by a feminist framework in which women can empower one another to cope with and eventually change adverse life situations (Kelly et al., 2004; Hébert & Bergeron, 2007).

Moreover, the participants experienced the intervention as a safe and explorative space for gendered identity work and personal integrity, as well as an explorative bodily space to discover embodied resources such as strength, stability and relaxation. Within this space, their corporeality gradually became associated with well-being instead of suffering. This way of gently exploring symptoms and uncomfortable sensations has been found to be a powerful treatment principle in stress and trauma therapy (Mattsson et al., 1998). Elements of awareness and nonjudgemental acceptance of one's experiences have been shown to have positive effects on distress and psychosomatic conditions (Keng et al., 2011). On an abstract level, the intervention— when understood as a breathing space—can serve as a metaphor representing both a safe place and a space for reflection. On a material and intraindividual level, breathing is essential for human life and vitality, and can therefore also play an important role in recovery and well-being (Skjaerven et al., 2003). Furthermore, breathing rhythm is directly interwoven with tensions and emotions in the body, and is thus responsive to stressors and strain in life (Gyllensten et al., 2010). It is clear that participants experienced excessive pressure on their time and a problematic relationship with the forced tempo of life (Wiklund et al., 2010). However, the thematic of the group sessions encouraged them to influence this negative experience by slowing down the pace. The participants started to prioritize time in a slightly different way.

In addition, within this safe space for gendered and embodied empowerment, the young women could challenge their social positions and stance towards life by upgrading and protecting themselves and their needs and setting limits. Likewise, Einberg et al. (2015) argue that if teenage girls feel 'connected' and secure, protective factors such as *manageability* and *meaningfulness* can work to relieve high demands and experienced unfairness in everyday life. However, our findings also illustrate participants' still ongoing struggles with personal burdens of responsibility and their negotiations around handling internal and external pressures. In line with findings from other studies, the young women in this study struggled to relate to or resist conflicting ideals and feminine subject positions (Oinas, 2001; Wiklund et al., 2010; Gustafsson et al., 2011). Already, during adolescence, girls find it difficult to defend themselves against media images of what women should look like (Einberg et al., 2015). Even 'feminist' women, despite their consciousness of gendered ideals and expectations, may have difficulties protecting and defending themselves from feeling dissatisfied with their bodies (Liimakka, 2011b). Therefore young women need to develop 'bodily empowerment' and 'embodied agency', understood as a power to act, grounded in embodied trust and acceptance of self.

However, it is important to acknowledge that young women themselves cannot be expected to change all the outer conditions that have to be acted upon politically and collectively. There is a need to further develop gender-sensitive group interventions to decrease this individualization of health problems among youth, and instead encourage spaces for collective support, action and change.

To conclude, we have identified a potential space for youth mental health within physiotherapy, as well as for context- and gender-sensitive approaches.

Acknowledgement

We thank the participants. We thank our colleague, Eva-Britt Malmgren-Olsson, also an author of the original publication, for her valuable engagement and competence in Umeå SHY.

REFERENCES

Aapola, S., Gonick, M., Harris, A., 2005. Young Femininity: Girlhood, Power and Social Change. Palgrave, New York.

Annandale, E., Kuhlmann, E., 2010. The Palgrave Handbook of Gender and Healthcare. Palgrave Macmillan, Basingstoke.

Connell, R., 2012. Gender health and theory: Conceptualizing the issue, in local and world perspective. Soc. Sci. Med. 74, 1675–1683.

Danielsson, U.E., Bengs, C., Samuelsson, E., Johansson, E.E., 2011. My greatest dream is to be normal': The impact of gender on the depression narratives of young Swedish men and women. Qual. Health Res. 21 (5), 612–624.

Davison, K.P., Pennebaker, J.W., Dickerson, S.S., 2000. Who talks? The social psychology of illness support groups. Am. Psychol. 55 (2), 205–217.

Einberg, E.L., Lidell, E., Clausson, E.K., 2015. Awareness of demands and unfairness and the importance of connectedness and security: Teenage girls' lived experiences of their everyday lives. Int. J. Qual. Stud. Health Well-being 10, 27653.

Frisén, A., Lunde, C., Kleiberg, A.N., 2013. Body esteem in Swedish children and adolescents: relationships with gender, age, and weight status. Nord. Psychol. 65, 65–80.

Gillander Gådin, K., Hammarström, A., 2005. A possible contributor to the higher degree of girls reporting psychological symptoms compared with boys in grade nine? Eur. J. Public Health 15, 380–385.

Gustafsson, S.A., Edlund, B., Davén, J., et al., 2011. How to deal with sociocultural pressures in daily life: Reflections of adolescent girls suffering from eating disorders. J. Multidiscip. Healthc. 4, 103–110.

Gustafsson, M., Ekholm, J., Öhman, A., 2004. From shame to respect: Musculoskeletal pain patients' experience of a rehabilitation programme—A qualitative study. J. Rehabil. Med. 36 (3), 97–103.

Gyllensten, A.L., Ekdahl, C., Hansson, L., 2009. Long-term effectiveness of basic body awareness therapy in psychiatric outpatient care: a randomized controlled study. Adv. Physiother. 11 (1), 2–12.

Gyllensten, A.L., Skär, L., Miller, M., Gard, G., 2010. Embodied identity – A deeper understanding of body awareness. Physiother. Theory Pract. 26 (7), 439–446.

Hagquist, C., 2009. Psychosomatic health problems among adolescents in Sweden – Are the time trends gender related? Eur. J. Public Health 19 (3), 331–336.

Hébert, M., Bergeron, M., 2007. Efficacy of a group intervention for adult women survivors of sexual abuse. J. Child Sex. Abus. 16 (4), 37–61.

Johnsen, R.W., Råheim, M., 2010. Feeling more in balance and grounded in one's own body and life: Focus group interviews on experiences with basic body awareness therapy in psychiatric healthcare. Adv. Physiother. 12 (3), 166–174.

Kelly, P.J., Bobo, T., Avery, S., McLachlan, K., 2004. Feminist perspectives and practice with young women. Issues Compr. Pediatr. Nurs. 27 (2), 121–133.

Keng, S.L., Smoski, M.J., Robins, C.J., 2011. Effects of mindfulness on psychological health: A review of empirical studies. Clin. Psychol. Rev. 31 (6), 1041–1056.

Lager, A., Berlin, M., Heimerson, I., Danielsson, M., 2012. Young people's health: health in Sweden: The National Public Health Report 2012. Chapter 3. Scan. J. Publ. Health 40 (Suppl. 9), 42–71.

Landstedt, E., Asplund, K., Gillander Gådin, K., 2009. Understanding adolescent mental health: The influence of social processes, doing gender and gendered power relations. Sociol. Health Illn. 31 (7), 962–978.

Liimakka, S., 2011a. I am my body: Objectification, empowering embodiment, and physical activity in women's studies students' accounts. Sociol. Sport J. 28, 441–460.

Liimakka, S., 2011b. Cartesian and corporeal agency: Women's studies students' reflections on body experience. Gend. Educ. 23, 811–823.

Malmgren-Olsson, E.-B., Bränholm, I.-B., 2002. A comparison between three physiotherapy approaches with regard to health-related factors in patients with non-specific musculoskeletal disorders. Disabil. Rehabil. 24 (6), 308–317.

Mattsson, M., Wikman, M., Dahlgren, L., et al., 1998. Body awareness therapy with sexually abused women. Part 2: Evaluation of body awareness in a group setting. J. Bodyw. Mov. Ther. 2 (1), 38–45.

Maclean, A., Sweeting, H., Hunt, K., 2010. Rules' for boys, 'guidelines' for girls: Gender differences in symptom reporting during childhood and adolescence. Soc. Sci. Med. 70 (4), 597–604.

McLean, S.A., Paxton, S.J., Wertheim, E.H., 2013. Mediators of the relationship between media literacy and body dissatisfaction in early adolescent girls: Implications for prevention. Body Image 10, 282–289.

Moksnes, U.K., Rannestad, T., Byrne, D.G., Espnes, G.A., 2011. The association between stress, sense of coherence and subjective health complaints in adolescents: sense of coherence as a potential moderator. Stress Health 27 (3), e157–e165.

Muir, K., Powell, A., McDermott, S., 2012. 'They don't treat you like a virus': Youth-friendly lessons from the Australian National Youth Mental Health Foundation. Health Soc. Care Community 20 (2), 181–189.

Oinas, E., 2001. Making Sense of the Teenage Body: Sociological Perspectives on Girls, Changing Bodies, and Knowledge. Åbo Akademi University Press, Åbo.

Öhman, A., 2001. Profession on the Move: Changing Conditions and Gendered Development in Physiotherapy. Umeå University, Umeå.

Patel, V., Flisher, A.J., Hetrick, S., McGorry, P., 2007. Mental health of young people: A global public-health challenge. Lancet 369 (9569), 1302–1313.

Patton, G.C., Coffey, C., Cappa, C., et al., 2012. Health of the world's adolescents: A synthesis of internationally comparable data. Lancet 379 (9826), 1665–1675.

Skjaerven, L.H., Gard, G., Kristoffersen, K., 2003. Basic elements and dimensions to the phenomenon of quality of movement – A case study. J. Bodyw. Mov. Ther. 7 (4), 251–260.

Strömbäck, M., 2014. Skapa rum. Ung femininitet, kroppslighet och psykisk ohälsa – Genusmedveten hälsofrämjande intervention [Create space. Young femininity, body, and mental health – A gender-sensitive and health promoting intervention]. Umeå University, Umeå.

Strömbäck, M., Formark, B., Wiklund, M., Malmgren-Olsson, E.-B., 2014. The corporeality of living stressful femininity – A gender theoretical analysis of young Swedish women's stress experiences. Young 22 (3), 271–287.

Strömbäck, M., Malmgren-Olsson, E.-B., Wiklund, M., 2013. Girls need to strengthen each other as a group': Experiences from a gender-sensitive stress management intervention by youth-friendly Swedish health services – A qualitative study. BMC Public Health 13, 907.

Strömbäck, M., Wiklund, M., 2015. Från genusblind till genusmedveten – Teordriven interventionsutveckling i ungdomsvänlig miljö [From gender-blind to gender-sensitive]. Fysioterapi, Stockholm, pp. 3, 24–31.

Strömbäck, M., Wiklund, M., Salander Renberg, E., Malmgren-Olsson, E.-B., 2015. Complex symptomatology among young women who present with stress-related problems. Scand. J. Caring Sci. 29 (2), 234–247.

Strömbäck, M., Wiklund, M., Salander Renberg, E., Malmgren-Olsson, E.-B., 2016. Gender-sensitive and youth friendly physiotherapy: Steps towards a stress management intervention for girls and young women. Physiother. Theory Pract. 32 (1), 20–33.

Sweeting, H., West, P., Young, R., Der, G., 2010. Can we explain increases in young people's psychological distress over time? Soc. Sci. Med. 71 (10), 1819–1830.

Thoits, P.A., 2011. Mechanisms linking social ties and support to physical and mental health. [Review]. J. Health Soc. Behav. 52 (2), 145–161.

Tylee, A., Haller, D.M., Graham, T., et al., 2007. Youth-friendly primary-care services: How are we doing and what more needs to be done? Lancet 369 (9572), 1565–1573.

Wängqvist, M., Frisén, A., 2013. Swedish 18-year-olds' identity formation: Associations with feelings about appearance and internalization of body ideals. J. Adolesc. 36, 485–493.

West, C., Zimmerman, D.H., 1987. Doing gender. Gend. Soc. 1 (2), 125–151.

World Health Organization, 2010. Youth-friendly Health Policies and Services in the European Region: Sharing Experiences. WHO, Copenhagen.

Wiklund, M., 2010. Close to the Edge: Discursive, Gendered and Embodied Stress in Modern Youth. Umeå University, Umeå.

Wiklund, M., Bengs, C., Malmgren-Olsson, E.-B., Öhman, A., 2010. Young women facing multiple and intersecting stressors of modernity, gender orders and youth. Soc. Sci. Med. 71 (9), 1567–1575.

Wiklund, M., Malmgren-Olsson, E.B., Öhman, A., et al., 2012. Subjective health complaints in older adolescents are related to perceived stress, anxiety and gender—A cross-sectional school study in Northern Sweden. BMC Public Health 12, 993.

Wiklund, M., Öhman, A., Bengs, C., Malmgren-Olsson, E.-B., 2014. Living close to the edge: Embodied dimensions of distress during emerging adulthood. SAGE Open 4.

Winzer, R., Brucefors, A.B., 2007. Does a short-term intervention promote mental and general health among young adults?—An evaluation of counselling. BMC Public Health 7, 319.

Wright, J., O'Flynn, G., Macdonald, D., 2006. Being fit and looking healthy: Young women's and men's constructions of health and fitness. Sex Roles 54, 707–716.

5.3.3   Physiotherapy for Children With Intellectual Disabilities

BEELEKE BREDERO ■ MICHEL PROBST

SUMMARY

Intellectual disability must be present before the age of 18 years. It can be characterized by limitations in daily life, with physical and mental impairments. Owing to these impairments and a decreased cognitive ability, social interaction is very hard for such children. Several factors are important in optimal treatment. First, it is recommended to increase physical fitness and decrease comorbidity due to a sedentary lifestyle, but keep in mind the physical condition of the child. Second, patients should be treated in groups, because this will enhance social capabilities. Third, the progression of the therapy should be discussed with colleagues, preferably of several disciplines, and family members or other significant persons should be involved in the therapy.

KEY POINTS

■ Intellectual disability leads to impairments in mental and physical functioning.

■ Consider the child's physical impairments when designing a treatment plan.

■ Choose activities that are sufficiently challenging for the child.

LEARNING OBJECTIVES

■ Which factors hinder the motor development of people with intellectual disability?

■ What are the cornerstones of the treatment for people with intellectual disability?

■ Which components of physical fitness will improve by doing regular sports activities?

INTRODUCTION

Intellectual disability (ID), or intellectual developmental disability (IDD), is diagnosed when a person has significant impairment in mental functioning and limitations in adaptive behaviour, which covers many daily practical and social skills. The disability must have an onset before 18 years (Hocking et al., 2016). There are several forms of ID or developmental delay (DD), but the most well known is Down syndrome (DS).

Mentally handicapped people are limited in their ability to learn, and they learn more slowly than average. They often struggle with their daily activities. Their ability to understand someone else's behaviour and to respond in a social way is less than their peers. The group of people with ID is very heterogeneous. Additional impairments and disabilities determine how much support and guidance they needed for living, self-care and leisure activities. The level of disability is based on an individual's intelligence quotient (IQ) level and can be divided into three different categories: light (IQ 50–70), moderate (IQ 35–50) or severe (IQ lower than 35) mental handicap. However, several organizations have recommended another system: the World Health Organization International Classification of Diseases (WHO ICD) Group on the Classification of Intellectual Disabilities conceptualized IDD as a metasyndromic health condition, parallel to other metasyndromic conditions such as dementia, which may be related to a variety of specific etiologies.

Persons with ID often have physical and/or comorbid disorders. Frequently occurring physical conditions are cardiovascular disorders, infections, leukaemia, thyroid dysfunction, intestinal problems, musculoskeletal disorders (low muscle tone, hypermobility of joints resulting in postural and orthopaedic problems) and obesity (De Winter et al., 2011).

Common psychiatric disorders in people with ID include psychosis, schizophrenia, anxiety disorders and personality disorders. The most frequently seen mental problems are excessive dependency on others, low self-esteem and low aspiration level (Pulver et al., 1994). People with ID frequently suffer from problem behaviour such as aggression, self-injury, anxiety, and maladaptive and antisocial behaviour; this is seen in 20% to 40% of cases. With behavioural problems, mood disorders or psychotic reactions, it is important to determine whether the living environment is adapted to the capabilities of the individual (Emerson, 2003; Hurdley, 2006; Owen, 2012).

MOTOR DEVELOPMENT

During the first 6 years of a child's life, gross motor skills (GMS) are learned, such as running, sitting, rolling, standing, walking and ball skills. The level of GMS is lower in children with ID in comparison to their peers. This is caused by a low IQ level and somatic problems, and is also due to a decreased ability to learn and having a poor physical condition (Vuijk et al., 2010).

These motor skills are necessary for daily functioning, so that children with ID face problems with daily activities. It is stated that the more complex a task, the harder it is to execute. A complex motor skill is: 'An open skill, which is more dependent on factors in the environment, for example, external objects and other players, than simple motor skills' (Capio et al., 2015). Moreover, if cognitive information is required to complete a motor task and/or if arms and legs are involved in the movement, it is hard for these children to execute the movement adequately because of their ID and restricted motor abilities.

Rintala & Loovis (2013) have shown that children with a disability perform significantly worse on several subtests of the Test of Gross Motor Development 2 (TGMD-2), compared with a group of children without an ID. Specifically, they scored worse on the subtests Gross Motor Quotient, Locomotor, and Object Control. In almost 50% of the subtests, the children with ID had no mastery of that skill and, in comparison with the Finnish normative group, they had a delay in their gross motor development of 3 years. Therefore the authors advise that children with ID need additional fundamental motor skills training in their active schooling or spare time.

MENTAL HEALTH PROBLEMS IN PEOPLE WITH INTELLECTUAL DISABILITY

Given that individuals with ID have difficulties in, inter alia, communication, processing skills and understanding others behaviour, they are more vulnerable to developing a mental disorder when compared with those of average intelligence (Cooper et al., 2007). This corresponds with the results of a British study by Emerson & Hatton (2007). The prevalence of a psychiatric disorder among children with an ID was 36%, compared with 8% among normally developing children. The most frequently seen disorders are autism spectrum disorder and conduct disorders. According to the authors, several factors play a role in the increased prevalence of mental health disorders in children with ID: child characteristics, family characteristics, stressful life events and educational setting.

Child Characteristics

The age of the child is important in relation to the type of psychiatric disorder a child can develop. The younger the child, the more likely it is that they will have a pervasive developmental disorder. Conduct disorders are seen more often in boys than in girls. From the age of 11 years mood disorders are more present in both boys and girls.

Family Characteristics

If a child grows up in a family with a low socioeconomic status, there is an increased risk of developing a conduct disorder; the higher the social class of the family, the lower the likelihood of developing conduct disorders or pervasive developmental disorders. However, there is an increased risk of developing mood disorders (depression, anxiety, etc.).

In addition to the financial state of the family, other characteristics may have an impact on the mental development of the child: being in a single-parent family, dysfunctional family patterns, a caregiver with mental health problems and punitive parenting. These factors make the child more vulnerable to the development of psychiatric disorders.

GENERAL GUIDELINES FOR PHYSICAL ACTIVITY

As mentioned earlier, children with ID experience problems in their motor development. Often they have balance and coordination disorders, and problems with lateralization. Furthermore, their physical fitness is limited and they have lower cardiorespiratory parameters. Therefore cardiovascular training can ensure improvement of these parameters (Lotan et al., 2004). For optimal rehabilitation it is recommended to provide psychomotor therapy to motivate these individuals optimally and, furthermore, to take their decreased learning ability into account.

Next to cardiovascular condition, strength must be taken into account as well. Measurements with isokinetic equipment show a decreased level of strength development. These differences in strength will have been present at a young age and are measured in the quadriceps muscles (Van de Vliet et al., 2006). People with DS perform more poorly on strength tests than their mentally retarded peers (Chia et al., 2002).

Several studies have shown that people with ID have significantly lower levels of physical activity in comparison with healthy peers (Temple & Walkley, 2003; Bartlo & Klein, 2011; Heller et al., 2011). The daily amount of physical activity is associated with the level of impairment: severe impairment corresponds with a low level of daily physical activity. However, despite the level of impairment, even a slight increase in energy expenditure due to physical activity is beneficial for people with ID (Bartlo & Klein, 2011).

It is important to be active, as a lack of movement has negative health outcomes. A lower rate of physical activity is associated with an increased body mass index (BMI), elevated blood sugar level, and an increased risk of cardiovascular diseases, cancer, diabetes mellitus and other chronic diseases. Moreover, it affects muscles and bone structures in a negative way, leading to a higher risk of osteoporosis, sarcopenia and osteoarthritis. Several mental health problems are associated with a lack of movement, including depression, anxiety disorders and sleep problems (Warburton et al., 2006).

A positive relationship has been shown between participation in sports and GMS (Fransen et al., 2012; Wagner et al., 2013; Lloyd et al., 2014). This applies to typically developing children as well as children with an ID (Westendorp et al., 2011). Participating in sports affects the child positively in several domains: physical fitness will increase, overall well-being will be enhanced and social skills will improve. Children with DS who regularly participate in sports activities have an increase in endurance and greater muscle strength in comparison to nonparticipating children with or without a disability (Murphy & Carbone, 2008).

Precautions in Sports Participation for Children With Disabilities

Before a child with mental or physical disability starts a sport, it is advisable to make sure that the activity is adapted to the child's needs and that the necessary precautions are taken. A participation chart is available, which has been developed by the American Academy of Orthopedic Surgeons, in which more information may be found (Wind et al., 2004).

Children with DS may have atlantoaxial instability; therefore it is recommended to obtain radiographs to determine whether this instability is present or not. If it is present, contact sports or sports with the risk of collision are not advisable. Epileptic seizures may also occur in children with disabilities. Therefore it is important to ensure that a child is never alone in water and to monitor a child closely if they are known to have these attacks.

It is important not to exclude children from certain activities, but to try to adapt the situation in such a way that the child is able to participate. Promote the message that child can do sports and motivate the child to be active (Murphy & Carbone, 2008).

Children with DS should be screened for possible heart diseases, because these can be hidden during their daily life. Before a child starts their sport, they should see a cardiologist who can obtain an echocardiogram and if necessary give specialist advice regarding sports participation (Roizen & Patterson, 2003).

Other aspects that must be taken into account are the duration and intensity of the sport. It is recommended that atypically developing children do exercises that are longer in duration, with a greater frequency and with a lower intensity compared with the guidelines for healthy age-matched controls (Durstine et al., 2000).

It is important to be aware of the consequences of some disabilities. Some children have a restricted aerobic capacity, osteoporosis, osteopenia or inefficient thermoregulation (risk of hyperthermia). These factors can cause musculoskeletal injuries. Therefore pay attention to the clothing and equipment of the child and adjust the sports programme to the child's capabilities.

In addition to physical aspects, environmental circumstances are important to consider. A child with an autism spectrum disorder, for example, may have problems with verbal instructions due to a lack of communication skills. Therefore it is advisable to give nonverbal instructions to the child. Take into account the fact that children with ID may not understand what is happening on the field during a team sport. For example, during a game of soccer, much information has to be processed, which is difficult for some children. In addition, the motor skills required are often too complicated for some children to conduct.

IMPROVING PHYSICAL FITNESS

Murphy and Carbone (2008) have designed general guidelines to increase components of health-related fitness: general strength, aerobic endurance, flexibility, bone strength and body composition. These principles are stated on evidence-based findings.

Strength

In people with DS in particular, muscle weakness is a frequently occurring problem. Decreased strength of the quadriceps is associated with reduced functional mobility. The aim of a training programme is to increase muscle mobility and endurance capacity. Calders et al. (2011) have shown that combined training (endurance and strength) has more of an effect than endurance only.

Aerobic Endurance

For children with or without disabilities, aerobic exercises are advisable. This will enhance physical fitness (aerobic capacity) and will influence mood in a positive way, by the release of specific neurotransmitters. In children with specific disabilities it may be necessary to use adapted fitness equipment. These improvements can only be achieved if the child trains sufficiently a minimum of three times a week. Aerobic exercise can be conducted individually or in group sessions, and may include various activities such as walking, running, dancing or swimming (Stanish & Frey, 2008).

It is important to motivate children and young people to be active, as it has been shown that, after an intervention period, participants did not continue their exercise programme (Lotan et al. 2004). In particular, people with ID are externally motivated, and most improvement may be achieved by the use of a token system (Stanish & Frey, 2008). Another option to ensure that children do not stop their sport is to provide physical education classes that are adapted to the child's needs. These classes are important for the maintenance and improvement of a child's physical fitness. In special education schools, physiotherapists can give advice to teachers regarding the optimization and adaptation of sports classes (Murphy & Carbone, 2008).

Flexibility

Muscle tightness and the development of muscle contractures are common problems for people with disabilities. These are generally caused by lack of movement and genetic predisposition. Specific stretching exercises can improve flexibility and decrease muscle tightness. These exercises may be divided into static and dynamic exercises. At the start of training, dynamic stretching is advised, and to finish the session it is recommended that the child perform static stretching exercises. In patients with severe muscle tightness and the presence of muscle contracture, specific equipment is required: splints, orthoses and/or specific chairs (Rimmer et al., 2010).

Bone Strength

People with intellectual and/or somatic disabilities have a low bone mineral density (Dreyfus et al., 2014; Geijer et al., 2014; Gregory et al., 2016). This is due to lack of movement, malnutrition, use of antiepileptic medication, low vitamin D levels and irregularities in skeletal maturation. According to the Physical Activity Guidelines for Americans (US Department of Health and Human Services, 2015), bone-strengthening activities are of great importance for young people. Such exercises can increase bone density and bone mass, and the greatest effect of these sports activities occurs in the years before and during puberty. However, they will also influence bone mineral density and bone mass after puberty.

All the exercises described in the guidelines can be adjusted to the capabilities of an individual child. Elastic stretch bands come in different colours, each representing the resistance of the band. Medicine balls are available in different models (size, weight, etc.). Other high-impact exercises for bone strengthening include rope skipping, basketball, volleyball and running.

When choosing the activity for a particular patient, keep in mind which activity will have the most influence on functioning in daily life. The focus can be on improving either balance, coordination, power or agility. High-impact activities are safe for children with good bony alignment; for those with severe disabilities a paediatrician should be consulted to decide which activities can be performed or which adjustments must be made.

Although some studies have shown promising results, more research is required. Because intervention studies involving high-impact activities are scarce, it is not yet possible to design an optimal training programme and to write clinical recommendations with specific parameters for the type, frequency and duration of an exercise programme (Li et al., 2013).

Gonzalez-Aguero et al. (2010) studied the effects of a twice-weekly exercise programme lasting 21 weeks for children with DS in the age range of 10–19 years. The results of this randomized clinical trial showed that the group that participated in an exercise programme that consisted of resistance training and plyometric exercises had an increase in hip and total bone mineral density. For further information about training programmes, please see Appendix A.

BENEFITS OF SPORTS PARTICIPATION IN CHILDREN WITH INTELLECTUAL DISABILITIES

As mentioned earlier, the execution of object-control skills is assumed to be more complex and require more

cognitive functioning than locomotor skills (Westendorp et al., 2011). While playing sports, the child has to react continuously to the changing situation. During sports, more complex skills are required. In order to react adequately, a certain level of executive functioning is required. For an effective execution of goal-directed plans, a child must have a certain level of executive functioning (Jurado & Roselli, 2007). Because children with borderline and mild ID show deficits in their executive functioning (Vuijk et al., 2010), performance in complex situations is assumed to be difficult for children with ID. It may be, therefore, that children with ID have more problems with object-control skills than with locomotor skills.

To determine a child's motor capabilities, the level of GMS can be assessed by using specific psychomotor measurement tools: Test Gross Motor Development 2 (TGMD-2) or Movement Assessment Battery for Children (Movement ABC). The GMS level is compiled from the results of a physical test, an observational assessment process and an interview regarding sport participation and recreation (Frey & Chow, 2006). The results of these tests can be used either as a starting point for therapeutic goals or as a follow-up during therapy.

TREATMENT APPROACHES

Recent literature primarily addresses ID in children. Most research has been done on developing early-intervention programmes for children with disabilities. For example, in a study by Wang & Ju (2002), physiotherapy interventions were used to improve GMS in young people with ID. The participants undertook balance exercises on balls and air pillows twice a week. The results showed that exercises on unstable surfaces improved deep sensibility in people with mild mental retardation. Furthermore, GMS and quality of life were improved in comparison with the control group. These results imply that physiotherapy interventions are indeed beneficial for people with ID.

Another type of rehabilitation programme for such patients is aimed at improving physical fitness and functional ability, which is, inter alia, described by Lotan et al. (2004) and Li et al. (2013).

In the limited available literature concerning treatment modalities for children with ID, the Treatment and Education of Autistic and Communication Handicapped Children (TEACCH) programme is recommend. This is based on a study by Panerai et al. (2002), in which the effectiveness of the TEACCH programme was compared with that of the classic Italian approach for the integration of children with disabilities in regular schools with support teachers. Based on the results, it can be concluded that the TEACHH programme has more of an effect on GMS and hand–eye coordination than the classic approach. According to the study by Panerai et al. (2002), the TEACCH programme is more effective because it is specifically developed for children with autism and handicapped children. Further research is required to investigate how the improvements can be transferred to daily life skills.

The treatment of mentally disabled children is primarily development orientated and is aimed towards the systematic development of their capabilities, knowledge and personal qualities. The mentally disabled must learn how to live in society. Therefore the main treatment goal is to improve physical fitness and psychological functioning. Adapted sports and exercise programmes are recommend, and team sports in particular will improve physical fitness and enrich the social life of the child.

Treatment Principles

According to the TEACCH programme, there are some cornerstones in treatment for people with ID, of which the first is safety. The environment should be safe for the child, there should be no risk of injury and the patient must have a real chance of success. Environmental factors such as noise, light and temperature play an important role. A cold room will cause hyperactivity, decreased attention and muscle stiffness; hot areas will cause lethargy (sleepiness, indifference). Furthermore, people with learning disabilities are especially sensitive to the factor of space, and especially their interpersonal space. Smaller spaces and a limited number of players are preferred. Because the learning capabilities are restricted, many repetitions are preferred, combined with feedback from the therapist. However, the patient must not be underestimated, because this will lead to a lack of confidence in the therapist and a decrease in the patient's motivation.

Furthermore, attention should be paid to following treatment modalities; for example, adjusting the rules if the game is too complicated or too simple. If the game is not at the level of the patient, they will be easily distracted. The senses may be stimulated by adjusting the material, for example by using sounds, bright colours, very tiny balls or very large balls.

As mentioned earlier, the improvement of physical fitness is important for people with ID, both for the physical condition as well social cohesion. The treatment should be adjusted to the needs of the individual. General principles in the treatment include: exercise to correct their posture, muscle strengthening, stretching and practising gross and fine motor skills. Children with ID should be encouraged to move a lot, as this is important for their psychomotor, psychological, physiological, cognitive and affective development. Furthermore, exercise contributes to the development of their intellectual and social abilities, and helps them to discover and get to know their bodies.

The role of the therapist is important in the treatment: they must be enthusiastic, happy, motivated and willing to make time to help the mentally handicapped. Every relationship has to be at the maximum level, because the mentally handicapped person will only consider the therapist as a partner and a friend if they show personal interest in them. How a mentally handicapped person learns new things depends on their past experiences, which may be only failures; this means that if a new situation is presented, the person will expect to fail. Motivation comes rather from the desire to avoid failures than from the will to succeed. In practice, people with ID require four times more motivation than the general population.

CONCLUSION

In the rehabilitation of children with ID, attention should be paid to the adjustment of the treatment room (with regard to temperature, light, noise, etc.). Furthermore, the treatment should be adjusted to the patient's needs and the goals should be established in consultation with the patient or caregiver.

REFERENCES

Bartlo, P., Klein, P.J., 2011. Physical activity benefits and needs in adults with intellectual disabilities: Systematic review of the literature. Am. J. Intellect. Dev. Disabil. 116 (3), 220–232.

Calders, P., Elmahgoub, S., de Mettelinge, T.R., et al., 2011. Effect of combined exercise training on physical and metabolic fitness in adults with intellectual disability: A controlled trial. Clin. Rehabil. 25 (12), 1097–1108.

Capio, C.M., Sit, C.H., Eguia, K.F., et al., 2015. Fundamental movement skills training to promote physical activity in children with and without disability: A pilot study. J. Sport Health Sci. 4 (3), 235–243.

Chia, Y.H.M., Lee, K.S., Teo-Koh, S.M., 2002. High intensity cycling performances of boys with and without intellectual disability. J. Intellect. Dev. Disabil. 27 (3), 191–200.

Cooper, S.A., Smiley, E., Morrison, J., et al., 2007. Mental ill-health in adults with intellectual disabilities: Prevalence and associated factors. Br. J. Psychiatry 190 (1), 27–35.

De Winter, C.F., Jansen, A.A.C., Evenhuis, H.M., 2011. Physical conditions and challenging behaviour in people with intellectual disability: A systematic review. J. Intellect. Disabil. Res. 55 (7), 675–698.

Dreyfus, D., Lauer, E., Wilkinson, J., 2014. Characteristics associated with bone mineral density screening in adults with intellectual disabilities. J. Am. Board. Fam. Med. 27 (1), 104–114.

Durstine, J.L., Painter, P., Franklin, B.A., et al., 2000. Physical activity for the chronically ill and disabled. Sports Med. 30 (3), 207–219.

Emerson, E., 2003. Prevalence of psychiatric disorders in children and adolescents with and without intellectual disability. J. Intellect. Disabil. Res. 47 (1), 51–58.

Emerson, E., Hatton, C., 2007. Mental health of children and adolescents with intellectual disabilities in Britain. Br. J. Psychiatry 191 (6), 493–499.

Fransen, J., Pion, J., Vandendriessche, J., et al., 2012. Differences in physical fitness and gross motor coordination in boys aged 6–12 years specializing in one versus sampling more than one sport. J. Sports Sci. 30 (4), 379–386.

Frey, G.C., Chow, B., 2006. Relationship between BMI, physical fitness, and motor skills in youth with mild intellectual disabilities. Int. J. Obes. 30 (5), 861–867.

Geijer, J.R., Stanish, H.I., Draheim, C.C., Dengel, D.R., 2014. Bone mineral density in adults with Down syndrome, intellectual disability, and nondisabled adults. Am. J. Intellect. Dev. Disabil. 119 (2), 107–114.

González-Agüero, A., Vicente-Rodríguez, G., Moreno, L.A., et al., 2010. Health-related physical fitness in children and adolescents with Down syndrome and response to training. Scand. J. Med. Sci. Sports 20 (5), 716–724.

Gregory, C.R., Stedge, H.L., Brandenburg, R.K., 2016. Effects of antiepileptic medications on bone density in individuals with intellectual and developmental disabilities. April 20, 2016. The Research and Scholarship Symposium, Paper10. <http://digital-commons.cedarville.edu/research_scholarship_symposium/2016/poster_presentations/10>.

Heller, T., McCubbin, J.A., Drum, C., Peterson, J., 2011. Physical activity and nutrition health promotion interventions: What is working for people with intellectual disabilities? Intellect. Dev. Disabil. 49 (1), 26–36.

Hocking, J., McNeil, J., Campbell, J., 2016. Physical therapy interventions for gross motor skills in people with an intellectual disability aged 6 years and over: A systematic review. Int. J. Evidence Based Healthcare 14 (3), 102–103.

Jurado, M.B., Roselli, M., 2007. The elusive nature of executive functions: A review of our current understanding. Neuropsychol. Rev. 17, 213–233.

Li, C., Chen, S., How, Y.M., Zhang, A.L., 2013. Benefits of physical exercise intervention on fitness of individuals with Down syndrome: A systematic review of randomized-controlled trials. Int. J. Rehabil. Res. 36 (3), 187–195.

Lloyd, M., Saunders, T.J., Bremer, E., Tremblay, M.S., 2014. Long-term importance of fundamental motor skills: A 20-year follow-up study. Adapt. Phys. Activ. Q. 31 (1), 67–78.

Lotan, M., Isakov, E., Kessel, S., Merrick, J., 2004. Physical fitness and functional ability of children with intellectual disability: Effects of a short-term daily treadmill intervention. Sci. World J. 4, 449–457.

Murphy, N.A., Carbone, P.S., 2008. Promoting the participation of children with disabilities in sports, recreation, and physical activities. Pediatrics 121 (5), 1057–1061.

Owen, M.J., 2012. Intellectual disability and major psychiatric disorders: A continuum of neurodevelopmental causality. Br. J. Psychiatry 200 (4), 268–269.

Panerai, S., Ferrante, L., Zingale, M., 2002. Benefits of the Treatment and Education of Autistic and Communication Handicapped Children (TEACCH) programme as compared with a non-specific approach. J. Intellect. Disabil. Res. 46 (4), 318–327.

Pulver, A.E., Nestadt, G., Goldberg, R., et al., 1994. Psychotic illness in patients diagnosed with velo-cardio-facial syndrome and their relatives. J. Nerv. Ment. Dis. 182 (8), 476–477.

Rimmer, J.H., Chen, M.D., McCubbin, J.A., et al., 2010. Exercise intervention research on persons with disabilities: What we know and where we need to go. Am. J. Phys. Med. Rehabil. 89 (3), 249–263.

Rintala, P., Loovis, E.M., 2013. Measuring motor skills in Finnish children with intellectual disabilities 1, 2. Percept. Mot. Skills 116 (1), 294–303.

Roizen, N.J., Patterson, D., 2003. Down's syndrome. Lancet 361 (9365), 1281–1289.

Stanish, H.I., Frey, G.C., 2008. Promotion of physical activity in individuals with intellectual disability. Salud Pública de México 50, s178–s184.

Tanaka, H., Monahan, K.D., Seals, D.R., 2001. Age-predicted maximal heart rate revisited. J. Am. Coll. Cardiol. 37 (1), 153–156.

Temple, V.A., Walkley, J.W., 2003. Physical activity of adults with intellectual disability. J. Intellect. Dev. Disabil. 28 (4), 342–353.

US Department of Health and Human Services, 2015. Physical Activity Guidelines for Americans: Be Active, Healthy, and Happy! Physical Activity Guidelines Advisory Committee, Physical Activity Guidelines Advisory Committee Report 2008, Washington, DC.

Van de Vliet, P., Rintala, P., Fröjd, K., et al., 2006. Physical fitness profile of elite athletes with intellectual disability. Scand. J. Med. Sci. Sports 16 (6), 417–425.

Vuijk, P.J., Hartman, E., Scherder, E., Visscher, C., 2010. Motor performance of children with mild intellectual disability and borderline intellectual functioning. J. Intellect. Disabil. Res. 54 (11), 955–965.

Wagner, M.O., Haibach, P.S., Lieberman, L.J., 2013. Gross motor skill performance in children with and without visual impairments—Research to practice. Res. Dev. Disabil. 34 (10), 3246–3252.

Wang, W.Y., Ju, Y.H., 2002. Promoting balance and jumping skills in children with Down syndrome. Percept. Mot. Skills 94 (2), 443–448.

Warburton, D.E., Nicol, C.W., Bredin, S.S., 2006. Health benefits of physical activity: the evidence. Can. Med. Assoc. J. 174 (6), 801–809.

Westendorp, M., Houwen, S., Hartman, E., Visscher, C., 2011. Are gross motor skills and sports participation related in children with intellectual disabilities? Res. Dev. Disabil. 32 (3), 1147–1153.

Wind, W.M., Schwend, R.M., Larson, J., 2004. Sports for the physically challenged child. J. Am. Acad. Orthop. Surg. 12 (2), 126–137.

APPENDIX A

Strength Training

The weight of the strength exercise is based on one repetition maximum (1 RM). As a start position, 70% of 1 RM is used, and as soon this is established there will be an increase of 10% each week. Each strength exercise consists of 1–3 sets of 7–8 repetitions.

Seven basic strength exercises were used during session: knee extension, knee flexion, ankle plantar flexion, hip extension, hip abduction, trunk flexion (abdominals), and trunk extension (erector spine).

Aerobic Endurance

The aerobic training programme is based on the ventilator anaerobic threshold (VAT), which can be assessed during an aerobic exercise test. Be aware that the rule of thumb to measure maximum heart rate (220–age) is not applicable for children with Down syndrome. For children, following formula can be used: $[208 - (0.7 \times \text{Age})]$ (Tanaka et al. 2001). At the start of the training, the patient will train at 90% of VAT and this will increase to 100% after 10 sessions and to 110% after 20 sessions.

To perform aerobic exercises correctly, the training intensity is important. A commonly used method is the Borg Scale of perceived exertion. For training with children, the Children's OMNI Scale of Perceived Exertion (OMNI Scale) or Perceived Exertion Index with Faces (PEIF) can be used.

According to American guidelines, deconditioned young people who cannot sustain aerobic activity for more than 10 minutes should work at an exercise intensity of 5–6 on the Children's OMNI Scale of Perceived Exertion (OMNI Scale). After the physical performance of the child has improved, the amount of training sessions can increase from 2 to 4 or more days per week.

The Progressive Aerobic Cardiovascular Endurance Run (PACER) or shuttle-run tests have been developed specifically for young people without disabilities, as well as for young people with intellectual disabilities, visual impairments or other disabilities with mild physical impairment.

Flexibility

These exercises can be divided into static and dynamic exercises. At the start of the training session dynamic exercises are advised, and to finish the training it is recommended to perform static exercises. In patients with severe muscle tightness and the presence of muscle contracture, specific equipment is required: splints, orthoses and/or specific chairs.

The dynamic stretching exercises are as follows:

Joint Rotation

Standing loose and flexed, extend and rotate the joints: wrists, elbows, shoulders and shoulder blades, hips, knees, ankles, feet and toes. In patients with balance problems, assistance is recommended. This can be by support of a physiotherapist or using a chair to maintain balance.

Shoulder Circles

While standing with knees slightly bent and feet shoulder width apart, raise the shoulder towards the ear and rotate it clockwise and counterclockwise. Make sure that the shoulder muscles are relaxed and the movement is smooth. Repeat with the other shoulder.

Arm Swings

Use the same standing position as with the shoulder circles. Move the arms over the head, down and back. After repeating 6–10 times, bring the arms in front of the chest and swing the arms across the body and away from the body.

Side Bends

Stand tall with the knees slightly bent and move the bodyweight from one leg to the other leg. Pull the trunk up and away from the hips and bend to the side with the weight-bearing leg. After repeating 6–10 times, repeat the movement in the other direction. Make sure that the movement is going in one direction, without leaning forwards or backwards, only moving sideways.

Hip Twists

Extend the arms out to the sides, and twist the torso and hips to the left, shifting the bodyweight onto the left foot. Twist the torso to the right while shifting the bodyweight to the right foot. Do 6–10 repetitions on each side.

Half Squats

Stand steady with the feet pointing forward and bring the hands in front of you at shoulder width. Bend the knees until the thighs are making an angle of 45° with the floor. Keep the back long throughout the movement and look straight forwards. Make sure that the knees are not beyond the toes. Once reaching the lowest point, fully straighten the legs to return to the starting position. This movement should be repeated 12–16 times; breathe in while descending and breathe out while ascending.

Bone Strengthening

The training consists of:

- Jumps: standing vertical jump, jump with run-in, drop jump (height between 40 and 50 cm) drop jump + horizontal jump (height jumped between 40 and 50 cm)
- Push-up against the wall (3 sets of 10 repetitions)
- Exercises with elastic-fitness bands:
  (a) lateral row
  (b) biceps curls: 3 sets of 12 repetitions
  (c) frontal row
- Exercises with medicine balls: while standing, throwing and catching medicine balls.

PHYSIOTHERAPY FOR ELDERLY

5.4.1 Physical Activity in People With Dementia: Clinical Recommendations for Physiotherapists

DAVY VANCAMPFORT ■ ANDREW SOUNDY ■ BRENDON STUBBS

SUMMARY

Dementia *is an umbrella term for a number of progressive brain disorders that affect memory, thinking, behaviour and the ability to perform everyday activities. Recent evidence shows that there is a consistent relationship between higher physical activity levels and a reduced risk of developing dementia, and for those already suffering with dementia physical activity may have a significant impact on improving cognitive functioning and the ability to perform activities of daily living. In this chapter, we aim to clarify why physical activity is beneficial for this vulnerable population and provide specific recommendations for the daily clinical practice.*

KEY POINTS

- Physical activity is beneficial in the prevention and management of dementia.
- Fall prevention is crucial in the multidisciplinary treatment of dementia.
- Research is needed to be able to develop physical activity guidelines that would be helpful to physiotherapists in advising patients with dementia at earlier and later stages of the disease.

LEARNING OBJECTIVES

- Be able to explain why physical activity is important for people with dementia.
- To gain insight in potential mechanisms for the benefits of physical activity on cognition in patients with dementia.
- Understand why motivating people with dementia towards an active lifestyle is challenging.

DEMENTIA: THE FACTS

Dementia is an umbrella term for a number of progressive brain disorders that affect memory, thinking, behaviour and the ability to perform everyday activities (American Psychiatric Association, 2013). It is a heterogeneous condition with many different subcategories of which Alzheimer disease is the most common form and may contribute towards 60%–80% of cases (Fratiglioni et al., 1999). Other major forms include vascular dementia, dementia with Lewy bodies (abnormal aggregates of protein that develop inside nerve cells) and a group of diseases that contribute to fronto-temporal dementia (degeneration of the frontal lobe of the brain) (American Psychiatric Association, 2013). The boundaries between the different forms of dementia are indistinct and mixed forms often coexist (Schneider et al., 2007).

In 2010, the global number of individuals with dementia was estimated at 35.6 million (Prince et al., 2013). This number is estimated to increase to 115.4 million by 2050, unless effective reductions of the incidence of dementia can be implemented (Alzheimer's Disease International, 2010). The World Alzheimer Report 2010 also estimates that ageing of the global population will make the economic effect of dementia greater than that of cancer, heart disease and stroke combined (Alzheimer's Disease International, 2010). This is not surprising since the inherent cognitive decline observed in all forms of dementia is associated with profound loss of independence, increased falls risk, a reduction in the capacity to undertake activities of daily living, nursing home admission and increased premature mortality (Pitkälä et al., 2013; Prince et al., 2013; Smith et al., 2013). For these reasons, the prevention and management of dementia is an international health priority (Prince et al., 2013). Nevertheless, no effective pharmaceutical treatment of dementia is currently available (Cooper et al., 2013). Epidemiological work has, however, identified a number of modifiable factors that are associated with increased risk of dementia (Weinstein et al., 2013). Cardiovascular risk factors such as hypertension, hypercholesterolaemia, a high body mass index and a sedentary lifestyle have been associated with incidence of dementia (Gorelick et al., 2011; Weinstein et al., 2013). Moreover, in total, up to half of all dementia cases may be attributable to physical inactivity and associated cardiovascular factors (Barnes &Yaffe, 2011).

THE IMPORTANCE OF PHYSICAL ACTIVITY IN THE TREATMENT OF DEMENTIA

Epidemiological research shows a consistent relationship between higher physical activity levels and a reduced risk of developing dementia (Yaffe et al., 2001; Sattler et al., 2011; Buchman et al., 2012). In a meta-analysis of 16 prospective, epidemiological studies on the incidence of neurodegenerative disease, engaging in more physical activity reduced the risk of developing all-cause dementia by 28% and of developing Alzheimer disease by 45%, even after controlling for confounding variables (Hamer & Chida, 2009). Future studies should examine the optimal dose of physical activity to induce protection, which presently remains unclear. Considering the protective effects of physical activity, it is not a surprise that within recent years interest has risen in physical activity as an effective nonpharmacological intervention in the prevention and management of dementia (Ahlskog et al., 2011). A recent systematic review and meta-analysis (Forbes et al., 2013) suggests that physical activity may have a significant impact on improving cognitive functioning and the ability to perform activities of daily living in people with dementia. Other recent research established that physical activity interventions can reduce falls among people with cognitive impairment (Guo et al., 2013) and also reduce total healthcare costs (Pitkälä et al., 2013). This has strengthened the need to promote physical activity in this population although this is often complex and requires skilled individuals to lead this (Malthouse & Fox, 2014).

POTENTIAL MECHANISMS FOR THE BENEFITS OF PHYSICAL ACTIVITY ON COGNITION IN PATIENTS WITH DEMENTIA

The potential mechanisms by which physical activity may improve cognitive function are likely through changes at systemic and molecular levels (Ratey & Loehr, 2011). Higher levels of physical activity and greater fitness tend to have greater hippocampal volume that may contribute to the reported improvements in attention and memory-related cognitive tasks (Erickson et al., 2009). Physical activity may also help to protect dementia disease through increasing cerebral blood flow. Recent evidence has shown a strong association between lower central carotid artery stiffness, an improved cognitive function and a higher aerobic fitness (Tarumi et al., 2013). On a molecular level, physical activity may improve cognitive function through its ability to increase neurotrophins and growth factors in the brain, notably brain-derived neurotropic factor, insulin-like growth factor-1 and vascular endothelial growth factor, all of which help to facilitate cognitive function through changes at the cellular level, including synaptic plasticity, neurogenesis and vascular function (Voss et al., 2013). In Alzheimer disease itself, the strongest evidence for the beneficial brain effects of physical activity is the research showing that physical activity results in a marked decrease in the cortical accumulation of amyloid-β peptides, which is considered one of the hallmark signs of Alzheimer disease (Stranahan et al., 2012). Taken together, there are strong indications that physical activity provides a powerful stimulus that can counteract systemic and molecular changes underlying the progressive loss of hippocampal function in dementia.

CHALLENGES WHEN MOTIVATING PATIENTS WITH DEMENTIA TOWARDS PHYSICAL ACTIVITY

Despite the beneficial findings for incorporating physical activity in the multidisciplinary treatment of dementia, there remain concerns that people with dementia are physically inactive (James et al., 2012). Therefore there is a need to identify the factors affecting the uptake of physical activity within this population (Forbes et al., 2013). Understanding the barriers and facilitators to participation in physical activity in people with dementia is essential in order to ensure that people with dementia obtain any health benefits. A recent review (Stubbs et al., 2014) demonstrated that within dementia factors such as polypharmacotherapy, difficulties in activities of daily living and the functional decline might be more pertinent barriers than an impaired cognition. There is also evidence that a history of falls was negatively associated with physical activity participation. This highlights the challenge that clinicians face when people with dementia start to develop slow walking speed, their falls risk increases and they actually start falling. Clearly the promotion of physical activity in this group requires careful consideration, and skilled clinicians and physiotherapists are ideally placed to lead in the promotion

of physical activity in people with dementia. Physiotherapists have the necessary skills to consider the typical mental and physical health barriers seen in this group.

GENERAL RECOMMENDATIONS FOR PRESCRIBING PHYSICAL ACTIVITY TO ELDERLY WITH DEMENTIA

It is recommended that people with dementia who are confronted with chronic conditions develop an activity plan in consultation with a physiotherapist so that the plan adequately takes into account therapeutic and risk-management issues related to chronic conditions (Stubbs et al., 2014). The plan should be tailored according to chronic conditions and activity limitations, risk for falls, individual abilities and the current physical fitness status. With sufficient skill, experience, fitness, and training, people with dementia can achieve considerable levels of physical activity and thus achieve the multiple benefits. The observation that increasing age is not a barrier to physical activity participation (Stubbs et al., 2014) indicates that, regardless of age, all people with dementia can engage in physical activity. The promotion of physical activity in people with dementia should therefore avoid ageism that discourages older adults from reaching their potential. In some long-term care facilities there is often an ingrained attitude among healthcare workers that sitting down and resting is the best thing for older adults with dementia. This is particularly the case for those who are at risk of falls and physiotherapists may also have to work with other healthcare professionals (such as nursing staff and occupational therapists) and caregivers to optimize the promotion of physical activity in this group. At the same time, physiotherapists should take into account that it is difficult or even impossible for some people with dementia to attain high levels of activity and the physiotherapists should use their clinical skills to develop appropriate adaptations. There is, however, substantial evidence that people with dementia who do less than the recommended levels of physical activity still achieve some health benefits. Physical activity should be increased or maintained gradually (Rimmer, 2003) and caregivers should form an important part of the plan in order to make this successful (Malthouse & Fox, 2014). This advice minimizes risk of overuse injury, makes increasing activity more pleasant and allows positive reinforcement for small steps that lead to the attainment of intermediate goals. It can be appropriate for people with dementia to spend a longer time at one step (e.g., attending exercise, yoga and/or tai chi classes 2 or 3 days per week) to gain experience, fitness and self-confidence. Very deconditioned people with dementia may need to exercise initially at less effort and may need to perform activity in multiple bouts (for example 5–10 minutes) rather than in a single continuous bout. In addition, physical activity plans need to be reevaluated when there are changes in health status and need to be tailored considering the disease stage.

EXAMPLES OF PHYSICAL ACTIVITIES THAT CAN BE IMPLEMENTED IN THE EARLIER STAGES OF DEMENTIA

Outdoor Activities

Physiotherapists can support people with dementia in the earlier stages of the disease to participate in local community or sports centres, which often provide a range of organized exercise and physical activity sessions suitable for deconditioned elderly. Barriers for participation in these local settings should be explored and strategies to cope with barriers should be implemented in a clinical action plan. In addition to community activities, walking and gardening provide good forms of physical activity (Alzheimer's Society, 2013). Walking and gardening are also physical activities that provide an opportunity to get outdoors (Stern & Konno, 2009; Littbrand et al., 2011). Gardening can be varied to suit the person's abilities from general tidying to weeding, raking up leaves and watering plants. It has been reported previously that gardening is enjoyed by many people with dementia (Stern & Konno, 2009; Littbrand et al., 2011). If a person with dementia does not have a garden, tending to indoor plants or flowers can be enjoyable for dementia sufferers also (Lee & Kim, 2008).

Indoor Activities

Next to outdoor activities, indoor ball games also show beneficial psychosocial effects. For example, a study by Graessel et al. (2011) indicates that people with dementia may retain their bowling skills or continue to participate in other ball games such as croquet, and so may enjoy indoor carpet bowls or skittles. Physiotherapists could also use dance as a therapeutic medium. Dancing to music in dementia can range from structured dances, and couple or group sessions, to more improvised movement involving ribbons, balloons or balls (Alzheimer's Society, 2013). Dancing to music can also be done in a seated position. Music can trigger past memories and emotions, which can be shared (Mc Dermott et al., 2014). Dancing is a very social activity and an enjoyable way to participate in exercise. Dancing may also improve gait, balance and reduce the risk of falls in people with dementia (Granacher et al., 2012). Finally, sufficient evidence is available for the use of tai chi and qigong in the treatment of dementia (Tadros et al., 2013). Both are gentle forms of Chinese martial arts that combine simple physical movements and meditation. These forms of physical activity focus on balance and stability, which are important in staying agile, and may reduce the risk of falls (Guo et al., 2013).

Structured Exercise Programmes

Patients with dementia will experience many health benefits when participating in a regular structured exercise programme. These exercises are aimed at building or maintaining muscle strength and balance and can also be performed in a seated position, which is less strenuous than exercises in a standing position. Some examples of seated exercises include marching, turning the body from side to side, raising the heels and toes, bending the arms, bending the legs, clapping under the legs, bicycling the legs, making circles with the arms, raising the opposite arm and leg and practising moving from sitting to standing (Alzheimer's Society, 2013). The promotion of structured exercise programmes may help to prevent the inherent progression of frailty and ultimately dependence. Current exercise recommendations for patients with Alzheimer disease (Rimmer, et al. 2003) are based on clinical experiences and practicality. These include aerobic exercise on 5 days per week at 10 minutes per session at a slow intensity. Progression should aim for 10 to 15 minutes per day and 5 to 7 days per week. Strength and resistance should be considered 3 days per week with one set of 10 to 12 repetitions using a theraband, and all exercises should be completed within 10 to 15 minutes. Progression from a seated position to a standing position should be an aim and an increase to three sets of 12 repetitions over 3 to 6 weeks is recommended (Rimmer, 2003). Further research is, however, highly needed in order to identify the optimal physical activity modalities, particularly in terms of frequency, intensity, type and duration for patients with different types and severity of dementia.

EXAMPLES OF PHYSICAL ACTIVITIES THAT CAN BE IMPLEMENTED IN THE LATER STAGES OF DEMENTIA

Physical activity can also be beneficial in the later stages of dementia. It may help to reduce the need for more supported care and minimize the adaptations needed to the home or surroundings. Exercises can range from changing position from sitting to standing, walking a short distance into another room or moving to sit in a different chair at each mealtime throughout the day. Some suggested exercises in the later stages of dementia are (Alzheimer's Society, 2013):

- When getting up or going to bed, the patient could move along the edge of the bed, in the sitting position, until the end is reached. This helps exercise the muscles needed for standing up from a chair.
- Balance in a standing position. This can be done holding onto a support if necessary. This exercise helps with balance and posture and can form part of everyday activities such as when showering or doing the washing up.
- Sit unsupported for a few minutes each day (under supervision of the physiotherapist in order to reduce the risk of falling). This exercise helps to strengthen the stomach and back muscles used to support posture.
- Stand up and move regularly. Moving regularly helps to keep leg muscles strong and maintain good balance.

People in the later stages of dementia should be encouraged to move about regularly and change chairs, for example, when having a drink or a meal. There should be opportunities to sit unsupported with supervision on a daily basis. A daily routine involving moving around the home can help to maintain muscle strength and joint flexibility. Muscle-strengthening exercises are particularly important in people with dementia in a later stage of their disease, given its role in preventing a loss of muscle mass, bone and its beneficial effects on functional limitations and reducing the risk for falling.

PHYSIOTHERAPISTS SHOULD HAVE A PIVOTAL ROLE IN THE ASSESSMENT AND MANAGEMENT OF CLINICAL PAIN IN PEOPLE WITH DEMENTIA

It is estimated that at least of 50% of individuals with dementia experience clinical pain, although the prevalence may be substantially higher in people living in long-term institutions (Achterberg et al., 2013). This may be a gross underestimate as there are great difficulties in conducting accurate pain assessment in this population. Physiotherapists may help in the multidisciplinary assessment of pain and can draw upon a range of physiotherapeutic techniques to provide non-pharmacological pain relief from any pain that individuals may experience.

CONCLUSION

There is scientific evidence that suggests that physical activity could have a significant impact on improving cognitive functioning and ability to perform activities of daily living in people with dementia. Physiotherapists who work with people with dementia should feel confident in promoting physical activity among this population, as decreasing the progression of cognitive decline and dependence in activities of daily living will have significant mental and physical health benefits, and possibly delay the need for placement in long-term care settings. However, there is currently insufficient scientific evidence to determine which type of physical activity (aerobic, strength training, balance) and what frequency and duration is most beneficial for specific types and severity of dementia. Clearly further research is needed to be able to develop best practice guidelines that would be helpful to physiotherapists in advising patients with dementia at earlier and later stages of the disease.

REFERENCES

Achterberg, W.P., Pieper, M.J., van Dalen-Kok, A.H., et al., 2013. Pain management in patients with dementia. Clin. Interv. Aging 8, 1471–1482.

American Psychiatric Association, 2013. Diagnostic and Statistical Manual of Mental Disorders, fifth ed. American Psychiatric Association, Washington DC.

Alzheimer's Disease International, 2010. World Alzheimer Report 2010. *The global economic impact of dementia.* Alzheimer's Disease International, London.

Alzheimer's Society, 2013. Exercise and physical activity for people with dementia. Alzheimer's Society, London.

Ahlskog, J.E., Geda, Y.E., Graff-Radford, N.R., Petersen, R.C., 2011. Physical exercise as a preventive or disease-modifying treatment of dementia and brain aging. Mayo Clin. Proc. 86 (9), 876–884.

Barnes, D.E., Yaffe, K., 2011. The projected effect of risk factor reduction on Alzheimer's disease prevalence. Lancet Neurol. 10, 819–828.

Buchman, A.S., Boyle, P.A., Yu, L., et al., 2012. Total daily physical activity and the risk of AD and cognitive decline in older adults. Neurology 78, 1323–1329.

Cooper, C., Mukadam, N., Katona, C., et al., 2013. Systematic review of the effectiveness of pharmacologic interventions to improve quality of life and well-being in people with dementia. Am. J. Geriatr. Psychiatry 21 (2), 173–183.

Erickson, K.I., Prakash, R.S., Voss, M.W., et al., 2009. Aerobic fitness is associated with hippocampal volume in elderly humans. Hippocampus 19, 1030–1039.

Forbes, D., Thiessen, E.J., Blake, C.M., et al., 2013. Exercise programs for people with dementia. Cochrane Database Syst. Rev. (12), CD006489.

Fratiglioni, L., De Ronchi, D., Agüero-Torres, H., 1999. Worldwide prevalence and incidence of dementia. Drugs Aging 15, 365–375.

Gorelick, P.B., Scuteri, A., Black, S.E., et al., 2011. Vascular contributions to cognitive impairment and dementia: a statement for healthcare professionals from the american heart association/ american stroke association. Stroke 42 (9), 2672–2713.

Graessel, E., Stemmer, R., Eichenseer, B., et al., 2011. Non-pharmacological, multicomponent group therapy in patients with degenerative dementia: a 12-month randomized, controlled trial. BMC Med. 9, 129.

Granacher, U., Muehlbauer, T., Bridenbaugh, S.A., et al., 2012. Effects of a salsa dance training on balance and strength performance in older adults. Gerontology 58 (4), 305–312.

Guo, J.L., Tsai, Y.Y., Liao, J.Y., et al., 2013. Interventions to reduce the number of falls among older adults with/without cognitive impairment: an exploratory meta-analysis. Int. J. Geriatr. Psychiatry.

Hamer, M., Chida, Y., 2009. Physical activity and risk of neurodegenerative disease: a systematic review of prospective evidence. Psychol. Med. 39, 3–11.

James, B.D., Boyle, P.A., Bennett, D.A., Buchman, A.S., 2012. Total daily activity measured with actigraphy and motor function in community-dwelling older persons with and without dementia. Alzheimer Dis. Assoc. Disord. 26 (3), 238–245.

Lee, Y., Kim, S., 2008. Effects of indoor gardening on sleep, agitation, and cognition in dementia patients-a pilot study. Int. J. Geriatr. Psychiatry 23 (5), 485–489.

Littbrand, H., Stenvall, M., Rosendahl, E., 2011. Applicability and effects of physical exercise on physical and cognitive functions and activities of daily living among people with dementia: a systematic review. Am. J. Phys. Med. Rehabil. 90 (6), 495–518.

Malthouse, R., Fox, F., 2014. Exploring experiences of physical activity among people with Alzheimer's disease and their spouse carers: a qualitative study. Physiotherapy 100 (2), 169–175. doi: 10.1016/j.physio.2013.10.002.

Pitkälä, K., Savikko, N., Poysti, M., et al., 2013. Efficacy of physical exercise intervention on mobility and physical functioning in older people with dementia: a systematic review. Exp. Gerontol. 48 (1), 85–93.

Prince, M., Bryce, R., Albanese, E., et al., 2013. The global prevalence of dementia: a systematic review and meta-analysis. Alzheimers Dement. 9 (1), 63–75.

Ratey, J.J., Loehr, J.E., 2011. The positive impact of physical activity on cognition during adulthood: a review of underlying mechanisms, evidence and recommendations. Rev. Neurosci. 22, 171–185.

Rimmer, J.H., 2003. Alzheimer's Disease. In: Durstine, J.L., Moore, G.E. (Eds.), ACSM's exercise management for persons with chronic diseases and disabilities, second ed. Human Kinetics, Champaign, USA.

Sattler, C., Erickson, K.I., Toro, P., Schröder, J., 2011. Physical fitness as a protective factor for cognitive impairment in a prospective population-based study in Germany. J. Alzheimers Dis. 26, 709–718.

Schneider, J.A., Arvanitakis, Z., Bang, W., Bennett, D.A., 2007. Mixed brain pathologies account for most dementia cases in community dwelling older persons. Neurology 69, 2197–2204.

Smith, J.C., Nielson, K.A., Woodard, J.L., et al., 2013. Physical activity and brain function in older adults at increased risk for Alzheimer's disease. Brain Sci. 3, 54–83.

Stern, C., Konno, R., 2009. Physical leisure activities and their role in preventing dementia: a systematic review. Int. J. Evid. Based Healthc. 7 (4), 270–282.

Stranahan, A.M., Martin, B., Maudsley, S., 2012. Anti-inflammatory effects of physical activity in relationship to improved cognitive status in humans and mouse models of Alzheimer's disease. Curr. Alzheimer Res. 9 (1), 86–92.

Stubbs, B., Eggermont, L., Soundy, A., et al. (2014). What are the factors associated with physical activity (PA) participation in community dwelling adults with dementia? A systematic review of PA correlates. Arch. Gerontol. Geriatr 59 (2), 195–203.

Tadros, G., Ormerod, S., Dobson-Smyth, P., et al., 2013. The management of behavioural and psychological symptoms of dementia in residential homes: does Tai Chi have any role for people with dementia? Dementia 12 (2), 268–279.

Tarumi, T., Gonzales, M.M., Fallow, B., et al., 2013. Central artery stiffness, neuropsychological function, and cerebral perfusion in sedentary and endurance-trained middle-aged adults. J. Hypertens. 31 (12), 2400–2409.

Voss, M.W., Erickson, K.I., Prakash, R.S., et al., 2013. Neurobiological markers of exercise-related brain plasticity in older adults. Brain Behav. Immun. 28, 90–99.

Weinstein, G., Wolf, P.A., Beiser, A.S., et al., 2013. Risk estimations, risk factors, and genetic variants associated with Alzheimer's disease in selected publications from the Framingham Heart Study. J. Alzheimers Dis. 33 (Suppl. 1), 439–445.

Yaffe, K., Barnes, D., Nevitt, M., et al., 2001. A prospective study of physical activity and cognitive decline in elderly women: women who walk. Arch. Intern. Med. 161, 1703–1708. doi:10.1001/archinte.161.14.1703.

5.4.2   Pain Assessment in People With Dementia

LAUREN FORDHAM

SUMMARY

This chapter is concerned with the recognition of pain in people with dementia and aims to provide a balanced presentation of the evidence available. The chapter will examine issues relating to the British national guidelines for pain assessment. Topics will also include concepts of pain and dementia, models of care and outcome measures.

KEY POINTS

■ Dementia

■ Cognitive impairment

■ Pain

■ Assessment

BACKGROUND

The term *dementia* has been described as pertaining to 'loss of memory, mood changes and problems with communication and reasoning' (Alzheimer's Society, 2012a, p. 4). In the United Kingdom, 800,000 people have been diagnosed with dementia and this is predicted to increase to over a million by 2025 (Dementia Action Alliance, 2010; Alzheimer's Society, 2012a). The incidence of dementia increases with age and so the population with dementia also frequently experience physiological pain as a result of physical ailments common to older people, such as stiffness in the joints (Zekry et al., 2008). The research indicates that between 47% and 66% of people with dementia also experience pain (Ferrell, Ferrell et al., 1995; Feldt et al., 1998; Zwakhalen et al., 2009). The International Association for the Study of Pain (2012) defines pain as 'an unpleasant sensory and emotional experience', and Kaasalainen offers the following definition, pertaining to pain in people with dementia, 'an unpleasant subjective experience that can be communicated to others either through self-report, when possible, or through a set of pain-related behaviours' (Kaasalainen, 2007, p. 571). The most common causes of pain in older people include osteoarthritis, osteoporotic vertebral fracture, peripheral neuropathy, cancer, polymyalgia and rheumatic and peripheral vascular disease (BPS & BGS: British Pain Society and British Geriatrics Society, 2007). There is evidence that pain can cause agitation, depression, poor sleep, reduced satisfaction with life, impaired movement ability and can also be associated with a greater risk of falling and disability in people with dementia (Forsyth, 2007; Lin et al., 2011b).

There are different types of pain and these can occur in the short term (*acute pain*), or in the long term (*persistent pain*) (BPS & BGS, 2007). The majority of the literature on pain assessment does not differentiate among different types of pain and so it is not feasible to segregate assessment for the different types of pain in this chapter. The literature on pain assessment also evaluates people with dementia as a homogeneous group and does not differentiate among different causes or presentations of dementia, consequently this chapter is also unable to differentiate among different types of dementia.

DRIVERS FOR EFFECTIVE PAIN ASSESSMENT

The BPS and BGS (2007) are responsible for publishing the British National Guidelines for Pain in Older People, which form the benchmark for this chapter. The main issue is that the research suggests that these guidelines are not being adhered to by healthcare professionals (Allcock et al., 2002; Herr et al., 2004; Williams, et al., 2005; Stolee et al., 2007). The commonly cited reason is that the advocated gold standard for pain assessment is to ask the person whether they are in pain, and this can be challenging when pertaining to a person with dementia because their symptoms often include difficulties with speech and expression, impaired recall and difficulty interpreting experiences (Buffum et al., 2007). People with dementia form a significant population for whom physiotherapy services are needed, including in association with orthopaedics and community rehabilitation. It should be noted at this point, that no research studies have been identified that evaluate pain assessment approaches for people with dementia who live at home, and this population is increasing secondarily to local service changes, motivated by national drivers, to help people to remain at home longer (Department of Health: DOH, 2009). Unidentified pain in people with dementia living at home has resulted in inappropriate admissions to the mental health inpatient unit. This is because the behavioural signs of pain can mimic other behaviours that might be secondary to the process of dementia and it can also temporarily increase cognitive impairment (BPS & BGS, 2007; Alzheimer's Society, 2012b). An example of this is Mrs. P, whose circumstances are illustrated in Box 1.

According to some organizations, dementia should be recognized as a terminal condition (Alzheimer's Society, 2012b), and palliative care recommendations specify that pain assessment is undertaken. If the person cannot verbalize their pain, it is specified that their behaviour is observed (National Institute of

---

BOX 1
CASE EXAMPLE

Mrs P is a lady who was admitted to hospital from a nursing home where she was reported to have been resisting staff when being helped to move for personal care. When assessed on the ward it was identified that this lady had a painful condition and was only resisting movement because the interventions by staff to help her move were causing her pain. The conflict ceased when her pain was treated. Inappropriate admissions are costly for an organization, at approximately £264 per person per excess bed days (DOH, 2012). In this case, better pain assessment in the community setting may help to prevent unnecessary hospital admission, which has a high financial cost and is detrimental to the well-being of the person with dementia.

BOX 2
REFLECTIVE QUESTIONS

- Does a failure to manage pain amount to professional neglect? (Parliamentary and Health Service Ombudsman, 2011)
- Could inadequate pain management result in litigation? (Schofield et al., 2007)
- Is pain management a fundamental human right? (Brennan et al., 2007)

Health and Care Excellence: NICE, 2006). The Alzheimer's Society supports this notion and recommends that 'all people with dementia should be free from pain at the end of their lives, with training and systems designed to detect and manage pain even if communication is diminished' (Alzheimer's Society, 2012b, p. 19). In light of this, for a comprehensive palliative care policy to be implemented, it is essential to ensure that the training and management systems are in place for effective pain assessment and it is not possible to do this until information is available about the existing approaches and their consistency with national guidelines. Organizational barriers will be discussed towards the end of this chapter.

MODELS OF CARE FOR PAIN ASSESSMENT

This section will discuss the literature that pertains to models of care that may form a foundation for pain assessment practices. The literature indicates that debates exist in the literature regarding the use of a standardized approach versus a person-centred care approach. A standardized approach is one that follows the same process systematically for every person, whereas the person-centred approach aims to uphold the individuality of the person and provide tailored care (Kitwood, 1997). Organizations often strive to provide a person-centred approach, although the procedures involved in care are often standardized, such as regulatory assessment forms. The national guidelines advise that pain should be treated as an individual phenomenon, suggesting that a person-centred approach is preferable, but the guidelines also contain an algorithm procedure for practice methods which suggests a standardized approach (BPS & BGS, 2007). Given this lack of clarity, the wider literature was consulted and is discussed under the relevant model of care.

The Standardized Model

Epperson & Bonnel (2004) and Schofield et al. (2008) present a standardized approach to pain assessment in their portrayal of algorithms of best practice. The recommendations in the algorithms can be seen in Table 1. The algorithm of Schofield et al. (2008) is purported to be generic to any setting and although it offers a template for pain assessment, it does not specify a timescale for assessment frequency or recommend a particular assessment scale. Conversely, Epperson & Bonnel (2004) specify that the frequency of pain assessment should differ in different settings. The advantages of the standardized approach for management purposes may be that it is easy to measure adherence and it may also be a system that ensures that pain assessment is not overlooked. Snow & Shuster (2006) also recommend a standardized approach to pain assessment through hypothesis testing. When their proposed method was evaluated in a sample of 114 nursing home residents, the hypothesis-testing group showed significantly fewer discomfort behaviours than the group who received a nonstandardized approach to pain assessment ($p < .001$), with the discomfort behaviours of 84% of the residents being ameliorated (Kovach et al., 2001). In summary, some authors advocate a standardized approach to pain assessment, but there is a lack of consistent specifications about when to assess and which assessment scale to use, and there is a paucity of clinical testing of the standardized processes.

The Person-Centred Model

The Picker Institute Europe (2002) and Smith (2007) suggest that organizations adopt a person-centred approach to pain assessment for people with dementia. Malloy & Hadjistavropoulos (2004) reference the work of Kitwood (1997) and assert that the prerequisite of person-centred care is to know the person with

TABLE 1
A Summary of the National Guidelines of Pain Assessment Relevant to People With Dementia

Guideline	The BPS and BGS (2007)	American Geriatrics Society (2002)	The Alzheimer's Society (2012b)	The National Council for Palliative Care (2012)
Pain to be assessed at every health assessment	✓	X pain to be assessed on initial visit	X 'routine practice' (p. 18)	
Try to ask about pain	✓	✓	✓	✓
Observe for behavioural signs of pain	✓	✓	✓	✓
Observe for behavioural signs of pain during movement and rest	✓	✓		✓
Use a standardized pain assessment scale	✓	✓	✓	✓
Consult with carers and family	✓	✓		
Be aware of pain-producing diagnosis, e.g., arthritis	✓	✓		

Key: ✓ = guideline features in publication. If blank the publication does not specify details about this guideline.

dementia. Smith (2007) develops this concept within the context of pain assessment and reports that, in practice, person-centred care pertains to understanding the history of the person's pain and its treatments, knowing their usual reactions to pain, and knowing what had triggered pain in the past and whether they tended to stoicism. The BPS and BGS (2007) also assert that familiarity with a person's usual patterns of behaviour may improve the ability to identify pain because the experience of pain, as well as the experience of dementia, is described as being unique to each person. McAuliffe et al. (2009) assert that this approach may not be practical clinically because it can take between 1 week and 3 months to get to know a person sufficiently to provide person-centred care, but their assertion may have different implications for different clinical settings. For example, in a long-term care setting, spending up to 3 months learning about a person with dementia may be achievable. Person-centred approaches are acknowledged in the literature as advantageous when working with people with dementia (Kitwood, 1997; Perrin et al., 2008), but the findings of this review suggest there is little evidence for their use in models of pain assessment. Organizational barriers need to be considered when examining the practice of person-centred care as, for example, Smith (2005) notes that person-centred care approaches rely on getting to know the person and this is unlikely to be realized if there is a high turnover of staff or early discharge policies.

THE NATIONAL GUIDELINES FOR PAIN ASSESSMENT

The BPS and BGS (2007) guidelines have geographical relevance to the United Kingdom and purport to be a product of the best evidence available from a literature search and a multiprofessional working group. The literature search for this chapter highlighted three additional national guidelines for pain assessment practices, and Table 1 summarizes the recommendations and compares the similarities and differences between them. The guideline statements in Table 1 were extracted from the BPS and BGS (2007) guidelines and the other publications did not include any additional recommendations in this area.

Frequency of Pain Assessment

The BPS and BGS (2007) recommend that pain is assessed at every visit, but there is disagreement about this in the wider literature, as illustrated in Table 1. Four of the papers are not specific in their recommendations and use terms such as *routine* and *monitor* (Herr & Garand, 2001; Herr et al., 2006a; Hadjistavropoulos et al., 2007; Schofield et al., 2008). Epperson & Bonnel (2004) suggest that the frequency of pain assessment depends on the clinical setting for the person with dementia, recommending 8-hourly assessments for the person in hospital and assessments every visit for people at home. The latter does concur with the BPS and BGS (2007) guidelines although no explanation is given for the difference in expectation of frequency. Bachino et al. (2001) added that pain should be assessed if the person's condition changes or if new symptoms arise, and both of these require sufficient knowledge of the person's usual behaviours, which the clinician may not have.

The Assessment of Pain Through Behavioural Observation

The gold standard recommendation for pain assessment is to ask the person if they are in pain (BPS & BGS, 2007), but the national guidelines state that 'in people with difficulty in communicating including cognitive impairment… an observational assessment is additionally required' (BPS & BGS, 2007, p. 11). The BPS & BGS (2007) report that people express pain through a common set of behaviours: autonomic changes, such as sweating; facial expressions, such as grimacing; body movements, such as rocking; vocalizations, such as groaning; changes in interpersonal interactions, such as aggression; changes in activity patterns, including sleep; and changes in mental status. Stolee et al. (2007) argue that behaviour is not just a proportionate reaction to pain intensity but can be reflective of other factors related to the pain experience, such as fear and anxiety. This chapter will adopt the assumption that the behaviours described by the BPS and BGS (2007) are valid, but this should be acknowledged as a possible limitation because there is a lack of consensus in the literature about which behavioural signs are valid indicators of pain (Bachino et al., 2001).

PAIN ASSESSMENT SCALES

The BPS and BGS (2007) assert that a pain assessment scale should be used to help observe for pain behaviours, but they do not recommend one particular scale, stating that further research is needed. The literature search identified a number of assessment scales, which are listed in Table 2 with the supporting evidence referenced. It is beyond the remit of this chapter to review the evidence for each scale, but there are a number of literature reviews on existing evidence of the effectiveness of pain scales and the conclusions of these will be discussed in the next section.

Smith (2005), Herr et al. (2006b), Stolee et al. (2005) and Thuathail & Welford (2011) completed systematic reviews of the literature on behavioural assessment scales and concluded that most scales were still under development and needed more testing. Despite this, some authors have recommended assessment scales within the current evidence base; for instance, Zwakhalen et al. (2006) propose that the Pain Assessment Checklist for Seniors with Limited Ability to Communicate (PASCLAC) and DOLOPLUS2 scales were most clinically useful and sensitive. The PASCLAC has items that are scored 0 or 1 if they are not present or present, respectively, whereas the DOLOPLUS2 scores 0 to 3, which allows for some measurement of pain intensity. A recommendation by an expert group also acknowledges PASCLAC, but favours the Pain Assessment in Advanced Dementia (PAINAD) as most clinically relevant (Herr et al., 2010). The PAINAD requires a 5-minute observation of the person in any one position, whereas the PASCLAC requires a more lengthy and dynamic observation. Herr et al. (2010) focused on assessment scales for use in nursing homes, whereas Zwakhalen et al. (2006) did not specify a clinical setting, which might explain the disparity in recommendations. On the other hand, Cunningham et al. (2010) also investigated the care home setting, but recommended The Abbey Scale and the Discomfort in Dementia Scale because they measure the six behaviours set out by their relevant national guidelines (American Geriatrics Society, 2002). Cunningham et al. (2010) further acknowledge the advantages of the NOPPAIN in that it requires the person to be observed during daily activities, but suggest it needs more psychometric testing. While and Jocelyn (2009) make

some clinically pertinent observations about the importance of applying the context of the setting when selecting an assessment scale. They note a number of setting-specific factors including the time available to complete the scale and the skills and training required to complete the scale. An example of this is given by Chatterjee (2012), who recommends the Disability Distress Assessment Tool (DisDAT) assessment scale because it meets the environmental needs of a hospice setting. In conclusion, the evidence does not advocate a gold standard pain assessment scale and this makes it difficult to evaluate whether an organization is meeting a recommendation. This chapter, in accordance with the BPS and BGS (2007) guidelines, proposes the standard that clinicians use an assessment scale.

The assessment scales previously discussed differ in whether they require the person with dementia to be static or moving during pain assessment. The advantage of an assessment scale that specifies that the person with dementia is observed during dynamic activities, such as walking and eating, means that the scale encourages adherence to the BPS and BGS (2007) recommendation that pain should be assessed during movement and at rest. No other findings in the literature review discussed the issue of assessment during movement, but given that it is a recommendation of the BPS and BGS (2007), it remains relevant for evaluation in this project. Any physiotherapist will be familiar with the arthritic knee that only causes pain when the person is weight bearing.

The literature search identified a small number of studies that examine the popularity of the use of pain assessment scales in practice. Abbey (2007) surveyed 2523 Australian residential facilities and found that the most popular scales were The Abbey Pain Scale (63%), followed by DS-DAT (10%), CNPI (32%) and PAINAD (5%); locally designed scales were used by 21% of facilities. The survey only had a 24% response rate, but this equates to a sample of 598 facilities. Smith & Kennerley (2012) also completed a survey of care homes, to which they received 33 responses and found that the most popular scale was the Abbey (42%), followed by DisDAT (27%), PACSLAC (12%) and DOLOPLUS2 (3%). The participants reported that the Abbey was appealing because of the ease of use and PACSLAC and DisDAT because of their person-centred design. The

TABLE 2

Pain Assessment Scales and Their Sources Identified in the Literature Search

Name of Assessment Scale	Featured Publication
The Discomfort Behaviour Scale	Stevenson et al., (2006); Monroe et al. (2012)
Pain Assessment Checklist for Seniors with Limited Ability to Communicate (PACSLAC)	Fuchs-Lacelle & Hadjistavropoulos (2004); Zwakhalen et al. (2006)[a]; Fuchs-Lacelle (2007); Zwakhalen et al. (2012)
Pain Assessment in Advanced Dementia (PAINAD)	Costardi et al. (2007); Lane et al. (2003); Warden et al. (2003); Hutchison et al. (2006); Leong et al. (2006); van Iersel et al. (2006)[a]; Zwakhalen et al. (2010); Jordan et al. (2011)[a]; Lin et al. (2011a)[a]; Garre-Olmo et al. (2012); Jordan et al. (2012); Liu et al. (2012); Mosele et al. (2012)
Disability Distress Assessment Tool (DisDAT)	Zieber et al. (2005); Dello Russo et al. (2008); Jordan et al. (2012)[a]
The Discomfort Scale for Patients with Advanced Dementia of the Alzheimer's Type (DS-DAT)	Hurley et al. (1992)
DOLOPLUS-2	Hølen et al. (2005); Hadjistavropoulos et al. (2008); Chen et al. (2010); Zwakhalen et al. (2012)
Mobilization Observation Behaviour Intensity Dementia Pain Scale (MOBID)	Husebo et al. (2007); Husebo (2008)[a]; Husebo et al. (2009)[a]; Husebo et al. (2010)[a]
Mobilization Observation Behaviour Intensity Dementia Pain Scale 2 (MOBID-2)	Husebo (2008)[a]
Checklist of Nonverbal Pain Indicators (CNPI)	Scherder & van Manen (2005); Ersek et al. (2011)
Certified Nursing Assistant Pain Assessment Tool (CPAT)	Cervo et al. (2007); Cervo et al. (2009)
The Abbey Pain Scale	Abbey (2003); Abbey et al. (2004)[a]; van Iersel et al. (2006)[a];
The Non-Communicative Patient's Pain Assessment Instrument (NOPPAIN)	Snow et al. (2004); Horgas et al. (2007)
Pain Assessment for the Dementing Elderly (PADE)	Villanueva et al. (2003)
The Assessment of Discomfort in Dementia (ADD) Protocol	Kovach et al. (2002)
The Hospice Approach Discomfort Scale	Krulewitch et al. (2000)[a]
Davies et al. (2004) pain assessment tool	Davies et al. (2004a); Davies et al. (2004b)
The Aged Care Pain Chart	Edvardsson et al. (2008)
The Behaviour Checklist	Baker et al. (1996)
The Facial Grimace Scale	Baker et al. (1996)
The Pain Behaviours for Osteoarthritis Instrument for Cognitively Impaired Elders (PBOICIE)	Tsai et al. (2008)
The Face, Legs, Activity, Cry and Consolability Pain Assessment Tool (FLACC)	Herr et al. (2006b); Voepel-Lewis et al. (2010)
Pain Assessment in the Communicatively Impaired (PACI)	Kaasalainen et al. (2011)
The Pain Assessment Tool in Confused Older Adults (PATCOA)	Decker & Perry (2003)
Amy's Guide	Galloway & Turner (1999)
The Simons and Malabar Pain Scale	Simons & Malabar (1995)
The Nonverbal Pain Assessment Tool	Klein et al. (2010)
Facial Action Coding System	Lints-Martindale et al. (2007)
Elderly Pain Caring Assessment 2 (EPCA-2)	Morello et al. (2007)
Pain Behaviour Checklist (PBC)	van der Putten & Vlaskamp (2011)

[a]Indicates that the study included two assessment scales and has been referenced in both categories

assessment scales in use amongst mental health physiotherapists featured as a thread discussion on The Chartered Society of Physiotherapy's website, and the NOPPAIN, Abbey and DisDAT were identified as most commonly in use (Fordham, 2011). In conclusion, studies show the Abbey Scale (2007) is popular and that other assessment scales are also in use, but that no clear trends are apparent.

INVOLVING CARERS WHEN ASSESSING FOR PAIN IN PEOPLE WITH DEMENTIA

The BPS and BGS (2007) recommend that clinicians consult with the carers and families of the person with dementia when assessing for pain. The reason for this recommendation is that those who know the person with dementia are best placed to know their usual pain behaviours and whether the person's behaviour has changed over a period of time. Conversely, the findings of Thun-Boyle et al. (2010) challenge this reasoning because 20 relatives were unable to interpret significant information pertinent to pain; for example, carers were aware that their loved one had a pain-producing condition, such as a pressure sore, arthritis or acute infection, and yet reported that the person was not in pain. The sample in this study was small and it is difficult to discuss medical cases with limited information but, despite this, the authors assert that having these at-risk factors should be sufficient to trigger an assumption of pain (Thun-Boyle et al., 2010).

AWARENESS OF PAIN-PRODUCING DIAGNOSES

The BPS and BGS guidelines state that 'a full medical history should be taken' (2007, p. 12) and this allows for an awareness of possible pain-producing diagnoses, such as the presence of arthritis. Other publications on the care of people with dementia have highlighted the importance of obtaining knowledge about physical health needs (NICE, 2006). This section forms the standard part of the physiotherapist's assessment as 'past medical history', though it is noted here because, in the case of someone with memory impairment, more diligence may be needed to obtain the medical history from other sources. The clinical experience of the author suggests that the introduction of electronic patient records gives physiotherapists the opportunity to have a better awareness of all the person's medical history and information. In certain counties in the United Kingdom the primary care and mental health services have opted for different electronic systems, which inhibits information sharing for the physiotherapist who often bridges this gap. It is recommended that physiotherapists are proactive in seeking liaison agreements where this occurs.

BARRIERS TO EFFECTIVE PAIN ASSESSMENT

Table 3 summarizes the barriers to pain assessment for people with dementia identified in the literature. Only organizational barriers are highlighted here, rather than barriers related to the individual therapist.

The Voice of the Person With Dementia in Pain Assessment Literature

An acknowledged barrier to effective pain assessment for people with dementia is that the research often excludes people with dementia (Bachino et al., 2001). One of the primary assertions of the 2012 World Alzheimer Report is that people with dementia should be given a voice, and the report exemplified this by surveying 2500 people with dementia and their families in the development of their publication (Alzheimer's Disease International, 2012). The Alzheimer's Society (2012b) surveyed 306 people with early dementia living at home to produce collective statements for their report, one of which was 'I will die free from pain and fear, and with dignity, cared for by people who are trained and supported in high quality palliative care' (p. 14, outcome one). In her book, Bryden wrote about her experiences of having dementia and implores people to 'look behind our behaviour to its meaning', (2005, p. 141), which could relate to the concept of interpreting the behaviour of the person with dementia for signs of pain, though she does not specifically address pain issues. The author of this chapter has been unable to identify any literature that explores the person with dementia's experience of pain assessment methods and this information would greatly inform this topic for future projects.

TABLE 3	
The Organizational Barriers to Effective Pain Assessment for People With Dementia Featured in the Findings of the Literature Search	
Barrier Identified	**Source**
The service users have impairments in verbal communication	Bachino et al. (2001); Frampton (2003); Sachs et al. (2004);
The evidence for the validity of assessment scales is insufficient	Frampton (2003); Bachino et al. (2001); McAuliffe et al. (2009)
Some assessment scales are completed at rest and so may miss movement-related pain	Bachino et al. (2001)
The pain assessment scales are not appropriate clinically	Cook et al. (1999); Frampton (2003); Stolee et al. (2007); McAuliffe et al. (2009)
Assessment scales are not easy to administer	Stolee et al. (2007)
Research into pain assessment has methodological flaws	Frampton (2003)
Assessment scales need further testing	Frampton (2003)
Healthcare clinicians are not using pain assessment scales	McAuliffe et al. (2009)
There is a lack of training or knowledge in healthcare professionals about pain assessment	Cook et al. (1999); Frampton (2003); Sachs et al. (2004); McAuliffe et al. (2009); Thun-Boyle et al. (2010)
There is a lack of collaboration between dementia care, palliative care and older adult care	Frampton (2003)
Carer's knowledge of pain assessment is insufficient	Frampton (2003); Sachs et al. (2004)
Lack of encouragement to involve the family	Frampton (2003)
Pain assessment is poorly documented	Frampton (2003); Stolee et al. (2007); McAuliffe et al. (2009)
Dementia is not seen as a terminal illness appropriate for a palliative care approach	Sachs et al. (2004); Thun-Boyle et al. (2010)
People with dementia are excluded from pain research	Bachino et al. (2001)
There is disagreement about the relevance of physiological changes as indicators of pain	Bachino et al. (2001)
Pain behaviour is misinterpreted as indicative of other problems or as a symptom of dementia	Stolee et al. (2007); McAuliffe et al. (2009); DOH (2009); Alzheimer's Society (2012a)
There is a belief that some people with dementia do not experience pain	McAuliffe et al. (2009)
There is not enough time to learn people's normal behaviours	Cook et al. (1999); Malloy & Hadjistavropoulos (2004)
There is a belief that pain is a normal part of ageing	Malloy & Hadjistavropoulos (2004)
Institutionalized and inauthentic relationships are adopted between the carer and the person with dementia	Malloy & Hadjistavropoulos (2004)
The organization requires staff to work in a way that achieves operational efficiency and has an inauthentic caring culture	Malloy & Hadjistavropoulos (2004)
Clinicians lack a proactive approach to pain assessment	Kaasalainen et al. (2006)
There is an erroneous assumption that someone who is in bed is comfortable	Kaasalainen et al. (2006)
Pain assessment is treated as a paper exercise and information is not interpreted	Thun-Boyle et al. (2010)

Now Test Yourself With This Questionnaire

1. When you are visiting a person with dementia, how often do you consider whether they experience pain?

Never   **Almost never**   **Occasionally/sometimes**   **Almost every time**   Frequently

Other (please specify):

2. Do you try to ask the person with dementia about their pain (verbally)?

Never   **Almost never**   **Occasionally/sometimes**   **Almost every time**   Frequently

Other (please specify):

3. Do you observe for behavioural signs of pain (bracing, restlessness, rubbing part of body, etc.)?

Never   **Almost never**   **Occasionally/sometimes**   **Almost every time**   Frequently

4. Do you observe for behavioural signs of pain when the person is moving as well as at rest?

Never   **Almost never**   **Occasionally/sometimes**   **Almost every time**   Frequently

5. Do you use a standardized pain assessment scale (for example, The Abbey Pain Scale)?

Never   **Almost never**   **Occasionally/sometimes**   **Almost every time**   Frequently

6. If you DO use pain assessment scales please indicate which ones below
   ☐ Discomfort Behaviour Scale
   ☐ Elderly Pain Caring Assessment 2 (EPCA-2)
   ☐ Facial Action Coding System
   ☐ Pain Behaviour Checklist (PBC)
   ☐ The Nonverbal Pain Assessment Tool
   ☐ Pain Assessment Checklist for Seniors with Limited Ability to Communicate (PACSLAC)
   ☐ Pain Assessment in Advanced Dementia (PAINAD)
   ☐ Disability Distress Assessment Tool (DisDAT)
   ☐ Discomfort Scale for Patients with Dementia of the Alzheimer's Type (DS-DAT)
   ☐ DOLOPLUS-2
   ☐ Mobilization Observation Behaviour Intensity Dementia Pain Scale (MOBID)
   ☐ Mobilization Observation Behaviour Intensity Dementia Pain Scale 2 (MOBID-2)
   ☐ Checklist of Nonverbal Pain Indicators (CNPI)
   ☐ Certified Nursing Assistant Pain Assessment Tool (CPAT)
   ☐ The Abbey Pain Scale (The Abbey)
   ☐ The Non-Communicative Patient's Pain Assessment Instrument (NOPPAIN)
   ☐ Pain Assessment for the Dementing Elderly (PADE)
   ☐ The Assessment of Discomfort in Dementia (ADD) Protocol
   ☐ The Hospice Approach Discomfort Scale
   ☐ Davies et al. (2004) pain assessment tool
   ☐ The Aged Care Pain Chart
   ☐ The Behaviour Checklist
   ☐ The Facial Grimace Scale
   ☐ The Pain Behaviours for Osteoarthritis Instrument for Cognitively Impaired Elders (PBOICIE)
   ☐ The Face, Legs, Activity, Cry and Consolability Pain Assessment Tool (FLACC)
   ☐ Pain Assessment in the Communicatively Impaired (PACI)
   ☐ The Pain Assessment Tool in Confused Older Adults (PATCOA)
   ☐ Amy's Guide
   ☐ The Simons and Malabar Pain Scale
Other (please specify)

7. When assessing for pain, do you ask the person with dementia's loved ones or carers for their insight?

Never   **Almost never**   **Occasionally/sometimes**   **Almost every time**   **Frequently**

8. Do you obtain information about the person's possible pain-producing diagnosis (for example, arthritic conditions)?

Never   **Almost never**   **Occasionally/sometimes**   **Almost every time**   **Frequently**

9. This question aims to produce information about any organizational barriers to identifying pain in people with dementia. These are barriers that you perceive apply to your area of work, not necessarily to your personal practice. Please tick any of the following that you perceive apply to your place of work.
   ☐ There is not enough time to assess for pain
   ☐ The assessment scales are not appropriate for my place of work
   ☐ Healthcare clinicians are not using pain assessment scales
   ☐ There is a lack of collaboration between dementia care, palliative care and older adult care
   ☐ Pain assessment is poorly documented in my organization
   ☐ In my organization, dementia is not seen as a terminal illness appropriate for a palliative care approach
   ☐ Pain behaviour is misinterpreted as indicative of other problems related to dementia
   ☐ There is a belief that some people with dementia do not feel pain
   ☐ There is not enough time to learn people's normal behaviours
   ☐ There is a belief that pain is a normal part of ageing
   ☐ The healthcare clinicians tend to be reactive to pain rather than proactive
   ☐ There is a tendency to treat pain assessment as a paper exercise where the information is not interpreted
   ☐ The knowledge of pain assessment in carers and loved ones of people with dementia is insufficient
   ☐ There is no training about pain assessment techniques
   ☐ There is not enough training about pain assessment techniques
   ☐ There is a belief that someone who is in bed is comfortable

Other (please specify):

CONCLUSIONS

Effective pain assessment in the person with dementia can have significant positive effects for their well-being. There is much consensus about the majority of the BPS and BGS (2007) national guidelines, but there remains inconsistency in the recommendations for a model of pain assessment, when to assess for pain, the usefulness of consulting carers and which assessment scale to use. Practice-based research has also shown that there are organizational barriers to pain assessment which may also be relevant to the reader.

REFERENCES

Abbey, J., 2003. Ageing, dementia and palliative care. In: O'Connor, M., Aranda, S. (Eds.), Palliative Care Nursing. A guide to practice, second ed. Radcliffe Medical Press, Oxford, pp. 313–328.

Abbey, J., 2007. Putting pain scales to the test. Aust. Nurs. J. 14, 43.

Abbey, J., Piller, N., De Bellis, A., et al., 2004. The Abbey pain scale: a 1-minute numerical indicator for people with end-stage dementia. Int. J. Palliat. Nurs. 10, 6–13.

Allcock, N., McGarry, J., Elkan, R., 2002. Management of pain in older people within a nursing home: a preliminary study. Health Soc. Care Community 10, 464–471.

Alzheimer's Disease International, 2012. World Alzheimer report 2012: Overcoming the Stigma of Dementia. Alzheimer Disease International, London.

Alzheimer's Society, 2012a. Dementia 2012: A National Challenge. Alzheimer's Society, London.

Alzheimer's Society, 2012b. My Life until the End. Dying Well with Dementia. Alzheimer's Society, London.

Alzheimer's Society, 2013. Low expectations: Attitudes on choice, care and community for people with dementia in care homes. Alzheimer's Society, London.

American Geriatrics Society Panel on Persistent Pain in Older Persons, 2002. The management of persistent pain in older persons. J. Am. Geriatr. Soc. 50, s205–s224.

Bachino, C., Snow, A., Kunik, M.E., et al., 2001. Principles of pain assessment and treatment in non-communicative demented patients. Clin. Gerontol. 23, 97–115.

Baker, A., Bowring, L., Brignell, A., Kafford, D., 1996. Chronic pain management in cognitively impaired patients: a preliminary research project. Perspectives (Montclair) 20, 4–8.

Brennan, F., Carr, D.B., Cousins, M., 2007. Pain management: a fundamental human right. Anesth. Analg. 105, 205–221.

British Pain Society and British Geriatrics Society, 2007. Guidance on: The Assessment of Pain in Older People. The Royal College of Physicians of London, London.

Bryden, C., 2005. Dancing with Dementia. Jessica Kingsley Publishers, London.

Buffum, M.D., Hutt, E., Chang, V.T., et al., 2007. Cognitive impairment and pain management: reviews of issues and challenges. J. Rehabil. Res. Dev. 44, 315–330.

Cervo, F.A., Bruckenthal, P., Chen, J.J., et al., 2009. Pain assessment in nursing home residents with dementia: psychometric properties and clinical utility of the CNA Pain Assessment Tool (CPAT). J. Am. Med. Dir. Assoc. 10, 505–510.

Cervo, F.A., Raggi, R.P., Bright-Long, L.E., et al., 2007. Use of the certified nursing assistant pain assessment tool (CPAT) in nursing home residents with dementia. Am. J. Alzheimers Dis. Other Demen. 22, 112–119.

Chatterjee, J., 2012. Improving pain assessment for patients with cognitive impairment: development of a pain assessment toolkit. Int. J. Palliat. Nurs. 18, 581–590.

Chen, Y.H., Lin, L.C., Watson, R., 2010. Validating nurses' and nursing assistants' report of assessing pain in older people with dementia. J. Clin. Nurs. 19, 42–52.

Cook, A.K., Niven, C.A., Downs, M.G., 1999. Assessing the pain of people with cognitive impairment. Int. J. Geriatr. Psychiatry 14, 421–425.

Costardi, D., Rozzini, L., Costanzi, C., et al., 2007. The Italian version of the pain assessment in advanced dementia (PAINAD) scale. Arch. Gerontol. Geriatr. 44, 175–180.

Cunningham, C., McClean, W., Kelly, F., 2010. The assessment and management of pain in people with dementia in care homes. Nurs. Older People 22, 29–37.

Davies, E., Male, M., Reimer, V., et al., 2004a. Pain assessment and cognitive impairment: Part 1. Nurs. Stand. 19, 39–42.

Davies, E., Male, M., Reimer, V., Turner, M., 2004b. Pain assessment and cognitive impairment: Part 2. Nurs. Stand. 19, 33–40.

Decker, S.A., Perry, A.G., 2003. The development and testing of the PATCOA to assess pain in confused older adults. Pain Manag. Nurs. 4, 77–86.

Dello Russo, C., Di Giulio, P., Brunelli, C., et al., 2008. Validation of the Italian version of the discomfort scale—dementia of Alzheimer type. J. Adv. Nurs. 64, 298–304.

Dementia Action Alliance, 2010. National dementia declaration for England. A call to action. Dementia Action Alliance. <http://www.dementiaaction.org.uk/assets/0000/1157/National_Dementia_Declaration_for_England.pdf.>

Department of Health, 2009. Living Well with Dementia: A National Dementia Strategy. Department of Health, London.

Department of Health, 2012. Reference Costs 2011–2012. Department of Health, London.

Edvardsson, D., Katz, B., Nay, R., 2008. Innovations in aged care. The aged care pain chart: an innovative approach to assessing, managing and documenting pain in older people. Australas. J. Ageing 27, 93–96.

Epperson, M.D., Bonnel, W., 2004. Pain assessment in dementia: tools and strategies. Clin. Excell. Nurse Pract. 8, 166–171.

Ersek, M., Polissar, N., Neradilek, M.B.J., 2011. Development of a composite pain measure for persons with advanced dementia: exploratory analyses in self-reporting nursing home residents. J. Pain Symptom Manage. 41, 566–579.

Feldt, K.S., Warne, M.A., Ryden, M.B., 1998. Examining pain in aggressive cognitively impaired older adults. J. Gerontol. Nurs. 24, 14–22.

Ferrell, B.A., Ferrell, B.R., Rivera, L., 1995. Pain in cognitively impaired nursing home patients. J. Pain Symptom Manage. 10, 591–598.

Fordham, L., 2011. Pain assessment in advanced dementia. Interactive CSP. Chartered Society of Physiotherapy, 11 May. <http://http://www.csp.org.uk/icsp/topics/pain-assessment-advanced-dementia-0.>

Forsyth, D., 2007. Pain in patients with cognitive impairment. In: Crome, P., Main, C.J., Lally, F. (Eds.), Pain in Older People. Oxford University Press, Oxford, 21–29.

Frampton, M., 2003. Experience assessment and management of pain in people with dementia. Age. Ageing 32, 248–251.

Fuchs-Lacelle, S.K. (2007). Pain and Dementia: The Effects of Systematic Assessment on Clinical Practices and Caregiver Stress. PhD Thesis. University of Regina.

Fuchs-Lacelle, S., Hadjistavropoulos, T., 2004. Development and preliminary validation of the pain assessment checklist for seniors with limited ability to communicate (PACSLAC). Pain Manag. Nurs. 5, 37–49.

Galloway, S., Turner, L., 1999. Pain assessment in older adults who are cognitively impaired. J. Gerontol. Nurs. 25, 34–39.

Garre-Olmo, J., López-Pousa, S., Turon-Estrada, A., et al., 2012. Environmental determinants of quality of life in nursing home residents with severe dementia. J. Am. Geriatr. Soc. 60, 1230–1236.

Hadjistavropoulos, T., Fitzgerald, T.D., Marchildon, G.P., 2010. Practice guidelines for assessing pain in older persons with dementia residing in long-term care facilities. Physiother. Can. 62, 104–113.

Hadjistavropoulos, T., Voyer, P., Sharpe, D., et al., 2008. Assessing pain in dementia patients with comorbid delirium and/or depression. Pain Manag. Nurs. 9, 48–54.

Hadjistavropoulos, T., Herr, K., Turk, D.C., et al., 2007. An interdisciplinary expert consensus statement on assessment of pain in older persons. Clin. J. Pain 23 (1 Suppl.), s1–s43.

Herr, K., Bjoro, K., Decker, S., 2006b. Tools for assessment of pain in nonverbal older adults with dementia: a state-of-the-science review. J. Pain Symptom Manage. 31, 170–192.

Herr, K.A., Bursch, H., Miller, L.L., Swafford, K., 2010. Use of pain-behavioural assessment tools in the nursing home. Expert consensus recommendations for practice. J. Gerontol. Nurs. 36, 18–29.

Herr, K.A., Coyne, P.J., Key, T., et al., 2006a. Pain assessment in the nonverbal patient: position statement with clinical practice recommendations. Pain Manag. Nurs. 7, 44–52.

Herr, K.A., Garand, L., 2001. Assessment and measurement of pain in older adults. Clin. Geriatr. Med. 17, 457–478.

Herr, K.A., Titler, M.G., Schilling, M.L., et al., 2004. Evidence-based assessment of acute pain in older adults. Clin. J. Pain 20, 331–340.

Hølen, J.C., Saltvedt, I., Fayers, P.M., et al., 2005. The Norwegian Doloplus-2, a tool for behavioural pain assessment: translation and pilot-validation in nursing home patients with cognitive impairment. Palliat. Med. 19, 411–417.

Horgas, A.L., Nichols, A.L., Schapson, C.A., Vietes, K., 2007. Assessing pain in persons with dementia: relationships among the non-communicative patient's pain assessment instrument, self-report, and behavioural observations. Pain Manag. Nurs. 8, 77–85.

Hurley, A.C., Volicer, B.J., Hanrahan, P.A., et al., 1992. Assessment of discomfort in advanced Alzheimer patients. Res. Nurs. Health 15, 369–377.

Husebo, B.S. (2008). Assessment of Pain in People with Dementia. Development of a Staff-Administered Behavioural Pain Assessment Tool. PhD Thesis. University of Bergen.

Husebo, B.S., Strand, L.I., Moe-Nilssen, R., et al., 2009. Pain behaviour and pain intensity in older persons with severe dementia: reliability of the MOBID pain scale by video uptake. Scand. J. Caring Sci. 23, 180–189.

Husebo, B.S., Strand, L.I., Moe-Nilssen, R., et al., 2010. Pain in older persons with severe dementia. Psychometric properties of the mobilization-observation-behaviour-intensity-dementia (MOBID-2) pain scale in a clinical setting. Scand. J. Caring Sci. 24, 380–391.

Husebo, B.S., Strand, L.I., Moe-Nilssen, R., et al., 2007. Mobilization-observation-behaviour-intensity-dementia pain scale (MOBID): development and validation of a nurse-administered pain assessment tool for use in dementia. J. Pain Symptom Manage. 34, 67–80.

Hurley, A.C., Volicer, B.J., Hanrahan, P.A., et al., 1992. Assessment of discomfort in advanced Alzheimer patients. Res. Nurs. Health 15, 369–377.

Hutchison, R.W., Tucker, W.F., Jr., Kim, S., Gilder, R., 2006. Evaluation of a behavioural assessment tool for the individual unable to self-report pain. Am. J. Hosp. Palliat. Care 23, 328–331.

International Association for the Study of Pain, 2012. 2011 IASP Taxonomy Update on Merskey, H., Bogduk, N. (eds) (1994) Part III: Pain Terms, A Current List with Definitions and Notes of Usage. [Online]. IASP Press, Washington. <http://www.iasp-pain.org/AM/Template.cfm?Section=Pain_Definitions.>

Jordan, A., Hughes, J., Pakresi, M., et al., 2011. The utility of PAINAD in assessing pain in a UK population with severe dementia. Int. J. Geriatr. Psychiatry 26, 118–126.

Jordan, A., Regnard, C., O'Brien, J.T., Hughes, J.C., 2012. Pain and distress in advanced dementia: choosing the right tools for the job. Palliat. Med. 26, 873–878.

Kaasalainen, S., 2007. Pain assessment in older people with dementia: using behavioural observational methods in clinical practice. J. Gerontol. Nurs. 33, 6–10.

Kaasalainen, S., Stewart, N., Middleton, J., et al., 2011. Development and evaluation of the pain assessment in the communicatively impaired (PACI) tool: Part II. Int. J. Palliat. Nurs. 17, 431–438.

Kitwood, T., 1997. Dementia Reconsidered. The Person Comes First. Open University Press, Buckingham.

Klein, D.G., Dumpe, M., Katz, E., Bena, J., 2010. Pain assessment in the intensive care unit: development and psychometric testing of the nonverbal pain assessment tool. Heart Lung 39, 521–528.

Kovach, C.R., Logan, B.R., Noonan, P.E., et al., 2001. Effects of the serial trial intervention on discomfort and behaviour of nursing home residents with dementia. Am. J. Alzheimers Dis. Other Demen. 21, 147–155.

Kovach, C.R., Noonan, P.E., Griffie, J., et al., 2002. The assessment of discomfort in dementia protocol. Pain Manag. Nurs. 3, 16–27.

Krulewitch, H., London, M.R., Skakel, V.J., et al., 2000. Assessment of pain in cognitively impaired older adults: a comparison of pain assessment tools and their use by nonprofessional caregivers. J. Am. Geriatr. Soc. 48, 1607–1611.

Leong, I.T., Chong, M.S., Gibson, S.J., 2006. The use of a self-reported pain measure, a nurse-reported pain measure and the PAINAD in nursing home residents with moderate and severe dementia: a validation study. Age Ageing 35, 252–256.

Lane, P., Kuntupis, M., MacDonald, S., et al., 2003. A pain assessment tool for people with advanced Alzheimer's and other progressive dementias. Home Healthc. Nurse 21, 32–37.

Lin, P.C., Lin, L.C., Shyu, Y.I., Hua, M.S., 2011a. Chinese version of the pain assessment in advanced dementia scale: initial psychometric evaluation. J. Geriatr. Psychiatry 26, 118–126.

Lin, P.C., Lin, L.C., Shyu, Y.I.L., Hua, M.S., 2011b. Predictors of pain in nursing home residents with dementia: a cross-sectional study. J. Clin. Nurs. 20, 1849–1857.

Lints-Martindale, A.C., Hadjistavropoulos, T., Barber, B., Gibson, S.J., 2007. A psychophysical investigation of the facial action coding system as an index of pain variability among older adults with and without Alzheimer's disease. Pain Med. 8, 678–689.

Liu, J.Y.W., Pang, P.C.P., Lo, K.S.L., 2012. Development and implementation of an observational pain assessment protocol in a nursing home. J. Clin. Nurs. 21, 1789–1793.

Malloy, D.C., Hadjistavropoulos, T., 2004. The problem of pain management among persons with dementia, personhood, and the ontology of relationships. Nurs. Philos. 5, 147–159.

McAuliffe, L., Nay, R., O'Donnell, M., Fetherstonhaugh, D., 2009. Pain assessment in older people with dementia: literature review. J. Adv. Nurs. 65, 2–10.

Monroe, T., Carter, M., Feldt, K., et al., 2012. Assessing advanced cancer pain in older adults with dementia at the end-of-life. J. Adv. Nurs. 68, 2070–2078.

Morello, R., Jean, A., Alix, M., et al., 2007. A scale to measure pain in non-verbally communicating older patients: the EPCA-2 study of its psychometric properties. Pain 133, 87–98.

Mosele, M., Inelmen, E.M., Toffanello, E.D., et al., 2012. Psychometric properties of the pain assessment in advanced dementia scale compared to self-assessment of pain in elderly patients. J. Am. Dir. Assoc. 13, 384–389.

National Institute for Health and Care Excellence, 2006. Dementia. Supporting people with dementia and their carers in health and social care. CB042. National Institute for Health and Care Excellence, London.

Parliamentary and Health Service Ombudsman, 2011. Care and compassion? Report of the Health Service Ombudsman on ten investigations into NHS care of older people. HC 778. The Stationery Office, London.

Perrin, T., May, H., Anderson, E., 2008. Wellbeing and Dementia. Churchill Livingstone, Edinburgh.

Sachs, G.A., Shenga, J.W., Cox-Hayley, D., 2004. Barriers to excellent end-of-life care for patients with dementia. J. Gen. Intern. Med. 19, 1057–1063.

Scherder, E., van Manen, F., 2005. Pain in Alzheimer's disease: nursing assistants' and patients' evaluations. J. Adv. Nurs. 52, 151–158.

Schofield, P., Aveyard, B., Black, C., 2007. The Management of Pain in Older People: A Workbook. Skills for Caring no. 3. M&K Publishing, Keswick.

Schofield, P., O'Mahony, S., Collett, B., Potter, J., 2008. Guidance for the assessment of pain in older adults: a literature review. Br. J. Nurs. 17, 914–918.

Simons, W., Malabar, R., 1995. Assessing pain in elderly patients who cannot respond verbally. J. Adv. Nurs. 22, 663–669.

Smith, D., Kennerley, D., 2012. Enhancing dementia care. David Smith and Dorothy Kennerley put the case for a single tool to help care staff distinguish pain from behavioural symptoms. Nurs. Manage. 19, 11.

Smith, M., 2005. Pain assessment in nonverbal older adults with advanced dementia. Perspect. Psychiatr. Care 41, 99–113.

Smith, S.D.M., 2007. Assessing pain in people with dementia 2: the nurse's role. Nurs. Times [online] 103 (30), 26. <http://www.nursingtimes.net/assessing-pain-in-people-with-dementia-2-the-nurses-role/197737.article.>

Snow, A.L., Weber, J.B., O'Malley, K.J., et al., 2004. Nursing assistant-administered instrument to assess pain in demented individuals (NOPPAIN). Dement. Geriatr. Cogn. Dis. 17, 240–246.

Snow, L.A., O'Malley, K.J., Cody, M., et al., 2004. A conceptual model of pain assessment for noncommunicative persons with dementia. Gerontologist 44, 807–817.

Snow, A.L., Shuster, J.L., 2006. Assessment and treatment of persistent pain in persons with cognitive and communicative impairment. J. Clin. Psychol. 62 (11), 1379–1387.

Stevenson, K.M., Brown, R.L., Dahl, J.L., et al., 2006. The discomfort behaviour scale: a measure of discomfort in the cognitively impaired based on the minimum data set 2.0. Res. Nurs. Health 29, 576–587.

Stolee, P., Hillier, L.M., Esbaugh, J., et al., 2005. Instruments for the assessment of pain in older persons with cognitive impairment. J. Am. Geriatr. Soc. 53, 319–326.

Stolee, P., Hillier, L.M., Esbaugh, J., et al., 2007. Pain assessment in a geriatric psychiatry program. Pain Res. Manag. 12, 273–279.

The National Council for Palliative Care, 2012. How would I know? What can I do? How to help someone with dementia who is in pain or distress. The National Council for Palliative Care, London.

The Picker Institute Europe, 2002. Relieving the Pain: Bringing about Improvements in Pain Management. [online]. The Picker Institute Europe, Oxford. <http://www.nhssurveys.org/Filestore/documents/news_letter_3.pdf.>

Thuathail, A., Welford, C., 2011. Pain assessment tools for older people with cognitive impairment. Nurs. Stand. 26, 39–46.

Thun-Boyle, I.C.V., Sampson, E.L., Jones, L., et al., 2010. Challenges to improving end of life care of people with advanced dementia in the UK. Dementia 9, 259–284.

Tsai, P.F., Beck, C., Richards, K.C., et al., 2008. The pain behaviours for osteoarthritis instrument for cognitively impaired elders (PBOICIE). Res. Geontol. Nurs. 1, 116–122.

van der Putten, A., Vlaskamp, C., 2011. Pain assessment in people with profound intellectual and multiple disabilities: a pilot study into the use of the pain behaviour checklist in everyday practice. Res. Dev. Disabil. 32, 1677–1684.

van Iersel, T., Timmerman, D., Mullie, A., 2006. Introduction of a pain scale for palliative care patients with cognitive impairment. Int. J. Palliat. Nurs. 12, 54–59.

Villanueva, M.R., Smith, T.L., Erickson, J.S., et al., 2003. Pain assessment for the dementing elderly (PADE): reliability and validity of a new measure. J. Am. Med. Dir. Assoc. 4, 1–8.

Voepel-Lewis, T., Zanotti, J., Dammeyer, J.A., Merkel, S., 2010. Reliability and validity of the face, legs, activity, cry, consolability behavioural tool in assessing acute pain in critically ill patients. Am. J. Crit. Care 19, 55–62.

Warden, V., Hurley, A.C., Volicer, L., 2003. Development and psychometric evaluation of the pain assessment in advanced dementia (PAINAD) scale. J. Am. Med. Dir. Assoc. 4, 9–15.

While, C., Jocelyn, A., 2009. Observational pain assessment scales for people with dementia: a review. Br. J. Community Nurs. 14, 438–442.

Williams, C.S., Zimmerman, S., Sloane, P.D., Reed, P.S., 2005. Characteristics associated with pain in long-term care residents with dementia. Gerontologist 45, 68–73.

Zekry, D., Herrmann, F.R., Grandjean, R., et al., 2008. Demented versus non-demented very old inpatients: the same comorbidities but poorer functional and nutritional status. Age Ageing 37, 83–89.

Zieber, C.G., Hagen, B., Armstrong-Esther, C., Aho, M., 2005. Pain and agitation in long-term care residents with dementia: use of the Pittsburgh Agitation Scale. Int. J. Palliat. Nurs. 11, 71–78.

Zwakhalen, S.M.G., Hamers, J.P.H., Abu-Saad, H.H., et al., 2006. Pain in elderly people with severe dementia: a systematic review of behavioural pain assessment tools. BMC Geriatr. 6 (3). <http://www.biomedcentral.com/1471-2318/6/3.>

Zwakhalen, S.M.G., Koopmans, T.C.M., Geels, P.J.E.M., et al., 2009. The prevalence of pain in nursing home residents with dementia measured using an observational pain scale. Eur. J. Pain 13, 89–93.

Zwakhalen, S.M., van der Steen, J.T., Najim, M.D., 2010. Which score most likely represents pain on the observational PAINAD pain scale for patients with dementia? (Chinese version). J. Adv. Nurs. 66, 2360–2368.

Zwakhalen, S.M., van't Hof, C.E., Hamers, J.P., 2012. Systematic pain assessment using an observational scale in nursing home residents with dementia: exploring feasibility and applied interventions. J. Clin. Nurs. 21, 3009–3017.

INDEX

Page numbers followed by "*f*" indicate figures, "*t*" indicate tables, and "*b*" indicate boxes.

Printed and bound by CPI Group (UK) Ltd, Croydon, CR0 4YY

03/10/2024

01040349-0007